[redacted]

Health Behavior

Emerging Research Perspectives

Health Behavior

Emerging Research Perspectives

Edited by

David S. Gochman

Raymond S. Kent School of Social Work
University of Louisville
Louisville, Kentucky

PLENUM PRESS • NEW YORK AND LONDON

Library of Congress Cataloging in Publication Data

Health behavior: emerging research perspectives / edited by David S. Gochman.
p. cm.
Includes bibliographies and index.
ISBN 0-306-42874-1
1. Health behavior. I. Gochman, David S.
RA776.9.H43 1988 88-19672
613—dc19 CIP

10 9 8 7 6 5

Printed in the United States of America

This book is dedicated to the cherished memory of my parents, Edward B. and Vesta Gabriel Gochman, who early in my life encouraged me to persevere, to seek quality, and to pursue scholarship; and to Esselyn C. Rudikoff, a psychologist and treasured friend, whose example and insights inspired me to understand behavior.

Contributors

Arnold Arluke Department of Sociology and Anthropology, Northeastern University, Boston, Massachusetts

Alice J. Baumgart School of Nursing, Queen's University, Kingston, Ontario, Canada

Zeev Ben-Sira School of Social Work, The Hebrew University of Jerusalem, Mount Scopus, Jerusalem, Israel

Philip K. Berger Martin School of Public Administration, University of Kentucky, Lexington, Kentucky

John G. Bruhn School of Allied Health Sciences, University of Texas Medical Branch, Galveston, Texas

Patricia J. Bush Laboratory for Children's Health Promotion, Department of Community and Family Medicine, Georgetown University School of Medicine, Washington, D.C.

Henry P. Cole Department of Educational and Counseling Psychology, University of Kentucky, Lexington, Kentucky

Edith A. Costello School of Nursing, Queen's University, Kingston, Ontario, Canada

Robert E. Davidson Department of Social Science, Illinois Institute of Technology, Chicago, Illinois

Alice E. Fusillo U.S. Department of Health and Human Services

Eugene B. Gallagher Departments of Behavioral Science and Sociology, University of Kentucky, Lexington, Kentucky

Thomas F. Garrity Department of Behavioral Science, University of Kentucky, Lexington, Kentucky

Reed Geertsen Department of Sociology, Utah State University, Logan, Utah

David S. Gochman Raymond A. Kent School of Social Work, University of Louisville, Louisville, Kentucky

James R. Greenley Department of Sociology, University of Wisconsin, Madison, Wisconsin

Marie R. Haug Center on Aging and Health, Case Western Reserve University, Cleveland, Ohio

Ronald J. Iannotti Laboratory for Children's Health Promotion, Department of Community and Family Medicine, Georgetown University School of Medicine, Washington, D.C.

Stephen Kaplan Department of Psychology, University of Michigan, Ann Arbor, Michigan

John P. Kirscht School of Public Health, University of Michigan, Ann Arbor, Michigan

Lloyd J. Kolbe Office of School Health and Special Projects, Division of Health Education, Center for Health Promotion and Education, U.S. Centers for Disease Control, Atlanta, Georgia

Richard R. Lau Department of Social and Decision Sciences, Carnegie–Mellon University, Pittsburgh, Pennsylvania

Philip R. Nader Department of Pediatrics, University of California at San Diego, La Jolla, California

Christian Ritter Department of Sociology and Anthropology, Kent State University, Kent, Ohio

Debra L. Roter Department of Behavioral Sciences and Health Education, Johns Hopkins University School of Hygiene and Public Health, Baltimore, Maryland

James F. Sallis Department of Pediatrics, University of California at San Diego, La Jolla, California

Alexander Segall Department of Sociology, University of Manitoba, Winnipeg, Manitoba, Canada

Ingrid Waldron Department of Biology, University of Pennsylvania, Philadelphia, Pennsylvania

Hazel H. Weidman Office of Transcultural Education and Research, Department of Psychiatry, University of Miami School of Medicine, Miami, Florida

Bruce A. Whitehead College of Information Studies, Drexel University, Philadelphia, Pennsylvania

Fredric D. Wolinsky Department of Sociology, Texas A & M University, College Station, Texas

Preface

HEALTH BEHAVIOR AS BASIC RESEARCH

Health behavior is not a traditional discipline, but a newly emerging interdisciplinary field. It is still in the process of establishing its identity. Few institutional or organizational structures, i.e., departments and programs, reflect it, and few books and journals are directed at it.

The primary objective of this book is thus to identify and establish health behavior as an important area of basic research, worthy of being studied in its own right. As a basic research area, health behavior transcends commitment to a particular behavior, a specific illness or health problem, or a single set of determinants.

One way of achieving this objective is to look at health behavior as an outcome of a range of personal and social determinants, rather than as a set of risk factors or as targets for intervention strategies directed at behavioral change. The book is thus organized primarily in terms of the size of the determinants of concern, rather than in terms of specific health behaviors, or specific health problems or conditions. With the first part of the book establishing working definitions of health behavior and health behavior research as basic frameworks, the second part moves from smaller to larger systems, informing the reader about basic research that demonstrates how health behavior is determined by personal, family, social, institutional, and cultural factors. These distinctions reflect some arbitrariness: the family, organizations, and institutions, for example, are social units. Moreover, families, social groupings, and organizations reflect elements of the culture in which they exist. Furthermore, the categorizing and sequencing of sections and chapters in no way reflects an attempt to exclude material that deals with other levels of determinants; it serves primarily to facilitate focusing more on one of these determinants than on others.

Because so much of health behavior is determined by encounters with the care delivery system, particularly with health professionals, the third part of the book examines the way such encounters determine health behaviors, and how health behaviors and the care delivery system affect one another. This part includes a section on perceptions and interactions, and a section on power, compliance, and control. The final part considers the relevance of knowledge generated by health behavior research in the training of health professionals, in health promotion and education, and in clinical applications, as well as future research directions and issues.

To emphasize and ensure the basic research commitment, contributors were advised that the book was not intended to be yet another volume on behavioral aspects of treatment, or on behavior and the medical model. They were asked to describe current knowledge relevant to their topics, to focus heavily on research dealing with basic concepts, and to include critical discussion of research and theoretical issues, together with their thoughts about future research directions. At appropriate stages, outlines and manuscripts were monitored carefully to encourage contributors to refer as much as possible to empirical data, and to ensure that there was no inappropriate emphasis on interventions and programmatic descriptions.

THE STATE OF THE ART

A second objective of the book is to present a representative selection of current health behavior research findings in a single volume. Although texts and books of readings are available in related areas, such as medical sociology (e.g., Mechanic, 1978, 1980; Wolinsky, 1988), health psychology (e.g., Sanders & Suls, 1982; Stone, Cohen, & Adler, 1979), and behavioral health (e.g., Matarazzo, Weiss, Herd, Miller, & Weiss, 1984), none of these were intended to address health behavior systematically. Accordingly, none present a broad spectrum of basic, representative health behavior research. The present volume thus presents the reader with "the state of the art" in health behavior research.

DIVERSITY OF PERSPECTIVES

A third objective is to ensure that the reader is exposed to varied perspectives in conceptual models, disciplines, populations, and methods, as well as to nonmedical frames of reference. This book exposes the reader to role theories, the health belief and locus of control models, sociology of knowledge frameworks, path analyses, organizational theory, concepts related to physical space, "health culture," as well as other conceptual paradigms. The contributors have training or professional involvements in anthropology, education, health education and health promotion, information sciences, nursing, medicine, psychology, public health, social work, and sociology.

DIVERSITY OF READERS

This book is intended for persons in a number of fields who are interested in issues related to research in health behavior. These include researchers in the social and behavioral sciences who want to know more about health behavior in general, or particular aspects of it, or who want to develop their own health behavior research; students in courses that integrate social and behavioral science and health, in disciplines such as anthropology, psychology, and sociology, and in professional programs in dentistry, medicine, nursing, public health, and social work; professionals who provide, plan, implement, and evaluate health services and programs: health eductors and promoters; health planners; public health dentists, nurses, and physicians; physicians in community and family practice; social workers; family planners; and hospital administrators.

DELIBERATE OMISSIONS

Notably absent from this book are chapters devoted to research on topics such as "Type A" personality, psychosomatics, and stress. While these are closely linked to health status, and sometimes to health behavior, they have been omitted because they are more generally models for understanding the etiology of disease and illnesses. Furthermore, although *wholism* has become a catchword among many who disavow the traditional medical model, the term has come to include charlatanism and cultism, as well as some impressive approaches to treatment. Presently, it remains more a statement of faith suggesting future research alternatives, than a body of well-thought-through, rigorously conducted research. Moreover, caution against a reverse "ethnocentrism," and overly romanticized views of non-high-technology medicine is cogently provided by Eisenberg and Kleinman (1981, p. 10): "Healing ceremonies can be efficacious, but hardly substitute for antibiotics or surgery." Accordingly, a section on "wholism," "wholistic medicine," or "wholistic health" does not appear in this book.

THE PRACTICAL RELEVANCE OF HEALTH BEHAVIOR

The practical value of increasing knowledge about, and understanding of, health behavior through rigorous, systematic research is implicit in the grave concern with health status in many contemporary societies (e.g., Knowles, 1977). Improvements in health status are less likely to be found in high-technology medicine than in environmental and psychosocial factors (e.g., Dubos, 1959/1977; Matarazzo, 1984; Powles, 1974/1980). Although solutions to an appreciable number of health problems require large-scale efforts at local, regional, and national levels to develop and enforce policies to control, minimize, and ultimately reduce the air, land, and water pollution; the hazards of transportation; and the risks of the workplace environment, solutions to other health problems require policies, programs, and processes that involve the personal health behavior of individuals and the population at large, in their family, social, and community milieus (e.g., LaLonde, 1974; *Preventive Medicine*, 1976).

Attempts to change individual health behaviors, either through individual therapeutic interventions or through larger-scale health promotion or health education programs, have been less than impressive. Many attempts are purely programmatic, hastily conceived, and lacking in theoretical rationale or empirical foundation. A major reason for this is the lack of *basic* knowlege about the target behaviors, about the contexts in which they occur, and about the factors that determine and stabilize them. Basic research in health behavior, aside from being worthy of study in its own right, may very well increase the effectiveness of interventions and programs designed to bring about behavioral change. Although demonstrations of the practical relevance of health behavior research are not a *major* objective of this book, the potential applications of such research to interventions and programs add to its value as a basic area of study.

REFERENCES

Dubos, R. (1977). The mirage of health. In J. H. Knowles (Ed.), *Doing better and feeling worse: Health in the United States*. New York: Norton. (Reprinted from R. Dubos, *Mirage of health: Utopias, progress, and biological change*, 1959, pp. 17–23, New York: Harper & Row)

Eisenberg, L., & Kleinman, A. (Eds.). (1981). *The relevance of social science for medicine*. Dordrecht: Reidel.

Knowles, J. H. (1977). The responsibility of the individual. In J. H. Knowles (Ed.), *Doing better and feeling worse: Health in the United States*. New York: Norton.

LaLonde, M. (1974). *A new perspective on the health of Canadians: A working document*. Government of Canada.

Matarazzo, J. D. (1984). Behavioral health: A 1990 challenge for the health sciences professions. In J. D. Matarazzo, S. M. Weiss, J. A. Herd, N. E. Miller, & S. M. Weiss (Eds.), *Behavioral health: A handbook of health enhancement and disease prevention*. New York: Wiley.

Matarazzo, J. D., Weiss, S. M., Herd, J. A., Miller, N. E., & Weiss, S. M. (Eds.). (1984). *Behavioral health: A handbook of health enhancement and disease prevention.* New York: Wiley.

Mechanic, D. (1978). *Medical sociology: A comprehensive text* (2nd ed.). New York: Free Press.

Mechanic, D. (Ed.). (1980). *Readings in medical sociology.* New York: Free Press.

Powles, J. (1980). On the limitations of modern medicine. In D. Mechanic (Ed.), *Readings in medical sociology.* New York: Free Press. (Reprinted from R. L. Kane (Ed.), *The challenge of community medicine*, 1974, pp. 89–122, Berlin: Springer)

Preventive medicine, USA: Health promotion and consumer health education. (1976). A task force report sponsored by the John E. Fogarty International Center for Advanced Study in the Health Sciences, National Institutes of Health; and the American College of Preventive Medicine. New York: Prodist.

Sanders, G. S., & Suls, J. (Eds.). (1982). *Social psychology of health and illness.* Hillsdale, NJ: Erlbaum.

Stone, G. C., Cohen, F., & Adler, N. E. (Eds.). (1979). *Health psychology—A handbook: Theories, applications, and challenges of a psychological approach to the health care system.* San Francisco: Jossey–Bass.

Wolinsky, F. D. (1988). *The sociology of health: Principles, practitioners, and issues* (2nd ed.). Belmont, CA: Wadsworth.

Acknowledgments

Over a period of years, many persons helped in the preparation of this book. I owe all of them my thanks. But some helped in such appreciable ways that they deserve acknowledgment here. I especially wish to thank Linda A. Exton for her excellent secretarial assistance, particularly in the timely and responsible preparation of formal invitations to contributors, and letters acknowledging receipt of materials and manuscripts; Charlotte A. Ford for her coordination of a variety of support activities; Jane Isert and Mary Ann Ostertag for their expeditious and careful photocopying of what must have seemed like tons of edited material; Professor Joan ten Hoor of the Ekstrom Library at the University of Louisville, for her invaluable assistance in generating computer searches relevant to my own chapters and to the editorial material introducing different sections of the book; Fr. Donald Duffy for his efforts in helping secure reprints; and Professor Donald W. Beless, Director, for the Kent School of Social Work's generosity in the use of its material and personnel resources, and for facilitating the approval of the sabbatical leave that enabled me to complete the editorial tasks in a timely way.

A great debt is owed each of the contributors for the care they devoted to their chapters and for their receptivity and constructive responses to the high density of editorial suggestions made throughout their chapters' progress. Moreover, the suggestions of Eugene B. Gallagher and Thomas F. Garrity in response to my inquiries about potential contributors are particularly appreciated.

Most of all, I want to thank Professor Helen G. Deines for her insightful suggestions, and for her continuous encouragement and enthusiasm for the book's basic conception and focus.

David S. Gochman

Contents

PART I

CONCEPTIONS OF HEALTH BEHAVIOR

CHAPTER 1

Health Behavior

Plural Perspectives

David S. Gochman

What "health behavior" means, and how it is treated in this book, are the basic topics of the first part of this chapter, which begins with a working definition of health behavior, discusses some related terms, and provides a definition of "health behavior research." The chapter continues with a discussion of conceptions of health, illness, and disease, and concludes by identifying some research issues that relate to these conceptions.

HEALTH BEHAVIOR

A Working Definition

Although health behavior's boundaries have not yet been rigidly or categorically set, and its definition has not yet been hardened in concrete, a working definition emerging from an earlier task (Gochman, 1981) establishes health behavior as

> those personal attributes such as beliefs, expectations, motives, values, perceptions, and other cognitive elements; personality characteristics, including affective and emotional states and traits; and overt behavior patterns, actions and habits that relate to health maintenance, to health restoration and to health improvement. (Gochman, 1982, p. 169)

This definition provides the focus for this book. "Behavior," moreover, denotes something that people *do* or *refrain from doing,* although not always consciously or voluntarily. It is not something *done to them.* A treatment is not a behavior. Furthermore, mending of broken bones, healing of wounds, immunity against disease, and resistance to infection are reflections of bodily states rather than behaviors. Health behavior thus does not embrace clinical improvement or physiological recovery, as such, but it does include analyses of specific behaviors that have an impact on improvement or recovery. Health status is not a behavior, but a person's perceptions of health status or of improvement, recovery, or other changes in health status are health behaviors. Finally, the working definition's broad construction of behavior includes not only directly observable, overt actions, but also those mental events and feeling states that are "observed" or measured indirectly.

DAVID S. GOCHMAN • Raymond A. Kent School of Social Work, University of Louisville, Louisville, Kentucky 40292.

Such a definition of health behavior recognizes in addition "that these personal attributes are influenced by, and otherwise reflect family structure and processes, peer group and social factors, and societal, institutional, and cultural determinants" (Gochman, 1982, p. 169).

Preventive and Protective Behavior, Illness Behavior, and Sick-Role Behavior

The working definition comprehensively embraces several others, including those delineated by Kasl and Cobb in their seminal articles (1966a,b) defining specific categories of health-related behavior.

Preventive and Protective Behavior. For Kasl and Cobb (1966a), health behavior denotes those actions undertaken by persons who believe they are well, and who are not experiencing any signs or symptoms of illness, for the purpose of remaining well. This usage confines "health behavior" to preventive actions. Among these are behaviors that have *primary* preventive value, including, but not limited to, a number of daily "nonmedical" activities. Breslow and his colleagues (e.g., Belloc & Breslow, 1972) have provided systematic evidence of the impact of six categories of "everyday" nonmedical behaviors upon health status and health risk. These behaviors are duration of sleep; eating habits, including regularity, frequency, amount eaten, and eating breakfast; weight management; physical recreational activity, including active sports, swimming or walking, working in the garden, doing exercises, taking weekend trips, and hunting or fishing; consumption of alcoholic beverages, including frequency and amount; and not smoking.

Other everyday preventive behaviors include wearing seat belts and motor cycle helmets; obeying traffic laws; and following health and safety regulations at work. A survey of physicians (Sobal, Valente, Muncie, Levine, & DeForge, 1985) found strong professional consensus about the preventive importance of these everyday behaviors, particularly about eliminating smoking and using protective equipment and clothing. Medical or technological behaviors with primary preventive value include making systematic use of immunizations known to be effective in preventing infectious diseases.

Other health behaviors encompass those that have *secondary* preventive value, i.e., they do not decisively prevent a condition from occurring, but they facilitate the early detection of a condition and thus minimize its impact. Such behaviors include—but are not limited to—undergoing periodic examinations for the early signs of cancer, heart disease, or dental conditions.

Supplementing those primary and secondary preventive behaviors that have empirical linkages to health status, are what Harris and Guten (1979) term "health protective behaviors." These are actions that people engage in "to protect their health whether . . . medically approved or not" (Harris & Guten, 1979), and are embraced under the concept of health behavior independently of their objective effectiveness. Such health protective behaviors might include praying; fixing things around the house; taking laxatives, emetics, enemas, cold showers, and hot baths; and consuming massive doses of vitamins.

Illness Behavior. For Kasl and Cobb (1966a), illness behavior comprises those actions undertaken by persons who are uncertain about whether they are well; who are troubled or puzzled by bodily sensations or feelings that they believe may be signs or symptoms of illness; who want to clarify the meaning of these experiences and thus determine whether they are well; and who want to know what to do if they are not. In the context of explaining the "help-seeking" behavior of such persons, Mechanic (1966/1972; 1978, Chapter 9) and Suchman (1965/1972) have developed major analyses of illness behavior.

Mechanic's model of illness behavior embraces "an individual's recognition that he needs advice, his decision whether to seek it, his choice of counsellor" (1966/1972, p. 128). Suchman's phrasings are different but the behaviors are similar. Both models examine the personal determinants of these illness behaviors, as well as how these behaviors are socially and culturally conditioned. Illness behaviors include—but are not limited to—responses to bodily signs and symptoms; seeking opinions and advice from persons who are believed to have health expertise, whether they are officially recognized by the larger society (health care professionals) or not (folk practitioners, lay therapists); seeking opinions and advice from relatives, friends, neighbors, colleagues; as well as doing nothing but waiting to see whether the unusual signs or symptoms go away.

Sick-Role Behavior. For Kasl and Cobb (1966b) and others (e.g., Parsons, 1951), sick-role behavior denotes those actions undertaken by persons who have already been designated as being sick, either by others or by themselves. Such behaviors include—but are not limited to—acceptance of a medically prescribed regimen; limitation of activity and of personal, family, and social responsibilities; and actions related to recovery and rehabilitation.

The critical distinctions that Kasl and Cobb and others make between various types of health behaviors are nonetheless important and should not be minimized. For example, it remains for future research to determine empirically whether there are commonalities or underlying unities among the behaviors embraced within each of the categories of "health behaviors," or whether the categories are uniformly and differentially related to diverse levels of determinants. However, it is their common presumed relationship to health that brings the several categories together.

HEALTH BEHAVIOR RESEARCH

Health behavior research, the systematic scientific examination of the aforementioned behaviors and their determinants, is an emerging area of interdisciplinary study. Because of the relative "youth" of the area, the term *research* necessarily includes not only empirical–experimental investigations and the data they generate, but scholarly—albeit nonempirical—analyses and conceptual frameworks that invite and stimulate future investigation.

Antecedent or Consequent; Input or Outcome

Health behavior can be analyzed in at least three ways. One way analyzes health behaviors as antecedents or causes of diseases, illnesses, and health status (e.g., Belloc & Breslow, 1972). A second way analyzes health behaviors as targets for systematic interventions directed at producing behavioral changes and ultimately at generating changes in health status (e.g., Breslow, 1978/1980). Such an approach is taken by health educators, by health promotion campaigns, and by public health programs. A third way, and the one that is the primary focus of this book, examines health behaviors as interesting in their own right, as personal and social phenomena that are inherently worthy of serious scientific investigation. As such, health behaviors are analyzed as consequences or outcomes of a variety of diverse personal and social processes.

A perspective that considers health behaviors as phenomena worthy of being understood on their own terms, and not studied simply because they affect health or because they can be modified to improve health, is more likely to generate basic, conceptually derived, rigorous, systematic scientific investigations, and thus be more likely to lead to greater understanding of these behaviors than perspectives that place health behaviors in an ancillary position.

What Health Behavior Research Is Not

A good definition states clearly not only what something is, but what it is not. Health behavior is conceptually distinct from treatment, and from physiological/biological/pharmacological responses to treatment. It is also conceptually distinct from health care, and from the organization or structure of the health delivery system. Health behavior as an area of research is thus not primarily concerned with the technology of health care, with medical procedures, with psychotherapy, or with other interventions. And it is not primarily concerned with the delivery of health care or services or with the organization of the health delivery system. Yet it touches profoundly upon all of these. Health behavior research *is* concerned with the way such interventions and institutional structures affect the health behavior of individuals. Health behavior research is not primarily concerned with health status. Yet a person's perceptions of health status and social and cultural definitions of health and health status are assuredly important health behaviors.

Health Behavior Research Is Not Behavioral Medicine. Health behavior research is not identical with behavioral medicine, which has been defined as the "field concerned with the *development* of *behavioral science* knowledge and techniques relevant to the understanding of *physical health* and *illness* and the *application* of this knowledge and these techniques to prevention, treatment and rehabilitation" (Schwartz & Weiss, 1978, p. 4). While some areas within behavioral medicine are also contained by health behavior, behavioral medicine deals with tension, stress, or anxiety and other "nonphysical" disorders that are importantly related to total well-being, *only* as these impinge upon specific "physical" disorders. The basic paradigm proposed for behavioral medicine (Schwartz & Weiss, 1978, p. 7) reflects the medical model's systematic concern with the prevention, etiology, pathology, diagnosis, treatment, and rehabilitation of specific disorders rather than with a broader range of health-relevant actions that do not relate to specific diseases or problems. Health behavior is defined independently of pathology, diagnosis, and treatment of specific disorders. It includes a concern for general health maintenance and wellness (e.g., Bruhn & Cordova, 1977, 1978) in addition to behaviors that are problem specific.

Moreover, health behavior research does not automatically begin with a medical framework and its assumptions. It does not accept uncritically the basic premises of the medical model in which physicians and other societally sanctioned health care practitioners establish and reify implicit norms of function and dysfunction. Health behavior embraces both mental and nonmental disorders and recognizes the interaction between them. It questions the traditional philosophical mind–body dualism that has led to separation and fragmentation of research in the health area, to say nothing of the separation and fragmentation of training and delivery of care and services.

Health Behavior Research Is Not Behavioral Health. Health behavior research is not "behavioral health," which Matarazzo (1980) defines as

> an interdisciplinary field dedicated to promoting a philosophy of health that stresses *individual responsibility* in the application of behavioral and biomedical science knowledge and techniques to the *maintenance* of health and the *prevention* of illness and dysfunction by a variety of self-initiated individual or shared activities. (p. 813)

"Behavioral health" is committed to the *application* of knowledge, and as inferred from Matarazzo's definition, it is not committed to seeking and establishing basic knowledge. Furthermore, behavioral health (Matarazzo, 1984) emphasizes an ideology aimed at improving health status by the combination of applied knowledge and individual responsibility. Although health behavior research accepts the importance of increasing knowledge, as an area of basic inquiry it must remain value-free about how persons ought to behave, and thus must pursue neutrality about individual responsibility. Furthermore, the knowledge it generates may well call attention to larger system factors that mediate health behaviors, or that present barriers to individual action, or that are greater health-risk factors than personal habits. More important, it is the *nonmedical* and *basic science* perspective of health behavior research that will be most likely to generate this knowledge.

HEALTH, ILLNESS, AND DISEASE

This discussion begs the question, "What is health?" and the corollary questions, "What is illness?" and "What is disease?" How these are defined, perceived, or conceptualized are important areas of health behavior research. As Wylie cautions, "Any attempt to define what health means lays the definer open to attack by critics armed with heavy reference books. Fortunately, this phenomenon has not prevented many groups and individuals from suggesting definitions . . ." (Wylie, 1970, p. 100). Diaz-Guerrero (1984), addressing the issue of whether there is a universal conception of health, analyzed the Semantic Differential responses of large samples representing 30 different cultures. The data revealed that health is looked at similarly across cultures in many ways. There is apparently cross-cultural agreement that health is characterized as "good," "potent," and "active," but Diaz-Guerrero recognizes that the meanings of these adjectives vary from one culture to another.

Even "disease," which can be given a very narrow meaning as "a medical hypothesis that implies particular pathological processes underlying a specific clinical syndrome" (Mechanic, 1978, p. 25), usually involving specific agents, nutritional deficiency, or biological inadequacy, is increasingly used to refer to behavioral and social processes for which no such specificity can be demonstrated (e.g., conditions such as anorexia, or antisocial behaviors).

Lewis cautions that it is virtually impossible "to recognize disease, or health, as an absolute" (Lewis, 1953/1980, p. 115), and it is beyond the scope of this chapter to discuss health, illness, and disease in depth, or to provide simple, categorical definitions for them. But it is important to show the pluralism of perspectives that are applied to these phenomena. Moreover, such pluralism, or diversity, is itself an important domain of health behavior research. There is thus an intellectual paradox inherent in the definitional process: the *process* of defining these terms has an impact on the *substance* of the definition.

Six elements, at least, contribute to the complexity and difficulty of definition. The first is the simultaneous existence of lay and professional, or scientific, definitions. Although these definitions overlap appreciably, they are nonetheless different and their differences have important implications for health behavior and health behavior research. Whereas differences between lay and professional definitions exist in relation to other phenomena (e.g., the chemical and physical universes, human nature, religion), the disparities between the two types of definitions have greater life-or-death relevance for the human condition in the area of health. To extend Hayes-Bautista's sociology of knowledge paradigm (Hayes-Bautista, 1978), professional definitions, like other aspects of professional knowledge, are more formal, i.e., more likely to be explicit and recorded in identifiable documents, and produced by specific acknowledged sources; emerge from a greater depth of knowledge; are acquired in a more structured, uniform way; and have fewer contradictions and greater clarity than lay definitions.

A second element contributing to the difficulty of definition is the existence of multiple professional or scientific definitions. Physicians, sociologists, anthropologists, and psychologists themselves offer different definitions of health and illness. For example, medical definitions emphasize the presence or absence of "pathology"; psychological definitions emphasize perceptions, feelings of well-being, and equilibrium.

A third element is the existence of plural definitions within each of these professions or sciences. Depending on theoretical or ideological commitments, persons working within the same field may view the terms differently. For example, Alonzo (1984) points out that within sociology, the structural–functional perspective views health in terms of the homeostasis or equilibrium of society, and disease as dysfunctional because it disrupts social equilibrium by impairing the expected performance of individuals. Alternatively, according to Alonzo, the ideational or interactional perspective in sociology views disease independently of—or as not inherent in—social behavior or performance, and emphasizes instead the importance of social interaction and social labeling in the determination of what is considered disease.

A fourth element contributing to the difficulty of defining these terms is the acknowledgment that at least three dimensions must be taken into account. As Levine and Sorenson note, there is consensus among varied cultural groups that both professional and lay definitions of health include an absence of symptoms or signs of illness, a sense or feeling of well-being, and the capacity to perform (Levine & Sorenson, 1984, p. 224). For convenience, these can be thought of as biomedical, personal, and sociocultural components. "Biomedical" subsumes a host of biological, biochemical, and physiological processes; "personal," a variety of affective, perceptual, behavioral, and other psychological components; and "sociocultural," myriad performance, interactional, social structure, and cultural components.

For example, the World Health Organization's (WHO) common denominator definition—"Health is a state of complete physical, mental and social well-being and is not merely the absence of disease or infirmity" (WHO, 1946/1948, p. 100)—recognizes the multifaceted nature of health, and that health involves these three components. Furthermore, although health and disease may have some link, this definition acknowledges that health has a reality that is independent of disease. However, this consensual definition does not say much about what health is, or about what is meant by "well-being."

Analyses of health, illness, and disease as dramatic parts of the human experience have continued through recorded history. Herzlich's thoughtful yet concise narrative of the history of medicine stresses that thinking about health and illness has always reflected a mixture of biological or medical components, together with components that are personal, social, and cultural (Herzlich, 1973). Despite what might be termed the emerging dominance of the "body orientation" (p. 2; Herzlich's quotation marks), which was facilitated and reinforced by advances in anatomy, physiology, and the other sciences, there has always been an appreciation of the personal, social, and environmental factors that generate disease or support its absence. Herzlich points out (p. 2) that Hippocrates, who is regarded as the founder of medicine because of his systematic concern for the body and its symptoms, recognized the effect of environmental factors in disease. A strictly "medical" definition of health, or a totally medical perspective on illness and disease, thus has no productive place in this discussion.

Granting the importance of considering these three interacting dimensions, a fifth element contributing to the complexity of defining these basic terms is the variety of phenomena that have been used as focal points. Different definitions of health and illness present varying degrees of juxtaposition, conflict, and equilibrium among the medical, personal, and social perspectives. Some common themes in the analyses leading to these definitions are: whether health and disease exist along a continuum, or whether they reflect a dichotomy; whether health is just the absence of some pathology, or whether it is something positive—what Herzlich contrasts as "health-in-a-vacuum" versus "health in reserve" (Herzlich, 1973, p. 56); the relative validity of scientific/professional/medical definitions in relation to folk/layperson/phenomenological definitions; the role of equilibrium and homeostasis concepts in defining health and illness; the use of "normative" standards (and if so, which ones); how health and illness are related to various types of social conflict; and whether health is an asymptotic, elastic, or open-ended concept (Polgar, 1968; Wylie, 1970).

Finally, a sixth element contributing to the difficulty is the simultaneous existence of several different health practice systems. Analyses of the organization of a society's health care practices provide a context in which these plural perspectives can be observed. Kennedy demonstrated, for example, that perceptions of health and illness vary with the mixture in any culture of "scientific" medicine, religious or "primitive" medicine, public health practice, folk medicine, and public safety practice (Kennedy, 1973). Gran (1979) also showed similar mixtures of health practice systems in preindustrial Arabic societies.

Many useful paradigms exist for examining, comparing, and integrating the plural perspectives on health and illness. Wolinsky's tridimensional conception (e.g., 1988, Chapter 4) is a good illustration of these. Wolinsky first identifies the medical model perspective, which emphasizes physiological malfunctioning, germ theory, and clinical signs and symptoms of malfunctioning as indicators of illness, and the absence of these as a definition of "what is not disease" rather than of "what is health." He examines the history of this model and critically evaluates its assumptions and its implications. A second perspective, the sociocultural approach, emphasizes an individual's capacity to perform expected roles and tasks and to function socially. Health in these terms is defined relative to a person's role enactments and participation in social processes. Persons who do not perform roles and tasks as expected, and who do not participate in expected ways in social processes are considered as deviant (e.g., Twaddle, 1973). Illness and "sick-role" behavior become ways of accounting for, explaining, and controlling such deviance. The third perspective, the psychological approach, considers health as the personal experience of general well-being. Persons who "feel" well are considered healthy; those who "feel" distressed or impaired or not at ease are considered ill.

For the purposes of this chapter, the diverse perspectives of health and illness are considered as examples of two broad approaches: the personal and the sociocultural. *Personal perspectives* are those that focus primarily on the person existing within a social environment; *sociocultural perspectives* are those that focus primarily on the social, societal, and cultural influences upon the individual.

Personal Perspectives

For convenience, representative examples of personal perspectives are grouped under three headings: functioning and equilibrium; breakdown; and personal construction.

Functioning and Equilibrium. Where functioning is smooth and unimpaired, equilibrium or homeostasis exists. Health has often been identified with such equilibria, with an organism functioning smoothly within its environment, continually adapting to it and readily restoring equilibrium when it has been disrupted. Elkes has identified the historical importance of equilibrium or homeostatic concepts to the field of medicine, and the importance of self-regulation as a component of health and well-being (Elkes, 1981). Polgar's scholarly analysis (1968) shows that contemporary equilibrium concepts have their origins in Indo-European history, predating the Galenian concepts of "four fluids"; and that the concept of equilibrium was inherent in the ancient Oriental notion of yin and yang.

Engel (1962/1975) urges a movement away from considering disease in terms of cell pathology, toward considering it in terms of "failures or disturbances in the growth, development, functions and adjustments of the organism as a whole or of any of its systems" (1975, p. 185), and argues that "there is no sharp dividing line between health and disease" (p. 191), that they "are relative concepts which do not easily lend themselves to simple definition" (p. 185). Health is defined as a state in which the organism is "functioning effectively, fulfilling needs, successfully responding to the requirements or demands of the environment, whether internal or external, and pursing its biological destiny, including growth and reproduction." Wylie (1970) suggests that "health is the perfect, *continuing* adjustment of an organism to its environment," and that "disease would be an imperfect continuing adjustment" (p. 103).

Patrick, Bush, and Chen, recognizing the functional dimensions of health as well as the social norms that define these functions, developed a complex and comprehensive formula for operationalizing health into mathematical terms (Patrick, Bush, & Chen, 1973). Their formula includes the performance of social and physical activities and mobility in relation to age, the value or preference that society attaches to these activities, together with physical symptoms and prognoses.

Blaxter and Paterson's analyses of lay models of disease in three generations of working-class Scottish women (1982; Blaxter, 1983) show clearly that they define health not so much in terms of the presence or absence of specific structural or anatomical conditions (Blaxter & Paterson, 1982, p. 27), but rather in terms of being able to carry out normal work, household, and social functions. "Good health was being able to work, being healthy enough 'for all practical purposes' " (p. 28). Moreover, the respondents clearly distinguish between illness and disease, acknowledging that persons could have a disease without being ill, that disease and health could coexist (p. 34).

Breakdown. When functioning is more than casually or routinely disrupted, and equilibrium is not readily reestablished, disequilibrium exists. Such imbalances or disequilibria are presumed to be stressful to the organism, and considered eventually to lead to disease and illness (e.g., Bahnson, 1974; Borysenko, 1984; Cassel, 1974). Increasingly, however, serious questions have been raised about the causal link between stress and illness (e.g., Kobasa, Maddi, & Kahn, 1982). Moreover, evidence is accumulating (e.g., Wiebe & McCallum, 1986) that part of the relationship between stress and health status may be attributable to health behaviors.

Breakdown is the failure of functioning and equilibrium. Polgar's historical analysis (1968) reveals that such departures from harmony were thought to result from becoming "civilized," a function of the way people live, of their moving away from nature. Antonovsky's innovative thinking about the failure of functioning and equilibrium moves in the direction of a generic disease model, the "breakdown concept," and away from conceptions of specific diseases (Antonovsky, 1973). The breakdown concept avoids dichotomizing persons as sick or well, but considers them along a continuum.

The breakdown concept assumes that it is possible to classify any condition along four dimensions: degree of pain; prevention of role and task performance; threat to life; and external recognition that the condition requires care. The degree to which persons are located along these four dimensions is a measure of the degree of their "breakdown." For example, regardless of the specific nature of a condition, a person who is not experiencing pain, whose role and task performance is only mildly impaired, whose condition is in no way life-threatening, and who is not readily recognized by others as needing professional care, has a much lower degree of breakdown than a person in great pain, who cannot perform social tasks and roles, whose condition—if not life-threatening—is "urgent," and who is readily recognized by others as needing professional care.

Antonovsky's scale to measure breakdown demonstrated not only that a small number of breakdown profiles could accommodate the health status of a large sample of Israeli women, but that some degree of breakdown, rather than complete health, was normative for this sample. Moreover, different ethnic groups had characteristically different breakdown profiles.

Personal Construction. Researchers moving away from scientifically and medically correct descriptions of the disease process, toward increasing understanding of personal or phenomenological definitions or conceptions of the disease process, are beginning to explore "commonsense" views or schemata of disease (Bishop & Converse, 1987; Lau & Hartman, 1983; Leventhal, Prohaska, & Hirschman, 1983). Lau and Hartman, for example, explored the variability of lay conceptions of common illnesses. Their observations revealed that the simple "germ" model of disease—in which people uniformly and sequentially experience unusual and/or unpleasant symptoms, define themselves as sick, are thus motivated to visit a physician, and are cured by virtue of the physician's killing the germs with drugs or medicine—is an inadequate representation of how diseases are personally experienced. Lau and Hartman found that commonsense representations of diseases vary considerably, and that this variability reflects five different dimensions: the condition's identity; its short- or long-term consequences; the timing of its course; its cause(s); and its cure. Lau and Hartman reason that it is when these commonsense individual "lay schemes" for evaluating or interpreting signs and symptoms no longer provide an adequate "fit," i.e., when they no longer can account for what people are experiencing, that people are inclined to believe they have something serious and take some appropriate action.

Closely related to such representations is the concept of attribution of illness (e.g., Campbell, 1975a,b; Mechanic, 1978, pp. 254–255). Mechanic points out that people vary in how they make sense out of their bodily experiences; how they attribute illness to events that disrupt their functioning; and how they define health in relation to total functioning as well as to experiences of specific symptoms (p. 254). They also vary in how they attribute causes to their conditions.

Moreover, personal constructions of health-related definitions have been shown to vary developmentally and with the life cycle (e.g., Gochman, 1985). Campbell (1975a,b) has shown both similarities and differences between youngsters' and parents' definitions of health and illness. Whereas youngsters and their mothers show strong consensus about the relative importance of specific signs and symptoms as indicators of illness (e.g., fever, vomiting), mothers were more likely to attribute illness to these signs and symptoms when they occurred in their children, than when they occurred in themselves.

Furthermore, as might be expected from developmental theories, youngsters' health-related definitions and health-related concepts are more concrete, more egocentric, and less abstract than those of adults, and demonstrate developmental changes that are congruent with Piagetian as well as Lewinian models (e.g., Burbach & Peterson, 1986; Gellert, 1962, 1978; Gochman, 1985; Natapoff, 1982; Rashkis, 1965; Simeonsson, Buckley, & Monson, 1979).

Sociocultural Perspectives

Representative examples of social, societal, and cultural perspectives on health, illness, and disease can similarly be grouped under three parallel headings: functioning and equilibrium in social contexts; social breakdown; and social constructions of health and illness.

Social Functioning and Equilibrium. Smooth social functioning and societal equilibrium presume that individual members will actively participate in the society's processes and activities, and will satisfactorily perform the roles and tasks required of them (e.g., Parsons, 1951; Twaddle, 1979). Alonzo's analyses (1984) bridge the gap between the personal and sociocultural perspectives. Avoiding some of the rigidity of the "structural" view of homeostasis in which society rather than the person attempts to maintain equilibrium, and in which disease is viewed as dysfunctional because it disturbs expected social behavior and thus threatens social equilibrium, Alonzo proposes an interactional or situational–adaptation model which recognizes that social situations vary in the degree to which they permit "adaptation." Alonzo's framework envisions people as generally active and continually striving for equilibrium within an environment that is constantly in flux. He reasons that it is necessary to examine the way in which bodily experiences (biophysical sensations) having the potential to be signs and symptoms of illness are continually evaluated in relation to social "objectification," or labeling. Moreover, adaptation is defined in terms of how well people can "contain" or limit the impact of such signs and symptoms so that their social functioning remains unaffected. Such containment may involve minor modifications or compromises of role performance in order that the persons may continue to be active in their social situation. Containment of such signs and symptoms is Alonzo's major theoretical construct.

Most daily situations allow for the easy containment of everyday signs and symptoms, and do not routinely produce such signs and symptoms. But some situations themselves produce such signs and symptoms and/or do not permit their ready containment. Health and illness are then viewed in terms of how readily signs and symptoms are containable within any situation or context.

Social Breakdown. Societal breakdown occurs when individual members do not behave or perform as the norms of the society require. To prevent this from occurring, societies attempt to place limits on, or otherwise control, such departures from expected behaviors. As Parsons noted, "health is intimately involved in the functional prerequisites of the social system" (1951, p. 430), and disease and illness are considered to be conditions which may impair individual members' abilities to perform as expected. While it was recognized that illness in many instances was "something which merely 'happened to people' " (p. 430) and was not something they could control, in other instances disease and illness could be considered to reflect personal and motivational determinants. To the degree that this latter view is valid, society provides and institutionalizes mechanisms of social control to avoid breakdown and thus society assures continuity of normative functioning. One such mechanism involves the conditional granting of the sick role and release from role and task responsibilities (pp. 312–313), which not only insulates the "deviant" person from society but has the further function of reintegrating the deviant through therapeutic intervention and cure. Thus, concepts of health and illness are used as mechanisms of control to reestablish the normative "healthy" state and prevent social breakdown.

Another perspective related to social breakdown is found in Shuval, Antonovsky, and Davies's (1973) analysis of illness as a mechanism for coping with failure. Although failure to perform as expected is recognized as existing in all societies, if such failure can be attributed to illness, then illness can become a legitimate rationale for a person's not behaving in a socially expected way, i.e., not succeeding or achieving.

Social Construction. Herzlich's anthropological–sociological investigation in France revealed that lay definitions of health consistently demonstrated a "social construction," involving an interplay between personal experiences and social and cultural norms and values. A predominant social or cultural "theme" observed among Herzlich's respondents is that "the way of life," i.e., living in a large, urban setting, is the primary source of illness, while the major pathogenic factor within the individual is primarily whether the person is or is not "a defender" against illness, i.e., whether the person exhibits a variety of mechanisms and skills to ward off the pathogenic effect of the environment and the way of life. These observations are parallel to the historical view that Polgar (1968) mentions, in which illness is ascribed to moving away from nature.

Herzlich further demonstrates that medical definitions of health and illness also involve "social construction" in that they often reflect the effects of prevailing social and cultural values upon what is considered "scientifically known" about biology and physiology. Moreover, Herzlich notes consistencies and regularities in these "social constructions" of health and illness, as well as in the lay beliefs about causality of illness and disease. Paradoxically, she notes (Chapter 8) that illness, at times, is viewed positively—as a liberator that enables a person to get away from the demands of everyday life and to be freed to pursue reading or other intellectual activities!

CONSENSUS AND CONFUSION

Remaining amid, and underlying this diversity, is a strong consensus among both professionals—physicians and scientists—and laypersons that health and the related concepts of illness and disease involve—in varying degrees—biomedical, personal, and sociocultural dimensions. Confusion, or lack of convergence, exists primarily in relation to the relative importance of each of these dimensions, and which among the many facets of each should be entered into any definition. Although lack of consensus around precise definitions is an important issue where attempts are made to evaluate the success of health interventions, programs, or systems of care (e.g., Wylie, 1970), it is not a barrier to conducting health behavior research.

Furthermore, any present or future research findings showing increased consensus or unanimity in how professionals believe these terms should be defined would not by themselves establish the validity or acceptability of such definitions. Wylie (1970) cautions that such definitions are tentative and evolutionary in character. It is *not* a goal for health behavior research to define these terms "definitively," but rather to determine what definitions exist in populations. However, the value for health behavior research of increased consensus would lie in the greater precision that would be afforded when such professional beliefs and definitions are compared with lay beliefs and definitions in studies of professional–client interactions, of compliance, and of responsiveness to health promotion programs. It follows that additional investigation of lay definitions, and how these either resemble or differ from those held by professionals form an agenda for future health behavior research.

Issues for Future Research

Both the consensus and the confusion provide incentives and impetus for future research. Among the important issues to be resolved by such research are those related to the confounding of method, discipline, and perspective; to generalizability; to population diversity; and to the search for meaning.

Confounding Effects. Currently available findings reflect a diversity of methods, from the systematic questionnaire techniques and self-reports of psychology (e.g., Bishop & Converse, 1987), to the focused, structured interviews of sociology (e.g., Blaxter, 1983), to the open, fluid, field observations of anthropology (e.g., Herzlich, 1973). Behind these diverse methods are a range of theoretical perspectives, ideologies, purposes, and rationales. Although the reported findings make sense intuitively, and the divergences are not difficult to accept, it remains impossible to separate the diversity of observations from the diversity of the research process. It is thus difficult to determine whether the lack of consensus about what health means is genuine or an artifact. One challenge for future health behavior research would be to bring diverse methods and frames of reference together in a systematic, interdisciplinary way in order to determine more rigorously what these lay definitions are.

Generalizability. The findings reported in this chapter represent the literature available through standard search activities (e.g., systematic reviews of selected journals, computer searches, awareness of what others are doing, and use of relevant bibliographical material). It is hard to escape the conclusion that definitions of health and illness have not been systematically examined on a large number of diverse populations. Questions thus arise about whether one can generalize beyond the French, Scottish, Israeli, and United States samples. Diaz-Guerrero's (1984) findings represent one attempt at a cross-national, cross-cultural effort, but conducting the interdisciplinary research identified in the previous section on a large number of randomly selected populations would be a second important task for future health behavior research.

An additional generalizability issue arises from questions about the validity of models proposed to measure health and illness, e.g., Antonovsky's (1973) breakdown model and Alonzo's (1984) containment model, for populations at large, and for demographic groups within such populations. Health behavior research into these promising and intellectually stimulating models, using varied populations, is a third important task for the future.

Population Diversity. The other side of the "consensus coin" is the existence of consistent, coherent differences within demographic segments of a population. A fourth task for future health behavior research is the determination of how various groups within a population differ in their definitions. Systematic study of diverse samples, of persons with different ethnic, educational, socioeconomic, or age characteristics, might reveal demographic diversity that would have important practical value in increasing the success of programs and improving communication between professionals and clients, for example.

Search for Meaning. Most of the research on definitions of health, illness, and disease has dealt with the "denotative" aspects of a definition. Ben-Sira's conception of "involvement with a disease" (1977) is one of the few studies that has dealt with "connotative" aspects: the personal impact or salience of health, illness, and disease. Determining the "effective meaning" of these phenomena for populations and population subgroups, in contrast to their "intellectual" meaning, is yet a fifth task for future health behavior research.

REFERENCES

Alonzo, A. A. (1984). An illness behavior paradigm: A conceptual exploration of a situational–adaptation perspective. *Social Science and Medicine, 19,* 499–510.

Antonovsky, A. (1973). The utility of the breakdown concept. *Social Science and Medicine, 7,* 605–612.

Bahnson, C. B. (1974). Epistomological perspectives of physical disease from the psychodynamic point of view. *American Journal of Public Health, 64,* 1034–1039.

Belloc, N. B., & Breslow, L. (1972). Relationship of physical health status and health practices. *Preventive Medicine, 1,* 409–421.

Ben-Sira, Z. (1977). Involvement with a disease and health-promoting behavior. *Social Science and Medicine, 11,* 165–173.

Bishop, G. D., & Converse, S. A. (1987). Illness representations: A prototype approach. *Health Psychology, 5,* 95–114.

Blaxter, M. (1983). The causes of disease: Women talking. *Social Science and Medicine, 17,* 59–69.

Blaxter, M., & Paterson, E. (1982). *Mothers and daughters: A three-generational study of health attitudes and behaviour*. London: Heinemann.

Borysenko, J. (1984). Stress, coping, and the immune system. In J. D. Matarazzo, S. M. Weiss, J. A. Herd, N. E. Miller, & S. M. Weiss (Eds.), *Behavioral health: A handbook of health enhancement and disease prevention.* New York: Wiley.

Breslow, L. (1980). Risk factor intervention for health maintenance. In D. Mechanic (Ed.), *Readings in medical sociology*. New York: Free Press. (Reprinted from *Science,* 1978, *200,* 908–912)

Bruhn, J. G., & Cordova, F. D. (1977). A developmental approach to learning wellness behavior. Part 1: Infancy to early adolescence. *Health Values, 1,* 246–254.

Bruhn, J. G., & Cordova, F. D. (1978). A developmental approach to learning wellness behavior. Part II: Adolescence to maturity. *Health Values, 2,* 16–21.

Burbach, D. J., & Peterson, L. (1986). Children's concepts of physical illness: A review and critique of the cognitive-developmental literature. *Health Psychology, 5,* 307–325.

Campbell, J. D. (1975a). Attribution of illness: Another double standard. *Journal of Health and Social Behavior, 16,* 114–126.

Campbell, J. D. (1975b). Illness is a point of view: The development of children's concepts of illness. *Child Development, 46,* 92–100.

Cassel, J. (1974). An epidemiological perspective of psychological factors in disease etiology. *American Journal of Public Health, 64,* 1040–1043.

Diaz-Guerrero, R. (1984). Behavioral health across cultures. In J. D. Matarazzo, S. M. Weiss, J. A. Herd, N. E. Miller, & S. M. Weiss (Eds.), *Behavioral health: A handbook of health enhancement and disease prevention.* New York: Wiley.

Elkes, J. (1981). Self-regulation and behavioral medicine: The early beginnings. *Psychiatric Annals, 11,* 48–57.

Engel, G. L. (1975). A unified concept of health and disease. In T. Millon (Ed.), *Medical behavioral science.* Philadelphia: Saunders. (Reprinted from G. L. Engel, *Psychological development in health and disease,* 1962, Philadelphia: Saunders)

Gellert, E. (1962). Children's conceptions of the content and functions of the human body. *Genetic Psychology Monographs, 61,* 293–405.

Gellert, E. (1978). What do I have inside me? How children view their bodies. In E. Gellert (Ed.), *Psychosocial aspects of pediatric care*. New York: Grune & Stratton.

Gochman, D. S. (1981). On labels, systems, and motives: Some perspectives on children's health behavior. In *Self-management educational programs for childhood asthma, 2,* Conference Manuscripts. Sponsored by Center for Interdisciplinary Research in Immunologic Diseases, University of California at Los Angeles; National Institute of Allergy and Infectious Diseases; Asthma and Allergy Foundation of America.

Gochman, D. S. (1982). Labels, systems and motives: Some perspectives for future research. In D. S. Gochman & G. S. Parcel (Eds.), Children's health beliefs and health behaviors [Special issue]. *Health Education Quarterly, 9,* 167–174.

Gochman, D. S. (1985). Family determinants of children's concepts of health and illness. In D. C. Turk & R. D. Kerns (Eds.), *Health, illness, and families: A life-span perspective*. New York: Wiley.

Gran, P. (1979). Medical pluralism in Arab and Egyptian history: An overview of class structures and philosophies of the main phases. *Social Science and Medicine, 13B,* 339–348.

Harris, D. M., & Guten, S. (1979). Health protective behavior: An exploratory study. *Journal of Health and Social Behavior, 20,* 17–29.

Hayes-Bautista, D. E. (1978). Chicano patients and medical practitioners: A sociology of knowledges paradigm of lay–professional interaction. *Social Science and Medicine, 12,* 83–90.

Herzlich, C. (1973). *Health and illness: A social psychological analysis* (D. Graham, Trans.). London: Academic Press.

Kasl, S. V., & Cobb, S. (1966a). Health behavior, illness behavior, and sick-role behavior: I. Health and illness behavior. *Archives of Environmental Health, 12,* 246–266.

Kasl, S. V., & Cobb, S. (1966b). Health behavior, illness behavior, and sick-role behavior: II. Sick-role behavior. *Archives of Environmental Health, 12,* 531–541.

Kennedy, D. A. (1973). Perceptions of illness and healing. *Social Science and Medicine, 7,* 787–805.

Kobasa, S. C., Maddi, S. R., & Kahn, S. (1982). Hardiness and health: A prospective study. *Journal of Personality and Social Psychology, 42,* 168–177.

Lau, R. R., & Hartman, K. A. (1983). Common sense representations of common illnesses. *Health Psychology, 2,* 167–185.

Leventhal, H., Prohaska, T. R., & Hirschman, R. S. (1983). Preventive health behavior across the life-span. In J. C. Rosen & L. J. Solomon (Eds.), *Preventing health risk behaviors and promoting coping with illness* (Vol. 8). Vermont Conference on the Primary Prevention of Psychopathology. Hanover, NH: University Press of New England.

Levine, S., & Sorenson, J. R. (1984). Social and cultural factors in health promotion. In J. D. Matarazzo, S. M. Weiss, J. A. Herd, N. E. Miller, & S. M. Weiss (Eds.), *Behavioral health: A handbook of health enhancement and disease prevention.* New York: Wiley.

Lewis, A. (1980). Health as a social concept. In D. Mechanic (Ed.), *Readings in medical sociology.* New York: Free Press. (Reprinted from *British Journal of Sociology,* 1953, *2,* 109–124)

Matarazzo, J. D. (1980). Behavioral health and behavioral medicine: Frontiers for a new health psychology. *American Psychologist, 35,* 807–817.

Matarazzo, J. D. (1984). Behavioral health: A 1990 challenge for the health sciences professions. In J. D. Matarazzo, S. M. Weiss, J. A. Herd, N. E. Miller, & S. M. Weiss (Eds.), *Behavioral health: A handbook of health enhancement and disease prevention.* New York: Wiley.

Mechanic, D. (1972). Response factors in illness: The study of illness behavior. In E. G. Jaco (Ed.), *Patients, physicians and illness: A sourcebook in behavioral science and health* (2nd ed.). New York: Free Press. (Reprinted from *Social Psychiatry,* 1966, *1,* 11–20)

Mechanic, D. (1978). *Medical sociology* (2nd ed.). New York: Free Press.

Natapoff, J. N. (1982). A developmental analysis of children's ideas of health. In D. S. Gochman & G. S. Parcel (Eds.), Children's health beliefs and health behaviors [Special issue]. *Health Education Quarterly, 9,* 34–45.

Parsons, T. (1951). *The social system.* Glencoe, IL: Free Press.

Patrick, D. L., Bush, J. W., & Chen, M. M. (1973). Toward an operational definition of health. *Journal of Health and Social Behavior, 14,* 6–23.

Polgar, S. (1968). Health. In D. L. Sills (Ed.), *International encyclopedia of the social sciences.* New York: Macmillan Co. and Free Press.

Rashkis, S. R. (1965). Children's understanding of health. *Archives of General Psychiatry, 12,* 10–17.

Schwartz, G. E., & Weiss, S. M. (Eds.). (1978). *Proceedings of the Yale conference on behavioral medicine.* Department of Health, Education and Welfare Publication (NIH) 78-1424.

Shuval, J. T., Antonovsky, A., & Davies, A. M. (1973). Illness: A mechanism for coping with failure. *Social Science and Medicine, 7,* 259–265.

Simeonsson, R. J., Buckley, L., & Monson, L. (1979). Conceptions of illness causality in hospitalized children. *Journal of Pediatric Psychology, 4,* 77–84.

Sobal, J., Valente, C. M., Muncie, H. L., Levine, D. M., & DeForge, B. R. (1985). Physicians' beliefs about the importance of 25 health promoting behaviors. *American Journal of Public Health, 75,* 1427–1428.

Suchman, E. A. (1972). Stages of illness and medical care. In E. G. Jaco (Ed.), *Patients, physicians and illness: A sourcebook in behavioral science and health* (2nd ed.). New York: Free Press. (Reprinted from *Journal of Health and Human Behavior,* 1965, *6,* 114–128)

Twaddle, A. C. (1973). Illness and deviance. *Social Science and Medicine, 7,* 751–762.

Twaddle, A. C. (1979). *Sickness behavior and the sick role.* Boston: G. K. Hall.

Wiebe, D. J., & McCallum, D. M. (1986). Health practices and hardiness as mediators in the stress-illness relationship. *Health Psychology, 5,* 425–438.

Wolinsky, F. D. (1988). *The sociology of health: Principles, practitioners, and issues* (2nd ed.). Belmont, CA: Wadsworth.

World Health Organization. (1948). *Official records of the World Health Organization. No. 2. Proceedings and final acts of the international health conference held in New York from 19 June to 22 July 1946*. United Nations: WHO Interim Commission. (Meeting held in 1946; *Proceedings* published in 1948)

Wylie, C. M. (1970). The definition and measurement of health and disease. *Public Health Reports, 85*, 100–104.

PART II

DETERMINANTS OF HEALTH BEHAVIOR

Personal Determinants

Cognitive Determinants

Research on the personal determinants of health actions is covered in two sections. The first section deals with cognitions; the second, with other personal characteristics and components of life-style. As cognitions, cognitive structures, or cognitive systems are themselves personal characteristics, the division of this section is arbitrary. However, health behavior research has been considerably enriched by two cognitive approaches: the health belief model and the locus of control model. The division of the section thus facilitates a greater focus on such models.

Cognition is the generic term for those personal thought processes that serve as frames of reference for organizing and evaluating experiences. Beliefs, expectations, perceptions, values, motives, and attitudes all provide the person with ways of filtering, interpreting, understanding, and predicting events. Cognitive approaches to human behavior emphasize phenomenology—events as they are psychologically experienced: the world as it is perceived by the person, in contrast to the world of physical "reality." Major cognitive approaches to predicting health behavior are the health belief model, the locus of control model, and the theory of behavioral intentions. Health as a motive or value, and those motives relevant to health behavior, represent another important cognitive determinant.

THE HEALTH BELIEF MODEL

The health belief model, often considered to be the major frame of reference in this area, and at one time referred to "in virtually every dissertation related to health behavior" (Green, 1974, p. 324), has been generating health behavior research since the 1950s. In its original form, developed to explain and predict why people engage in specific preventive behaviors such as accepting a vaccine or participating in a tuberculosis screening procedure (e.g., Rosenstock, Derryberry, & Carriger, 1959), the model stated that perceptions of being susceptible to some condition, the perceived seriousness of that condition, and perceptions of the availability of behaviors that prevent or treat the condition, were all related to the likelihood that an individual would engage in some specific preventive behavior. To the degree that people believe that (1) they are highly susceptible or vulnerable to some health problem such as tuberculosis or hypertension, (2) the problem is a serious or severe one, and (3) specific actions such taking as a chest X ray or a blood pressure test will be of benefit in preventing its occurrence or minimizing its risks—and that these benefits outweigh the social and monetary costs or barriers presented by these actions, such people will be more likely to take those specified health actions than if they believe (1) they are in no way susceptible or vulnerable to the problem, (2) the problem is not serious or major, and (3) the specific actions would have no net benefits to them in preventing or minimizing the problem. The health belief model thus is an essentially cognitive, rational view of health activities.

Numerous examples exist of research generated by the model. Urberg and Robbins (1984) demonstrated that perceived vulnerability to the risks of smoking was associated with lower likelihoods that adolescents would begin to smoke. Manfredi, Warnecke, Graham, and Rosenthal (1977) showed that beliefs about the benefits of early detection and treatment of breast cancer were related to knowledgeability about breast self-examinations. Chen and Tatsuoka (1984) showed that several beliefs derived from the model predicted preventive dental behaviors—brushing, flossing, and regular dental visits—in a sample of American women; and that perceptions of barriers and the salience of dental care were the strongest predictors. Ben-Sira and Padeh's study of participation in a Tays–Sachs screening program in Israel (1978) showed that pregnant women were less likely than nonpregnant women to believe that they were susceptible to being carriers of the condition. Ben-Sira and Padeh interpret this as a defense mechanism to reduce the emotional threat of carrying the disease, and suggest that where such risks are involved, there may be cross-pressures that influence the levels of the health belief model variables. Furthermore, a series of assessments of health-related expectations in young populations derived from the model (e.g., Gochman, 1986; Gochman & Saucier, 1982) demonstrated that beliefs about vulnerability are remarkably consistent and stable during childhood and adolescence.

Systematic compendia of research generated by the model, together with critical analyses, have been provided by Becker (1974) and Janz and Becker (1984). Janz and Becker, for example, used a "significance ratio" (p. 36) to compare the predictive value of the several variables encompassed by the model, and to show historical changes in the way the variables were conceptualized and measured, and in their relative effectiveness. For studies published prior to 1974, "perceived susceptibility" was the best overall predictor. For studies published during the years 1974–1984, "perceived barriers" was the best predictor, followed by "perceived benefits" and "perceived susceptibility." "Perceived seriousness" was far less valuable as a predictor. Yet, in a prospective study, Eckert and Goldstein (1983) observed that perceived severity played a role as a trigger to seeking medical care, as well as a role in the choice of source of care. However, the magnitude of its importance was influenced by income level. Neighbors (1984) also found perceived severity to be related to care seeking.

Janz and Becker's observations are congruent with the increased attention paid to conceptualizing and measuring perceived benefits and barriers in later work, particularly in studies that attempted to develop measures of benefits and barriers that were congruent with the phenomenological world of respondents (e.g., Eisen, Zellman, & McAlister, 1985), in contrast to the presumptive reality of medical technology.

Kirscht's chapter provides insights into the model's current use as a predictor of a variety of health actions, as well as an assessment of its complexity and status. It also reveals how the model has become less involved in the prediction of "medically" determined or medically specified behaviors, and more involved in the prediction of a broad spectrum of health-relevant, but nonmedically specified behaviors. Moreover, Kirscht's discussion of ways of dimensionalizing behaviors (e.g., habitual or nonhabitual; repetitive or one-time; initiating or stopping) and how differences along these dimensions have important implications for the predictive value of the model, is a critically important conceptual contribution.

LOCUS OF CONTROL

The second major cognitive approach stems from Rotter's conception of locus of control (1966). The degree to which persons perceive themselves as being in control over events in their lives (internal locus of control), in contrast to perceiving that events or outcomes in their lives are capricious or subject to control by others (external locus of control), has been found to be related to the likelihood that they will engage in selected health behaviors, although the evidence is not uniformly conclusive. Wallston and Wallston (1978) provided one of the earliest systematic reviews of this literature, and Seeman and Seeman's longitudinal analysis (1983) shows that persons who believe that they are more "in control" in relation to health and illness are more likely to engage in health-promoting behaviors than those who believe that they are less "in control."

Very much related to locus of control are Pill and Stott's observations of working-class British women (1985), in whom strong beliefs about personal responsibility for health and illness coexist with strong beliefs about external causes of disease, e.g., germs, heredity, and environmental factors. Moreover, women who had strong beliefs about personal responsibility for health and illness were more likely to engage in beneficial health behaviors (e.g., not smoking, proper eating).

Lau's chapter on beliefs about control systematically identifies a variety of health behaviors that have been successfully predicted by locus of control, in addition to providing a critical assessment of the model. Lau also identifies a number of issues related to the measurement of locus of control, which is probably the cognitive dimension related to health that has been most widely studied from a psychometric or instrument-construction perspective. As his chapter reveals, such beliefs are found to be multidimensional. In addition to the scales discussed in Lau's chapter, a children's health locus of control scale has been developed by Parcel and Meyer (1978) for use with young populations.

BEHAVIORAL INTENTION THEORY

The theory of behavioral intentions (e.g., Fishbein & Ajzen, 1975), a third cognitive model with implications for health behavior, is less widely employed and less well known. According to behavioral intention theory, a person's attitude toward some act, moral beliefs related to the act, and perceptions of social norms relevant to the act determine the person's intention to engage in the act. The concept of "specificity of intention" is critical to this theory. General attitudes toward an object appear less powerful as predictors of behavior in relation to that object, than is an intention to engage in a specific behavior. Moreover, unlike the health belief or locus of control models, behavioral intention theory systematically includes normative pressures and factors that facilitate or deter the specified behavior.

Pomazal and Brown (1977) demonstrated how the components of behavioral intention theory are related to the intention to use a controlled substance (marijuana). They reasoned that the model's three components are necessary and probably sufficient to predict the behavior, and that additional variables do not contribute appreciably to the prediction. Ajzen and Fishbein (1980) showed how intentions to engage in specific behaviors are successful predictors of changes in eating behavior and dieting. In addition, protection motivation theory, which integrates components of the health belief and locus of control models, has been successful in predicting intentions to exercise (Wurtele & Maddux, 1987).

While Kirscht's chapter on the health belief model alludes to behavioral intention theory, Ritter's chapter on social supports and social networks discusses explicitly and in some detail how behavioral intention theory mediates between social interaction and personal beliefs and health behaviors, and Cole, Berger, and Garrity's chapter critically analyzes the theory in relation to compliance.

HEALTH AS A VALUE OR MOTIVE

The importance of another type of cognition, health as a motive or value, has received little systematic research attention, although it relates to these cognitive models. Although the original health belief model assumed that high levels of perceived susceptibility and perceived severity were themselves motivational, subsequent research showed that health as a motive is independent of perceived susceptibility (Gochman, 1977), and that health motivation is a factor in organizing health-related beliefs and intentions (Gochman, 1972). Lau, Hartman, and Ware (1986) provided a systematic analysis of health as a value, devised a way of measuring it, and successfully incorporated that measure in predictions derived from the locus of control model.

The question of the role of health as a value in the prediction of health behaviors can be transformed into the question, What are the values that are relevant to health behavior? Research (Gochman, 1975) has shown that health may be less salient in the population than is presumed, and less salient than other values, such as concern for appearance. Concern for appearance, moreover, was one of several cognitive and social factors that was observed to be related to sun exposure behaviors among sunbathers (Keesling & Friedman, 1987).

Kristiansen (1984) observed that health as a value contributed to the prediction of preventive health behaviors, but that other values contributed as well. On the other hand, Smith, Wallston, Wallston, Forsberg, and King (1984) observed that value of control in relation to health care processes was not a significant predictor of health-related behaviors, among those facing terminal illness.

OTHER COGNITIVE APPROACHES

Other approaches not identified with any of the major cognitive models are reflected in: Minkler's (1978) examination of health-relevant beliefs and attitudes in the elderly and the incongruity between their cognitions and behaviors, and between their cognitions and "reality"; McKee's (1975) observation of large attitudinal differences between users and nonusers of nonprescription or "recreational" drugs; Kahn, Anderson, and Perkoff's (1973) analysis of the perceptions of need for care held by users of emergency rooms; Mburu, Smith, and Sharpe's (1978) report of how attitudes toward modern medicine determine use of health services among the Matungulu people of Kenya; Crandall and Duncan's (1981) comparison of attitudinal and situational factors as predictors of physician use, as well as their observations that attitudes and beliefs about physicians, personal health, and health care were better predictors of physician use among low-income persons than were financial resources; Selstad, Evans, and Welcher's (1975) observations that females who had undergone an abortion and who a year later were not regular users of contraception were more likely than regular users to believe that premarital sex activity was wrong; and Wagenfeld, Vissing, Markle, and Petersen's observations (1979) of attitudinal and ideological differences between participants in the laetrile movement and the general population. Those in the laetrile movement, for example, were less likely to be convinced of the importance of regular physical examinations, and more likely to use chiropractors and other alternatives to "orthodox" medical care.

In an effort to improve predictions about "self-management" of asthma in youngsters and adolescents, Matus, Kinsman, and Jones (1978) attempted to systematize the measurement of related attitudes. Their factor analyses showed seven clearly defined and stable clusters of attitudes to chronic asthma and hospitalization: minimization of severity; passive observance of illness; bravado; expectation of staff rejection; moralistic authoritarianism; stigma; and external control. It remains for further research to relate these promising attitudes to patient behavior.

REFERENCES

Ajzen, I., & Fishbein, M. (1980). *Understanding attitudes and predicting social behavior*. Englewood Cliffs, NJ: Prentice–Hall.

Becker, M. H. (Ed.). (1974). The health belief model and personal health behavior [Special issue]. *Health Education Monographs, 2*(4).

Ben-Sira, Z., & Padeh, B. (1978). "Instrumental coping" and "affective defense": An additional perspective in health promoting behavior. *Social Science and Medicine, 12,* 163–168.

Chen, M.-S., & Tatsuoka, M. (1984). The relationship between American women's preventive dental behavior and dental health beliefs. *Social Science and Medicine, 19,* 971–978.

Crandall, L. A., & Duncan, R. P. (1981). Attitudinal and situational factors in the use of physician services by low-income persons. *Journal of Health and Social Behavior, 22,* 64–77.

Eckert, J. K., & Goldstein, M. C. (1983). An anthropological approach to the study of illness behavior in an urban community. *Urban Anthropology, 12,* 125–139.

Eisen, M., Zellman, G. L., & McAlister, A. L. (1985). A health belief model approach to adolescents' fertility control: Some pilot program findings. *Health Education Quarterly, 12,* 185–210.

Fishbein, M., & Ajzen, I. (1975). *Belief, attitude, intention and behavior: An introduction to theory and research*. Reading, MA: Addison–Wesley.

Gochman, D. S. (1972). The organizing role of motivation in health beliefs and intentions. *Journal of Health and Social Behavior, 13,* 285–293.

Gochman, D. S. (1975). The measurement and development of dentally relevant motives. *Journal of Public Health Dentistry, 35,* 160–164.

Gochman, D. S. (1977). Perceived vulnerability and its psychosocial context. *Social Science and Medicine, 11,* 115–120.

Gochman, D. S. (1986). *Youngsters' health cognitions: Cross-sectional and longitudinal analyses*. Louisville, KY: Health Behavior Systems.

Gochman, D. S., & Saucier, J.-F. (1982). Perceived vulnerability in children and adolescents. In D. S. Gochman & G. S. Parcel (Eds.), Children's health beliefs and health behaviors [Special issue]. *Health Education Quarterly, 9,* 46–59.

Green, L. W. (1974). Editorial. In M. H. Becker (Ed.), The health belief model and personal health behavior [Special issue]. *Health Education Monographs, 2,* 324–325.

Janz, N. K., & Becker, M. H. (1984). The health belief model: A decade later. *Health Education Quarterly, 11,* 1–47.

Kahn, L., Anderson, M., & Perkoff, G. T. (1973). Patients' perceptions and uses of a pediatric emergency room. *Social Science and Medicine, 7,* 155–160.

Keesling, B., & Friedman, H. S. (1987). Psychological factors in sunbathing and sunscreen use. *Health Psychology, 6,* 477–493.

Kristiansen, C. M. (1984, August). *Using the value of health to predict health behavior*. Paper presented at the 92nd annual convention of the American Psychological Association, Toronto.

Lau, R. R., Hartman, K. A., & Ware, J. E., Jr. (1986). Health as a value: Methodological and theoretical considerations. *Health Psychology, 5,* 25–43.

Manfredi, C., Warnecke, R. B., Graham, S., & Rosenthal, S. (1977). Social psychological correlates of health behavior: Knowledge of breast self-examination techniques among black women. *Social Science and Medicine, 11*, 433–440.

Matus, I., Kinsman, R. A., & Jones, N. F. (1978). Pediatric patient attitudes toward chronic asthma and hospitalization. *Journal of Chronic Diseases, 31*, 611–618.

Mburu, F. M., Smith, M. C., & Sharpe, T. R. (1978). The determinants of health services utilization in a rural community in Kenya. *Social Science and Medicine, 12*, 211–217.

McKee, M. R. (1975). Drug abuse knowledge and attitudes in 'Middle America.' *American Journal of Public Health, 65*, 584–591.

Minkler, M. (1978). Health attitudes and beliefs of the urban elderly. *Public Health Reports, 93*, 426–432.

Neighbors, H. W. (1984). Professional help use among Black Americans: Implications for unmet need. *American Journal of Community Psychology, 12*, 551–566.

Parcel, G. S., & Meyer, M. P. (1978). Development of an instrument to measure children's health locus of control. In K. A. Wallston & B. S. Wallston (Eds.), Health locus of control [Special issue]. *Health Education Monographs, 6*, 149–159.

Pill, R., & Stott, N. C. H. (1985). Choice or change: Further evidence on ideas of illness and responsibility for health. *Social Science and Medicine, 20*, 981–991.

Pomazal, R. J., & Brown, J. D. (1977). Understanding drug use motivation: A new look at a current problem. *Journal of Health and Social Behavior, 18*, 212–222.

Rosenstock, I. M., Derryberry, M., & Carriger, C. K. (1959). Why people fail to seek poliomyelitis vaccination. *Public Health Reports, 74*, 98–103.

Rotter, J. B. (1966). Generalized expectancies for internal versus external control of reinforcement. *Psychological Monographs, 80*(1).

Seeman, M., & Seeman, T. E. (1983). Health behavior and personal autonomy: A longitudinal study of the sense of control in illness. *Journal of Health and Social Behavior, 24*, 144–160.

Selstad, G. M., Evans, J. R., & Welcher, W. H. (1975). Predicting contraceptive use in postabortion patients. *American Journal of Public Health, 65*, 708–713.

Smith, R. A., Wallston, B. S., Wallston, K. A., Forsberg, P. R., & King, J. E. (1984). Measuring desire for control of health care processes. *Journal of Personality and Social Psychology, 47*, 415–426.

Urberg, K., & Robbins, R. (1984). Perceived vulnerability in adolescents to the health consequences of cigarette smoking. *Preventive Medicine, 13*, 367–376.

Wagenfeld, M. O., Vissing, Y. M., Markle, G. E., & Petersen, J. C. (1979). Notes from the cancer underground: Health attitudes and practices of participants in the laetrile movement. *Social Science and Medicine, 13A*, 483–485.

Wallston, K. A., & Wallston, B. S. (Eds.). (1978). Health locus of control [Special issue]. *Health Education Monographs, 6*(2).

Wurtele, S. K., & Maddux, J. E. (1987). Relative contributions of protection motivation theory components in predicting exercise intentions and behavior. *Health Psychology, 6*, 453–466.

CHAPTER 2

The Health Belief Model and Predictions of Health Actions

John P. Kirscht

INTRODUCTION

An important role of applied social science in health has been the promulgation of theory designed to account for health behaviors of individuals and groups. Efforts to model various health-related actions have multiplied and become increasingly sophisticated. Stone (1979), in his comprehensive review of psychology and the health system, noted that "the questions of why people behave as they do and how they may be induced to behave differently have represented the core of American psychology throughout this century" (p. 70). Recent growth in the study of health behavior has significant roots in the pioneering efforts of applied psychologists and sociologists, represented in the frameworks outlined in the seminal article by Kasl and Cobb (1966). As noted by Leventhal, Zimmerman, and Gutmann (1984) in their critical review, "the health belief model is the cognitive model most frequently used in studies of health behavior and compliance" (p. 384).

Because of its historical and contemporary role, the present chapter aims to evaluate the nature of the evidence for the explanatory value of the health belief model and to raise issues related to that evidence. Citations are intended to cover significant research without attempting to be comprehensive. Several other reviews of the health belief model literature exist (Becker, 1974; Becker *et al.*, 1977; and especially Janz & Becker, 1984). A further aim is to suggest areas of applicability and to note where and why the model may be less functional. While the model has been dynamic, as well as controversial, and several versions have appeared over the years (see Cummings, Becker, & Maile, 1980), it is much simpler to discuss the model in the singular, noting some evolutionary features.

THE MODEL

As Rosenstock (1974a) made clear, the original model grew out of the need to solve practical problems, but in the context of a Lewinian view of practicality. Thus, the model reflected a combination of a "naive" (i.e., phenomenological) psychological approach and

JOHN P. KIRSCHT • School of Public Health, University of Michigan, Ann Arbor, Michigan 48109-2029.

the attempt to formulate a few basic dimensions that could account for health behaviors. It is instructive to note that the health belief model grew from applied research in health education problems rather than within the confines of academic psychology.

At the core of the formulation is a set of health cognitions concerned with personal susceptibility to a condition, the perceived severity of that condition, the efficacy of a behavior, and barriers to the behavior. Severity and barriers are respective aggregates of all of the disutilities of the health threat, and all of the costs of actually engaging in the behavior. Susceptibility, representing the personal probability of the threat, was never thought to satisfy formal probability theory, but was regarded as meaningful across situations. Although not clearly dealt with, the concept implies the likelihood of the threat in the absence of special actions to deal with it. Efficacy represents the perceived value of the action for reducing the threat.

While the theoretical structure of the model has never been well-specified, writers suggest that the belief elements together produce some degree of psychological readiness to act in the face of a threat. If these beliefs are above some threshold, action is likely if environmental conditions permit it. Haefner (1974) noted the lack of specification, pointing out that some proponents postulated a complex interaction among the factors, without spelling out how such relationships might be structured. Most studies, however, treated the model as additive (e.g., Becker, Drachman, & Kirscht, 1972; Cummings, Jette, Brock, & Haefner, 1979). In addition to the basic beliefs, health belief theorists have added other elements, most notably "modifying factors"; these comprised personal and social characteristics such as age, sex, culture, and knowledge, and were regarded as modifying the belief elements. Although the theoretical place of such diverse factors is not clear, they can be regarded as exogenous variables. Behavioral differences among groups (e.g., age groups of SES levels) may reflect different levels and combinations of beliefs, which are the final pathway.

A number of suppositions underlie the health belief model, some of which are generic to the models of this type, while others are peculiar to the subject matter. Several years ago, Rosenstock (1974b) noted that a cue was necessary to trigger action; this factor, calling the beliefs into a salient position, is an assumption that seems characteristic of cognitive models of many sorts. Causal direction is assumed to run from beliefs to behavior (without excluding the very real possibility of the other direction). Since the model deals with avoidance of health threats, it appears axiomatic that such threats arouse behavioral tendencies representing attempts to cope with the situation. No one thought, however, that the beliefs correspond to some objective reality, and wishful thinking can readily enter the system.

The health belief model developed as a theory of specific actions, although the time frame was not always explicit. As the domains of applicability of the model widened, however, more general beliefs and behaviors were studied. For example, beliefs about an array of health threats, or general beliefs about vulnerability to disease were studied. As dependent variables, "health protective actions" or "taking prescribed medications" were studied. Such extensions raised the question of whether these were studies of the same model. It can, of course, be assumed that more abstract, general beliefs are formed from concrete, specific beliefs, events, and situations.

PREDICTIONS OF HEALTH ACTIONS

While there are many ways to structure discussion of research relating to the health belief model, we will use the types of behavior studied as the major mode of classification. Within each category, major findings will be noted and interpreted.

Prevention

Preventive health behavior involving medical professionals was the original focus of the health belief model (Rosenstock & Kirscht, 1979), and included an array of behaviors, such as voluntary checkups and immunizations. This research has been reviewed elsewhere (Rosenstock, 1974b; Janz & Becker, 1984). Most early studies were retrospective. Prospective evidence for the role of health beliefs in relation to an asymptomatic checkup by a physician came from an experimental study on the effects of educational films about heart disease, TB, and cancer (Haefner & Kirscht, 1970). An aim of the messages was to increase appropriate beliefs and to persuade viewers to take actions—a checkup was a common theme in all messages. Beliefs were assessed after the films were shown. Compared to controls, the experimental groups increased beliefs about health threats and about the benefits of actions. Higher levels of intention to act were associated with these beliefs and more of the experimental subjects subsequently obtained a voluntary checkup. Belief changes were shown to be associated with checkups. In this study, more general beliefs, i.e., summed over the different health conditions, were better predictors than disease-specific items. However, a checkup is a multipurpose behavior.

Rundall and Wheeler (1979a), using path analysis, attempted to compare three models for predicting preventive medical visits: financial constraints, health beliefs, and system barriers. Data were obtained retrospectively from a cross-sectional survey of adults. Indices were formed for susceptibility to and severity of four diseases, and benefits of professional intervention for preventing them. Of these indices, susceptibility was the only significant bivariate correlate of preventive visits; "having a usual source of care," however, was the single best predictor, one that could be regarded as an indirect measure of barriers to care. In the path model, the investigators found that each of the health belief measures had a significant, but small, direct effect on preventive visits (the effect of severity was negative), and that the effects of income were mediated through susceptibility and having a usual source of care.

Immunizations have offered unusually good opportunities to test the health belief model because of the specificity of the threat, and the definitive but relatively simple action required. Health beliefs concerning swine flu were assessed via telephone interviews with some 300 adults in Michigan prior to the availability of the vaccine (Cummings *et al.*, 1979). Reinterviews were conducted after the immunization campaign ended. Each of the belief measures—susceptibility, severity, benefits of vaccine, barriers to obtaining the shot, including perceived vaccine safety—yielded significant relationships to intention to be vaccinated and to the behavior itself. A multiple correlation of .5 between beliefs and behavior was found. A measure of intention, however, was the best predictor of the behavior. In a path model, beliefs concerning susceptibility, severity, and efficacy were important predictors of intention. In addition, the authors noted that past experience with flu shots and social influence were determinants of beliefs concerning efficacy.

Generally similar findings were reported by Oliver and Berger (1979). Their prospective study of swine flu vaccination was done on community and student samples, with rather low response rates. Vaccination status was subsequently checked against health department records. Although the belief measures were different from those ordinarily used, the investigators developed indices of threat and of benefits–barriers. Behavior was principally a function of intention, but the belief variables predicted intention ($R^2 = .35$). As part of a survey of senior citizens in a New York county, Rundall and Wheeler (1979b) collected information by mail (retrospectively) concerning swine flu. Using logistic regression analysis with the dichotomous dependent variable, the investigators found that susceptibility and perceived danger of the vaccine were significant predictors in a model that also included demographic characteristics and physician visits.

Because of the repeated measure design of the study reported by Cummings *et al.* (1979), Brock (1984) used the data to examine belief stability and behavior–belief relationships after the immunization campaign. Beliefs were more stable for those who did not obtain the shot than for those who did, as might be expected. Further, perceived susceptibility to swine flu was significantly reduced for the shot-takers. At the same time, behavior predicted the beliefs somewhat better than the reverse, indicating that people rationalized their behavior.

An extended study of influenza vaccination was carried out at the Seattle Veterans Administration Medical Center (Carter, Beach, Inui, Kirscht, & Prodzinski, 1986). While a major purpose was to develop a decision model in which specific benefits and costs of flu versus vaccination were assessed, the investigators also gathered information on health beliefs and intentions. Two separate prospective studies of chronically ill patients were done in successive years. In the first, some 350 patients were questioned prior to the immunization program, plus 165 additional patients afterwards. In the following year, 359 patients were interviewed prior to vaccine availability; of these, 231 had previously participated. Flu shots were recommended for all of these patients. While the decision model, based on weighted utilities, was the best predictor of both intent and vaccination, the health belief variables also performed respectably: measures of susceptibility, severity, and benefits were significantly associated with immunization. In regression analyses, efficacy and susceptibility were significant predictors for both intention (R^2 = .5) and behavior (R^2 = .25). Results were very similar whether assessment of beliefs was made prospectively or retrospectively (susceptibility was measured conditional on no immunization), although the relationships were somewhat exaggerated in the group assessed after the fact. Outcomes in the second study were very similar. Beliefs about benefits were by far the major belief predictor.

Health belief variables have been investigated in relation to hepatitis B vaccination among hospital workers (Palmer & King, 1983; Bodenheimer, Fulton, & Kramer, 1986). Vaccination programs have been somewhat controversial, in part because of fears about AIDS, and rates of acceptance by health workers were lower than expected. Bodenheimer *et al.* (1986) did a prospective study of health beliefs about the vaccine among 1500 hospital employees. Utilizing an extensive questionnaire, they examined health beliefs and other factors in relation to acceptance of the vaccine (intent to take the shot). The latter measure was a good predictor of actual vaccination and only 4% of those who initially *rejected* the vaccine subsequently received it. A regression analysis showed susceptibility, beliefs about safety and effectiveness (a combined index), and severity to be significant predictors (R^2 = .2) of acceptance. Objective "risk group" was a major predictor of susceptibility, and susceptibility itself predicted severity.

Taken together, the findings of research on preventive medical behavior yield some of the strongest evidence for the predictive usefulness of health beliefs, both singly and in combination. Research has progressed to testing of more complex models, although model specification is still at relatively simple levels.

Screening and Detection

As Hochbaum (1958) noted long ago, the perceived value of a screening test must include beliefs about the difference in outcomes from detection than from nondetection. Earlier work indicated that beliefs in benefits and in susceptibility to conditions were important for TB, Tay–Sachs disease, and breast cancer screening; more recently, belief about benefits was associated with screening for cervical cancer (see King, 1982). In King's prospective study of screening for high blood pressure, a health center in England sent invitations for hypertension screening to all patients 35–65 years old. Questionnaires including a number of health belief items were sent to a sample prior to the screening. Measures of susceptibility and benefits with respect to hypertension (but not severity or general health beliefs) predicted attendance. These measures were also significant in a discriminant function analysis, along with perceptions of barriers and other factors. As has been found in a number of studies, a measure of intention was the best predictor of attendance; in turn, perceptions of severity and of benefits predicted intention. By contrast, in a retrospective study of a cardiovascular screening clinic, where all residents in the community had been invited to be screened as part of a heart disease intervention program, health beliefs concerning severity, susceptibility, benefits, and barriers were not related to participation (Pirie *et al.*, 1986).

Returning to a clinic for a reading on a TB skin test was studied by Wurtele, Roberts, and Leeper (1982). Some 550 screenees took the test and responded to a questionnaire that assessed health beliefs. Returning for the test result was associated with perceived personal concern about TB (but not with "how serious is TB"), and with benefits and barriers. Although there was no difference on personal susceptibility to TB, *nonreturners* believed more people got TB than did returners. Except for personal susceptibility, all of the belief measures were significant in a stepwise discriminant analysis. Again, intention was the strongest predictor of attendance.

Calnan and Moss (1984) reviewed a number of studies relating health beliefs to breast self-examination (BSE). Grady, Kegeles, Lund, Wolk, and Farber (1983), for example, studied women patients who had been offered BSE instruction. Beliefs regarding the effectiveness of the procedure and about barriers to practicing it differentiated participants from nonparticipants, whereas susceptibility and "salience" (an index of thinking about, or discussing, breast cancer) did not. Calnan and Moss (1984) interviewed a group of women from among the population of women 45–64 years old in a city in the United Kingdom, all of whom were invited to attend a BSE class. A follow-up assessed BSE practice a year later. Attending the class was predicted by perceived vulnerability to breast cancer and more concern about it, an indicator of severity. General vulnerability to disease was not a factor, nor were beliefs concerning costs and benefits, although these were predictive of practice a year later. In a discriminant analysis, the major predictors of attendance were vulnerability, general control over health, and personal health behaviors. Among studies done retrospectively on the *practice* of BSE, Howe (1981) found relationships to "attitude" questions that appeared to measure efficacy and barriers, but not to perceived risk among a group of high-risk women. However, both Hallal (1982) and Kelly (1979) reported that belief about benefits and susceptibility were associated with BSE. Perhaps the most sophisticated treatment of health beliefs and BSE is that by Ronis and Harel (1986). Subjective expected utility (SEU) was combined with the health belief model. In SEU, actions are evaluated in terms of the product of perceived probabilities and utilities, and the alternative chosen that maximizes the payoff. Ronis and Harel created a model in which the valences for performance of BSE versus inaction were introduced. Causally, they regard the relative utility of the action to be directly influenced by perceived benefits and costs, and benefits to be influenced by susceptibility and severity for earlier and later detection. If detecting cancer has value (benefits), it must lie in earlier treatment; such treatment must affect the severity of the disease. In a probability sample of 619 women in Detroit, Ronis and Harel found that beliefs about benefits and costs both had reliable direct effects on the practice of BSE. Perceptions of severity affected benefits in the ways hypothesized and had no direct effects on behavior. Susceptibility, however, had significant direct effects and did not, as hypothesized, interact with severity. The authors speculate that they might not have met the conditions for an interaction to occur, given the high levels of perceived susceptibility and severity.

diff elements usefulness to overall model; radars measuring same & diff concepts.

Healthy and Risky Behaviors

Of major interest to those in the field of health are personal habits and characteristics that are related to the development of chronic conditions; such "life-style" features as smoking, diet, weight, exercise, safety practices, and use of alcohol are included. Note that these are repeated actions, nonmedically oriented. Much of the emphasis on health promotion and disease prevention has shifted toward control of risks, and the health belief model has been applied both to the behaviors themselves and, more importantly, to the prediction of change in behavior.

Two widely cited retrospective studies, both involving cross-section surveys, examined health beliefs and personal behaviors. Langlie (1977) assessed 11 different behaviors, ranging from nutrition to immunizations, in a sample of adults. Harris and Guten (1979) surveyed "health protective behaviors" in adults. Both studies found that different behaviors were not highly interrelated. Both also found some relationships between health beliefs and indexes of behavior, but that vulnerability was negatively associated with health behavior (Langlie) or nonlinearly related to it (Harris and Guten).

Weinberger, Greene, Mamlin, and Jerin (1981) compared smokers and ex-smokers on perceptions of susceptibility to, and severity of, health problems. Former smokers were discriminated from current smokers in their beliefs about personal vulnerability. Heavier smokers evaluated the consequences of smoking as less severe. While many current smokers appear to recognize the potential harm from smoking, personal vulnerability may be low. In previously unpublished data from a cohort of Michigan adults surveyed in 1980 and 1982, we found that beliefs concerning the healthful effects of not smoking differed significantly between nonsmokers and smokers. Prospectively, however, the perceived health value of not smoking failed to predict cessation although an initial desire to quit was a significant predictor. Conversely, however, those who started smoking during the study period initially had lower levels of beliefs concerning the health benefits of not smoking.

In a study of smoking cessation (Kirscht, Janz, & Becker, 1986) involving 250 patients attending an internal medicine clinic, health beliefs were assessed after an initial visit and follow-up information was obtained 6 months later. The major factor predicting cessation was a measure of intention. However, intention was predicted by baseline beliefs concerning the value of quitting (a measure of the *reduction* in vulnerability to health problems), and perceived vulnerability if smoking continued. Perceived difficulty in quitting, a measure of barriers, also predicted cessation and was related to perceptions of value. Beliefs about susceptibility to health problems, both for continued smoking and for not smoking, were assessed by Strecher, Becker, Kirscht, Eraker, and Graham-Tomasi (1985) in a group of over 200 Veterans Administration patients, as part of a smoking cessation trial. Difficulties resisting urges to smoke were also measured. Neither index was directly related to reduction in smoking 3 months later, but the interaction of the two was a significant predictor, with higher susceptibility plus lower difficulty yielding the greatest reduction. Actually, the difference between the two susceptibility measures was utilized, which can be interpreted as a measure of perceived benefits.

Velicer, DiClemente, Prochaska, and Brandenburg (1985) developed a "decisional balance" measure for assessing reasons for and against smoking. This scale, based on the Janis and Mann (1977) conceptualization of decision-making, yielded two major factors: reasons for, and reasons against smoking. The latter has items reflecting elements of the health belief model, as well as other types of belief. Scale scores differentiated classes of smokers and ex-smokers, such as those who are thinking about change, relapsers, and recent quitters, cross-sectionally in a large group of volunteers. Scores also prospectively predicted change in smoking status at a 6-month follow-up.

Smoking prevention is quite a different matter. Common wisdom in the field is that youngsters, who are the prime candidates for the initiation of cigarette use, are quite unmoved by longer-term health considerations (Flay, 1985). Major theories of initiation of smoking emphasize peer pressure, deviance, and the influence of family smoking patterns. A prospective study of smoking in adolescents (Bauman & Chenoweth, 1984) did not find expected health consequences related to subsequent behavior, whether it was initiation or maintenance. It appears that starting cigarette use is a function of more immediate conditions, such as social approval, than of concern about future health effects.

It is probably true that cognitive factors, such as health beliefs, exert little influence on the daily flow of habitual behavior. Rather, they are of more consequence when signals for change are noted (Kirscht, 1983). Thus, when change is contemplated, or a decision taken about participation in a systematic effort at change, health beliefs may come to the fore and guide behavior, as well as be affected by the course of the effort. For example, Oldridge's review (1982) of exercise in relation to primary and secondary prevention of heart disease, suggests that health considerations play a part in decisions to participate, but appear unimportant in day-to-day activity levels.

Children's Health Beliefs

Two studies carried out by Kegeles and his colleagues with junior high school students represent sophisticated and thorough efforts to test the model prospectively with respect to oral health behaviors (Kegeles & Lund, 1982; Weisenberg, Kegeles, & Lund, 1980). In both studies, health beliefs of the youngsters were assessed prior to the introduction of the dental program, and again following the introduction. Measures of the beliefs were taken at both the specific and general levels, using the format developed by Gochman (1972). Multiplicative indexes were formed, as well as simple additive measures of susceptibility, severity, and effectiveness of actions. Some 250 participants from six schools were involved in each study. In the first study, only beliefs about susceptibility were consistently associated with topical fluoride treatment, and the direction was negative. In the second study, dealing with use of a fluoride mouth rinse, very few relationships were found between any beliefs and any measures of behavior; those found were negative in direction.

The results of these studies raise questions about the applicability of the health belief model to adolescents' health-related behavior. While the behaviors studied were novel, the opportunity for health beliefs to operate was certainly present and no obvious artifact of the situation appeared to determine the outcomes. It might be noted that a retrospective survey of children in Washtenaw County, Michigan (Dielman, Leech, Becker, Rosenstock, & Horvath, 1982), yielded virtually no relationships between health belief model factors and any behavior. We are left with a problem of little support for the model as it applies to the behavior of youngsters.

model of no use to predict adolescents & children health behaviour

Sickness Behavior

A significant extension of the health belief model beyond prevention took place when explanations were constructed for both illness and sick-role behavior (Becker, 1974). Work with the model in relation to illness led to efforts to specify relationships of the model to other conceptual frameworks (see Kirscht, 1974). With these explanations, the nature of the events underlying beliefs about health problems was extended, as the presence of symptoms or of a diagnosed condition reflected a different type of threat.

Research on symptom occurrence and response to symptoms has provided a much richer picture of how people interpret bodily states and act selectively (Mechanic, 1978).

Such information provides a basis for interpreting symptom attributions in terms of health belief model variables. Personal representations of illnesses involve beliefs concerning risk, etiology, and treatment (see also the "common sense" approaches to health and illness: Leventhal, Meyer, & Nerenz, 1980; Lau and Hartman, 1983). Safer, Tharps, Jackson, and Leventhal (1979) divided the process of illness behavior into three stages: symptom appraisal, illness decision, and seeking care. Different processes were hypothesized to come into play at each stage; for example, sensory events and perceptions were thought to be most important in the first stage. Health belief model components (characterized as "abstract") were regarded as contributing to the second stage, but less so in the other stages. An exploratory study on 93 patients who were seeking medical care for symptoms sought to identify what factors contributed to the speed of movement through each stage. The overall supposition that a variety of factors affect delay at the different stages was confirmed, but health belief model variables were important predictors at each stage.

Leavitt (1979) conducted a combined retrospective and prospective study of members of a prepaid health care plan. For each of 25 symptoms, data were obtained on beliefs concerning vulnerability, severity, and the utility of medical care; in addition, beliefs about the benefits of a set of preventive actions were assessed. Use of services was extracted from records for periods of 12 months before and 12 months after the administration of questionnaires. The indexes of vulnerability and of benefits of preventive actions were consistently related to utilization for both periods.

Seeking medical care for symptoms was the subject of a major prospective study of a sample of 1200 adults in Los Angeles (Berkanovic, Telesky, & Reeder, 1981). After an initial face-to-face interview, participants were called about every 6 weeks to gather information on symptom occurrence, evaluation, and actions taken. General beliefs about susceptibility, costs, and efficacy were obtained, plus, in each telephone contact, the judged severity, recurrence, and need for care of the symptoms reported. By far the largest correlations came from symptom-specific beliefs, especially about efficacy ($r = .69$) and severity ($r = .56$), whereas likelihood of recurrence was negatively related ($r = -.14$). These measures, plus barriers, remained significant through a hierarchical multiple regression analysis. Similar findings came from a statewide survey of 600 adults in Illinois (Tanner, Cockerham, & Spaeth, 1983) in which physician utilization was best predicted by the occurrence of symptoms and the respondent's evaluation of the severity of the symptoms. Turk, Litt, Salovey, and Walker (1985) found that mothers' interpretation of symptoms and of the child's behavior were critical factors in decisions to seek urgent care. Although suggestive of the value of a health belief model interpretation of illness behavior, these studies cannot definitively establish causal direction.

Compliance with medical advice became a major area of study regarding sickness behavior in recent years. The health belief model was applied to a number of different conditions, both among adult patients themselves and among parents of children under medical care. Patients' (or parents') beliefs about the threat of an illness, the value and costs of the prescribed regimen were presumed to be factors in the level of compliance. Although the majority of these studies have been retrospective, some prospective research has also been done. Because the review by Janz and Becker (1984) is rather thorough in this area, we will restrict comments to a few considerations.

Evidence of the predictive value of health beliefs for compliance appears strongest when the beliefs of parents, particularly mothers, are examined in relation to a regimen prescribed for a child. This applies particularly where actions of the parent determine the "behavior"; yet there is also evidence of applicability to habits, such as diet, where the child's own behavior plays more of a part. Becker, Maiman, Kirscht, Haefner, and Drachman (1977) found that both general and specific beliefs concerning vulnerability, severity, benefits, and barriers on the part of the mother were related to subsequent weight loss by the child. Kirscht, Becker, Haefner, & Maiman (1978) noted that, in the same data, the major beliefs were all significant predictors in multiple regressions, although the variance accounted for declined over four follow-up visits.

Among adults under medical treatment, however, the evidence for health beliefs as causal factors in compliance is much less clear, particularly in relation to ongoing treatment of chronic disease. Even some retrospective studies have not yielded relationships. Hershey, Morton, Davis, and Reichgott (1980) assessed compliance among 132 hypertensive patients attending a hypertension clinic. None of the health belief model indexes differentiated levels of adherence to prescribed medications, with the exception of a six-item measure of barriers. The study by Cummings, Becker, Kirscht, and Levin (1982) on compliance among a group of 115 hemodialysis patients included thorough assessment of beliefs specific to various parts of the regimen. In general, beliefs about benefits and barriers were associated with compliance measures, particularly those self-reported; among the other beliefs, only susceptibility showed an association and only for dietary restriction. In conclusion, Cummings *et al.* said, "The assumption (proposed by the HBM) that an individual decides to comply, or not comply, with a treatment regimen based on beliefs . . . was generally not supported by these data" (p. 578). Thus, the health belief model has not clearly demonstrated predictive validity in relation to compliance with medical recommendations. Some reasons for difficulty in the application include, first, the habit basis for many aspects of regimens, especially in chronic disease and, second, the fairly common finding that different aspects of regimens are unrelated (e.g., medication and appointment-keeping) (Kirscht & Rosenstock, 1979). In a very important study, Inui, Carter, Pecoraro, Pearlman, and Dohan (1980) found considerable variation in compliance with medications for hypertension within individual patients both for a given drug and across different drugs. It is possible that most assessments of compliance have not been sufficiently specific.

THREATENING HEALTH COMMUNICATIONS

Communications about health-related events carry content and association that are potentially distressing, since ill health threatens our well-being and portends pain, suffering, and, possibly, the termination of life. Even a positive and upbeat message about health may intimate that negative possibilities lurk in the background. Research dealing with the effects of threat in communications has a long and very checkered history (Leventhal, 1971; Sutton, 1982; Sutton & Eiser, 1984); health-related content was widely used in the procession of studies dealing with relationships between fear and action. Although the health belief model does not deal explicitly with emotional states of the individual or with the relationships between perceptions of threat and the arousal of fear, negative emotion may well be a part of the appraisal process. Various conceptualizations of threat and fear have been put forward (see the review by Beck and Frankel, 1981) that recognize ties to the health belief model. Most explicit is Rogers's theory of protection motivation (1975) in which the message factors of noxiousness, probability, and efficacy of response affect beliefs regarding severity, susceptibility, and effectiveness of coping. Appraisal of the threat, rather than emotion itself, is emphasized.

In attempting to integrate the fragmented and conflicting research on threatening communications, Beck and Frankel (1981) gave a central role to the controllability of a threat. Controllability has two aspects: response efficacy, equivalent to perceived benefits, and personal efficacy, identified with Bandura's theory (1977) of self-efficacy. Beck and Lund (1981) noted that personal efficacy beliefs were the most important predictors of flossing behavior among a group of dental patients exposed to communications about periodontal disease. Self-efficacy beliefs as related to health behaviors have been thoroughly reviewed by Strecher, DeVellis, Becker, and Rosenstock (1986). Among others, Beck and Lund suggest incorporating beliefs about efficacy into the health belief model. This raises a question of whether a distinct concept is being added, and, if so, with what structural position in the model.

As Kegeles (1980) pointed out, attempts to add concepts to the health belief model have not been particularly fruitful. Such attempts may dilute the model to a theoretical pastiche. One can consider, however, a broader conception of barriers, in which major perceived facilitators and hindrances are included. Facilitators can include beliefs about help from others, conveniences of various sorts, existing skills, and other resources that make the behavior easier to accomplish; barriers would continue to reflect all salient costs, including lack of skills and the presence of fears regarding the behavior. In this way, efficacy beliefs can be viewed as related to the present model without invoking additional concepts.

Research on fear arousal developed in the context of studying the effects of communication on cognitive and behavioral change. Although the health belief model *per se* is not a theory about change, it has often been utilized in interventions involving health messages. In reality, the model may have its greatest utility in developing and testing interventions. The components can serve as dimensions for defining the nature of a health threat in terms of different types of impact, risk for people, possible actions to take and their value, and what such actions might entail in terms of resources and skills. In addition, other parts of the communication process may be facilitated through health belief considerations: the attentional steps necessary for the process to occur can be affected by the way in which a health threat is presented and dramatized; the nature of existing beliefs about a health problem may also determine the value of different types of information. Reassurance about the value of acting can be used to offset a threat.

Interventions arising more or less explicitly from the health belief model include communications about influenza (Larson, Bergman, Heidrich, Alvin, & Schneeweiss, 1982; Carter *et al.*, 1986), childhood obesity (Becker *et al.*, 1977), treatment of hypertension (Inui, Yourtee, & Williamson, 1976), smoking cessation (Janz *et al.*, 1986), VD education (Simon & Das, 1984), and adolescent sex education (Eisen & Zellman, 1986). In each case, health beliefs were not the only considerations that entered into development of message content, but they did provide an organizing framework for the communications.

CONCEPTUAL ISSUES

Are there aspects of health beliefs and behavior that may help explain some of the diversity of findings? It may be useful to consider the nature of the behaviors, the specificity of the belief concepts, and the ways they are operationalized. The evidence suggests that the model fits some types of behavior better than others. Some behaviors are nearly continuous, some sporadic, and some occur rarely. Compliance with a long-term medication regimen entails repetitive behaviors; so does an exercise program, toothbrushing, and taking vitamin pills. Immunizations are more prototypic one-time actions.

A related dimension is that of initiating desirable versus discontinuing undesirable ones. Starting and stopping appear to reflect different processes; in particular, giving up a risky behavior is often not subject to the effects of simple reinforcement from the environment as the addition of a healthy behavior may be. Repetitive behaviors tend to become habitual, one meaning of which is ''controlled by automatic processes'' (Hunt, Matarazzo, Weiss, & Gentry, 1979). These processes are the very opposite of complex decision-making in which a behavior is the end result of conscious ruminations concerning pros and cons. While there is a continuum between full-blown habit and formal decision-making, cognitive models are more appropriate for the latter domain. Thus, the health belief model should fit best in the less repetitive realm where health considerations are clearly linked to the action; it is also appropriate in the context of a decision about starting or stopping a repetitive behavior. The health belief model is less likely to predict initiating the elimination of a habit because risky habits are often tied to a number of nonhealth considerations.

Another conceptual issue is that of belief specificity. Fishbein and colleagues (e.g., Fishbein & Ajzen, 1975) have repeatedly called for testing the relationship between attitudes and behaviors that are at the same level of specificity. Typically, where a specific action for an identified and limited health purpose is predicted, the beliefs that are specific to that purpose should be the best predictors, rather than general, abstract beliefs.

Some behaviors, or measures of behavior, however, are more general. For example, a "checkup" is seen by many as a general-purpose health-related behavior. It may be appropriate to look at beliefs concerning a number of conditions or a global sense of vulnerability and severity in relation to the behavior. A number of daily living behaviors, such as diet and stress, are regarded as having widespread, nonparticularized effects on health. Parental behaviors on behalf of children seem to be as well predicted by general health concerns, as by specific threats that occur; this may reflect the caretaking role that is generalized well beyond the episodes of daily living. At least, the issue of specificity-generality requires consideration in testing the predictive value of components of the model with respect to behavior.

In several places, we noted that the relationship between measures of susceptibility and behavior was sometimes negative. Such findings raise problems of the conceptual and operational status of beliefs about susceptibility, and about the direction of effects between beliefs and behavior. For example, if an action is regarded as effective in relation to a health problem, then taking the action should reduce the perceived likelihood of the problem. On the other hand, if no action is taken, perceived susceptibility should remain the same, or even increase, unless there is new information about the threat itself. If one receives a vaccine judged to be totally effective against hepatitis, perceived susceptibility to hepatitis should drop to zero, while the level of susceptibility would not be expected to change in the absence of the vaccine. Unfortunately, in a number of studies, a distinction between such conditional and unconditional likelihoods was not made, leading to possible confusion.

With behaviors requiring repeated performance, relationships of gross susceptibility to action will depend on the degree of performance or at what point in a performance cycle observations are made. Again, however, susceptibility should not change in the absence of action. Even a detective action may show a difference. A negative outcome ("You don't have high blood pressure") provides information about susceptibility and may yield a cyclic effect that depends on the time since the procedure occurred. These considerations should make it possible to specify more clearly the expected relationship between beliefs about susceptibility and behavior.

Without doubt, the health belief model will continue to be employed in an explanatory mode, with emphasis on predicting behavior. In this connection, there are considerations that need to be addressed. First, as Janz and Becker (1984) noted, retrospective studies are of very limited value. Not only is predictive research needed but small-scale experiments are necessary to determine whether modification of the beliefs leads to the expected effects. Further, the temporal course of particular types of belief (e.g., concerning preventive behavior and susceptibility) needs to be explored. Second, explicit consideration must be given to what benefits and costs are perceived in different health-related behaviors and how they can be made commensurate for purposes of assessment. For example, do costs reduce, or simply balance off, perceived efficacy? Finally, at this rather late date, the structure of the model itself should be specified in ways that permit testing of the formulation *qua* model, in contrast to examining a hodgepodge of elements. Such probing will be more useful if done on an array of different types of behaviors to establish some sense of areas in which applications are more or less successful. In conclusion, the health belief model is complex and variable in its history, yet surprisingly robust and useful.

REFERENCES

Bandura, A. (1977). Self-efficacy: Toward a unifying theory of behavioral change. *Psychological Review, 84,* 191–215.

Bauman, K., & Chenoweth, R. (1984). The relationship between the consequences adolescents expect from smoking and their behavior: A factor analysis with panel data. *Journal of Applied Social Psychology, 14,* 28–41.

Beck, K., & Frankel, A. (1981). A conceptualization of threat communications and protective health behavior. *Social Psychology Quarterly, 44,* 204–217.

Beck, K., & Lund, A. (1981). The effects of health threat seriousness and personal efficacy upon intentions and behavior. *Journal of Applied Social Psychology, 11,* 401–415.

Becker, M. (Ed.). (1974). *The health belief model and personal health behavior.* Thorofare, NJ: Charles B. Slack.

Becker, M., Drachman, R., & Kirscht, J. (1972). Predicting mothers' compliance with pediatric medical regimens. *Journal of Pediatrics, 81,* 843–854.

Becker, M., Haefner, D., Kasl, S., Kirscht, J., Maiman, L., & Rosenstock, I. (1977). Selected psychosocial models and correlates of individual health-related behaviors. *Medical Care, 15* (Suppl.), 27–48.

Becker, M., Maiman, L., Kirscht, J., Haefner, D., & Drachman, R. (1977). The health belief model and dietary compliance: A field experiment. *Journal of Health and Social Behavior, 18,* 348–366.

Berkanovic, E., Telesky, C. & Reeder, S. (1981). Structural and social psychological factors in the decision to seek medical care for symptoms. *Medical Care, 19,* 693–709.

Bodenheimer, H., Fulton, J., & Kramer, P. (1986). Acceptance of hepatitis B vaccine among hospital workers. *American Journal of Public Health, 76,* 252–255.

Brock, B. (1984). *Factors influencing intentions and behavior toward swine flu vaccine.* Doctoral dissertation, University of Michigan.

Calnan, M., & Moss, S. (1984). The health belief model and compliance with education given at a class in breast self-examination. *Journal of Health and Social Behavior, 25,* 198–210.

Carter, W., Beach, L., Inui, T., Kirscht, J., & Prodzinski, J. (1986). Developing and testing a decision model for predicting influenza vaccination compliance. *Health Services Research, 20* (6, Pt. II), 897–932.

Cummings, K., Becker, M., Kirscht, J., & Levin, N. (1982). Psychosocial factors affecting adherence to medical regimens in a group of hemodialysis patients. *Medical Care, 20,* 567–580.

Cummings, K., Becker, M., & Maile, M. (1980). Bringing the models together: An empirical approach to combining variables used to explain health actions. *Journal of Behavioral Medicine, 3,* 123–145.

Cummings, K., Jette, A., Brock, B., & Haefner, D. (1979). Psychosocial determinants of immunization behavior in a swine influenza campaign. *Medical Care, 17,* 639–649.

Dielman, T., Leech, S., Becker, M., Rosenstock, I., & Horvath, W. (1982). Parental and child health beliefs and behaviors. *Health Education Quarterly, 9,* 156–173.

Eisen, M., & Zellman, G. (1986). The role of health belief attitudes, sex education, and demographics in predicting adolescents' sexuality knowledge. *Health Education Quarterly, 13,* 9–22.

Fishbein, M., & Ajzen, I. (1975). *Belief, attitude, intention, and behavior: An introduction to theory and research.* Reading, MA: Addison–Wesley.

Flay, B. (1985). Psychosocial approaches to smoking prevention: A review of findings. *Health Psychology, 4,* 449–488.

Gochman, D. (1972). Development of health beliefs. *Psychological Reports, 31,* 259–266.

Grady, K., Kegeles, S., Lund, A., Wolk, C., & Farber, N. (1983). Who volunteers for a breast self-examination program? Evaluating the bases for self-selection. *Health Education Quarterly, 10,* 79–94.

Haefner, D. (1974). The health belief model and preventive dental behavior. *Health Education Monographs, 2,* 420–432.

Haefner, D., & Kirscht, J. (1970). Motivational and behavioral effects of modifying health beliefs. *Public Health Reports, 85,* 478–484.

Hallal, J. (1982). The relationship of health beliefs, health locus of control, and self-concept to the practice of breast-self-examination in adult women. *Nursing Research, 31,* 137–142.

Harris, D., & Guten, S. (1979). Health protective behavior: An exploratory study. *Journal of Health and Social Behavior, 20,* 17–29.

Hershey, J., Morton, B., Davis, J., & Reichgott, M. (1980). Patient compliance with antihypertensive medication. *American Journal of Public Health, 70,* 1081–1089.

Hochbaum, G. (1958). *Participation in medical screening programs: A sociopsychological study.* U.S. Public Health Service Publication No. 572.

Howe, H. (1981). Social factors associated with breast self-examination among high risk women. *American Journal of Public Health, 71,* 251–255.

Hunt, W., Matarazzo, J., Weiss, S., & Gentry, W. (1979). Associative learning, habit, and health behavior. *Journal of Behavioral Medicine, 2,* 111–124.

Inui, T., Carter, W., Pecoraro, R., Pearlman, R., & Dohan, J. (1980). Variations in patient compliance with common long-term drugs. *Medical Care, 18,* 986–993.

Inui, T., Yourtee, E., & Williamson, J. (1976). Improved outcomes in hypertension after physician tutorials: A controlled trial. *Annals of Internal Medicine, 84,* 646–651.

Janis, I., & Mann, L. (1977). *Decision making: A psychological analysis of conflict, choice, and commitment.* New York: Free Press.

Janz, N., & Becker, M. (1984). The health belief model: A decade later. *Health Education Quarterly, 11,* 1–47.

Janz, N., Becker, M., Kirscht, J., Eraker, S., Billi, J., & Woolliscroft, J. (1986). *Evaluation of a minimal-contact smoking cessation intervention in an outpatient setting.* Unpublished manuscript.

Kasl, S., & Cobb, S. (1966). Health behavior, illness behavior, and sick role behavior. *Archives of Environmental Health, 12,* 246–266, 531–541.

Kegeles, S. (1980). The health belief model and personal health behavior. *Social Science and Medicine, 14C,* 227–229.

Kegeles, S., & Lund, A. (1982). Adolescents' health beliefs and acceptance of a novel preventive dental activity: Replication and extension. *Health Education Quarterly, 9,* 192–208.

Kelly, P. (1979). Breast self-examination: Who does them and why. *Journal of Behavioral Medicine, 2,* 31–38.

King, J. (1982). The impact of patients' perceptions of high blood pressure on attendance at screening: An extension of the health belief model. *Social Science and Medicine, 16,* 1079–1091.

Kirscht, J. (1974). The health belief model and illness behavior. *Health Education Quarterly, 2,* 387–408.

Kirscht, J. (1983). Preventive health behavior: A review of research and issues. *Health Psychology, 2,* 277–301.

Kirscht, J., Becker, M., Haefner, D., & Maiman, L. (1978). Effects of threatening communications and mothers' health beliefs on weight change in obese children. *Journal of Behavioral Medicine, 1,* 147–157.

Kirscht, J., Janz, N., & Becker, M. (1986). *Psychosocial predictors of change in cigarette smoking.* Unpublished manuscript.

Kirscht, J., & Rosenstock, I. (1979). Patients' problems in following recommendations of health experts. In G. Stone, F. Cohen, & N. Adler (Eds.), *Health psychology* (pp. 189–215). San Francisco: Jossey–Bass.

Langlie, J. (1977). Social networks, health beliefs, and preventive health behavior. *Journal of Health and Social Behavior, 18,* 244–260.

Larson, E., Bergman, J., Heidrich, F., Alvin, B., & Schneeweiss, R. (1982). Do postcard reminders improve influenza vaccination compliance? *Medical Care, 20,* 639–648.

Lau, R., & Hartman, K. (1983). Common sense representations of common illnesses. *Health psychology, 2,* 167–185.

Leavitt, F. (1979). The health belief model and utilization of ambulatory care services. *Social Science and Medicine, 13A,* 105–112.

Leventhal, H. (1971). Fear appeals and persuasion: The differentiation of a motivational construct. *American Journal of Public Health, 61,* 1208–1224.

Leventhal, H., Meyer, D., & Nerenz, D. (1980). The common sense representation of illness danger. In S. Rachman (Ed.), *Medical psychology* (Vol. II, pp. 7–29). New York: Pergamon Press.

Leventhal, H., Zimmerman, R., & Gutmann, M. (1984). Compliance: A self-regulation perspective. In D. Gentry (Ed.), *Handbook of behavioral medicine* (pp. 369–436). New York: Guilford Press.

Mechanic, D. (1978). *Medical sociology* (2nd ed.). New York: Free Press.

Oldridge, N. (1982). Compliance and exercise in primary and secondary prevention of coronary heart disease: A review. *Preventive Medicine, 11,* 56–70.

Oliver, R., & Berger, P. (1979). A path analysis of preventive health care decision models. *Journal of Consumer Research, 6,* 113–122.

Palmer, D., & King, R. (1983). Attitude toward hepatitis vaccination among high-risk hospital employees. *Journal of Infectious Diseases, 147,* 1120–1121.

Pirie, P., Elias, W., Wackman, D., Jacobs, D., Murray, D., Mittelmark, M., Luepker, R., & Blackburn, H. (1986). Characteristics of participants and nonparticipants in a community cardiovascular risk factor screening: The Minnesota Heart Health Program. *American Journal of Preventive Medicine, 2,* 20–25.

Rogers, R. (1975). A protection motivation theory of fear appeals and attitude change. *Journal of Psychology, 91,* 93–114.

Ronis, D., & Harel, Y. (1986). *Health beliefs and breast examination behaviors: Analyses of linear structural relations.* Unpublished manuscript.

Rosenstock, I. (1974a). Historical origins of the health belief model. *Health Education Monographs, 2,* 328–335.

Rosenstock, I. (1974b). The health belief model and preventive health behavior. *Health Education Monographs, 2,* 354–386.

Rosenstock, I., & Kirscht, J. (1979). Why people seek health care. In G. Stone, F. Cohen, & N. Adler (Eds.), *Health psychology* (pp. 161–188). San Francisco: Jossey–Bass.

Rundall, T., & Wheeler, J. (1979a). The effect of income on use of preventive care: An evaluation of alternative explanations. *Journal of Health and Social Behavior, 20,* 397–406.

Rundall, T., & Wheeler, J. (1979b). Factors associated with utilization of the swine flu vaccination program among senior citizens. *Medical Care, 17,* 191–200.

Safer, M., Tharps, Q., Jackson, T., & Leventhal, H. (1979). Determinants of three stages of delay in seeking care at a medical care clinic. *Medical Care, 17,* 11–29.

Simon, K., & Das, A. (1984). An application of the health belief model toward educational diagnosis for VD education. *Health Education Quarterly, 11,* 403–418.

Stone, G. (1979). Psychology and the health system. In G. Stone, F. Cohen, & N. Adler (Eds.), *Health psychology* (pp. 47–75). San Francisco: Jossey–Bass.

Strecher, V., Becker, M., Kirscht, J., Eraker, S., & Graham-Tomasi, R. (1985). Psychosocial aspects of changes in cigarette-smoking behavior. *Patient Education and Counseling, 7,* 249–262.

Strecher, V., DeVellis, B., Becker, M., & Rosenstock, I. (1986). The role of self-efficacy in achieving health behavior change. *Health Education Quarterly, 13,* 73–92.

Sutton, S. (1982). Fear-arousing communications: A critical examination of theory and research. In J. Eiser (Ed.), *Social psychology and behavioral medicine* (pp. 303–337). New York: Wiley.

Sutton, S., & Eiser, J. (1984). The effect of fear-arousing communications on cigarette smoking: An expectancy-value approach. *Journal of Behavioral Medicine, 7,* 13–33.

Tanner, J., Cockerham, W., & Spaeth, J. (1983). Predicting physician utilization. *Medical Care, 21,* 360–369.

Turk, D., Litt, M., Salovey, P., & Walker, J. (1985). Seeking urgent pediatric treatment: Factors contributing to frequency, delay, and appropriateness. *Health Psychology, 4,* 43–59.

Velicer, W., DiClemente, C., Prochaska, J., & Brandenburg, N. (1985). Decisional balance measures for assessing and predicting smoking status. *Journal of Personality and Social Psychology, 48,* 1279–1289.

Weinberger, M., Greene, J., Mamlin, J., & Jerin, M. (1981). Health beliefs and smoking behavior. *American Journal of Public Health, 71,* 1253–1255.
Weisenberg, M., Kegeles, S., & Lund, A. (1980). Children's health beliefs and acceptance of a dental preventive activity. *Journal of Health and Social Behavior, 21,* 59–74.
Wurtele, S., Roberts, M., & Leeper, J. (1982). Health beliefs and intention: Predictors of return compliance in a tuberculosis detection drive. *Journal of Applied Social Psychology, 12,* 128–136.

CHAPTER 3

Beliefs about Control and Health Behavior

Richard R. Lau

The desire to control one's environment and the events in one's life is a very general human motive. It plays a central role in several basic (although very different) theories of personality and social psychology (e.g., Bandura, 1977; de Charms, 1968; Fromm, 1941; Kelley, 1967; White, 1959). Because the desire for control is such a general motivation, beliefs about whether one has control over one's life have attracted much research interest. The research that is relevant to health falls into three main categories. The first addresses the question of the extent to which control reduces the stressfulness of an aversive event. The second type of research looks at the results of an attributional style known as "learned helplessness." The third category of research includes those studies that look at more generalized beliefs about control as an individual difference or personality factor. This chapter will briefly review the first two of these theoretical orientations before delving more deeply into the third individual difference or "locus of control" approach. A brief summary at the end of this chapter will attempt to tie these three orientations together again.

CONTROL AND STRESS

Stress can be said to exist when an individual is unable to respond adequately to an important environmental demand (Sells, 1970). A good deal of stress clearly has unhealthy consequences for most people (Cohen, 1980; Lazarus, 1966; Wolff, 1953), and many researchers have studied how different types of control reduce the aversiveness of a stressful event. This research is summarized by Averill (1973) and Thompson (1981).

According to Thompson (1981), there are three major reasons *why* control reduces stress. First, some types of control (i.e., informational control, which provides knowledge about the onset of an aversive stimulus) are confounded with predictability. Predictability of onset may reduce stress because it not only allows one to prepare for the aversive stimulus but also signals when one can relax and let down one's guard. Second, as Miller (1979) argues, some types of control (i.e., behavioral control, which allows the individual to regulate when an aversive stimulus occurs or to moderate its aversiveness) give one the assurance that an aversive situation will not get so aversive that one cannot handle it;

RICHARD R. LAU • Department of Social and Decision Sciences, Carnegie–Mellon University, Pittsburgh, Pennsylvania 15213.

control allows people to minimize the maximum noxious stimuli they will face. This is another type of predictability. Third, a lack of control may be stressful because it reflects negatively on the self, and control therefore reverses this process. Lack of control can lead to learned helplessness, as discussed below. None of these hypotheses by themselves can explain all of the beneficial effects of control in different situations, however.

LEARNED HELPLESSNESS

A great deal of research since the mid-1970s falls under the general rubric of "learned helplessness," a theory developed by Seligman and his colleagues (1975; Abramson, Seligman, & Teasdale, 1978). The basic idea underlying learned helplessness is that people (and animals, for that matter) may learn that they have no control over what happens to them in some situations. This learning usually comes about through a lack of contingency between past efforts to change one's situation and the outcomes associated with those efforts. This learned helplessness has motivational, cognitive, and emotional consequences. It can lead to an almost numbed acceptance of a negative situation, so that an individual no longer tries to change that situation for the better because he or she does not expect those efforts to make any difference. For the same reason, learned helplessness can lead to an inability to learn that new responses *are* available that do affect outcomes. As a result of both of these processes, learned helplessness can lead to lower self-esteem and depression. It may even lead to sudden death (Seligman, 1975).

A "reformulated" learned helplessness theory recognizes that the attributions people make for the noncontingency between efforts and outcomes are crucial, however (Abramson *et al.*, 1978). More specifically, *universal helplessness* (there is nothing anyone can do) can lead to cognitive and motivational deficits but not emotional ones. Only *personal helplessness* (there is nothing I can do, but there are things other people might be able to do) will lead to lower self-esteem. Moreover, attributions about the specificity (global versus specific) and chronicity (stable versus unstable) of the cause of the noncontingency should determine how generalized its results are, both over time and across situations.

Maier and Seligman (1976) and Peterson (1982) provide reviews of the vast learned helplessness literature. Two areas that have been addressed by this literature are most clearly health relevant. The first is the extent to which depression is the result of a general, chronic tendency or "style" of attributing positive outcomes to external sources and attributing negative outcomes to the self (Alloy & Abramson, 1982; Borthe & Hammen, 1981; Klein, Fencil-Morse, & Seligman, 1976; Martin, Abramson, & Alloy, 1984; Peterson & Seligman, 1984). Regularly making such attributions—which is analogous to a lack of contingency between one's *own* efforts and outcomes—could logically lead anyone into a depression (assuming people do not intentionally bring negative outcomes on themselves). Hence, these researchers are drawing direct analogies between learned helplessness and the process by which some people become depressed. Now certainly clinical depression is a very heterogeneous diagnosis, and no one believes that attributions and the resulting helplessness are the precursors of all types of depression (Depue & Monroe, 1978). Still there is accumulating evidence that the perception of lack of control over important outcomes in one's life can lead to serious depression in some instances (see Sweeney, Anderson, & Bailey, 1986).

A second research area examines the behavior of patients in hospitals in terms of learned helplessness. It is argued that hospitalized people have little control over their lives, particularly in areas over which people normally have a great deal of control; many experience learned helplessness and become apathetic and depressed as a result. Taylor (1979) refers to two types of hospitalized patients: those who willingly follow the dictates of the hospital staff (''good patients''), and those who react with anger and resistance to a perceived arbitrary removal of freedoms (''bad patients''). Taylor (1979) and Raps, Peterson, Jonas, and Seligman (1982) have analyzed ''good patient'' behavior in terms of learned helplessness. Certainly there are clear health risks for both ''good patients'' and ''bad patients,'' which can be alleviated, Taylor argues, by a more ''informed participant role'' for the patient (Tayor, 1979, p. 180). I will return to this point in the concluding section of this chapter.

HEALTH LOCUS OF CONTROL BELIEFS

Locus of Control as a Theoretical Construct

Locus of control refers to ''the degree to which individuals perceive events in their lives as being a consequence of their own actions, and thereby controllable (internal control), or as being unrelated to their own behavior, and therefore beyond personal control (external control)'' (Lefcourt, 1976). The best known figure in this field is Rotter, whose research on locus of control beliefs has inspired, directly or indirectly, most of the work that will be discussed in this section (Rotter, 1954, 1975). Derived from social learning theory, locus of control theory hypothesizes that behavior is a function of the expectancy that a certain action will lead to a particular goal, combined with the reinforcement value of that goal. This expectancy is conceptualized as a generalized, relatively stable aspect of personality that is applicable to many different situations, particularly situations in which more specialized expectancies, based on prior experience in this specific domain, have not developed. The concept has been applied to the area of health for at least 25 years, since Seeman and Evans's (1962) well-known study of alienation among hospitalized tuberculosis patients. After briefly reviewing past research on beliefs about control and health, the remainder of this chapter will summarize my own research in this area and present my current thoughts about health locus of control beliefs.

Review of Past Research

Several major reviews of the literature linking locus of control beliefs to health behaviors exist (e.g., Strickland, 1978; Wallston & Wallston, 1981, 1982). Their findings are summarized briefly here. The interested reader is urged to read these reviews (or the original research) for further detail.

Strickland's (1978) review is the most sanguine. Theoretically,

> . . . one would expect that internals, in contrast to externals, would be more sensitive to health messages, would have increased knowledge about health conditions, would attempt to improve physical functioning, and might even, through their own efforts, be less susceptible to physical and psychological dysfunction. (p. 1193)

Strickland reviews research supporting all of these claims. To mention only those studies dealing with health behaviors, internal beliefs have been linked to the desire for more information about a disease one is susceptible to or has already contracted (Seeman & Evans, 1962; Wallston, Maides, & Wallston, 1976; Wallston, Wallston, Kaplan, & Maides, 1976); they have been associated with following dietary restrictions and to keeping medical appointments among kidney patients on dialysis (Weaver, 1972); internal beliefs have been linked to the ability to lose weight (Balch & Ross, 1975) and to quit smoking after the health risks associated with smoking became more well known (James, Woodruff, & Werner, 1965; Steffy, Meichenbaum, & Best, 1970); and they have been linked to the performance of a variety of preventive health behaviors such as seat belt use (Williams, 1972a), physical exercise (Sonstroem & Walker, 1973), contraceptive use (Lundy, 1972; MacDonald, 1970), and engaging in preventive dental care (Williams, 1972b). There are also published accounts failing to replicate locus of control effects for most of these health behaviors, however, and Strickland warns that undoubtedly many negative findings were never published. She also warns that the magnitude of the effects is rarely reported in these studies.

As Wallston and Wallston (1978) point out in their earliest review of the literature, these inconsistent results could be due to a variety of factors, including, most prominently, the use of many different kinds of locus of control measures. To help alleviate this problem, both the Wallstons (Wallston, Wallston, Kaplan, & Maides, 1976; Wallston, Wallston, & De Vellis, 1978) and John Ware and I (Lau & Ware, 1981) have developed health-specific locus of control scales (see below). *A priori,* one would expect a health-specific locus of control scale to produce stronger results than a general locus of control measure, but this has not always been the case. In fact, a more recent review of the literature linking health-specific locus of control beliefs to health responses (Wallston & Wallston, 1981) paints a fairly negative picture. When health locus of control beliefs are used as independent variables, the Wallstons conclude that they are generally not related to information seeking except in the area of hypertension, where several studies have found that internal subjects seek out more information about that disease (Toner & Manuck, 1979; Wallston, Maides, & Wallston, 1976). Nor have health locus of control beliefs generally been linked to the performance of a variety of preventive health behaviors (e.g., exercise, losing weight, and wearing seat belts), with the exception that internals are better able to quit smoking successfully (Kaplan & Cowles, 1978; Wildman, Rosenbaum, Framer, Keane, & Johnson, 1979).

When groups that theoretically should differ in their locus of control beliefs are used to validate the scales (i.e., when health locus of control beliefs are used as dependent variables), the data are somewhat more promising. For example, nonsmokers and people who have been able to quit smoking are more internal than smokers; people who go to a health fair are more internal than the general population as a whole (Wallston & Wallston, 1981); birth control users and women who have chosen to have an abortion are more internal than unmarried pregnant women (Harkey & King, 1976, as reported in Wallston & Wallston, 1981). While these results are consistent with theory, we do not know if health-specific locus of control beliefs contributed to the different behavioral responses or if the behaviors influenced those beliefs. A crucial question that needs to be answered to interpret such "known group" studies is: how stable are health locus of control beliefs over time? If health locus of control beliefs are fairly ephemeral, changing with every illness and experience with doctors or self-care, then it is difficult to give much weight to any of the research cited above. If, on the other hand, health locus of control beliefs are relatively stable, then one can be more confident in interpreting known group differences as being caused by the locus of control beliefs, rather than the other way around.

How Should Health Locus of Control Beliefs Be Linked to Health Behaviors?

The optimism of Strickland's (1978) review contrasts sharply with the pessimism of Wallston and Wallston's review (1981; see also Wallston & Wallston, 1984). One explanation of this difference is that the Wallstons, as a "clearinghouse" for research using their scales, were aware of a higher proportion of all the relevant research—positive and negative, published and unpublished—than was Strickland. Certainly there will be a bias toward negative results in unpublished research; the more such research one is aware of, the more negative one would tend to be about the literature as a whole. On the other hand, the decision to publish (or to submit one's paper for publication) is based not just on the agreement of results with theory but also on the confidence that editors and researchers themselves have in how competently the research was conducted. We should probably give more weight to (the generally more positive) published research than to unpublished research. Another possibility is that the Wallstons, with so much invested in the area, have expectations that are too high. Several times in their review of the literature, they discount theoretically consistent and statistically significant results because the amount of variance explained by health locus of control beliefs is small.

More generally one must address the question of what sort of relationship one *should* find between health locus of control beliefs and any preventive health response. Of course the answer depends on the behavior under consideration and the particular situation. First, as the Wallstons are careful to point out, there is usually no reason to expect health locus of control beliefs *by themselves* to predict health behaviors (although the bulk of the literature reviewed above has examined just this relationship). Locus of control beliefs are generalized expectancies, but the underlying theory is an expectancy-*value* theory. Therefore, internal health locus of control beliefs, *in combination with a high value placed on health,* should predict preventive health behaviors; however, there is no theoretical reason for people with internal locus of control beliefs *who do not value health highly* to perform any health-relevant behavior. Now in certain situations, such as when people are sick (particularly when people are seriously ill), it is probably safe to assume that all people in that situation value health highly. But we cannot make that assumption about relatively healthy people in asymptomatic states (Lau, Hartman, & Ware, 1986). Hence, anyone using locus of control beliefs to study preventive health behaviors should examine the interaction between health value and health locus of control. Yet very few researchers have done this.

Another complication arising in the study of preventive health behaviors is that many of those behaviors are habits learned early in life. Brushing teeth, exercise, and healthy eating behavior are all things that most people have been doing (or not doing) since childhood. But the *reasons* that children perform these behaviors have little to do with health. Therefore, it is difficult to predict these same behaviors in adults from health beliefs if the behaviors are still habitual. Indeed, it is very difficult to predict habitual behaviors from anything except prior behavior. Hence, situations (or behaviors) should be sought in which there is a reasonable expectation that locus of control beliefs should predict some behavior. In such situations, however, locus of control beliefs should be important predictors of whether people perform some recommended behavior. By "important" I mean "widely generalizable" more than "powerfully linked." Locus of control beliefs are important because they should be moderately associated with a wide variety of different types of behaviors in different situations. Therefore, it is imperative for researchers in the health field to have reliable and valid locus of control scales specifically designed for the health area.

THE MEASUREMENT OF HEALTH LOCUS OF CONTROL BELIEFS

The first researchers to try to develop a health-specific locus of control scale were Dabbs and Kirscht (1971), although as they later admit their scale deals more with motivation for control (i.e., how strongly control is desired) than with perceptions of or beliefs about control (Kirscht, 1972). The Wallstons developed the first serious health-specific locus of control scale that is consistent with Rotter's theory (Wallston, Wallston, Kaplan,

& Maides, 1976). Their original measure was an 11-item unidimensional scale with 5 "internal" items and 6 "external" items.

From both the manifest content of the items and from a factor analysis of data resulting from an administration of the Wallston's scale to a small sample of patients admitted to emergency rooms of two Los Angeles hospitals, John Ware and I suspected that the "unidimensional" scale was actually made up of two separate subscales, an "efficacy of self-care" scale consisting of the five internal items, and a "chance" scale consisting of the six external items. Moreover, we had read, and disagreed with, Andersen's early conceptualization of beliefs in the efficacy of self-care as the *opposite* of beliefs in the efficacy of doctors and the professional medical care system (Andersen, Kravits, & Anderson, 1971; this same self-care-*versus*-doctors conceptualization is shared by the behavior subscale of the Krantz [Krantz, Baum, & Wideman, 1980] Health Opinion Survey). To one who believes strongly both in the efficacy of self-care and in doctors, the two beliefs seemed more like complements than opposites.

Collins's (1974) factor analysis of the original Rotter locus of control scale led to the conclusion that it too was multidimensional. Following Collins, we designed a multidimensional health locus of control scale that consisted of four subscales: beliefs in Self-Control Over Health, Provider Control Over Health, Chance Health Outcomes, and General Health Threat (Lau & Ware, 1981). The Wallstons were simultaneously developing a multidimensional health locus of control scale. Following Levenson (1974), they came up with three subscales: Internal Health Locus of Control, Powerful Others Health Locus of Control, and Chance Health Locus of Control (Wallston, Wallston, & DeVellis, 1978).

In manifest content and intent, the Wallstons' three subscales are very similar to Lau and Ware's Self-Control, Provider Control, and Chance Health Outcomes subscales. The Wallstons have always utilized a six-point Likert format, whereas Lau and Ware have used a seven-point format. The Wallstons' subscales have two equivalent forms, while Lau and Ware's has only one. All of the Wallstons' items are personally worded (i.e., they contain "I," "me," or "my"), while most of Lau and Ware's are phrased to reflect more general beliefs (i.e., beliefs about oneself *and* other people). Hence, it is conceivable that the Wallstons' subscales would predict a respondent's own health behaviors better than Lau and Ware's, while our subscales would better predict people's relevant behavior vis-à-vis other people (e.g., their children) and/or their expectations of what other people would do. (However, I know of no study comparing the predictive validity of the two scales, nor am I advocating one.) All of the items within the Wallstons' subscales are worded in the same direction, while Lau and Ware's subscales all contain a mix of positively and negatively worded items. Therefore, it is possible that the Wallstons' subscales will be contaminated with an acquiescent response set, a possibility that becomes increasingly likely when persons from lower socioeconomic classes are studied (Ware, 1978). In most situations, however, it is likely that a researcher would obtain equivalent results utilizing either scale.

The Carnegie–Mellon University Health Project

The Lau–Ware health locus of control scale has been used in scores of master's theses, doctoral dissertations, and similar published and unpublished research projects. It has also been translated into at least three languages. We have not had the opportunity to present scale norms from applications of the scale in different populations, an oversight that I would like to correct here (see Wallston & Wallston, 1981, for scale norms from both their unidimensional and multidimensional scales). I would like to do this in the context of my own most recent utilization of the four subscales. To do that I must briefly describe the study in which these data were collected.

I have just completed a 3-year longitudinal study of an entering freshman class at Carnegie–Mellon University. These students were initially contacted in the summer (of 1983) before they entered college. Of the 1129 students who had paid their preregistration fee on time and who actually enrolled at Carnegie–Mellon University (CMU) in the fall, baseline data were obtained from 1026 (or 91%). This baseline questionnaire included a variety of items about these students' health beliefs and health behaviors. That fall, after school had started, their parents were sent a similar questionnaire, asking about the parents' health beliefs and behaviors and about their attempts to teach various health behaviors to their children. Data were obtained from 947 (or 92%) of the parents. Both the students' baseline questionnaire and the parents' questionnaire contained the Lau–Ware health locus of control items. The students were then contacted to complete much shorter questionnaires twice a year for their first 3 years of college, once each semester. One of the short questionnaires each year asked about the performance of various health behaviors, while the other questionnaire asked primarily about health beliefs. The fourth questionnaire, sent out in the fall of the students' sophomore year, also contained the health locus of control items (532 students remained in the study at the end of 3 years).

Of the students, 69% were male and 31% female; 7% Asian American, 3% black, 1% Hispanic or Native American Indian, and the reminder white. Their age ranged from 15 to 27, but the great majority were 17, 18, or 19. All were single. The parents ranged in age from 34 to 74 (the mean age was 47); 80% were the student's mother, 19% were fathers, and a scattering of stepfathers, grandmothers, aunts, and uncles also responded.

Scale Norms for the Lau–Ware Health Locus of Control Measure

Table 1 presents the means, standard deviations, and reliabilities (when reported by the researcher) of the Lau–Ware health locus of control scale applied to eight different populations, including the baseline students and parents samples described above. In each case the four or eight items comprising a subscale have been averaged together so that that range is always 1.0–7.0. The items have been scored such that high values on the subscale indicate agreement with the subscale as it is named. People who score high on each of the subscales believe that people can control their own health, that doctors can control their health, that sickness and health are determined by luck (and hence are uncontrollable), and that there are many bad diseases that are not controllable by anyone. The reliabilities (internal consistencies) have always been in the 0.6–0.8 range except for the General Health Threat subscale, which is less internally consistent than the other three. Part of this lower reliability is due to the fact that this subscale contains only four items, and therefore a lower coefficient alpha must be expected relative to a longer scale. But in at least one application of this subscale (Lau, 1982) the items did not all cluster together, so the weakness may also stem from relatively few people thinking about health in terms of threat.

If the objective midpoint of these subscales is 4.0 (''Neither Agree Nor Disagree''), then it is clear that most people believe health is controllable. The means of the Self-Control Over Health and Provider Control Over Health are both well above 4.0 in almost all samples and therefore clearly on the ''Agree'' side of the continuum, while the mean for Chance Health Outcomes is clearly on the ''Disagree'' side of the response scale. Nonetheless, many people also believe that ''there are many diseases that can just wipe you out'' (presumably despite the efforts of self-care or doctors), because the mean of General Health Threat is moderately on the ''Agree'' side of 4.0. This latter belief is generally somewhat weaker than the others, however, as indicated by a mean usually closer to 4.0 than that of the other three subscales.

The data in Table 1 also provide some discriminant validity for the subscales. The

TABLE 1. Scale Norms for Lau–Ware Health Locus of Control Scale Reliability

N	Sample description	Mean	Standard deviation	Internal consistency	Test–retest
326	Introductory psychology students[a]				
	Self-control over health	5.22	0.68	0.65	0.71[b]
	Provider control over health	4.99	0.71	0.67	0.77
	Chance health outcomes	2.20	0.93	0.71	0.69
	General health threat	4.73	0.91	0.70	0.43
40	Pregnant women choosing home birth[c]				
	Self-control over health	5.90	0.69		
	Provider control over health	3.35	1.11		
	Chance health outcomes	2.60	0.91		
	General health threat	4.25	0.81		
40	Pregnant women choosing hospital birth[c]				
	Self-control over health	4.82	0.68		
	Provider control over health	5.53	0.81		
	Chance health outcomes	3.24	1.02		
	General health threat	4.94	0.80		
39	Insulin-dependent diabetics[d]				
	Self-control over health	5.11	0.84		
	Provider control over health	5.41	1.02		
	Chance health outcomes	3.05	1.13		
	General health threat	4.65	0.90		
711	Males in adult conditioning classes[e]				
	Self-control over health	5.43		0.62	
	Provider control over health	4.70		0.63	
	Chance health outcomes	3.11		0.62	
	General health threat	4.70		0.39	
719	Females in adult conditioning classes[e]				
	Self-control over health	5.42		0.62	
	Provider control over health	4.78		0.55	
	Chance health outcomes	2.88		0.66	
	General health threat	4.56		0.47	
1025	Entering college freshmen[f]				
	Self-control over health	5.44	0.64	0.62	0.53[g]
	Provider control over health	4.94	0.80	0.74	0.63
	Chance health outcomes	2.96	0.96	0.74	0.52
	General health threat	4.45	1.05	0.47	0.44
947	Parents of college students[f]				
	Self-control over health	5.14	0.71	0.57	
	Provider control over health	4.96	0.94	0.77	
	Chance health outcomes	3.05	1.17	0.77	
	General health threat	4.44	1.11	0.48	

[a] Data from Lau & Ware (1981).
[b] Stability over 6 weeks.
[c] Data from Johnson (1983).
[d] Data from Giles (1984).
[e] Data from Gottlieb & Baker (1985).
[f] Data from longitudinal study described in this chapter.
[g] Stability over 17 months.

samples in which beliefs in Provider Control Over Health are the highest are pregnant women choosing a hospital birth (Johnson, 1983) and the insulin-dependent diabetics (Giles, 1984), the two samples in which people's health most objectively *is* under the control of medical professionals. The group whose beliefs in Provider Control were the lowest, on the other hand, were pregnant women who had chosen to have their baby at home with a midwife rather than in a hospital with an obstetrician (Johnson, 1983). These same women also exhibited the highest levels of beliefs in Self-Control Over Health, as one would expect.

Table 2 shows the results of two confirmatory factor analyses of the Lau–Ware health locus of control items from the students' baseline and from the parents in the longitudinal study described above. The actual question wording of the 26 items is shown in Table 2, which presents standardized estimates that were calculated by the program LISREL VI (Joreskog and Sorbom, 1984). Each item was allowed to load only on its hypothesized factor. The four factors were allowed to correlate freely with each other, but no correlations among item error variances were allowed. In accordance with the hypothesized factor structure, all hypothesized factor loadings were highly significant (median t of 10.12). The χ^2 statistic associated with these two models was highly significant, as one would expect with sample sizes this large; but the adjusted goodness of fit statistics were a very respectable .89 for the students and .82 for their parents.

Health Locus of Control Beliefs and Health Behaviors: Some Representative Data

Having already reviewed past findings linking locus of control beliefs to health and discussing what sort of relationships should be expected, I will present some representative data from the CMU health project that illustrate these relationships. One "behavioral" measure described eight different sets of symptoms (e.g., "you had been feeling poorly and had a fairly high temperature every day for three days") and asked respondents how likely they were to consult a doctor about each of these. Beliefs in Provider Control Over Health correlated .19 ($p < .001$) with a measure summarizing these hypothetical intentions to visit a doctor. Provider Control beliefs also correlated significantly ($r = .14$, $p < .01$) with a measure of how recently respondents had visited a doctor and a dentist for a regular checkup. Provider Control beliefs did not correlate with actual visits to the CMU health center during the freshman year, however (women, students not from the Pittsburgh area, and people whose subjective health status was worse during the year, were more likely to have visited the health center numerous times). Provider Control beliefs should not interact with health value to predict either the behavioral intention to visit a doctor scale nor actual doctor visits because in both instances (the first hypothetically) the respondent is feeling ill, a time when virtually everyone is motivated to get better. Health value theoretically *should* interact with Provider Control beliefs to predict getting (asymptomatic) checkups from medical professionals, but they did not.

Of the various preventive health behaviors studied, breast self-examination (BSE) is the one behavior that is most likely to be linked to beliefs in Self-Control Over Health because BSE is not a well-learned habitual behavior for the majority of women in our sample. When the study began, few of the women were performing BSE correctly, if at all. Moreover, it is hard to think of any motivation for performing BSE other than maintaining good health. (In contrast, exercise or good eating habits could be performed for reasons that have little to do with health, such as appearance.)

Theoretically, beliefs in Self-Control Over Health should help determine the performance of BSE only in those women who place a high value on health. To be as conservative as possible, beliefs in Self-Control Over Health from the baseline questionnaire were cor-

TABLE 2. Confirmatory Factor Analysis of Lau–Ware Health Locus of Control Scale

Item placement	Item wording	Students sample	Parents sample
	Self-control over health		
1	If I get sick, it's usually my own fault.[a]	.32	.13
5	Healthwise, there isn't much you can do for yourself when you get sick.	.42	.36
7	Anyone can learn a few basic health principles which can go a long way in preventing illness.[a]	.43	.38
9	I have a lot of confidence in my ability to cure myself once I get sick.[a]	.29	.20
14	"Taking care of yourself" has little or no relation to whether you get sick.	.49	.54
18	In the long run, people who take care of themselves stay healthy and get well quick.[a]	.41	.46
24	There is little one can do to prevent illness.	.54	.68
28	People's ill health results from their own carelessness.[a]	.45	.28
	Provider control over health		
4	Doctors can rarely do very much for people who are sick.	.62	.61
8	Many times doctors do not help their patients to get well.	.48	.55
10	Recovery from illness requires good medical care more than anything else.[a]	.42	.38
12	Doctors can do very little to prevent illness.	.39	.39
15	Doctors relieve or cure only a few of the medical problems their patients have.	.58	.67
19	Most sick people are helped a great deal when they go to a doctor.[a]	.70	.68
23	Seeing a doctor for regular check-ups is a key factor in staying healthy.[a]	.43	.50
26	Doctors can almost always help their patients feel better.[a]	.54	.67
	Chance health outcomes		
3	Whether or not people get well is often a matter of chance.[a]	.47	.52
11	When it comes to health, there is no such thing as "bad luck."	.54	.59
16	People who never get sick are just plain lucky.[a]	.56	.62
21	Good health is largely a matter of fortune.[a]	.60	.64
25	Staying well has little or nothing to do with chance.	.67	.59
30	Recovery from illness has nothing to do with luck.	.60	.60
	General health threat		
2	Some kinds of illness are so bad that nothing can be done about them.[a]	.33	.33
13	In today's world, few diseases are totally debilitating (crippling).	.19	.31
22	No matter what anybody does, there are many diseases that can just wipe you out.[a]	.85	.75
29	There are a lot of medical problems that can be very serious or even fatal (can kill you).[a]	.43	.45

[a] Item was reversed for scoring. We have always used a seven-point Likert format, with Point 1 labeled "Strongly Agree," Point 4 labeled "Neither Agree Nor Disagree," and Point 7 labeled "Strongly Disagree."

related with self-reported performance of BSE in the last wave of data collection (spring of the junior year), separately for those women falling into the top and bottom halves of the distribution on a measure of Health Value that was also gathered in the baseline questionnaire. (The measure of health value was a four-item Likert scale; see Lau *et al.*, 1986.) Hence, this constitutes a *prospective* test of the ability of health locus of control beliefs to predict health behavior. For the 57 women who did not value health very highly, Self-Control beliefs correlated −.13 (n.s.) with performance of BSE. But for the 77 women who valued health most highly, Self-Control beliefs correlated .21 ($p < .05$) with BSE. The difference between these two correlations is also significant, $z = 2.48$, $p < .05$. The same results occur when an analysis of covariance is performed in which rate of BSE during the students' junior year is the dependent variable, Self-Control beliefs and Health Value are the independent variables, and BSE at baseline is the covariate. The crucial Self-Control by Health Value interaction is significant, $F(4, 137) = 2.54$, $p < .04$. (The covariate is also highly significant, $p < .001$.) The means indicate that those women who *improved* their BSE over the course of the study most were women who believed in Self-Control Over Health and who placed a high value on health.

How strong is this relationship between locus of control beliefs and BSE? The .21 correlation in the high health value group suggests that Self-Control beliefs alone predict little more than 4% of the variance in BSE performance. While appearing low, this 4% is a magnitude that would typically be observed between health locus of control beliefs and a preventive health behavior in most situations. Furthermore, one must also realize that *neither health locus of control beliefs nor any behavioral criterion is going to be measured with perfect reliability*. Hence, *any observed correlation between the two will be attenuated due to measurement error*. When the .21 correlation is corrected for attenuation (using the coefficient alpha of .63 as the reliability of Self-Control Over Health and a test–retest [1 year] correlation of .55 as the reliability of the single-item measure of BSE), the correlation rises to .36. This means that if both Self-Control Over Health and BSE performance could be measured perfectly, the former would predict about 13% of the variance in the latter.

Value Correlates of Health Behaviors

The same type of analysis was conducted on the other six health behaviors studied in the CMU health project (eating, drinking, exercise, sleeping, smoking, and wearing seat belts). For five of the six behaviors the differences were in the expected direction (i.e., a higher correlation between beliefs in Self-Control Over Health and performance of the health behavior in the high health value group than in the low health value group), but only twice were any of the individual correlations even close to statistical significance (Self-Control beliefs correlated .24 with exercising and .15 with good eating habits, $p <$ .01 and .06, respectively, in the high health value group), and never were the differences between the correlations observed in the high health value and low health value groups significant.

If these correlations were corrected for attenuation due to measurement error, they would certainly rise, but to nowhere near the level observed for BSE. One reason for the difference is that most of these health behaviors could be performed for reasons that have little or nothing to do with health (Lau *et al.*, 1986). Consider the data in Table 3, which shows the simple correlations between each of nine different values that were measured (in terms of a ranking) in the fall of the respondents' junior year, and performance of the six health behaviors as reported during the spring of that year, for men and women. The data in Table 3 illustrate how little those behaviors, at this time in these people's lives, have to do with valuing health. One should thus not *expect* health locus of control beliefs

TABLE 3. Values and the Performance of Health Behaviors

	Wearing seat belts	Proper exercise	Eating	Sleeping	Not smoking	Not drinking
Males (n = 287)						
Excitement	−.13**	.04	.02	−.10*	−.06	−.17***
Fellowship	.03	−.08	−.13**	.09	.05	−.08
Health	.12**	.27***	.14**	.16***	.23***	−.04
Individualism	.00	.03	.03	−.02	−.03	.00
Inner harmony	.03	−.04	.00	−.02	−.05	.10
Physical appearance	−.07	.07	.06	.03	.00	−.15**
Popularity	−.07	−.12**	−.11*	−.10*	−.02	−.04
Security	.11*	−.08	−.04	.09	−.02	.07
Wisdom	.01	−.02	.14**	−.06	−.07	.23***
Females (n = 142)						
Excitement	−.01	.26***	−.01	.06	.03	.03
Fellowship	.10	−.14*	−.13	−.03	−.11	.00
Health	.03	.13	.13	−.05	.00	−.02
Individualism	−.08	.11	−.14*	−.02	.02	−.09
Inner harmony	−.02	−.13	−.11	−.13	.05	.01
Physical appearance	−.17**	.02	−.03	.11	−.07	.01
Popularity	.03	−.04	.02	.03	.11	.04
Security	.06	−.18**	.12	.04	−.05	.07
Wisdom	.04	.03	.17**	−.01	.06	−.04

Note: Table entries are Pearson product-moment correlations.
* $p < .10$; ** $p < .05$; *** $p < .01$.

to be highly associated with the performance of a variety of health behaviors, at least in a college population.

For males, a high ranking of "health" is moderately associated with five of the six health behaviors, particularly exercise and not smoking. But several other values are associated with most of the health behaviors. For example, wearing seat belts has as much to do with ranking "security" high, and "excitement" low, as it does with health. And rejecting (or moderating) that favorite college pasttime of drinking apparently has little or nothing to do with valuing health for males; rather, ranking "wisdom" high, and "excitement" and "physical appearance" low, are the strongest value correlates of not drinking.

The pattern of observed correlations between values and each health behavior seems to make sense. Wearing seat belts is associated with "security" and rejecting "excitement" (these same two values would probably be associated with not driving at excessive speeds as well); proper eating habits are associated with ranking "health" and "wisdom" high, and "fellowship" and "popularity" low, presumably because the latter two values lead to occasions of "pigging out" and between-meal (junk food) snacks; getting sufficient sleep is positively associated with "health" and negatively associated with "excitement" and "popularity," presumably because the latter two values lead to staying up late partying; and so on.

The value correlates of health behaviors in females (shown in the bottom half of Table 3) are much less clear. In fact, three of the health behaviors did not correlate significantly with any of the values. Moreover, valuing "health" was not significantly correlated with any of the health behaviors (except BSE, which is not shown in Table 3). Exercise is associated with ranking "excitement" high and "security" low, which makes sense at least in terms of more vigorous and/or competitive activities. But it is difficult to explain why ranking "fellowship" low should be associated with exercise, or why proper eating habits are associated with rejecting "individualism," or why getting sufficient sleep should be associated with rejecting "physical appearance." Exercise and proper eating habits were expected to be associated with a high ranking of "physical appearance" and "popularity," but they were not, probably because these two values were ranked very low by almost everyone.

A summary scale was formed from the five health behaviors positively associated with a high ranking of "health" for males, and from the four health behaviors positively associated with "health" in females (including BSE), that were more reliable and valid indicators of a preventive orientation than any measure of an individual preventive health behavior. The correlation between beliefs in Self-Control Over Health and this summary measure of preventive health behaviors is .08 and −.02 for males and females who do not value health highly, and .14 and .34 for those who do value health highly. The latter two correlations (which theoretically should be the highest) increase to .34 and .71 when corrected for attenuation due to measurement error.

THE DEVELOPMENT AND STABILITY OF HEALTH LOCUS OF CONTROL BELIEFS

One question that has rarely been addressed is: how do these locus of control beliefs develop? What factors enter into their formation? And how stable are they over time? Some of these questions were addressed in a previous study (Lau, 1982) of college students. Early health training that focused on self-care (brushing one's teeth, getting enough sleep, and so on) was positively associated with beliefs in Self-Control Over Health, while regularly being taken to doctors and dentists for preventive checkups was associated with beliefs in Provider Control Over Health. Prior experience with illness in the family (both personal and vicarious experience) was positively associated with beliefs in Chance Health Outcomes and negatively associated with Self-Control and Provider Control Over Health. These three subscales were very stable over a 6-week period and were not affected by minor illness experiences during those 6 weeks. The weakness of this earlier study is that all of the family health history and parent training information came from the students themselves, and is therefore of questionable validity.

The CMU health project allowed a replication and extension of this earlier study by obtaining information directly from the parents. The model shown in Figure 1 was tested for each of the four health locus of control subscales. Only latent, unobserved constructs or factors are shown in Figure 1, but each of them had several manifest or observed indicators.

1. *Illness in the Family* had three indicators: counts of the number of family members (excluding the CMU student) with a chronic illness, the number of family members with arthritis, diabetes, or tuberculosis, and the number of family members who had experienced cancer, a heart attack, or some other "serious" disease.
2. *The Child's Illness Experience* was measured by a count of the number of common contagious childhood diseases the CMU student had experienced, a count of the number of "serious" illnesses the child had had (these last two were taken from the health records that students were required to provide the health center before enrolling), and a subjective report of how frequently the student had been sick as a child (the student's and parents' answers to this question were averaged together).

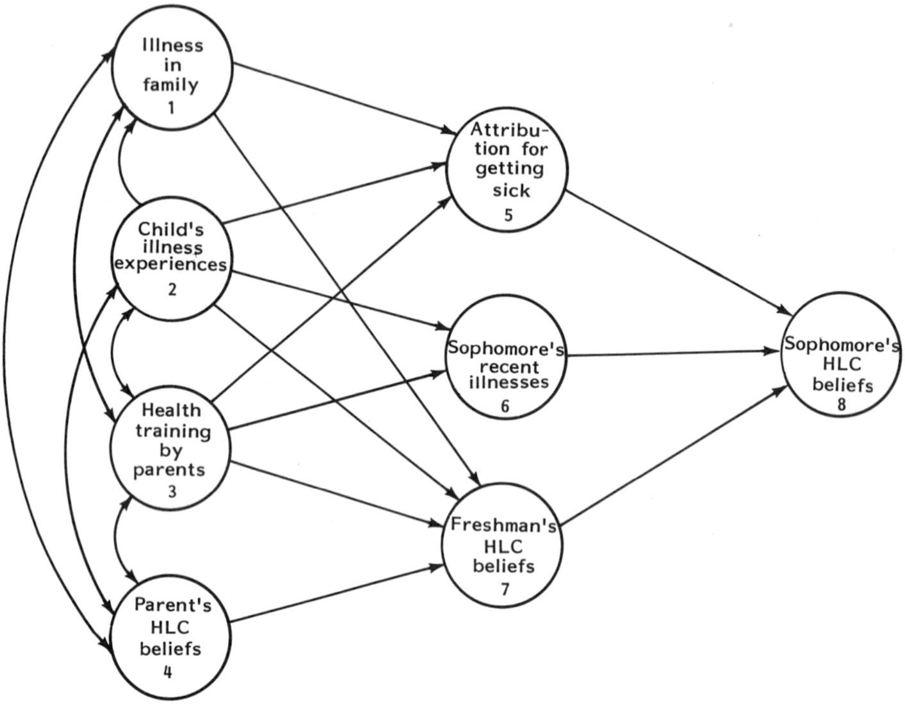

FIGURE 1. The development and stability of health locus of control beliefs in young adults.

3. *Health Training by Parents* was measured by items gathered from the parents' reporting of how strongly and consistently they tried to train their children about wearing seat belts, proper nutrition, the importance of physical exercise, and the dangers of smoking and drinking.
4. *Parent's HLC Beliefs* were the four or eight items comprising the different health locus of control subscales, as answered by the parents.
5. *Attributions for Getting Sick* came from a series of questions asking respondents about "the last time they had gotten sick" (see Lau & Hartman, 1983). After describing their most recent illness in their own words, students were asked how controllable was the reason they had gotten sick in this one particular instance, and how much their recovery was due to their own efforts. This set of questions was asked once during the freshman year and again in the fall of the sophomore year, so two distinct illnesses were almost always considered.
6. *The Sophomore's Recent Illness Experiences* were measured by subjective measures of the student's current health status, collected twice during the freshman year (these two were averaged together) and once during the fall of the sophomore year, a count of the number of times the student had actually visited the CMU health center during the freshman year, and a report of when (i.e., how long ago) the student had last been sick.
7. *The Freshman's HLC Beliefs* were the four or eight items comprising the different health locus of control subscales that were measured at baseline, before these students entered CMU.

8. *Sophomore's HLC Beliefs* were measured by the four or eight items of the different health locus of control subscales collected during the fall of the sophomore year.

The model is recursive, with causality flowing from left to right in Figure 1. In general, those factors hypothesized to be prior or causal variables are measured by items actually collected at an earlier time than those measuring caused or dependent variables. The one major exception to this general rule is that Parent's HLC Beliefs were actually measured 2–3 months after the Freshman's HLC Beliefs were collected from the baseline questionnaire. In this case it is assumed that (a) the health locus of control beliefs are fairly stable over time (which is empirically the case) and therefore if they had been measured in the parents before data were gathered from their children the responses would have been much the same, and (b) that causality goes primarily from the parents to their children (although undoubtedly there is some influence from the children to their parents as well).

The model was tested with LISREL VI (Joreskog & Sorbom, 1984), and data summarizing the important causal paths among the latent variables are shown in Table 4. (All of the factor loadings linking the hypothesized manifest indicators to the latent factors were highly significant.) None of the paths from Illness in the Family, Child's Illness Experiences, or Health Training by Parents were statistically significant, although in a few cases the estimates did exceed their standard errors. One important source of young adult's

TABLE 4. The Development and Stability of Health Locus of Control Beliefs

Paths common to all four models[a]		
Illness in family to attribution for getting sick	($\gamma_{1,5}$)	.019
Child's illness experiences to attribution for getting sick	($\gamma_{2,5}$)	.022
Child's illness experiences to sophomore's recent illnesses	($\gamma_{2,6}$)	.177**
Health training by parents to attribution for getting sick	($\gamma_{3,5}$)	.086
Health training by parents to sophomore's recent illnesses	($\gamma_{3,6}$)	−.041

Paths involving HLC beliefs		Self-control	Provider control	Chance health	General threat
Illness in family to freshman's HLC beliefs	($\gamma_{1,7}$)	−.294	−.014	−.259	−.152
Child's illness experiences to freshman's HLC beliefs	($\gamma_{2,7}$)	.232	.040	.365	.200
Health training by parents to freshman's HLC beliefs	($\gamma_{3,7}$)	.028	.041	−.087	.012
Parent's HLC beliefs to freshman's HLC beliefs	($\gamma_{4,7}$)	.196*	.220****	.191**	.130*
Attribution for getting sick to sophomore's HLC beliefs	($\beta_{5,8}$)	.459****	.015	−.302****	−.078
Sophomores recent illnesses to sophomore's HLC beliefs	($\beta_{6,8}$)	−.124**	−.133***	.050	.075
Freshman's HLC beliefs to sophomore's HLC beliefs	($\beta_{7,8}$)	.598****	.725****	.592****	.557****

Note: Table entries are standardized LISREL estimates.

[a] Coefficients in the top panel are actually averages of the estimates from the four separate models. These estimates differed slightly from model to model, but none of them ever differed significantly from 0 except $\gamma_{2,6}$, which was always significantly greater than 0.

* $p < .10$; ** $p < .05$; *** $p < .01$; **** $p < .001$.

health locus of control beliefs that was consistently identified by the models was their parent's health locus of control beliefs ($\gamma_{4,7}$). For all four subscales this path was positive and significantly greather than 0. But the model could explain only 5–10% of the variance in the Freshman's HLC Beliefs. Clearly the model does not capture all important determinants of health locus of control beliefs.

The path from Freshman HLC Beliefs to Sophomore HLC beliefs ($\gamma_{7,8}$) measures the stability of the health locus of control beliefs over a 17-month period. This path is quite large and highly significant in all four replications of the model (i.e., for each of the four subscales), which suggests that in general, health locus of control beliefs are, as theory dictates, fairly stable characteristics of personality. Recent Illness Experiences were related to changes in two of the health locus of control beliefs over time ($\gamma_{6,8}$). The poorer the students' health had been over the past year or so, the less strongly they believed in Self-Control and Provider Control Over Health. This does not replicate the earlier study, in which recent illness experiences were not observed to be related to changes in any of the health locus of control subscales (Lau, 1982). But the intervening time period here was much longer than in the earlier study (17 months versus 6 weeks), which could plausibly account for the difference. The greater time between measurements would allow many more illness experiences to occur, each of which could have influenced health locus of control beliefs slightly but, cumulatively, could have had a significant effect on those beliefs. Finally, and replicating a result first reported by Lau and Hartman (1983), internal and controllable Attributions for Getting Sick were positively associated with increased beliefs in Self-Control Over Health, while external and uncontrollable attributions were associated with increased beliefs in Chance Health Outcomes ($\beta_{5,8}$).

SUMMARY AND CONCLUSIONS

This chapter has reviewed relevant literature linking beliefs about control to health and health behavior. Three somewhat disparate research paradigms were examined, one exploring how different types of control moderate stress, a second looking at learned helplessness, and a third studying health locus of control beliefs. These three areas are related conceptually, for they all involve in one way or another the link between beliefs about control and some health-related response. Methodologically the paradigms are quite different, however, with the stress paradigm typically using experiments to manipulate control (and frequently employing animals as subjects), the learned helplessness literature more frequently using clinical studies, and the locus of control paradigm typically measuring control beliefs to predict some behavioral response.

Although these three literatures have progressed fairly independently, some studies have examined variables germane to more than one of them. For example, two different studies measured subjects' (general) locus of control beliefs before subjecting them to a standard learned helplessness manipulation. Hiroto (1974) used only extreme internals and externals (people scoring more than one standard deviation from the mean) and found a main effect for both locus of control and the helplessness manipulation (contingent or noncontingent reinforcement) on problem-solving tasks, with externals and those experiencing noncontingent reinforcement performing less well. Cohen, Rothbart, and Phillips (1976) studied a more general population (i.e., not just extreme internals and externals) and, not surprisingly (given their less extreme population), did not find a main effect of locus of control on either problem-solving or non-problem-solving tasks. But locus of control did interact with the helplessness manipulation in predicting performance on a non-problem-solving task: only externals who experienced noncontingent reinforcement performed more poorly than the other groups of subjects. The differences between these two studies suggest that extreme externals are in essence chronically in a state of learned helplessness, presumably because they have experienced noncontingent reinforcement situations many times in the past. If one draws an analogy between having no control over contracting disease and seeing recovery as having little to do with one's own efforts (which were the attributions that some of our respondents made about their recent illnesses) and a noncontingent reward situation, then it is possible to conceive of subjects who believe in Chance Health Outcomes and/or General Health Threat as experiencing learned helplessness whenever they are sick. This leads to the further hypothesis that externals will in general find an illness experience to be more stressful and more debilitating than internals.

Another important link between the different control literatures concerns how these findings can be applied to larger public health problems. If some people react to hospitalization with "good patient" behavior and others with "bad patient" behavior (Taylor, 1979), this suggests that certain hospital procedures could be modified to fit the control beliefs or preferences of patients. Such modification should reduce the stress associated with the "total institution" aspects of being in a hospital, should make "bad patients" more willing to comply with medical recommendations, and could result in improved health outcomes for all patients (see Cromwell, Butterfield, Brayfield, & Curry, 1977). More generally it has been suggested that designing behavioral change programs to "fit" the control beliefs or preferences of clients should make all such programs more effective, and there is some evidence to suggest that it does (Abramowitz, Abramowitz, Roback, & Jackson, 1974; Best, 1975; Best & Steffy, 1975; Friedman & Dies, 1974; Kilmann, 1974; Kilmann, Albert, & Sotile, 1975; Wallston, Wallston, Kaplan, & Maides, 1976). For example, Wallston, Wallston, Kaplan, & Maides, (1976) designed two different programs for weight reduction, one self-directed, the other more externally oriented with a greater reliance on group pressure. People whose health locus of control beliefs matched the orientation of their group (internals with the self-directed group, externals with the group pressure group) were more satisfied with the group and actually lost more weight during the course of the program.

This idea is one of the most promising avenues for health locus of control research. Health professionals with knowledge of their patient's health locus of control beliefs could design therapies or medical regimens consistent with those beliefs that would maximize compliance, thus helping to alleviate the very serious noncompliance problem (DiMatteo & DiNicola, 1982; Sackett & Haynes, 1976). Krantz has even developed two scales that specifically measure a preference for information and a preference for behavioral involvement in medical treatment (Krantz *et al.,* 1980) that might be more useful than a more general health locus of control scale.

A related idea is to design media messages aimed at changing behavior in a way that would differentially appeal to internals or externals. For example, of the various health behaviors studied in the CMU health project, the one that students were least likely to perform well was BSE. An experiment was conducted to try to improve this behavior (Jacobs & Lau, 1988). Women were randomly assigned to receive one of two different advertisements for a workshop teaching proper BSE. One advertisement was entitled "Control Breast Cancer" and stressed how women had to take control of their own health by performing BSE. The other advertisement was entitled "Don't Press Your Luck" and stressed that getting breast cancer was a matter of chance. All women also received a brochure from the American Cancer Society describing "How to Examine Your Breasts." Thus, there was reason to hope that BSE might improve even for people who did not come to the workshop, which was a one-time-only affair scheduled late in the fall semester and therefore could not be expected to attract many participants. (Indeed, only about a dozen women actually attended the workshop.)

At the beginning of the following semester, half of the subjects in each advertisement condition received a reminder about the importance of BSE and a second copy of the "how-to" brochure. Unlike the initial mailing, this second mailing was identical for all subjects, but it was intended to reinforce the earlier message. The workshop and mailings came from the university health center and thus had no apparent association with the health study.

Several months later, as part of the regular spring questionnaire, the women were asked about their BSE, as they had been the previous 2 years. The basic hypothesis was that locus of control beliefs should interact with the advertisement to predict changes in BSE. Preliminary analyses confirm this hypothesis: the women who improved their BSE most over the previous year were women in the self-care group who received the "Control Breast Cancer" advertisement plus the reminder, and women in the chance group who received the "Don't Press Your Luck" advertisement plus the reminder.

This finding supports the exciting idea that media health campaigns could be more effective if they aimed their message specifically at the locus of control beliefs of their audience, a possibility that is quite remote for any message aimed at a general population but might not be so remote for messages aimed at more specific populations. If this experiment is replicable, one could imagine large health maintenance organizations with an interest in improving the health of their members administering a health locus of control scale as a regular part of an intake interview. Subsequent communications about proper preventive health behaviors and proper utilization of medical professionals (that many HMOs send to all of their members indiscriminantly) could be designed specifically for and mailed directly to people with different types of locus of control beliefs.

Acknowledgments

I would like to thank Karen Hartman and Marilyn Jacobs for reading an earlier version of the manuscript.

REFERENCES

Abramowitz, C. V., Abramowitz, S. I., Roback, H. B., & Jackson, C. (1974). Differential effectiveness of directive and nondirective group therapies as a function of client internal–external control. *Journal of Consulting and Clinical Psychology, 42,* 849–853.

Abramson, L. Y., Seligman, M. E. P., & Teasdale, J. D. (1978). Learned helplessness in humans: Critique and reformulation. *Journal of Abnormal Psychology, 87,* 49–74.

Alloy, L. B., & Abramson, L. Y. (1982). Learned helplessness, depression, and the illusion of control. *Journal of Personality and Social Psychology, 42,* 1114–1126.

Andersen, R., Kravits, J., & Anderson, O. W. (1971). The public's view of the crisis in medical care: An impetus for changing delivery systems? *Economics and Business Bulletin, 24,* 44–49.

Averill, H. R. (1973). Personal control over aversive stimuli and its relationship to stress. *Psychological Bulletin, 80,* 286–303.

Bandura, A. (1977). Self-efficacy: Toward a unifying theory of behavioral change. *Psychological Review, 84,* 191–215.

Best, J. A. (1975). Tailoring smoking withdrawal procedures to personality and motivational differences. *Journal of Consulting and Clinical Psychology, 43,* 1–8.

Best, J. A., & Steffy, R. A. (1975). Smoking modification procedures for internal and external locus of control clients. *Canadian Journal of Behavioral Science, 7,* 155–165.

Balch, P., & Ross, A. W. (1975). Predicting success in weight reduction as a function of locus of control: A unidimensional and multidimensional approach. *Journal of Consulting and Clinical Psychology, 43,* 119.

Borthe, D. G., & Hammen, C. L. (1981). The attributional model of depression. *Personality and Social Psychology Bulletin, 7,* 53–58.

Cohen, S. (1980). Aftereffects of stress on human performance and social behavior: A review of research and theory. *Psychological Bulletin, 88,* 82–108.

Cohen, S., Rothbart, M., & Phillips, S. (1976). Locus of control and the generality of learned helplessness in humans. *Journal of Personality and Social Psychology, 34,* 1049–1056.

Collins, B. E. (1974). Four components of the Rotter internal-external scale: Belief in a difficult world, a just world, a predictable world, and a politically responsive world. *Journal of Personality and Social Psychology, 29,* 381–391.

Cromwell, R. L., Butterfield, E. C. Brayfield, F. M., & Curry, J. L. (1977). *Acute myocardial infarction: Reaction and recovery.* St. Louis: Mosby.

Dabbs, J. M., & Kirscht, J. P. (1971). Internal control and the taking of influenza shots. *Psychological Reports, 28,* 959–962.

de Charms, R. (1968). *Personal causation: The internal affective determinants of behavior.* New York: Academic Press.

Depue, R. A., & Monroe, S. M. (1978). Learned helplessness in the perspective of the depressive disorders: Conceptual and definitional issues. *Journal of Abnormal Psychology, 87,* 3–20.

DiMatteo, M. R., & DiNicola, D. D. (1982). *Achieving patient compliance.* Elmsford, NY: Pergamon Press.

Friedman, M. L., & Dies, R. R. (1974). Reactions of internal and external test-anxious students to counseling and behavior therapies. *Journal of Consulting and Clinical Psychology, 42,* 921.

Fromm, E. (1941). *Escape from freedom.* New York: Farrar & Rinehart.

Giles, S. L. (1984). *Relationship between locus of control expectancies and disease-related learning and disease control in diabetics.* Unpublished manuscript, Oregon Health Sciences University.

Gottlieb, N. H., & Baker, J. A. (1985). *Health beliefs, health locus of control and other cognitive factors in alcohol use, physical activity and smoking: Differences by university fitness program participation.* Unpublished manuscript, University of Texas, Austin.

Hiroto, D. S. (1974). Locus of control and learned helplessness. *Journal of Experimental Psychology, 31,* 311–327.

Jacobs, M. L., & Lau, R. R. (1988). The effect of locus of control beliefs on the success of health-related communications. Manuscript in preparation, Carnegie–Mellon University.

James, W. H., Woodruff, A. B., & Werner, W. (1965). Effect of internal and external control upon changes in smoking behavior. *Journal of Consulting Psychology, 29,* 184–186.

Johnson, S. E. D. (1983). *Internal–external control as one factor in the maternity client's choice of midwife/home birth versus obstetrician/hospital birth.* Unpublished master's thesis, University of Pittsburgh.

Joreskog, K. G., & Sorbom, D. (1984). *LISREL VI: Analysis of linear structural relationships by the method of maximum likelihood.* Chicago: National Educational Resources.

Kaplan, G. D., & Cowles, A. (1978). Health locus of control and health value in the prediction of smoking reduction. *Health Education Monographs, 6,* 129–137.

Kelley, H. H. (1967). Attribution theory in social psychology. In D. Levine (Ed.), *Nebraska symposium on motivation,* (Vol. 15, pp. 192–240). Lincoln: Nebraska University Press.

Kilmann, P. R. (1974). Direct and nondirect marathon group therapy and internal–external control. *Journal of Counseling Psychology, 21,* 380–384.

Kilmann, P. R., Albert, B. M., & Sotile, W. M. (1975). Relationships between locus of control, structure of therapy, and outcome. *Journal of Consulting and Clinical Psychology, 43,* 588.

Kirscht, J. P. (1972). Perceptions of control and health beliefs. *Canadian Journal of Behavioral Science, 4,* 225–237.

Klein, D. C., Fencil-Morse, E., & Seligman, M. E. P. (1976). Learned helplessness, depression, and the attribution of failure. *Journal of Personality and Social Psychology, 33,* 508–516.

Krantz, D., Baum, A., & Wideman, M. (1980). Assessment of preferences of self-treatment and information in health care. *Journal of Personality and Social Psychology, 39,* 977–990.

Lau, R. R. (1982). Origins of health locus of control beliefs. *Journal of Personality and Social Psychology, 42,* 322–334.

Lau, R. R., & Hartman, K. A. (1983). Common sense representations of common illnesses. *Health Psychology, 2,* 167–185.

Lau, R. R., Hartman, K. A., & Ware, J. E., Jr. (1986). Health as a value: Methodological and theoretical considerations. *Health Psychology, 5,* 25–43.

Lau, R. R., & Ware, J. E., Jr. (1981). Refinements in the measurement of health-specific locus-of-control beliefs. *Medical Care, 19,* 1147–1158.

Lazarus, R. S. (1966). *Psychological stress and the coping process.* New York: McGraw–Hill.

Lefcourt, H. M. (1976). *Locus of control: Current trends in theory and research.* Hillsdale, NJ: Erlbaum.

Lundy, J. R. (1972). Some personality correlates of contraceptive use among unmarried female college students. *Journal of Psychology, 80,* 9–14.

MacDonald, A. P. (1970). Internal–external locus of control and the practice of birth control. *Psychological Reports, 27,* 206.

Maier, S. F., & Seligman, M. E. P. (1976). Learned helplessness: Theory and evidence. *Journal of Experimental Psychology: General, 105,* 3–46.

Martin, D. J., Abramson, L. Y., & Alloy, L. B. (1984). Illusion of control for self and others in depressed and nondepressed college students. *Journal of Personality and Social Psychology, 46,* 125–136.

Miller, S. M. (1979). Controllability and human stress: Method, evidence and theory. *Behaviour Research and Therapy, 17,* 287–304.

Peterson, C. (1982). Learned helplessness and health psychology. *Health Psychology, 1,* 153–168.

Peterson, C., & Seligman, M. E. P. (1984). Causal explanations as a risk factor for depression: Theory and evidence. *Psychological Review, 91,* 347–374.

Raps, C. S., Peterson, C., Jonas, M., & Seligman, M. E. P. (1982). Patient behavior in hospitals: Helplessness, reactance, or both? *Journal of Personality and Social Psychology, 42,* 1036–1041.

Rotter, J. B. (1954). *Social learning and clinical psychology.* Englewood Cliffs, NJ: Prentice–Hall.

Rotter, J. B. (1975). Some problems and misconceptions related to the construct of internal vs. external control of reinforcement. *Journal of Consulting and Clinical Psychology, 43,* 56–67.

Sackett, D. L., & Haynes, R. B. (Eds.). (1976). *Compliance with therapeutic regimens.* Baltimore, MD: Johns Hopkins University Press.

Seeman, M., & Evans, J. W. (1962). Alienation and learning in a hospital setting. *American Sociological Review, 27,* 772–783.

Seligman, M. E. P. (1975). *Helplessness: On depression, development, and death.* San Francisco: Freeman.

Sells, S. B. (1970). On the nature of stress. In J. E. McGrath (Ed.) *Social and psychological factors in stress.* New York: Holt, Rinehart & Winston.

Sonstroem, R. J., & Walker, M. I. (1973). Relationship of attitude and locus of control to exercise and physical fitness. *Perceptual and Motor Skills, 36,* 1031–1034.

Steffy, R. A., Meichenbaum, D., & Best, J. A. (1970). Aversive and cognitive factors in the modification of smoking behavior. *Behaviour Research and Therapy, 8,* 115–125.

Strickland, B. R. (1978). Internal–external expectancies and health-related behaviors. *Journal of Consulting and Clinical Psychology, 46,* 1192–1211.

Sweeney, P. D., Anderson, K., & Bailey, S. (1986). Attributional style in depression: A meta-analytic review. *Journal of Personality and Social Psychology, 50,* 974–991.

Taylor, S. E. (1979). Hospital patient behavior: Reactance, helplessness, or control? *Journal of Social Issues, 35,* 156–184.

Thompson, S. C. (1981). Will it hurt less if I can control it? A complex answer to a simple question. *Psychological Bulletin, 90,* 89–101.

Toner, J. B., & Manuck, S. B. (1979). Health locus of control and health-related information seeking at a hypertension screening. *Social Science and Medicine, 13A,* 823.

Wallston, B. S., & Wallston, K. A. (1978). Locus of control and health: A review of the literature. *Health Education Monographs, 6,* 107–117.

Wallston, B. S., & Wallston, K. A. (1984). Social psychological models of health behavior: An examination and integration. In A. Baum, S. E. Taylor, & J. E. Singer (Eds.), *Handbook of psychology and health* (Vol. 4, pp. 23–53). Hillsdale, NJ: Erlbaum.

Wallston, B. S., Wallston, K. A., Kaplan, G. D., & Maides, S. A. (1976). Development and validation of the health locus of control scale. *Journal of Consulting and Clinical Psychology, 44,* 580–585.
Wallston, K. A., Maides, S., & Wallston, B. S. (1976). Health-related information seeking as a function of health-related locus of control and health value. *Journal of Research in Personality, 10,* 215–222.
Wallston, K. A., & Wallston, B. S. (1981). Health locus of control scales. In H. M. Lefcourt (Ed.), *Research with the locus of control construct,* (Vol. 1, pp. 189–243). New York: Academic Press.
Wallston, K. A., & Wallston, B. S. (1982). Who is responsible for your health? The construct of health locus of control. In G. S. Sanders & J. Suls (Eds.), *Social psychology of health and illness* (pp. 65–95). Hillsdale, NJ: Erlbaum.
Wallston, K. A., Wallston, B. S., & DeVellis, R. (1978). Development of the multidimensional health locus of control (MHLC) scales. *Health Education Monographs, 6,* 160–170.
Ware, J. E., Jr. (1978). Effects of acquiescent response set on patient satisfaction ratings. *Medical Care, 16,* 327–336.
Weaver, R. (1972). *Internality, externality, and compliance as related to chronic home dialysis patients.* Unpublished master's thesis, Emory University (cited in Strickland, 1978).
White, R. W. (1959). Motivation reconsidered: The concept of competence. *Psychological Review, 66,* 297–333.
Wildman, H. E., Rosenbaum, M. N. S., Framer, E. M., Keane, T. M., & Johnson, W. G. (1979). *Smoking cessation: Predicting success with the health locus of control scale.* Paper presented at the Association for the Advancement of Behavior Therapy, San Francisco.
Williams, A. F. (1972a). Factors associated with seat belt use in families. *Journal of Safety Research, 4,* 133–138.
Williams, A. F. (1972b). Personality characteristics associated with preventive dental health practices. *Journal of American College of Dentists, 39,* 225–234.
Wolff, H. G. (1953). *Stress and disease.* Springfield, IL: Thomas.

Personal Determinants

Personal Characteristics and Life-Style

Although a number of personal and life-style variables have been linked conceptually and empirically to health behavior, no personality models, factors, theories, or concepts have had as great and as pervasive an impact on health behavior research as have the health belief or locus of control models. Helsing and Comstock's observation (1977) that "psychosocial characteristics have not been studied as thoroughly as demographic factors" (p. 1044) remains as true of the larger area of health-related behaviors as it was originally in relation to seat belt use.

Discussion of research on personal characteristics can be considered under three headings, depending on the *primary* focus: discrete personal characteristics; trigger factors; and integration of these two.

DISCRETE PERSONAL CHARACTERISTICS

Discrete personal characteristics include not only those attributes that are traditionally thought of as personality variables, such as anxiety or dependency; but also demographic characteristics such as educational and income levels, which are often (usually inappropriately) considered as "social" or as components of socioeconomic status; health status; and life-style.

Personality Variables

A large portion of the research on personality variables was conducted to increase understanding of smoking behavior, and to evaluate the impact of antismoking campaigns. (Some of these studies also examined demographic and other characteristics in addition to personality variables.) Attempts have been made to relate smoking to extraversion (e.g., Cherry & Kiernan, 1976), to stimulation seeking (e.g., Eysenck, 1965), and to seeking positive affect (e.g., Leventhal & Avis, 1976; Tomkins, 1968), but the conclusions have been unclear.

Williams (1973) observed that smoking among teenagers was positively related to personality characteristics such as chance-taking, external control, and impulsivity, and negatively related to harm-avoidance and order. Williams also noted that teenagers who smoked were more likely to have a same-sex parent who smoked, and were more likely than nonsmokers to come from families with low occupational status, and low parental education. Moreover, Williams demonstrated gender differences in the way these variables were related to one another. In addition, he found that smoking was negatively related to seat belt use and getting adequate sleep.

Among college students, Arnett, Black, and McNeary (1974) found that a personal distaste for smoking, fear of cancer, and parental wishes were the most important reasons given for either not smoking or giving it up. They also noted that smokers tended to be less aware of the hazards of smoking, and more likely to have a same-sex parent who smoked than were nonsmokers.

In summarizing the literature on personal determinants of smoking behavior in youngsters, for example, Flay and his colleagues (Flay, d'Avernas, Best, Kersell, & Ryan, 1983) state that there are "few personality variables that discriminate consistently between adolescents who will begin to smoke regularly and those who will remain nonsmokers" (p. 138).

Radelet (1981) observed that nonusers of tranquilizers were less reluctant to admit to having unpleasant feelings and were less likely to have friends who used tranquilizers than were tranquilizer users.

In relation to other health behaviors, for example, Palfrey *et al.* (1983) observed that significantly more delinquent than nondelinquent youngsters were unable to identify a regular source of health care. Duckitt and Broll (1983) were unable to find consistent or appreciable personality differences, i.e., anxiety, extraversion, critical independence, sensitivity, shrewd pragmatism, inhibition, in illness behavior such as days spent in bed.

Murphy's analysis (1978) of differential use of a symptom checklist by two groups of Montreal women revealed that although the group that had higher scores was very similar to the group with lower scores on most personality dimensions, as a group they had higher ego ideals and higher levels of awareness of their own needs beyond basic security, and that the score differences could be accounted for in terms of differences in "self-actualization."

Helsing and Comstock's analysis of nonuse of seat belts (1977) revealed that nonusers were more likely to have more aggressiveness, and greater feelings of depressed mood, alienation, and general stress and unhappiness than were users. Nonuse was also associated with infrequency of church attendance, but not consistently related to aspects of preventive behaviors other than to lengthier time since their last dental visit, and (for females) since their last Pap smear. Nonusers were also more likely to be female than male, and to have fewer years of education and lower income.

Magarey, Todd, and Blizard's concise study (1977) of factors associated with breast self-examination and delay in reporting breast symptoms, demonstrated that conscious factors such as fear of breast loss, disease, or dying were of little relevance in contrast to the greater predictive value of unconscious uses of denial and other defense mechanisms.

Income, Education, Occupation, and Age

In addition to some of the demographic characteristics identified in the previous paragraphs, Salber and her colleagues (e.g., Salber, Freeman, & Abelin, 1968) observed that factors such as parental occupation, parental smoking, and student status (honor student or not), which distinguished smokers from nonsmokers at age 15, did not distinguish them at age 21.

Lave, Lave, Leinhardt, and Nagin (1979) found that low-income, unmarried males who are new to their communities and who are in good health, are less likely to have a regular source of health care than are women or married persons who have resided in their communities for a time and who have higher incomes or who may be in poorer health. Okada and Wan (1978) showed that when economic barriers to care are removed, poor persons still do not seek out dental care to the degree that the nonpoor do.

Luft, Hershey, and Morrell (1976) observed that use of physician services in a rural community is better predicted by health status and by having a regular source of care, than by income and insurance coverage. And Monteiro (1973) showed that income was increasingly less important as a determinant of care-seeking behaviors.

Christie and Lawrence (1978) observed that attitudes toward hospitalization were negatively correlated with age among men, and positively correlated with age among women.

Swigar, Quinlan, and Wexler (1977) observed that among women who apply for abortion, those who chose eventually not to have an abortion do not differ in age, race, marital status, occupation, partner's age, and partner's occupation from those who do have the abortion. The only distinguishing characteristics were the woman's and partner's educational levels. Those who had the abortion, and their partners, had more years of education. Okafor's (1983) report of hospitalization among rural Nigerians showed the impact of education in conjunction with perceptions of need.

Titkow's (1983) analysis of illness behavior in Warsaw showed that educational level was a determinant of utilization of sources of care beyond the district clinics, of selectivity in use of certain hospitals, and of seeking nongovernmental laboratory tests.

Health Status

The role of health status itself as a determinant of health behavior was examined by Kulik and Mahler (1987), who observed that acutely ill college students believed themselves to be more vulnerable to health problems in the future (even if these were unrelated to their present condition), and more interested in receiving preventive materials, than were apparently healthy students. Garrity, Somes, and Marx (1978) observed that perceived health status was primarily a function of recent life changes. Wan's discriminant analysis (1976) showed that perceived health status was a function of employment status; the severity of physical disability, including the need for assistance in mobility; and psychological well-being. Moreover, Wan concluded that measures of personal and social functioning are more valuable as predictors of perceived health than are socioeconomic status or psychological well-being. The discrepancies between the findings of Garrity *et al.* and those of Wan are attributable largely to the differences in the data they were analyzing.

Life-Style

Badura's analysis (1984) of the behavioral factors in illness led to an attempt at integrating the varied and diverse personal characteristics that underlie behaviors that place people at risk for diseases, and into a discussion of the concept of "life-style" as it relates to health and illness. Badura's model considers personal stressful experiences in conjunction with personality variables, particularly with self-concept and emotional equilibrium. Badura developed a critical analysis of the term *life-style* and pointed to the need for clarifying its meaning.

Bruhn's chapter identifies a number of behaviors that relate to health risks and discusses them in relation to life-style, paying particular attention to the way in which life-style is acquired. In addition, the chapter introduces the increasingly important concept of "wellness" and relates it to life-style.

TRIGGER FACTORS

Trigger factors, those events that seem to precipitate health behavior—particularly use of a service—were dramatically described by Zola (1973) who elaborated on how stressful events or experiences of personal or social disequilibrium "triggered" a medical care visit for symptoms that had existed for some time. Among the major triggers, Zola identifies interpersonal crises; and perceptions of interference with social or personal relations, or with vocational or physical activity.

Mechanic and his colleagues have documented the trigger role of psychological stress in determining perceptions of health status (Tessler and Mechanic, 1978), and in the seeking of care (Tessler, Mechanic, & Dimond, 1976).

Bloor (1985), building on Zola's work, noted that care-seeking, in a sample of boardinghouse residents in Scotland, was likely to occur when there was a break in the everyday accommodation that characterizes the way most people adapt to symptoms, at the same time when there was also a relevant external cue encouraging the seeking of care. Bloor suggests that work often promotes accommodation to symptoms and illness and allows persons suffering to temporize and postpone seeking care.

Verbrugge (1985) has provided systematic documentation of how daily events, in conjunction with bad moods, trigger medical drug use, medical and dental care-seeking, lay referral behaviors, and restricted activities.

INTEGRATIVE APPROACHES

Anderson (e.g., Anderson & Bartkus, 1973) has proposed a basic model that includes discrete personal characteristics together with triggering factors. Anderson's "behavioral model" identifies three categories of factors to be taken into account in predicting a number of health behaviors: predisposing; enabling; and need factors. The model has often been the basis for path analyses to predict or account for use of health services, but has implications for other health behaviors as well. In the context of developing a plan to provide services for older persons, Ward (1977) provides a concise literature review of research undertaken within this behavioral model.

Using this model, Wan and Soifer (1974) were able to demonstrate, for example, that need variables—health status and responsiveness to illness—were the most important predictors of physician visits, more so than the enabling factors of insurance coverage, costs of visits, and income (which had no effect at all). Selwyn (1978) has used this model to discriminate between users and nonusers of child health services among poor residents of a barrio in Colombia.

Moreover, a path analysis by Bush and Osterweis (1978) demonstrated that perceived morbidity—a need factor—is the best predictor of prescription medicine use, although age, race, and gender—predisposing factors—contribute appreciably, as does perceived availability of care, an enabling factor. Bush and Iannotti's chapter demonstrates how path analysis as a statistical tool is used to compare and contrast the predictive value of different levels of personal determinants.

REFERENCES

Anderson, J. G., & Bartkus, D. E. (1973). Choice of medical care: A behavioral model of health and illness behavior. *Journal of Health and Social Behavior, 14,* 348–362.

Arnett, J. H., Black, M. W., & McNeary, S. S. (1974). An 11-year study of cigarette smoking habits of students entering Drexel University, Philadelphia. *American Journal of Public Health, 64,* 120–123.

Badura, B. (1984). Life-style and health: Some remarks on different viewpoints. *Social Science and Medicine, 19,* 341–347.

Bloor, M. J. (1985). Observations of abortive illness behavior. *Urban Life, 14,* 300–316.

Bush, P. J., & Osterweis, M. (1978). Pathways to medicine use. *Journal of Health and Social Behavior, 19,* 179–189.

Cherry, M., & Kiernan, K. (1976). Personality scores and smoking behaviour: A longitudinal study. *British Journal of Preventive and Social Medicine, 30,* 123–131.

Christie, D., & Lawrence, L. (1978). Patients and hospitals: A study of the attitudes of stroke patients. *Social Science and Medicine, 12,* 49–51.

Duckitt, J., & Broll, T. (1983). Life stress, personality and illness behavior: A prospective study. *Psychological Reports, 53,* 51–57.

Eysenck, H. J. (1965). *Smoking, health and personality.* New York: Basic Books.

Flay, B. R., d'Avernas, J. R., Best, J. A., Kersell, M. W., & Ryan, K. B. (1983). Cigarette smoking: Why young people do it and ways of preventing it. In P. McGrath & P. Firestone (Eds.), *Pediatric and adolescent behavioral medicine.* New York: Springer.

Garrity, T. F., Somes, G. W., & Marx, M. B. (1978). Factors influencing self-assessment of health. *Social Science and Medicine, 12,* 77–81.

Helsing, K. J., & Comstock, G. W. (1977). What kinds of people do not use seat belts? *American Journal of Public Health, 67,* 1043–1050.

Kulik, J. A., & Mahler, H. I. M. (1987). Health status, perceptions of risk, and prevention interest for health and nonhealth problems. *Health Psychology, 6,* 15–27.

Lave, J. R., Lave, L. B., Leinhardt, S., & Nagin, D. (1979). Characteristics of individuals who identify a regular source of medical care. *American Journal of Public Health, 69,* 261–267.

Leventhal, H., & Avis, N. (1976). Pleasure, addiction, and habit: Factors in verbal report or factors in smoking behavior. *Journal of Abnormal Psychology, 85,* 478–488.

Luft, H. S., Hershey, J. C., & Morrell, J. (1976). Factors affecting the use of physician services in a rural community. *American Journal of Public Health, 66,* 865–871.

Magarey, C. J., Todd, P. B., & Blizard, P. J. (1977). Psycho-social factors influencing delay and breast self-examination in women with symptoms of breast cancer. *Social Science and Medicine, 11,* 229–232.

Monteiro, L. (1973). Expense is no object . . . : Income and physician visits reconsidered. *Journal of Health and Social Behavior, 14,* 99–115.

Murphy, H. B. M. (1978). The meaning of symptom-check-list scores in mental health surveys: A testing of multiple hypotheses. *Social Science and Medicine, 12,* 67–75.

Okada, L. M., & Wan, T. T. H. (1979). Factors associated with increased dental care utilization in five urban, low-income areas. *American Journal of Public Health, 69,* 1001–1009.

Okafor, S. I. (1983). Factors affecting the frequency of hospital trips among a predominantly rural population. *Social Science and Medicine, 17,* 591–595.

Palfrey, J. S., Karniski, W., Clarke, S., Tomaselli, M., Meltzer, L. J., & Levine, M. D. (1983). Health profiles of early adolescent delinquents. *Public Health Reports, 98,* 449–457.

Radelet, M. J. (1981). Health beliefs, social networks, and tranquilizer use. *Journal of Health and Social Behavior, 22,* 165–173.

Salber, E. J., Freeman, H. E., & Abelin, T. (1968). Needed research on smoking: Lessons from the Newton study. In E. F. Borgatta and R. R. Evans (Eds.), *Smoking, health and behavior.* Chicago: Aldine.

Selwyn, B. J. (1978). An epidemiological approach to the study of users and nonusers of child health services. *American Journal of Public Health, 68,* 231–235.

Swigar, M. E., Quinlan, D. M., & Wexler, S. D. (1977). Abortion applicants: Characteristics distinguishing dropouts remaining pregnant and those having abortion. *American Journal of Public Health, 67,* 142–146.

Tessler, R., & Mechanic, D. (1978). Psychological distress and perceived health status. *Journal of Health and Social Behavior, 19,* 254–262.

Tessler, R., Mechanic, D., & Dimond, M. (1976). The effect of psychological distress on physical utilization: A prospective study. *Journal of Health and Social Behavior, 17,* 353–364.

Titkow, A. (1983). Illness behavior and action: The patient-role. *Social Science and Medicine, 17,* 637–646.

Tomkins, S. (1968). A modified model of smoking behavior. In E. F. Borgatta & R. R. Evans (Eds.), *Smoking, health, and behavior*. Chicago: Aldine.

Verbrugge, L. M. (1985). Triggers of symptoms and health care. *Social Science and Medicine, 20,* 855–876.

Wan, T. T. H. (1976). Predicting self-assessed health status: A multivariate approach. *Health Services Research, 11,* 464–477.

Wan, T. T. H., & Soifer, S. J. (1974). Determinants of physician utilization: A causal analysis. *Journal of Health and Social Behavior, 15,* 100–108.

Ward, R. A. (1977). Services for older people: An integrated framework for research. *Journal of Health and Social Behavior, 18,* 61–70.

Williams, A. F. (1973). Personality and other characteristics associated with cigarette smoking among young teenagers. *Journal of Health and Social Behavior, 14,* 374–380.

Zola, I. K. (1973). Pathways to the doctor—from person to patient. *Social Science and Medicine, 7,* 677–689.

CHAPTER 4

Life-Style and Health Behavior

John G. Bruhn

The only way to keep your health
Is to eat what you don't want . . .
Drink what you don't like . . .
And do what you'd rather not.
Mark Twain

The heaviest burdens of illness in the United States today are related to aspects of individual behavior, especially long-term patterns of behavior often referred to as "life-style." The Centers for Disease Control (1980) of the United States Health Service have estimated that 50% of mortality from the 10 leading causes of death in the United States can be traced to life-style.

FACTORS AFFECTING THE LEARNING OF LIFE-STYLE AND PERSONAL HEALTH BEHAVIORS

A person's life-style or way of life and health behavior are closely interrelated. Health behavior refers to those actions (or inactions) we take that directly or indirectly affect our health status or well-being. The purposes of this chapter are to: (1) discuss the factors that influence the learning of life-style and personal health behaviors; (2) discuss the relationship between life-style and health behavior; (3) outline some of the intrinsic and extrinsic motivations for changing life-styles and health behaviors; (4) analyze the trade-offs and value choices that are involved in changing life-styles and health behaviors; and (5) discuss the theoretical development and further research needed to refine our understanding of the contribution of behavior to the burden of illness.

The Relationship between Life-Style and Health Behavior

Health behaviors are part of life-style, which is a broader concept encompassing not only behaviors and attitudes, but an outlook or philosophy of life. Health is associated with common habits and with social networks. Social ties appear to be associated with

JOHN G. BRUHN • School of Allied Health Sciences, University of Texas Medical Branch, Galveston, Texas 77550.

TABLE 1. Some Characteristics of Illness and Wellness Life-Styles

Illness life-style	Wellness life-style
Use of limited coping skills	Learns new or modifies old coping skills
Socially withdrawn, shy, minimal interaction	Open and receptive to others
Sees change as barrier, obstacle	Initiates and directs change
Perceives few choices and options in problem-solving	Perceives and exercises choices and options in problem-solving
No clear-cut goals or purpose to life	Has purpose to life and goals
Limited use of resources in adapting	Makes use of resources of all kinds in adapting
Relies on already acquired skills, limited skills	Enhances personal, social, and other skills
Black–white view of issues and problems	Integrating approach to issues and problems
Crisis-oriented approach to problems	Problem-solving/preventive attitude
Passive/reactive behavior	Active/initiating behavior
Minimal self-care activities	Maximal self-care activities
Socially isolated or weak social ties	Strong social ties
Risk-seeking health behavior	Risk-conscious health behavior
Pessimistic/fatalistic attitude	Optimistic/hopeful attitude
Stress-producing behavior	Stress-reducing behavior
External locus of control	Internal locus of control
Anger/depression common emotions	Frustration, anxiety, and compulsive behavior common
Negative self-image, low self-esteem	Positive self-image, high self-esteem

health status and mortality. High-risk health practices and weak social ties appear to precede illness. Life-style, therefore, involves some type of social network. Life-style can include the geographical area where one lives, the way a living area is decorated, the kind of car one drives, the kind of food one eats, the kind of clothes one wears, the kind of entertainment and leisure activities one engages in, and so on. Life-style is a person's way of life. Some aspects of life-style are chosen by the individual, while others may be determined, for example, by whom one marries. As a friend recently told me, "I would love to live in Denver, but Bill [her husband] homesteaded in Buffalo, Wyoming."

Health behaviors are learned during the process of growth and development through parental and peer modeling, information acquired through the mass media, and life changes. Life-style is also learned and modeled, but it has many components that are acquired and changed as one moves through the life cycle. Life-style and health behaviors are closely interrelated so changes in one usually affect the other. For example, a change in eating habits might influence where we buy groceries and which restaurants we eat at and even whether we order a special meal on an airplane. On the other hand, a job promotion will possibly affect not only where we eat, but what we eat. Therefore, as changes occur throughout the life cycle, modifications occur in both life-style and health behavior to accommodate the life change.

Table 1 lists some characteristics that are thought to be either illness enhancing or wellness enhancing. Some of these characteristics have been the focus of research, others are based on the experience of the author, and still others are speculative and need to be studied. The list of factors is meant to convey that one or more of the characteristics in combination tend to foster or enhance a person's vulnerability or susceptibility to either illness or wellness. As Berkman and Breslow (1983) have observed, ". . . the individual has the power to maintain his own health by the observance of simple prudent rules of behavior." Some of the characteristics listed in Table 1 are attitudes, others are behaviors, and still others relate to personality attributes. Table 1 reinforces the idea of the scope and complexity of the terms *illness* and *wellness* as two extreme conditions. Indeed, illness and wellness could be more accurately viewed as processes that extend along a continuum and that include a blend of the various characteristics, some of which may change with time and place.

A Developmental Conceptual Framework

One may reasonably start with the hypothesis that "wellness" is a life-style that can be taught, learned, and modified by humans throughout their life spans. The development of a wellness life-style may be conceived of as a cumulative process that can be influenced by physical, behavioral, psychological, and social factors (Ng, Davis, Manderscheid, & Elkes, 1981). Wellness can be defined as a philosophy that views individuals as having some influence on their degree of healthiness. Wellness further implies that individuals are actively engaged in the process of enhancing their healthiness, not just maintaining it. Therefore, wellness requires learning a point of view, specific tasks, and a means of supporting and reinforcing such a life-style. Sources of support and reinforcement will change throughout the life cycle, but the individual will make special efforts to seek out such a support system in order to live a wellness life-style. Bruhn and his colleagues have suggested that Erikson's typology of eight developmental stages of man offers a beginning in the search for an understanding of the wellness process (Bruhn, Cordova, Williams, & Fuentes, 1977; Bruhn & Cordova, 1977, 1978). These researchers have proposed an index for assessing wellness based upon the individual's completion of the minimal wellness tasks appropriate to each developmental stage. Children grow up in our society exposed to our concept of health as the absence of illness. There is no parallel concept available to a child to help learn about wellness, as there are concepts for developing such other positive values as honesty, industry, or kindness to animals. For this reason it is important to identify both the tasks that are appropriate for learning about wellness at various points along the developmental continuum and those tasks that will enhance an individual's motivation to work toward wellness.

Bibace and Walsh (1979, 1981) conducted studies of cognitive processes underlying children's responses to health, illness, and bodily functions in the developmental sequence. They found that children's conceptions of health and illness are correlated with marked differences in the degree of personal control over the cause and alleviation of illness. They argued that it is important from a cognitive-development perspective to carry out a series of studies that determine the shifts in these concepts from early childhood to adulthood. This approach also permits the examination of the influence of factors such as education, peer pressure, illness experience, and so forth in shaping and changing health behaviors.

A conference held in 1981 (Bruhn & Parcel, 1982), which proposed to produce a set of guidelines for researchers in the area of children's health behavior, found little consensus and large gaps in our knowledge of how health behavior develops. Developmental and learning theories were noted as being especially important to help identify factors that account for child health practices.

As noted in a government report,

> health-relevant behavior is an integral part of lifestyle, which starts forming in infancy. It is influenced by a wide variety of factors including the examples set and instruction given by parents, siblings, peers, schools, religious and community groups, and the media. Socialization—the combined effect of all of these factors—is more powerful than

> any single attempt to teach new behaviors. (U.S. Department of Health and Human Services, 1979, p. 5)

The better-known models of health-related behavior have been summarized by Becker and Maiman (1983). Although most of these models attempt to understand health and illness behavior from both the individual and social context perspective, they do not incorporate the influence of change as it occurs along the developmental continuum. Indeed, most research using these models has been concerned with the health behavior of adults. Nor do these models deal with the development of life-style.

Factors That Shape Life-Style and Health Behaviors

For discussion purposes, the many factors that can influence the development of life-style and health behaviors can be grouped into four major categories: personal, environmental, cultural, and group factors.

Environmental Factors. Although there are several aspects of our physical environment over which we can sometimes exert some direct control and choice (e.g., where we work and live), often such controlled choices are not possible. There are many more aspects of our physical environment that are influenced by public and organizational policies and policies over which we have little direct personal control, e.g., air, water, noise, pesticides, pollutants, and food preservatives (McKee, 1974; Milio, 1981). The quality of our physical environment has direct and indirect effects on our health. Some effects may be subtle, but nonetheless cumulative. In the United States, we have viewed the physical environment as something to be changed to accommodate our need for industrialization and modernization. Seldom are long-term plans made to anticipate the effects of the changes we make. As a result, health hazards in our physical environment are dealt with as they become a problem. As the speed of technology and industrialization has accelerated, environmental problems have become more numerous, complex, and not amenable to solitary solutions. The type and quality of the physical environment will also directly bear on the nutritional environment, i.e., the kinds of foods available and their cost. The physical environment will also influence the type, availability, and accessibility of health and social services. It might be expected that the more restrictive and hazardous the physical environment, coupled with a feeling of little personal control to change it, the more individual health behavior will be limited, inflexible, and of low value. Indeed, given certain physical conditions, behavioral options that influence health may not be known or considered important, especially if such behaviors have no immediate, observable effect. The physical environment is not only important in shaping children's life-styles as well as their attitudes, beliefs, values, and behaviors regarding health, but also continues to modify all aspects of health throughout life. The shaping process is also reciprocal: as our physical environment changes, we are changed, and as we change, we modify our physical environment.

Cultural Factors. What a society or group values establishes the goals that are considered important and worth working for and preserving. Values are reflected in all types of media and permeate all age and socioeconomic levels of society. From an early age in the United States, we learn that being independent and being able to satisfy personal needs are highly valued. Health is not highly valued. Health is considered by the public to be a commodity that can be purchased when needed. Individuals have delegated responsibility for the maintenance of their health, and with high expectations, to a variety of specialists (Knowles, 1977). Health behaviors are largely learned passively during the process of socialization. Because healthy life-styles and behaviors are not highly valued or systematically taught, unhealthy life-styles and behaviors that are learned take substantial effort to modify (Maccoby & Farquhar, 1975; Maccoby, Farquhar, Wood, & Alexander, 1977; Bernstein & McAlister, 1976). Indeed, as Warner (1985) has pointed out, marketing specialists in the tobacco industry have subtly changed their advertising tactics, e.g., eliminated smoke from ads, and are attempting to recruit women into the smoking population. Thus, individuals are continually confronted with messages in the mass media that minimize the health effects of certain behaviors. It is easier for individuals to receive and process information selectively to confirm the behavior they have chosen to pursue, than to change that behavior. Inconsistent and conflicting information in the media creates a formidable barrier to the recognition and acceptance of accurate information about health risks, especially as industries that have products with health risks, alter their marketing strategies to counter new health behavior modification strategies. Schenck, Runyan, and Earp (1985) suggested that to be more effective, for example, in the use of seat belts, health educators need to target their information toward certain critical beliefs. These authors pointed out that drivers' perceptions of their own risk of being injured in a car crash were associated with their opinions on the seat belt use laws. If the drivers had been exposed to personalized risk data, the observed influence of the data may have been greater. Adults' perceptions of risk are conveyed to children, and children, in turn, will select from the media information that fits what they see and hear from adults with whom they have frequent contact.

Group Factors. Although there have been few studies that have dealt directly with health learning, it would appear that a good share of life-style and health and illness behavior is acquired in the family setting (Mechanic, 1963). Litman (1974) found that parents, irrespective of generation, were the most frequently mentioned source of health attitudes and opinions, followed by the spouse, health personnel, and the mass media. There also appears to be some evidence that families' use of medical care services may be related to such factors as the parents' level of education, their concern about their own health (Mechanic, 1964), and feelings of powerlessness and alienation (Morris, Hatch, & Chipman, 1966), as well as the existence of a close-knit, nonscientific ethnic tradition (Suchman, 1965). In addition, parental attitudes and their relationship toward the child have been found to have a direct effect on the family's ability to manage and treat medical problems (Davis, 1963; Khurana & White, 1970; Lewis & Zeichner, 1960).

The significant role played by the wife-mother as a primary agent of health behavior in the family is becoming increasingly clear. In a survey of food habits and attitudes of school children, the mother was found to serve as a prominent influence in matters of health and nutrition (Litman, 1974). Mothers also tend to exert considerable control over the child's immunization and dental behavior. A mother's illness or prolonged incapacitation is also a serious threat to family functioning. Health and illness behavior are closely tied to family solidarity and the type of adjustment family members as individuals, and as a family, make to illness, hospitalization, and rehabilitation.

Parenting styles have been correlated with the development of social competence (Baumrind, 1979). Child-rearing attitudes that recognize the child as an individual, and foster the child's assumption of responsibility, were associated with positive health behavior in children (toothbrushing, sleep habits, exercise, nutritional practices, and refraining from smoking). In contrast, children raised in families with an autocratic style of child-rearing were not as likely to practice such behavior (Pratt, 1976). Certain kinds of families report that they practice a variety of positive health behaviors: families that are actively involved with the larger community, that show open internal communication patterns, that allow children to contribute to family decision-making, and in which husbands and wives share family responsibilities (Pratt, 1976).

Peer pressure is an important factor in learning health behavior. Students themselves report that peer pressure, especially influence from a "favorite" peer, appears to be the most potent of those pressures. Lewis and Lewis (1984) asked children in Grades 5–8 about the dares or challenges they received from other children. Peer pressure was reported most frequently by 8th grade students. About 50% of the dares encouraged problem behaviors that placed the children (or others) at risk of personal injury, or the potential development of habits hazardous to their health. With increasing age, more dares occurred in the school environment and fewer involved risk of personal injury. Among 7th and 8th graders, more boys were dared to perform acts of violence, and more girls were challenged to be sexually active.

The power of peer influences and conformity pressure among early adolescents to smoke cigarettes is well known (Severson *et al.,* 1981; Evans *et al.,* 1978). The pretext of pressure to smoke appears to be related to the way that smoking functions as a sign of independence from adult authority and of maturity. Correlates of tobacco use in early adolescence include not only peer behavior, but parental smoking as well. The exact mechanism for this relationship is uncertain, but includes peer pressure, identification with parents as role models, greater perceived or actual permissiveness regarding smoking, and increased opportunity for surreptitious smoking (McAlister, Perry, & Maccoby, 1979; McAlister, 1983).

Young adolescents tend to be the healthiest people in the population. They are sick less often than members of other age groups and many are never seriously sick or incapacitated. Despite the general state of good health at this time of life, the leading causes of death are from suicide, homicide, and vehicular accidents. Numerous theories have been advanced to explain the increase in violent deaths among the young—affluence, war, decline in religious belief, permissive parents, and so forth. The suspicion also exists that the self-destructiveness of the young is a symptom of more widespread problems in society at large. As people reach the age of 35, they are less likely to die violently—the more subtle, chronic processes of heart disease, hypertension, cancer, and the toll of excessive smoking, drinking, and eating begin to emerge as the major killers (The Surgeon General's Report, 1979). Fuchs (1974) has said the more education people have, the healthier they tend to be. People with more education tend to come from families with more money, who can afford better medical care. Good education may lead to more sensible work and living habits. Formal schooling may increase self-confidence and decrease stress. And it is possible that people who are sophisticated enough to see the benefits of a good education are also aware of the importance of a healthy way of life. Fuchs concluded that people determine much of their health status by the way they live.

Personal Factors. Personal life-style factors that relate to health behavior include beliefs about control, hardiness, and coping skills.

Beliefs are personally formed cognitive configurations that are often culturally determined and shared. They are preexisting notions about reality that serve as a perceptual "set." Beliefs determine what is fact, i.e., how things are in the environment, and they shape the understanding of its meaning. The extent to which people feel confident of their power of mastery over the environment affects whether an encounter will produce threats or challenges. Similarly, people develop beliefs about health and the degree to which they can influence their own health status. Beliefs about personal control have to do with feelings of mastery and confidence. There are several models for explaining the components of health beliefs, including personal control. Perhaps the best known is the "health belief model," which is discussed in detail elsewhere in this volume. A sense of coherence or being at one with the world should have supportive functions, as Antonovsky (1979) suggested, and is probably a positive factor in social and work functioning and health.

Control refers to our real or perceived ability to determine outcomes of an event. When our behavior is perceived as causally linked to outcomes, perceptions of control are possible. When the outcomes cannot be tied to behavior, it is more difficult to believe that we are in control (Gatchel & Baum, 1983). Much of the interest in control has dealt with two issues: (1) the effects of believing that one has control and that outcomes are contingent on responses and (2) the effects of believing that outcomes are not contingent on behavior and therefore not controllable. The first has been concerned most directly with the mediating effects of perceived control on response to aversive stimulation and stress. The second has been concerned with learned helplessness and the debilitating effects of believing that one cannot control what happens.

Although results are not altogether clear and convincing as one might hope, the bulk of research is consistent in implying that when faced with health problems, individuals who have an internal locus of control appear to engage in generally more adaptive responses than externally controlled individuals. These range from preventive health measures through remedial strategies when illness occurs. Findings suggest that the development of an internal orientation could lead to improved health practices for some individuals who have been inclined to believe that life events are beyond their responsibility and more a function of external control. However, internal beliefs may not always be facilitative. The readiness of internals to master behavior is appropriate when events are controllable. When internals persist in attempting to control events without results, they may exacerbate the undesirable situation they are attempting to relieve. Internal control is but one aspect of the personal life-style that needs to be considered.

Kobasa, Maddi, and Kahn (1982) examined "hardiness" as a personality construct comprised of three characteristics: commitment, the tendency to appraise demands as challenging rather than threatening, and having a sense of control over one's fate. It was found that people characterized as hardy were less prone to develop illness under stress. Hardiness appeared to function as a resistance resource in buffering the effects of stressful events. It is not yet clear how hardiness develops, nor its role with other resources such as social support. Of particular interest are possible interactions among the resistance resources. For example, one might expect an interaction showing that hardiness as a component of life-style is especially effective in preserving health when constitutional strengths are low. A possible mechanism for this might be health practices. Positive health practices may function to offset constitutional predispositions to some extent. Hardy persons might be more conscientious in positive health practices. In contrast, persons low in hardiness might engage in negative health practices. These interactions need further study.

Overall functioning is largely determined by the effectiveness with which a person appraises and copes with the events of day-to-day living. The effectiveness of appraisal within a specific encounter is determined in part by its match with the flow of events. Ambiguity and vulnerability, which are present in most encounters, can make this match difficult to achieve. Effective coping also depends on a match between appraisal of coping options and actual coping demands, and between a selected coping strategy and other personal agendas (Lazarus & Folkman, 1984). Social functioning over the long term is an extension of coping effectiveness in many specific encounters throughout life.

Risk, Responsibility, Reward, and Needs

An individual's perceptions, in addition to the numerous environmental, cultural, group, and personal factors previously discussed, can influence the development of health behavior. Individuals' perception of vulnerability or susceptibility, their perception of benefits and costs, and their perceptions and assessments of competing needs all influence, in various ways, health actions or inactions (Feuerstein, Labbé, & Kuczmierczyk, 1986).

In this regard, the conflict theory model of personal decision-making, unlike the health belief model, attempts to specify the conditions under which individuals will give priority to health matters and seek out medical information about the consequences of alternative courses of action. Janis and Mann (1977) delineated five stages individuals go through in order to arrive at a stable decision. These stages were identified by observing individuals who made health decisions they subsequently carried out successfully; these included giving up smoking, losing weight on a low-calorie diet, or contemplating a series of recommended medical treatments. Stage 1 takes the form of an event or communication that conveys a threat or opportunity. The individual must either ignore or repeat the challenge or accept it and progress to the next stage of decision-making. In Stage 2, the individual carefully considers the goals relevant to the decision and looks for alternatives. Throughout Stage 3, the individual evaluates the proposed cost of each alternative. Stage 4 sees the decision maker increasingly committed to a course of action. Finally, in Stage 5, the decision maker discards new challenges and continues with implementing the decision. Janis and Mann (1977) postulate that only when an individual's pattern is vigilant will the person be able to make a rational choice based on weighing the benefits or costs of taking an action. An advantage of this model is that it has testable implications that could counteract beliefs responsible for maladaptive behavior.

The perception and assessment of personal risk is an important, but, as yet, not fully understood, aspect of life-style and health behavior. The decision on whether or not to take an action depends on the kind of information received and also on the state in which the recipient of the information is at the time. Baric (1969) described four different states of health (healthy, "at risk," convalescent, and ill) and noted that people in each of these states will have a need for a different kind of health information. Baric explained that a healthy person who becomes aware of a health threat, will undergo a process similar to that of acquiring a sick role, i.e., the process of acquiring a "quasi-sick" or "at risk" role. Baric emphasized the limitations of efforts to modify health behavior if intervention is focused on the sick role or at the point at which a person has already made a health decision based on a perception and assessment of risk.

Finally, a person's perception of risk, possible benefits, and assessment of need, relate to an overall attitude of responsibility for one's health. Our health care system provides sophisticated, technological services for complex physical disease; it is not as effective in providing preventive services. The general public expects health care to be available, accessible, and affordable when they need it. Furthermore, the public has high expectations of medicine's ability to cure and rehabilitate. These expectations are reinforced by mass media and the publicity given to technological advances in health care. Providers of health services have helped to create high expectations and a dependency on technology to cure disease. The attitude that is still prevalent in our country is that you do not need to assume personal responsibility for your health. An individual's attitude toward responsibility for health is learned at an early age, modified and reinforced by the media, and often is unchangeable until a health crisis forces a reevaluation of attitude, behavior, and life-style. A life-threatening event is often a potent modifier of priorities and attitudes toward life (Cousins, 1979).

Knowles (1977) emphasized that the next major advances in the health of Americans will be determined by what individuals are willing to do for themselves and for society-at-large.

> If he is willing to follow Breslow's seven rules for healthy living, he can extend his life and enhance his own and the nation's productivity. If he is willing to reassert his authority with his children, he can provide for their optimal mental and physical development. If he participates fully in private and public affairs to reduce the hazards of the environment, he can reduce the causes of preventive death and disability. If he is unwilling to do these

things, he should stop complaining about the steadily rising costs of medical care and the disproportionate share of the GNP that is consumed by health care. (p. 78)

CHANGING LIFE-STYLES AND HEALTH BEHAVIOR

Life-style is the most important modifiable factor influencing health and illness today. It is difficult to stimulate the development of, or change to, a healthy life-style with traditional health education methods. For some problems, change may require legal means such as enforced speed limits, air bags, and increased taxes on tobacco and alcohol. For a few, education through social groups and mass media may be adequate. For other health problems, only supportive medical care will be available for some time to come. For most health problems, a combination of approaches using all methods to change life-style and appropriate use of medical care will be necessary. Finally, for some health problems, it may be decided that they must be endured in order to support values more important than health (Haggerty, 1977).

Barriers to Change

Table 2 lists several factors that can inhibit changes in life-style or health behavior. Some of these factors can also be facilitators of change, depending on the social situation and meaning to the individual.

Working with asymptomatic persons to alter life-style risk factors offers very different problems and therefore requires intervention models that go beyond those used in the traditional treatment of patients motivated by sickness (Hollis, Connor, & Matarazzo, 1982). Compliance is difficult to achieve when health produces little or no rewarding physical feedback, e.g., reduction of pain, and typically elicits only minimal or short-term acknowledgment and support by family, friends, and employer. Peer pressure or incentives offered by an employer, e.g., time off from a job for exercise, "health" days, and so on, can be important motivators for change. However, it has long been the contention of public health educators that health behaviors do not occur in isolation (Green, 1984). They are interrelated to form a cohesive pattern or life-style. Positive health habits could be viewed as constituting an effective life-style that reflects an ability to anticipate problems and to meet and cope with them actively. The individual's personal concept of risk and its links to specific behaviors affects decisions to modify life-style and assume responsibility for self-management. These actions, in turn, help shape positive changes in self-concept, which reinforce the process of self-management (WHO, 1986).

People are reluctant to alter patterns that represent powerful, predictable, and immediate sources of gratification which are deeply ingrained in social and cultural contexts. One possible impediment may be the lack of a comprehensive national health policy and the mixed messages the public receives about the health risks of certain substances. These inconsistencies may reinforce the ambivalence and resistance to change among many people. Furthermore, there is an apparent lack of real commitment to the concept of healthier living. The government continues tobacco subsidies, while the Surgeon General takes a strong stand on the health risks of smoking. Similarly, certain foods and alcohol are promoted by the mass media, while the health sector warns about their abuse. Perhaps one of the greatest barriers to change may be the "live for today and don't worry about tomorrow" attitude prevalent in our country, coupled with the high expectations that the sophisticated technology of medicine can mend almost any health malady that might occur. There is little incentive for individuals to assume responsibility for their health or to adopt a spartan pattern of living (Milio, 1981).

TABLE 2. Some Factors That Might Encourage or Discourage Life-Style and Health Behavior Change

Factors that might encourage change	Factors that might discourage change
Personal	Personal
Premature death of family member or friend from preventable disease	Negative attitude toward own age and aging
Health changes in self	Not a risk taker
Concern about own physical appearance	Health not a high personal priority
	State of health has been good to excellent
	Chronic illness
Job	Job
Employer support of healthy life-style activities at work	Shift work or irregular work hours
Work colleagues make health behavior changes	Negative attitudes of employer and co-workers
Flexibility in work hours	Change in jobs
Retirement	Frequent travel
Change in jobs	Unemployment or increased job responsibilities
Family	Family
Family encouragement and participation in healthy life-style	Divorce
Children become self-sufficient and independent	Marriage
Health change in family member	Move to new geographical area
Comments from children about smoking, drinking, diet, etc.	Addition of new members to family
Divorce	
Marriage	
Move to new geographical area	
Economic	Economic
Insurance premium reductions for healthy behaviors	Work at more than one job
Other	Other
Strong encouragement from physician	Little or no encouragement from physician

Facilitators of Change

Table 2 also lists some factors that can encourage changes in life-style and specific health habits. While educators and researchers have used different approaches to promote healthy life-styles, these approaches have been derived from various professional or theoretical orientations, or the personal interest of the interventionist, rather than appeal to the diversity of values and motivations of the target audience. We, therefore, know little about many of the possible facilitators of change.

VALUE CHOICES AND TRADE-OFFS OF A HEALTHY LIFE-STYLE

One reason for the difficulty in getting people to change their health behaviors is that preserving health is not our society's highest value. It competes with many other values, including wealth, power, security, knowledge, and social acceptance. Many studies have reported that people's knowledge of health and health risks has increased, and beliefs have changed as the result of interventions. However, efforts to mold or change values and influence behavior have been less successful. Health beliefs vary from disease to disease, person to person, and even in the same person over time. Thus, singular appeals to change health behavior or life-style have to be meaningful to an individual at a particular point in time. In other words, individuals have to be "ready" to change. Appropriate change times might be when there are fewer pressing or compelling priorities for an individual's personal resources.

Perhaps one of the more important aspects that dissuade people from changing their life-style or health behaviors is the *benefit* they derive from the life-style and behaviors with which they have become comfortable. It is difficult to persuade persons to give up a behavior or make major changes in the way they live when the benefits of these changes are unknown. Such substitutions are often viewed as a punishment or sacrifice. The trade-off between behaviors or life-styles is not seen as an equal one.

Another aspect of value change involves the *source* of values. Values are obtained from our culture, science, religion, and personal experience. Sometimes, information about values differs between these sources, requiring that individuals make choices to guide their behavior. Indeed, individuals may make behavioral choices that appear inconsistent with respect to their value of health; for example, an individual may exercise regularly, but not wear seat belts, or adhere to dietary restrictions, but smoke cigarettes. These inconsistencies may reflect conflicts in information between sources of values and, hence, the individual's ambivalence about how total health is valued.

A third aspect of value change relates to *how individuals learned* their values about health, i.e., through modeling, chance, or "moralizing." Attempts to change values using the same approach in which the values were learned may have an opposite effect, especially if the conditions that surrounded the initial learning are now different. Pratt (1976) suggested that it is simply not a number of separate factors that affect how health is valued, but the overall pattern of values, of which health is one part, that is important. To cause individuals to change how they value health taps a complex, deeply embedded belief system that is not easily modifiable, at least with simple, solitary means of intervention or modification.

Value change is one of the most formidable tasks in health education. Indeed, it would seem more prudent with respect to time, effort, and cost to teach and model healthy life-styles and health behaviors beginning in early childhood than to attempt to change deeply entrenched values in adulthood.

It is difficult to assess the personal benefits of healthy life-styles as what is considered beneficial will differ among individuals. Oster and Epstein (1986) suggested that cholesterol-lowering interventions, no matter what their cost, are unlikely to result in substantial direct savings to the health care system. However, the indirect benefits of intervention are quite high for young and middle-aged adults, as well as for those with severe elevations of cholesterol or with additional coronary risk factors. Often individuals assume that they will add years to their life. A recent follow-up of Harvard graduates showed that by the age of 80, the amount of additional life attributable to adequate exercise, as compared with sedentariness, was from 1 to more than 2 years (Paffenbarger, Hyde, Wing, & Hsieh, 1986). Most often, however, the personal benefits of health behavior are physiological, cognitive, and/or behavioral (Dubbert, Martin, & Epstein, 1986). Sime (1984), for example, described research showing reductions in anxiety and depression and increases in body attitude and self-confidence due to exercise.

An individual's choices and decisions about changing life-style and health behaviors will also be influenced by life events and stage of development. The death of a family member from a heart attack is likely to have a greater influence in motivating a middle-aged family member than an adolescent to change his/her life-style. On the other hand, wearing seat belts could be seen to have a positive benefit to all members of a family, irrespective of age, if they have lost a family member in an automobile accident where wearing a seat belt may have meant survival. Everyone, seemingly, has "times" or "points" in their life when they are more receptive to health information and perhaps more motivated to change. To capture and sustain these positive times is a continual challenge to health professionals. In this respect Pill and Stott (1987) have developed an index to measure the extent to which people perceive their daily decisions regarding diet, exercise, smoking, drinking, and so on as choices that determine future health. This index has the potential for identifying those segments of a population most ready to alter their lifestyle.

FUTURE RESEARCH DIRECTIONS

A primary emphasis in learning about health behavior has been to attempt to change persons' attitudes, beliefs, and behaviors with respect to health using techniques or approaches based on a variety of theoretical propositions about behavior. In other words, we have obtained some information about which health behaviors are changeable and under what conditions, and which behaviors are less susceptible to change. Although some studies have followed individuals over time to assess the durability of change, for the most part, longitudinal studies have been dependent upon funding periods, i.e., usually a maximum of 5 years. Frequently, the populations or samples chosen for study have had a malady that required life-style and other changes of the afflicted persons in order to enhance their compliance with a medical regimen to control the malady. While all of these approaches are necessary to understand both health and illness behavior fully, we know relatively little about health behavior among healthy individuals, how, and in what way health behaviors change throughout life, and factors that influence the limits of health behavior change, and factors that help to maintain healthy behaviors over time. Table 3 outlines some future directions for research in life-style and health behaviors that have, as yet, not been addressed.

One of the promising theoretical approaches to the study of health behavior is the developmental approach (Roberts, Maddux, & Wright, 1984). Given the frequent obstacles of time, money, and geographical mobility of study populations, a reasonable research design would be cross-sectional. Schulz and Rau (1985) pointed out that relatively little is known about social support through the course of life. Social support and health behavior should have important links throughout life. There have been relatively few attempts to examine health behavior in the context of the life span. Kahn and Antonucci's (1980) convoy model is one attempt to describe the structure and function of social networks and their relation to the individual throughout life. Convoys are the structure in which an individual performs certain roles. These roles are the basis for contact and interaction with others. Social relationships can grow beyond that of a specific role and be valued for other reasons. Convoy membership and its stability over time is important in learning health behaviors and life-style. Convoy membership is also crucial in affecting behavioral and life-style change. Knowledge of convoys and their functions has several direct applications to life-style and health behavior. In the case of individuals who do not have convoys or effective ones, interventions could be planned. People with successful convoys could be supported to prevent unnecessary disruptions and maintain important supportive relationships.

Pilisuk, Chandler, and D'Onofrio (1982–83) identified four levels of intervention that hold promise for embracing supportive relationships instrumental to better health, which need to be explored and used in future studies: (1) creating new supportive networks when

TABLE 3. Areas for Future Research in Life-Style and Health Behavior

Studies of the health behavior of healthy individuals and families

- We need to know how health behaviors are formed (learned) and maintained at different periods in life. This could be accomplished by more studies of children's health behaviors and by comparative studies of individuals at different age decades.
- We need to know more about trade-offs between health behaviors among healthy people, i.e., which ones they are likely to give up, which ones may be more susceptible to change as they progress through the life cycle, and what social situations present a "readiness" for trade-offs in behavior.
- We need to know more about the "clustering effect" of health behaviors among individuals at different stages of life and identify approaches to changing clusters of related behaviors rather than focus on individual behaviors.
- We need to know about the relationship of high-risk life stages, e.g., adolescence, to the learning of new behaviors and/or the giving up of certain behaviors.
- We need to know more about how "risk" is learned and its relationship to stage of life.
- We need to know more about family health behaviors that are shared and reinforced among "healthy families" at different generational levels.
- We need to know more about the "limits" or capability of change for individuals and families.
- We need to know more about how individuals and families maintain health behavior, whether healthy or unhealthy, i.e., the role and types of social support involved in the maintenance of health behavior.
- Develop new, or modify existing, theories based on information obtained from these data.

Studies of health behavior that involve primary health care providers

- We need to know more about the health and illness behavior of the same individuals over time. Family medicine, health maintenance organizations, industries, and businesses are natural laboratories in which to carry out "naturalistic" longitudinal observations of the changeability of habits and behavior of individuals when sick compared to when well. This would provide insights into intervention strategies and the timing of change in people's lives.

Studies of health behavior in different cultural groups

- We need to know more about types of health behaviors that are common or uncommon in different ethnic and cultural groups. Not all groups value the same things, nor are they receptive to interventions to promote change based on the health values of Caucasian culture.

Studies of techniques and tools to measure health behavior

- There are available instruments, scales, and indices to measure or assess health behavior, health beliefs, and health values. Not all of these techniques are appropriate across age, sex, or ethnic groups. There is a need to refine research methodologies for more accurate and replicable ways to measure health behavior.

Studies of how coping responses are transformed into life-style patterns

- Very little is known about the interactions between health beliefs, stress, coping, and the various aspects of life-styles. Eating, smoking, and drinking to excess are possible responses to stress. Once these responses are transferred from short-term coping reactions into life-style patterns, they become risk factors.

they do not exist, (2) promoting cohesion when linkages exist but are weak, (3) increasing the range and effectiveness of existing networks, and (4) providing indirect advocate services on behalf of supportive networks or groups with similar needs.

Although theory is important in organizing and testing knowledge, existing theory can inhibit creativity in seeking fresh approaches to study phenomena. We need to learn more about health behavior in a naturalistic sense before we can effectively intervene to change aspects of human behavior we, as yet, know little about. The future holds much challenge and calls for innovation in this fertile field for research.

REFERENCES

Antonovsky, A. (1979). *Health, stress and coping*. San Francisco: Jossey–Bass.

Baric, L. (1969). Recognition of the "at-risk" role: A means to influence health behavior. *International Journal of Health Education, 12,* 24–34.

Baumrind, D. (1979). Parental disciplinary patterns and social competence in children. *Youth and Society, 9,* 239–276.

Becker, M. H., & Maiman, L. A. (1983). Models of health-related behavior. In D. Mechanic (Ed.), *Handbook of health, health care, and the health professions* (pp. 539–568). New York: Free Press.

Berkman, L. F., & Breslow, L. (1983). *Health and ways of living: The Alameda County study*. London: Oxford University Press.

Bernstein, D. A., & McAlister, A. (1976). The modification of smoking behavior: Progress and problems. *Addictive Behaviors, 1,* 89–102.

Bibace, R., & Walsh, M. E. (1979). Developmental stages in children's conceptions of illness. In G. C. Stone, F. Cohen, & N. E. Adler (Eds.), *Health psychology* (pp. 285–301). San Francisco: Jossey–Bass.

Bibace, R., & Walsh, M. E. (Eds.). (1981). *Children's conceptions of health, illness, and bodily functions*. San Francisco: Jossey–Bass.

Bruhn, J. G., & Cordova, F. D. (1977). A developmental approach to learning wellness behavior. Part I: Infancy to early adolescence. *Health Values, 1,* 246–254.

Bruhn, J. G., & Cordova, F. D. (1978). A developmental approach to learning wellness behavior. Part II: Adolescence to maturity. *Health Values, 2,* 16–21.

Bruhn, J. G., Cordova, F. D., Williams, J. A., & Fuentes, R. G. (1977). The wellness process. *Journal of Community Health, 2,* 209–221.

Bruhn, J. G., & Parcel, G. S. (1982). Current knowledge about the health behavior of young children: A conference summary. *Health Education Quarterly, 9,* 142–166.

Centers for Disease Control. (1980). *Ten leading causes of death in the United States, 1977*. Washington, DC: U.S. Government Printing Office.

Cousins, N. (1979). *Anatomy of an illness as perceived by the patient*. New York: Norton.

Davis, F. (1963). *Passage through crisis: Polio victims and their families*. Indianapolis: Bobbs–Merrill.

Dubbert, P. M., Martin, J. E., & Epstein, L. H. (1986). Exercise. In K. A. Holroyd & T. L. Creer (Eds.), *Self-management of chronic disease: Handbook of clinical interventions and research* (pp. 127–161). New York: Academic Press.

Evans, R. I., Rozelle, R. M., Mittlemark, M. B., Hansen, W. B., Blane, A. L., & Davis, J. (1978). Deterring the onset of smoking in children: Knowledge of immediate physiological effects and coping with peer pressure, media pressures, and parent modelling. *Journal of Applied Social Psychology, 8,* 126–136.

Feuerstein, M., Labbé, E. E., & Kuczmierczyk, A. R. (1986). *Health psychology: A psychobiological perspective*. New York: Plenum Press.

Fuchs, V. R. (1974). *Who shall live? Health economics and social choice*. New York: Basic Books.

Gatchel, R. J., & Baum, A. (1983). *An introduction to health psychology*. Reading, MA: Addison–Wesley.

Green, L. W. (1984). Modifying and developing health behavior. *Annual Review of Public Health, 5,* 215–236.

Haggerty, R. J. (1977). Changing lifestyles to improve health. *Preventive Medicine, 6,* 276–289.

Hollis, J. F., Connor, W. E., & Matarazzo, J. D. (1982). Lifestyle, behavioral health, and heart disease. In R. J. Gatchel, A. Baum, & J. E. Singer (Eds.), *Handbook of psychology and health* (Vol. 1, pp. 465–502). Hillsdale, NJ: Erlbaum.

Janis, I. L., & Mann, L. (1977). *Decision-making: A psychological analysis of conflict, choice and commitment*. New York: Free Press.

Kahn, R. L., & Antonucci, T. C. (1980). Convoys over the life course: Attachment, roles, and social support. In P. B. Bates & O. G. Brim (Eds.), *Life-span development and behavior* (Vol. 3, pp. 253–286). New York: Academic Press.

Khurana, R. C., & White, P. (1970, August). Attitudes of the diabetic child and his parents toward illness. *Postgraduate Medicine, 48,* 72–76.

Knowles, J. H. (1977). The responsibility of the individual. In J. H. Knowles (Ed.), *Doing better and feeling worse: Health in the United States* (pp. 57–80). New York: Norton.

Kobasa, S. C., Maddi, S. R., & Kahn, S. (1982). Hardiness and health: A prospective study. *Journal of Personality and Social Psychology, 42,* 168–177.

Lazarus, R. S., & Folkman, S. (1984). *Stress, appraisal, and coping*. Berlin: Springer.

Lewis, C. E., & Lewis, M. A. (1984). Peer pressure and risk-taking behaviors in children. *American Journal of Public Health, 74,* 580–584.

Lewis, V., & Zeichner, A. (1960). Impact of admission to a mental hospital on the patient's family. *Mental Hygiene, 44,* 503–509.

Litman, T. J. (1974). The family as a basic unit in health and medical care: A social-behavioral overview. *Social Science and Medicine, 8,* 495–519.

Maccoby, N., Farquhar, J. W., Wood, P. D., & Alexander, J. (1977). Reducing the risk of cardiovascular disease: Effects of a community-based campaign on knowledge and behavior. *Journal of Community Health, 3,* 100–114.

Maccoby, N., & Farquhar, J. W. (1975). Communication for health: Unselling heart disease. *Journal of Communication, 25,* 114–126.

McAlister, A. L. (1983). Social psychological approaches. In T. Glynn, C. Leukefeld, & J. Ludford (Eds.), *Preventing adolescent drug abuse: Intervention strategies* (NIDA Research Monograph No. 47, DHHS Publication No. ADM 83-1280). Washington, DC: U.S. Government Printing Office.

McAlister, A. L., Perry, C., & Maccoby, N. (1979). Adolescent smoking: Onset and prevention. *Pediatrics, 63,* 650–658.

McKee, W. D. (Ed.). (1974). *Environmental problems in medicine*. Springfield, IL: Thomas.

Mechanic, D. (1963). Religion, religiosity and illness behavior—The special case of the Jews. *Human Organization, 22,* 202–208.

Mechanic, D. (1964). The influence of mothers on their children's health attitudes and behavior. *Pediatrics, 33,* 444–453.

Milio, N. (1981). *Promoting health through public policy*. Philadelphia: Davis.

Morris, N., Hatch, M. H., & Chipman, S. S. (1966). Deterrents to well-child supervision. *American Journal of Public Health, 56,* 1232–1241.

Ng, L. K. Y., Davis, D. L., Manderscheid, R. W., & Elkes, J. (1981). Toward a conceptual formulation of health and well-being. In L. K. Y. Ng & D. L. Davis (Eds.), *Strategies for public health: Promoting health and preventing disease* (pp. 44–58). Princeton, NJ: Van Nostrand–Reinhold.

Oster, G., & Epstein, A. M. (1986). Primary prevention and coronary heart disease: The economic benefits of lowering serum cholesterol. *American Journal of Public Health, 76,* 647–656.

Paffenbarger, R. S., Hyde, R. T., Wing, A. L., & Hsieh, C.-C. (1986). Physical activity, all-cause mortality, and longevity of college alumni. *New England Journal of Medicine, 314,* 605–613.

Pilisuk, M., Chandler, S., & D'Onofrio, C. (1982–83). Reweaving the social fabric: Antecedents of social support facilitation. *International Quarterly of Community Health Education, 3,* 45–66.

Pill, R., & Stott, N. C. H. (1987). Development of a measure of potential health behavior: A salience of lifestyle. *Social Science and Medicine, 24,* 125–134.

Pratt, L. (1976). Child rearing methods and children's health behavior. *Journal of Health and Social Behavior, 14,* 61–69.

Roberts, M. C., Maddux, J. E., & Wright, L. (1984). Developmental perspectives in behavioral health. In J. D. Matarazzo, S. M. Weiss, J. A. Herd, N. E. Miller, & S. M. Weiss (Eds.), *Behavioral health: A handbook of health enhancement and disease prevention* (pp. 56–68). New York: Wiley.

Schenck, A. P., Runyan, C. W., & Earp, J. L. (1985). Seat belt use laws: The influence of data on public opinion. *Health Education Quarterly, 12,* 365–377.

Schulz, R., & Rau, M. T. (1985). Social support through the life course. In S. Cohen & S. L. Syme (Eds.), *Social support and health* (pp. 129–149). New York: Academic Press.

Severson, H., Fallen, C., Nautel, C., Biglon, A., Ary, D., & Lichtenstein, E. (1981). Oregon Research Institute's smoking prevention program: Helping students resist peer pressure. *Oregon School Study Council Bulletin, 25,* 1–39.

Sime, W. E. (1984). Psychological benefits of exercise training in the healthy individual. In J. D. Matarazzo, S. M. Weiss, J. A. Herd, N. E. Miller, & S. M. Weiss (Eds.), *Behavioral health: A handbook of health enhancement and disease prevention* (pp. 488–508). New York: Wiley.

Suchman, E. (1965). Social patterns of illness and medical care. *Journal of Health and Human Behavior, 6,* 2–16.

The Surgeon General's Report on Health Promotion and Disease Prevention. (1979). *Healthy people* (DHEW(PHS) Publication No. 79-55071). Washington, DC: U.S. Government Printing Office.

U.S. Department of Health and Human Services. (1979). *Better health for our children: A national strategy, Vol. 1* (DHHS(PHS) Publication No. 79-55071). Washington, DC: U.S. Government Printing Office.

Warner, K. E. (1985). Tobacco industry response to public health concern: A content analysis of cigarette ads. *Health Education Quarterly, 12,* 115–127.

World Health Organization Office for Europe, (1986). Regional Office for Health Education, Copenhagen, Denmark. *Social Science and Medicine, 22,* 117–124.

CHAPTER 5

Pathways to Health Behavior

Patricia J. Bush and Ronald J. Iannotti

INTRODUCTION

As an analytic technique, *path analysis* is fortuitously named. Compared to others, e.g., LISREL, logit, probit, or discrimination, *path analysis* provides intuitive insight into its purpose and procedure, and on a level that nonstatisticians can readily appreciate. The word *path* suggests starting at one point and proceeding in one direction to another. It is only necessary to add the idea of causation, that having been caused to arrive at one point in the path, there is a nonzero probability of proceeding forward to another, to grasp the essence of path analysis. When the end point of the path is a health behavior and one wishes to test a theory about why that health behavior varies in a population, i.e., why some do it and some do not, or why some do it more often than others, the causal pathway is an attractive concept. Path analysis provides a mathematical way, through a series of equations, to test a hypothesized chain of events or conditions.

Suppose, for example, that one wishes to account for, as many health researchers have (e.g., Wan & Soifer, 1974; Berki & Kobashigawa, 1976; Markides, Levin, & Ray, 1985; Wolinsky, 1978), the number of times individuals in a defined population visited a physician in a 12-month period, and one has some theories about individual or system level characteristics that might explain variations in visit rates. The path approach is to specify these characteristics as variables, to categorize them, and to hypothesize a model in which the categories are arranged in a logical order of precedence, one in which the value of at least one variable in the first category is hypothesized to influence (account for, explain, cause, determine) the value of at least one variable in the second category, and so on from the second category to the third, until the dependent or terminal variable, the number of physician visits, is reached. The isomorphic mathematical representation that results is only as useful as the implicit theoretical sequence on which it rests. The researcher is responsible for making the schematic representation, hypothesizing, for example, that income level has a causal influence on illness level which in turn influences physician visits, and not the other way around (see Figure 1). The mathematical representation can reveal how much of the variation in physician visits is accounted for directly by income level and indirectly by income level through illness, and how much is accounted

PATRICIA J. BUSH and RONALD J. IANNOTTI • Laboratory for Children's Health Promotion, Department of Community and Family Medicine, Georgetown University School of Medicine, Washington, D.C. 20007.

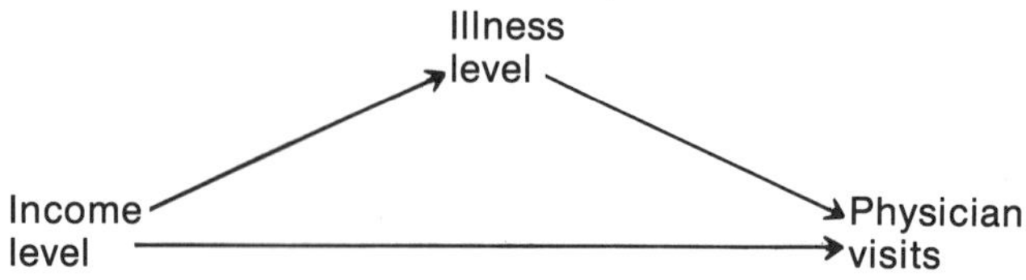

FIGURE 1. Three-variable path scheme.

for directly by illness level. The model reflects the complexity of the real world in comparison with simple correlations which neither imply causation nor allow for more than two variables at a time. Caution is necessary. While a causal relationship is inferred, the statistical basis for the relationship is covariance or correlation and the real cause of the covariance or correlation may not correspond with that which is hypothesized.

Path modeling has found a ready acceptance among those who recognize that health behaviors do not have single causes, but are the product of chains of predisposing influences. In the common vernacular, "One thing leads to another." Table 1 lists the health behaviors that have been the end points in path models, the final "thing" that the others lead to. As can be seen, health care services dominate the literature. In addition to the five attempts to predict physician visits, path analyses have been performed to predict hospital visits and days of hospitalization, dentist visits, use of home care services, and use of medicines, both prescribed and over-the-counter. Path analysis also has been applied to predict use of abusable substances, compliance with physician directives, satisfaction with health care services, and, recently, intentions to perform health behaviors. In addition to explaining the cause of a specified health behavior in a population, path analysis has been used to compare theoretical models in population subgroups (Markides *et al.,* 1985; Ritter & Taylor, 1980), longitudinally to predict behavior from one point in time to another (Kaplan, Martin, & Robbins, 1984) and to compare different theoretical models (Bush, Iannotti, Davidson, & Schneider, 1985).

The remainder of this chapter contains discussions of the advantages and disadvantages of using path analysis compared with other methods, comments on the success of path analysis in explaining health behavior, examples of the application of path analysis, and some suggestions for applications of path analysis in health behavior. Unless otherwise specified, health behavior refers to behaviors such as those listed in Table 1.

ADVANTAGES OF PATH ANALYSIS

The primary advantage of path analysis is that it permits testing hypothesized multivariate linear causal models. Other advantages are that it provides a breakdown of the covariance between variables into direct, indirect, and spurious or joint effects, an explanation of intervening variables as well as the terminal variable, and a parsimonious diagram of causal links with coefficients that indicate the association between determined and determining variables.

As discussed by Duncan (1966), Wright's application of path analysis to population genetics in a series of articles dating from 1918 was one of its earliest uses; Wright, however, used path coefficients to generate theoretical correlations. In subsequent work in which paths accounting for observed correlations among variables were estimated, Wright linked heredity and environment to intelligence, and in an econometric model, prices to farm production. Until the early 1970s, much of the interest in path analysis was theoretical

TABLE 1. Examples of Path Analysis in Health Behavior Research

Dependent variable	R^2 (%)	N^a	Study	Year
Health services use				
Physician visits (12 months)	18	2,168[C]	Wan & Soifer	1974
	09	10,000[N]	Berki & Kobashigawa	1976
	22	7,655[N]	Andersen & Aday	1978
	09–12	≥120,493[N]	Wolinsky	1978
	07–22	1,125[C]	Markides *et al.*	1985
Hospital days (12 months)	08–10	≥120,493[N]	Wolinsky	1978
Hospital/clinics use (12 months)	03–05	2,076[S]	Ritter & Taylor	1980
Dentist visits (12 months)	04–05	≥120,493[N]	Wolinsky	1978
Home care services (current)	77	524[S]	McAuley & Arling	1984
Satisfaction with hospitals/ clinics	8–12	2,076[S]	Ritter & Taylor	1980
Medicine use				
Prescribed (2 days)	29	2,378[C]	Bush & Osterweis	1978
	28	300[C]	Sharpe *et al.*	1985
OTC (2 days)	06	2,378[C]	Bush & Osterweis	1978
Psychotropics (12 months)	09	28,064[N]	Cafferata & Meyers	1985
Abusable substance use				
Marijuana (2 years)	25–36	445[N]	Ritter	1985
Marijuana (1 month/1 year)	09	3,052[C]	Kaplan *et al.*	1994
Cocaine (2 years)	35–42	445[N]	Ritter	1985
Alcohol (1 week)	07	3,052[C]	Kaplan *et al.*	1984
Other illicit (1 year)	24	3,052[C]	Kaplan *et al.*	1984
Compliance				
Weight change (2 weeks)	22–49	164[c]	Becker *et al.*	1977
Appointment keeping (12 months)	17	164[c]	Becker *et al.*	1977
Behavioral expectations				
Medicines	71	300[C]	Bush *et al.*	1985
	42	270[C]	Bush	1986
Marijuana	52–54	445[N]	Ritter	1985
Cocaine	53–54	445[N]	Ritter	1985

[a] Sampling frame: C = city/county; S = state; c = clinic; N = national (Wolinsky's study analyzes data from three separate years with *N*s of 120,493; 132,891; 134,502).

(e.g., Blalock, 1964). In 1968, Andersen explained the use of health services as a result of a three-stage sequence of predisposing, enabling, and need components. He hypothesized that some persons have a propensity to use more health services than others, which can be predicted by personal characteristics, i.e., predisposing factors existing prior to the onset of perceived need. However, having a greater propensity to use health services, he argued, is insufficient to account for greater use. Some means to attain the service and the perception that the service is available must also be present for the health service to be used. If both the predisposing and enabling conditions are met, then potential users of a health service must perceive illness or the need to prevent illness for use of a health service to ensue.

In subsequent years, a number of variations on the theoretical framework were offered for understanding health services use (e.g., Andersen & Aday, 1978; Wan & Soifer, 1974;

Bush & Osterweis, 1978). All of these, however, were based on Andersen's 1968 model, which assumes that use depends on: first, the predisposition of an individual as measured by demographic and social characteristics; next, the ability of the individual to obtain services, which depends on the individual's personal resources and the availability of resources in the community; and last, need, as determined by the individual's self-perception and/or the opinion of health professionals. In other words, predisposing factors lead to enabling factors which lead to need factors which lead to health services use. Prior to conceptualization of these models, health services use was viewed as a rather simple matter of supply and demand which derived from illness.

The development of the health belief model (HBM), conceived by Rosenstock and others (e.g., Rosenstock, 1966), paralleled the development of Andersen's health services utilization model (HSUM). Because the HBM is considered at length elsewhere in this volume, it is discussed only briefly here. The HBM, similar to the HSUM, is a linear causal model, thus making it equally attractive for the application of path analysis. The HBM differs from the HSUM in that, in its conception, it focused on individual characteristics that lead to preventive health behaviors including the following major "readiness to take action" elements: (1) the level of threat posed by the health problem as determined by an individual's perceived susceptibility to and severity of the health problem; (2) an individual's perception of benefit to be derived from engaging in a behavior to reduce the threat, weighed against (3) the perception of barriers (psychological, physical, social, economic) to performing the behavior; and (4) some type of external or internal trigger or cue to take action. Demographic and psychosocial factors were viewed as capable of modifying these relationships, but not of directly affecting preventive health behavior.

In recent years, as the HBM has been explored for its application to sick-role behavior, the distinction between the HSUM and the HBM has become blurred; the HSUM's predisposing, enabling, need, and use categories share variables with the HBM's modifying, readiness, and use categories. The HSUM's primary distinction is its emphasis on system level characteristics. Both are, however, suitable for path analysis, and dominate the health behavior literature. Only recently have different models suitable for path analysis begun to emerge, particularly longitudinal models emphasizing abusable substance use (Kaplan *et al.*, 1984; Ritter, 1985).

We have seen the advantage of path analysis over simply determining the covariance between a dependent and an independent variable. Path analysis provides a breakdown of the covariance into direct and indirect effects, producing a pattern of causal relations which can then be examined for its fit with a hypothesized model. In multivariate analysis to predict a health behavior, path analysis adds nothing statistically over simple regression expressed as a single equation. Therefore, if the researcher is interested only in predicting the dependent variable, there is no advantage over a simple regression equation. If the researcher has a unidirectional (recursive) model identifying the complex chain of relationships that lead to behavioral events, and is seeking a technique that is easy to interpret, then path analysis is advantageous. As a pattern based on a hypothesized causal model such as the HBM or the HSUM, path analysis makes "explicit the rationale for a set of regression calculations" (Duncan, 1966). Thus, in one diagram, path analysis explains not only the direct and indirect "causes" of a health behavior, but the direct and indirect "causes" of each intervening variable between the terminal variable and the most distal set of variables in the model. The path diagram, with its path coefficients for those links which are determined significant in the regression equations, is a parsimonious way to judge the fit of an entire model.

Path analysis cannot explain more of the variation in a health behavior than can regression analysis, nor increase the correlation between variables. In practice, there will always be unexplained variance in the system. In the Path model, exogenous variables are de-

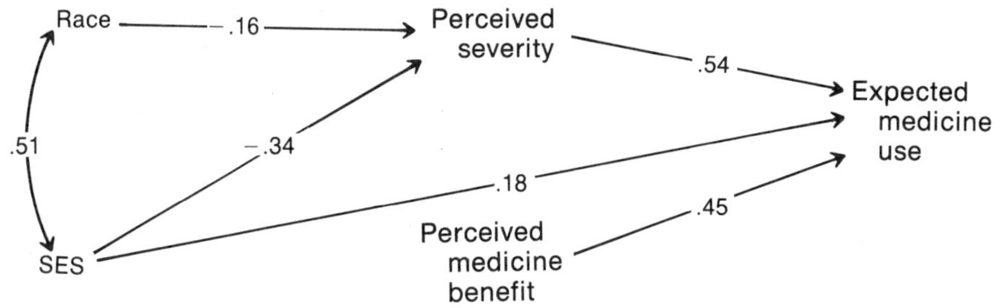

FIGURE 2. A three-stage path diagram predicting expected medicine use by children.

termined by causes outside of the hypothesized system. Endogenous variables are determined by the linear combination of the exogenous variables and other endogenous variables in the model. Residuals reflect variations in the system variables that are not explained by other variables. Residuals are assumed to be uncorrelated with each other and to be uncorrelated with immediately preceding determining variables. The total effect of one variable on another is the zero-order correlation coefficient between two variables. Path analysis decomposes this correlation into the direct effect (the path coefficient), the indirect effect, which is the effect of the exogenous or endogenous variable through one or more intervening variables in the system, and a noncausal component. The noncausal component is: (1) the joint effect of two or more exogenous variables which are correlated, e.g., Race and SES in Figure 2; or (2) the spurious effect which exists when the correlation between endogenous variables is the result of both having a common cause; for example, in Figure 2, Perceived Severity has a spurious effect on Expected Medicine Use because both are caused by SES.

The path coefficient (direct effect) linking a determining to a determined variable may be conveniently expressed in its standardized form (beta weight). The beta weight estimates the amount in standard deviation units of the determined variable that is associated with one standard deviation in the determining variable after controlling for the other determining variables, i.e., $p_{ij} = c_{ij}\, s_j/s_i$, where p_{ij} is the standard path coefficient, c_{ij} is the unstandardized path coefficient, s_j is the standard error of the determining variable, and s_i is the standard error of the determined variable.

The path coefficients or beta weights are placed along the paths in the diagram, thus presenting an immediate visual representation of the strengths of the significant causal paths. Those variables which have not reached the significance level or attained a minimal value for a path coefficient set *a priori* by the researcher are not included in the diagram. For large samples (several thousand), the significance level is frequently set at .01 or the beta weight required to be at least .10.

For the following discussion, refer to Figure 2 and Table 2, which illustrate a subset of the path model developed by Bush *et al.* (1985) to predict expected medicine use in children. The complete model is described later in this chapter.

In Figure 2, a straight line arrow represents causal covariation and the numbers on the arrows are beta weights. Unanalyzed covariation may exist between variables in the same column, e.g., between Perceived Severity and Perceived Medicine Benefit, but to preserve clarity in the diagram, only those in the most distal (first stage) column customarily are shown, e.g., between SES and Race. Relationships among variables in the same column are specified as nonexistent or flow in either direction. The system is, however, entirely recursive—no feedback or reverse arrows are permitted. There is an implied residual term ($\sqrt{1 - R^2}$) for each variable; the residuals are often not included in the diagram but, as in Figure 2, implied.

TABLE 2. Decomposition of Effects in Hypothesized Three-Stage Path Diagram Predicting Children's Expected Medicine Use

Dependent variable Independent variable	Covariance	Causal effects: Direct	Indirect	Total	Spurious or joint effects
Expected medicine use					
Perceived severity	66	54	—	54	12
Perceived medicine benefit	67	45	—	45	22
SES	−07	18	−18	0	−07
Perceived severity					
SES	−42	−34	—	−34	−08
Race	−33	−16	—	−16	−17

As illustrated in Figure 2, Expected Medicine Use was regressed on the independent variables and Perceived Severity and Perceived Medicine Benefit were each regressed on variables SES and Race. The regressions, usually ordinary least squares (OLS), determined that three variables (SES, Perceived Severity, and Perceived Medicine Benefit) had significant direct effects on Expected Medicine Use, i.e., explained a significant amount of the variance (R^2) of Expected Medicine Use. The beta weights (standardized path coefficients) are also shown as direct causal effects in Table 2. SES has an indirect effect on Expected Medicine Use through Perceived Severity as well as a direct effect. The amount of the indirect effect is attained by multiplying the beta weights along the paths. This indirect effect (−.18) is added to the direct effect (.18) to form the total effect (.00) of SES on Expected Medicine Use. This illustrates that, while the correlation between two variables is insignificant, there may indeed be significant paths between them. In this case, SES is not significantly correlated with Expected Medicine Use but there are significant paths between them: SES has a direct effect on Expected Medicine Use and an indirect effect through Perceived Severity. Although there is also an indirect effect of Race on Expected Medicine Use through Perceived Severity, this is not shown in Table 2. Also indicated in this analysis, neither Race nor SES have significant paths to Perceived Medicine Benefit, but both help explain the variance in Perceived Severity. The curved arrow between SES and Race simply indicates that these variables are significantly correlated with each other. Of course, other variables may have been in the original model at stage one or two, which do not appear in the path diagram or the table because they did not reach significance in any of the regression equations. Also, there are implied residuals to account for the variance unexplained in Perceived Severity, Perceived Medicine Benefit, and Expected Medicine Use by the set of three recursive regression equations.

As shown in Table 2, after the direct and indirect effects (if any) are summed, they are subtracted from the covariance (zero-order product moment correlations) to obtain the spurious or joint effects. To assist with the interpretation of diagrams and tables, a correlation matrix is usually shown as well. The explained variances may be shown on the diagram or included in the table. If there are many indirect paths, an additional table can reveal the most important complex relationships. Note that, unless the path coefficients are large, the multiplication along a pathway results in small indirect effects.

It is often the case that more variance in an intervening (midstage) variable is explained than in the dependent variable. It is this ability of path analysis to show the causes of the variation in intervening variables that makes it an especially attractive and unique approach for theoreticians.

DISADVANTAGES OF PATH ANALYSIS

The disadvantages of path analysis are associated with uncertainties in the formulation of the model, recursiveness of the equations, assumptions which are implicit in the statistical technique, and data interpretation.

The sequence, the causal path, the stages, are entirely specified in the mind (theory?) of the researcher. Nothing in the analytic technique will indicate, for example, that the order is wrong; that, for example, the variables in Figure 1 should be reversed so that a better causal path than "income affects physician visits directly and indirectly through illness" is one in which "physician visits affect illness via income." Once the order of elements in the model has been specified through some process of explicating deductive theory, that's it. The regression equations are run recursively, even though there may be plausible alternatives. For example, Bush and Osterweis (1978), using the HSUM to account for medicine use, hypothesized two "need" variables, perceived morbidity and anxiety; the researchers were not willing to say that one of these was more likely to "cause" the other than the reverse. Predisposing and enabling elements were both hypothesized to precede, to "cause," perceived morbidity and anxiety and these in turn to lead to medicine use. Sharpe, Smith, and Barbre (1985) used a similar model to predict prescribed medicine use, but hypothesized anxiety to be a predisposing variable along with various sociodemographic variables. The covariance between anxiety and perceived morbidity in both models was significant and positive. However, in the Sharpe *et al.* representation, anxiety has both a direct and an indirect effect on prescribed medicine use through four other variables (including perceived morbidity) which accounted for the total covariance between anxiety and prescribed medicine use. In the Bush–Osterweis model there was, of course, no possibility of indirect effects, and only part of the covariance between anxiety and prescribed medicine use is accounted for. Also the Bush–Osterweis model, in contrast to that of Sharpe *et al.,* allows for an explanation of the sources of anxiety. Because it lies in the most distal level of the Sharpe *et al.* model, there are no variables hypothesized to precede anxiety.

You may well ask which of these models is correct, the Bush–Osterweis or the Sharpe *et al.* representation. There is no right answer. Indeed, one might pose an alternative case that perceived morbidity causes anxiety. The hypothesized model depends entirely on the researcher. The statistical techniques will not, cannot, select the model. It is on the basis of theory alone that the sequence of variables in a model is judged correct.

Changing the order of the determining variables does not affect the amount of variance explained in the path, but may change the amount of variance explained in an intervening variable. For example, Bush *et al.* (1985) tested a configuration based on the HBM in which a behavioral intention, Expected Medicine Use, was the terminal variable, and Expected Physician Visits was conceived as a measure of perceived severity of illness at the preceding readiness stage, which also included other readiness variables, e.g., Perceived Vulnerability to Illness and Perceived Benefit of Medicines. The overall variance explained in Expected Medicine Use was 71%, and in expected Physician Use (Perceived Severity), 38%. An argument could be made that Expected Physician Visits should be conceived as a terminal variable itself, or as an intervening stage between readiness variables and Expected Medicine Use. If the model is hypothesized in the latter fashion, the variance explained in Expected Medicine Use remains at 71%, but with the readiness variables included in the regression equation to predict Expected Physician Visits, the variance explained in expected physician visits increases from 38% to 56%.

The statistical technique can only support a model which is entirely recursive, i.e., there is no feedback or reciprocal causation. The researcher is prohibited from posing a case in which, for example, anxiety influences perceived morbidity which feeds back to influence anxiety, even though this is a rational interpretation.

Despite its attractiveness, path analysis is not necessarily the path of least resistance. Given the assumption about the nature of the data, assumptions that are frequently very difficult to meet in the social sciences, it is difficult to judge how far one can stray from the straight and narrow without producing a meaningless maze.

It is assumed that relationships between variables are linear, additive, and, of course, causal. Each endogenous variable is to be measured without error on an interval scale and to be normally distributed. The residual (if any) of a variable is assumed to be uncorrelated with any other residual and with any variable immediately preceding the variable under consideration, and to have a mean of zero (Land, 1969). In general, the assumptions are the same as for least squares regression and pose the same problems because social science variables frequently do not meet the assumptions (Pedhazur, 1982). Social science variables are often measured on nominal and ordinal scales and they are often skewed. Consequently, assumptions are at risk of being violated. The challenge for the researcher is to get some sense of how much damage can be done by relaxing certain restrictions, and to find some support for these relaxations. One such support is Boyle (1970) who stated that treating an ordinal level scale like an interval one has little consequence for the results. Dichotomous nominal variables such as gender abound in health behavior research and are treated like interval data when they are determining variables, but with great caution when they are the terminal variable.

An additional problem that occurs in path analysis is the potential for excessive collinearity or multicollinearity which occurs when two or more of the independent variables are highly correlated with each other. There are a variety of methods available for assessing collinearity and multicollinearity (Pedhazur, 1982). Collinearity is of great concern when the correlation between two variables exceeds .80 in the same category of characteristics, and multicollinearity is highly problematic when the multiple correlation coefficient of a determining variable regressed on the other determining variables exceeds .80 (Farrar & Glauber, 1967). If collinearity or multicollinearity is high, the model may be underestimated, meaning that the coefficients of some variables will be unreliable or, if extreme, indeterminate. For example, if two variables such as income and education are highly correlated, their beta weights will be lower than each would be if only one were in the model.

Knowing that one or more assumptions have been violated does not mean that the problems are easily repaired, or that it is easy to judge the magnitude of distortion that can result. There are various tests that can be performed to search for violations of the assumptions of normal distributions of the variables, linearity, and lack of collinearity and multicollinearity. For variables measured on noninterval scales, dummy variables can be constructed for nominally scaled variables and ordinal scales may be treated like interval scales.

A visual examination of the variables will reveal those that have standard deviations larger than their means, and tests for kurtosis and skewness can be run. The use of non-normally distributed variables in the regression analysis will have conservative effects on the size of the estimated variance. Scattergrams of each independent variable with each dependent variable can be constructed to check for nonlinearity and various transforms of the independent variables performed until linear relationships are observed. Two methods of dealing with multicollinearity include selection of only one of the offending variables or using factor weights from a principal component factor analysis to create a new variable. Each of these solutions has attendant problems, so caution is necessary (Pedhazur, 1982).

A dichotomous variable is frequently the object of path analysis to predict a health behavior. With large samples, and the variable skewed no more than 15% toward one of the values, OLS regression is permissible. For large samples, OLS estimates are strongly correlated with logistic estimates, and the path coefficients and explained variance produced by OLS regressions are easier to interpret (Hanushek & Jackson, 1977).

The nature of OLS regression is to select the variable that explains the most variance in the dependent variable after controlling for the other variables that are in the model. If two correlated variables are significantly correlated with the dependent variable in bivariate analysis it is common to find that only one of the two variables appears in the model (see the earlier discussion of multicollinearity). When this happens, there is a tendency for the researcher to assume that the variables which drop out have no relationship to the dependent variable. The discussion tends to focus on the paths and path coefficients that result from the regression. This is unfortunate. The information revealed in the correlation matrix should be considered in association with the resultant path model. For example, in Bush's (1986) test of a hypothesized model to predict adult expected medicine use, the covariances between this end-point variable and four readiness variables were with X_5, .59, with X_2, .35, with X_1, .28, and with X_4, .26. The regression analysis selected three of these and dropped X_1. An examination of the correlation matrix revealed that X_1 was highly correlated with X_4 ($r = .78$), which probably accounted for the failure of X_1 to be included. If X_4 had not been available for inclusion or had not been hypothesized to be included, then it is likely that X_1 would have been selected. Conversely, relationships that have been suppressed and are not observed in bivariate correlations, may be selected by the regression analysis. The point is that the correlation matrix is a vital part of the analytic technique and should be examined in association with the resultant paths.

APPROACHES TO PATH ANALYSIS

Table 1 shows the variety of health behaviors, including behavioral intentions, satisfaction with care, and compliance with physician directives, that have been the object of path analysis and a measure of the success of the techniques in terms of the percentage of overall variance explained in the models. It also shows the size of the sample and an indication of its source—whether it is drawn from a national survey or a defined local population. As can be seen, except for McAuley and Arling's (1984) path analysis to predict the use of in-home care services by the very elderly (75+ years), in which 77% of the variance in use of this service was explained by four variables, the variance explained in the target variable tends to be rather low. No more than 22% of the variance has been explained in physician visits (Andersen & Aday, 1978; Markides *et al.*, 1985). Moreover, illness-morbidity characteristics contribute the greatest proportion of the explained variance in physician visits and to days spent in hospital as well (Wolinsky, 1978) with enabling and predisposing factors contributing relatively little in addition to the need factors.

Even when path analyses do not contribute substantially toward understanding dependent variables, they may offer insights regarding the intervening variables in a model. Wolinsky (1978), observing the small contributions of predisposing and enabling characteristics to explained variances in physician and hospital use measures, questioned their utility and by implication, the utility of HSUM and the use of path analysis to test it, stating ". . . any causal models derived from generic frameworks such as Andersen & Newman's (1973, which is basically of a sociocultural nature), are left unsupported by these data." Why then, one may ask, should path analysis be applied when a simple covariance statistic may serve almost as well to explain variation in health services use? There are, we suggest, several valid reasons, not the least being that we are forced to acknowledge that the model and/or the measurement techniques are not good enough. Second, path analysis provides the opportunity to explain the hypothesized causal "need" factors. For example, although

Wan and Soifer (1974) explained only 17% of the variance in their dependent variable, annual physician visits, by a hypothesized HSUM which included predisposing, enabling, and need-for-care variables, a more impressive 49% of the variance was explained in one of their need-for-care variables, response to illness, by enabling and predisposing variables, including health insurance and education level. Seventeen percent of the variance in another "need" variable, poor health, was explained by five enabling and predisposing variables. If the only goal of the model were to explain physician visits, one must agree with Wolinsky. If, however, the source of variation in need-for-care variables is also of interest, then the path approach offers a clear advantage over simple correlation or regression.

In other applications of the HSUM, e.g., medicine use, the utility of path analysis is more apparent. In two efforts to explain medicine use (Bush and Osterweis, 1978; Sharpe *et al.,* 1985), finding perceived morbidity to be the strongest predictor was not very interesting. Of greater interest is that anxiety was a significant predictor in both studies, and that the overall R^2 was remarkably similar (.29 and .28), despite a recall period of 2 days versus 2 weeks, data collection more than a decade apart, and very different populations (age 15–65 years versus 60+ years; Baltimore, Maryland versus Tupelo County, Mississippi). In the Sharpe *et al.* study, neither physician visits, sex, nor race had significant direct effects on prescribed medicine use as they did in the Bush–Osterweis study, suggesting that these variables are not as important in the elderly as in younger persons. An argument can be made that an important utility of path analysis is not only to provide insight into the source of intervening model variables, but to provide a means to compare the same models in different populations or population subgroups and at different times.

As seen in Table 1, path analysis has been more successful (explained more variance) when predicting behavioral intentions, i.e., medicine use intentions (Bush *et al.,* 1985; Bush, 1986) and abusable substance use intentions (Ritter, 1985) rather than actual use of medicines and abusable substances. In one of these efforts (Ritter, 1985), intentions to use abusable substances at one time have been used to predict use at a future time. These applications will be examined in greater detail in the following sections each of which contains an example of a different way in which path analysis has been applied to explain health behavior: path analysis to compare models among population subgroups, hierarchical path analysis, path analysis in longitudinal studies, and path analysis to compare models in the same and different populations.

Path Analysis to Compare Models among Subgroups

Markides *et al.* (1985) used Andersen's HSUM to compare the determinants of physician use among three generations of Mexican-Americans. The oldest generation was aged 65–80 years; the average age of their children was 49 years, and of their grandchildren, 26 years. The greatest amount of variance in the dependent variable, annual physician visits, was explained in the middle generation (R^2 = .22) and the least in the youngest generation (R^2 = .07). In the oldest generation (R^2 = .14), only two hypothesized "need" variables, physical symptoms and self-rated health, had significant direct effects on physician visits; in the youngest generation, only the predisposing variable, gender, had a positive direct effect, whereas in the middle generation, direct paths to physician visits were drawn from three "need-for-care" variables: physical symptoms, self-rated health, and worry-over-health. In the oldest and middle generations, a predisposing variable, chronic disease, had an indirect effect through physical symptoms and self-rated health.

As a final step in their analysis, Markides *et al.* added three variables measuring acculturation (language use, ethnicity of friends, traditional Mexican values) to all the equations for each age group and found no significant direct effects on physician visits for any of the acculturation variables. There was limited evidence to support a theory of acculturation affecting physician use indirectly through need variables. In the middle generation only, greater acculturation tended to decrease worry over health and thus to decrease physician visits, and having more traditional values tended to lower self-ratings of health which increased physician visits.

In none of the generations was a large proportion of the variation in physician visits explained. Nevertheless, the three-generation approach shows that influences on health behaviors can be different in population subgroups, as documented by differences in the total amount of variance explained in the dependent variable, and differences in the beta weights of the variables, even though the analysis cannot reveal whether the differences are related to age or are the result of social change. The models have gone beyond the classic HSUM to include components that have been hypothesized to account for differences in health services use among Mexican-Americans.

Hierarchical Path Analysis

In hierarchical path analysis, variables are added in groups sequentially to test the additional explanatory value of a block of variables such as the HSUM's "enabling" or "need" categories in a hypothesized model. Hierarchical path analysis, which assesses effects of an entire category of variables on subsequent variables, usually supplements traditional path analysis, which assesses the effects of each variable on subsequent variables.

An example of the application of hierarchical path analysis can be found in a study by Wolinsky (1978). Health Interview Survey data were used in a series of eight path analyses for each year, 1971 to 1973, to evaluate the HSUM's ability to account for the number of hospital days in 2 weeks and 12 months, total hospital episodes, dental visits in 2 weeks and 12 months, interval between dental visits, physician visits in 12 months, and interval between physician visits. In addition to assessing the effects of each hypothesized independent variable on the use variables in each of the three years, the categories of variables were evaluated as blocks, with the illness-morbidity (need) block as most proximal, the enabling block as next, and the predisposing block as most distal, in order to identify the additional variance explained by each block.

The amount of variance in the use variables explained by either approach is of course the same, and as shown by the three examples in Table 1, not very impressive. For 12-month dentist visits, only higher levels of education and income were associated with more visits and a shorter interval between visits. For hospital days in 12 months, the pattern shows that the more bed disability and restricted activity days in 2 weeks, the more chronic conditions and the fewer total conditions, the greater the probability of using hospital services. More frequent users of physician services tended to be younger, to perceive their health to be poorer, to have more days of limited activity, to have more total but fewer chronic conditions, to be married and to have smaller families than persons who use physician services less frequently. Comparing results suggests that chronic conditions are likely to lead to hospitalizations, and other conditions are likely to lead to physician visits.

In the hierarchical analysis by blocks, the illness-morbidity variables contributed the most to the small amounts of explained variance in hospital and physician use, raising questions about the utility of enabling and predisposing variables in the HSUM. However, in contrast, to predict dentist use, most of the explained variance was contributed by enabling and predisposing characteristics rather than "need" factors.

Although in Wolinsky's study, little of the variance was explained in any of the use variables (which may reflect variable measurement rather than a problem with the model), the hierarchical technique is an attractive one for comparing the efficiency of models in explaining variations in different health behavior variables, and provides insight into different processes associated with different health behaviors.

Path Analysis in Longitudinal Studies

Considering that path analysis offers the opportunity to test a model consisting of causal stages, it is surprising that greater use has not been made of it in longitudinal studies to evaluate whether characteristics at one time predict characteristics at a later time. It is less surprising that when path analysis has been used in longitudinal studies, it has been used most often to predict use of abusable substances (Kaplan *et al.,* 1984; Ritter, 1985), or intentions to use abusable substances (Ritter, 1985). There has, after all, been much more interest in identifying the *early* predictors of abusable substances than in identifying the *early* predictors of other health behaviors.

Kaplan *et al.* (1984) used path analysis in an innovative way to predict abusable substance use in terms of four explanatory perspectives: self-derogation, peer influence, social control, and early substance use. In brief, a theory integrating these constructs suggests that early self-devaluing experiences in membership groups leads to self-derogation which, in turn, leads to loss of motivation to conform to group norms and a disposition to adopt deviant behaviors and to associate with others who have adopted deviant behaviors.

Data were gathered in a three-wave panel of junior high students. The researchers posed a six-stage model incorporating 20 variables with the middle four stages (Stages 2 through 5) measured cross-sectionally at Time 2. Illicit drug use at Time 3 (Stage 6) was regressed on 10 variables measured at Time 2 (distributed among Stages 2 to 5) and 9 variables measured at Time 1 (Stage 1). Two of the nine Stage 1 variables represented early use of abusable substances (alcohol and marijuana), and the remainder were related to theories about the relationship of abusable substances use to self-derogation, perceived peer use, and social control relative to peers, family, and school. At Time 2, Stage 2 included three drug use variables (alcohol, marijuana, other illicit); Stage 3 included three social control variables; Stage 4 included two self-derogation variables; and Stage 5 included two perceived peer use variables.

In OLS regression, 7 of the 20 variables in the longitudinal model explained 24% of the variance in illicit drug use at Stage 6. The 7 variables were: alcohol and marijuana use at Stage 1, alcohol, marijuana, and other illicit drug use at Stage 2, self-derogation at Stage 4, and perceived friends' drug use at Stage 5. The significant paths supported a stage theory in which early use of alcohol and marijuana is associated with subsequent use of illicit drugs.

In addition to the OLS regression to predict illicit drug use at Time 3, the four theories supporting the Time 2 stages were evaluated by exploring each of the four theoretical paths separately to determine not only the contribution of an individual characteristic to illicit drug use, but also the sequence of stages associated with the individual characteristic which directly predicted illicit drug use. For example, 30% of the variance in perceived friends' drug use (Stage 5) was explained by five variables: perceived friends' drug use at Stage 1, alcohol and marijuana use at Stage 2, a social control variable at Stage 3, and a self-derogation variable at Stage 4.

As indicated, the four stages at Time 2 represent four predictive constructs: self-derogation, social control, peer influence, and early use. Of these, only the social control variable did not affect illicit drug use directly. All four formed logical indirect causal pathways which supported the theories and revealed complementarity among the constructs. For example, two constructs, peer influence and social control, help explain progression from use of alcohol to use of marijuana to use of other illicit drugs. Each construct initiates a causal chain of influence from Time 1 which complements the others and adds predictive power to the overall model. The research illustrates the value of path analysis in longitudinal research, and the value of testing constructs from complementary theoretical perspectives to build models.

Path Analysis to Compare Models in the Same and Different Populations

A children's health belief model (CHBM) based on the HBM postulated by Rosenstock (1966) was developed by Bush *et al.* (1985) to predict children's expectations of taking medicines for common health problems and tested in a population of 300 children in Grades 3–7. Three goals of the study were: to evaluate the ability of the CHBM to explain children's expectations of medicine use, to learn whether the addition of child-specific characteristics increased the variance explained in children's expectations of medicine use in the hypothesized CHBM, and to examine the influence of the children's primary caretakers as the source of the children's medicine use expectations.

A path sequence was conceived in four stages with sociodemographic characteristics at the first stage leading to other modifying factors (cognitive/affective, enabling, environmental) at the second stage; readiness factors (motivations, perceived threat of illness, perceived benefit of taking medicines, perceived barrier to taking medicines) at Stage 3, and expected medicine use as the terminal variable.

The four-stage CHBM was examined in three steps. In Step 1, a classic paradigm was tested which included variables that have previously been associated with health behaviors in the adult preventive and sick-role models. In Step 2, variables were added which are relevant only to a children's model, i.e., they are either measured differently than they would be in adults, e.g., children's health locus of control, or they are unlikely to be measured in adults at all, e.g., autonomy in medicine use, parental status. In Step 3, caretaker variables were added to test their explanatory power in the CHBM to suggest whether the child's primary caretaker influences the child's expected medicine use and readiness to take medicine factors.

In Step 1, the adult version (the classic HBM paradigm) of the CHBM explained 67% of the variance in children's Expected Medicine Use for five common health problems with two readiness factors (relative to the five health problems), Perceived Severity of Illness and Perceived Benefit of Medicines, predominating. Expected Medicine Use was also directly associated with greater Illness Concern (worry accompanying the five health problems), greater perception of Vulnerability to Illness (five health problems), higher SES, maleness, and fewer Physician Visits. Two demographic variables, Race and Age, had indirect effects.

In Step 2, the addition of the child-specific variables increased the explained variance in Expected Medicine Use by only 2%, to 69%. Although five child-specific variables had significant paths, all but one were indirect.

In Step 3, variables based on data obtained from the children's caretakers were added to those significant variables remaining in the CHBM after Step 2. These were hypothesized as modifying variables. They are parallel to the CHBM's readiness and use variables but were derived from questions asked of the caretaker on behalf of the child. The model suggested, for example, that a mother's illness concern for her child would be reflected in her child's own illness concern and in turn affect the child's Expected Medicine Use.

The addition of the caretakers' variables increased the explained variance in the CHBM only 2% to 71%, with Caretaker's Expected Child's Medicine Use having a positive direct effect on the child's Expected Medicine Use. However, the explained variance in each of the child's readiness variables was increased substantially, suggesting the importance of caretakers in the development of their children's health beliefs.

In a separate analysis, the classic (adult HBM) model was applied to the children's primary caretakers (93% mothers), to predict the caretakers' expected use of medicines. The children's and caretakers' models were then compared. The adult version was applied to predict Caretaker's Expected Medicine Use for the five common health problems and 42% of the variance was explained by three readiness variables, perceived vulnerability, perceived severity of illness, and perceived benefit of medicines, all three relative to the five health problems. Although the caretakers' model did not explain as much variance in Expected Medicine Use as the children's, there were more similarities in the models than differences. Of 15 variables which were measured the same way or were intended to represent the same construct, two-thirds appeared in both models. Developmental differences were suggested by different strengths of predictor variables. For example, Perceived Vulnerability to Illness was a better predictor in the caretakers' model whereas Perceived Severity was stronger in the children's model. Cognitive/affective and demographic variables played similar roles in both models but health status measures were stronger in the caretakers' model.

The use of path analysis to evaluate different representations of the CHBM suggested that child-specific and environmental variables add little to the prediction of Expected Medicine Use, and that the classic adult model represents children as well as adults. However, if the goal is to explain the origin of children's beliefs (readiness factors), then the addition of child-specific and caretaker variables and perhaps other environmental variables is worthwhile.

SUMMARY

Path analyses have been used successfully to predict use of health services, prescribed medicines, and abusable substances, to predict behavioral expectations regarding medicines and abusable substances, and to predict compliance with treatment. In areas where the prediction of the outcome variable has had limited success, valuable insights have been gained regarding influences on intervening variables of interest such as health attitudes, prior health behaviors, and prior use of medicines and abusable substances that lead to outcome variables. Causal paths toward intermediate variables are most evident in the work of Bush *et al.* (1985) and Kaplan *et al.* (1984). The intermediate variables of greatest interest in the HSUM have been "need" factors such as response to illness, physical symptoms, and various assessments of health status (Markides *et al.*, 1985; Wolinsky, 1978). Some applications of the HSUM have identified personality factors such as anxiety and worry over health (Bush & Osterweis, 1978; Markides *et al.*, 1985; Sharpe *et al.*, 1985), but personality factors have been more evident in attempts to explain use and intentions to use medicines and abusable substances (Bush *et al.*, 1985; Bush, 1986; Kaplan *et al.*, 1984). These models suggest the importance of individual characteristics such as health locus of control, risk-taking, autonomy, self-derogation, and social control. Path analyses have shed light on the role of these factors as well as providing some understanding as to their origin. The use of path analysis to identify paths toward intermediate steps could contribute substantially to the conceptualization of better models of the development and maintenance of health behaviors, and further work in this area should be encouraged.

Another promising use of path analysis is with longitudinal data. The temporal sequence of the data lends itself to causal analyses. Paths can be identified cross-sectionally to indicate the relationship between attitudes and behaviors in the same time period. Frequently more interesting, however, are longitudinal causal paths. The work of Kaplan *et al.* (1984) illustrates paths between early use of abusable substances by the subjects and their peers which leads to increased later use of abusable substances. Future studies applying similar models to use of medicines and health services should be encouraged.

Finally, it should be recognized that path analysis is a form of structural equation modeling which is experiencing a rapid growth in popularity. LISREL uses both measurement and structural equation models to address issues of measurement error. If multiple measures of constructs are planned and there are theoretical bases for a path model, structural equation models offer approaches to analysis of causality without the restrictive assumptions characteristic of traditional path analysis (Pedhazur, 1982).

REFERENCES

Andersen, R. (1968). *A behavioral model of families' use of health services* (Research Series No. 25). Chicago: Center for Health Administration Studies.

Andersen, R., & Aday, L. A. (1978). Access to medical care in the U.S.: Realized and potential. *Medical Care, 16,* 533–546.

Andersen, R., & Newman, J. F. (1973). Societal and individual determinants of medical care utilization in the United States. *Milbank Memorial Fund Quarterly, 44,* 94–124.

Becker, M. H., Maiman, L. A., Kirscht, J. P., Haefner, D. P., & Drachman, R. H. (1977). The health belief model and prediction of dietary compliance: A field experiment. *Journal of Health and Social Behavior, 18,* 348–366.

Berki, S. E., & Kobashigawa, B. J. (1976). Socioeconomic and need determinants of ambulatory care use: Path analysis of the 1970 Health Interview data. *Medical Care, 14,* 405–421.

Blalock, H. M. (1964). *Causal inferences in nonexperimental research.* Chapel Hill: University of North Carolina Press.

Boyle, R. P. (1970). Path analysis and ordinal data. *American Journal of Sociology, 75,* 461–480.

Bush, P. J. (1986). *Children, medicines and abusable substances; A longitudinal study.* Final report (R01 DA 02686) submitted to the National Institute on Drug Abuse.

Bush, P. J., Iannotti, R. J., Davidson, F. R., & Schneider, S. (1985). *A children's medicine belief model.* Paper presented at the annual meeting of the American Public Health Association, Washington, DC.

Bush, P. J., & Osterweis, M. (1978). Pathways to medicine use. *Journal of Health and Social Behavior, 19,* 179–189.

Cafferata, G. L., & Meyers, S. M. (1985). *Pathways to psychotropic drugs: Understanding the basis of sex differences.* Paper presented at the meeting of the American Sociology Association, Washington, DC.

Duncan, O. D. (1966). Path analysis: Sociological examples. *American Journal of Sociology, 72,* 1–16.

Farrar, D., & Glauber, R. (1967). Multicollinearity in regression analysis: The problem revisited. *Review of Economics and Statistics, 44,* 92–107.

Hanushek, E. A., & Jackson, J. E. (1977). *Statistical methods for social scientists.* New York: Academic Press.

Kaplan, H. B., Martin, S. S., & Robbins, C. A. (1984). Pathways to adolescent drug use: Self-derogation, peer influence, weakening of social controls, and early substance use. *Journal of Health and Social Behavior, 25,* 270–289.

Land, K. C. (1969). Principles of path analysis. In E. Borgatta (Ed.), *Sociological methodology* (pp. 3–37). San Francisco: Jossey–Bass.

Markides, K. S., Levin, J. S., & Ray, L. A. (1985). Determinants of physician utilization among Mexican-Americans: A three-generations study. *Medical Care, 23,* 236–245.

McAuley, W. J., & Arling, G. (1984). Use of in-home care by very old people. *Journal of Health and Social Behavior, 25,* 54–64.

Pedhazur, E. J. (1982). *Multiple regression in behavioral research.* New York: Holt, Rinehart, & Winston.

Ritter, C. (1985). *Behavioral intentions, marijuana and cocaine use: An assessment of the Fishbein model.* Paper presented at the annual meeting for the Study of Social Problems, Washington, DC.

Ritter, C., & Taylor, G. S. (1980). *Satisfaction with health services among the elderly and non-elderly: A comparison of two path models.* Paper presented at the annual meeting of the Mid-South Sociological Association, Little Rock, AR.

Rosenstock, I. (1966). Why people use health services. *Milbank Memorial Fund Quarterly, 44,* 92–107.

Sharpe, T. R., Smith, M. C., & Barbre, A. R. (1985). Medicine use among the rural elderly. *Journal of Health and Social Behavior, 26,* 113–127.

Wan, T. H., & Soifer, S. J. (1974). Determinants of physician utilization: A causal analysis. *Journal of Health and Social Behavior, 15,* 100–108.

Wolinsky, F. D. (1978). Assessing the effects of predisposing, enabling, and illness-morbidity characteristics on health service utilization. *Journal of Health and Social Behavior, 19,* 384–396.

Family Determinants

The family is presumed to be an important factor in the acquisition and support of health behavior, and presumably a fertile area for health behavior research. Yet relatively few empirical studies have carefully and systematically explored how, and to what degree, the family is a determinant of health behavior. Litman's review (1974) of the social and behavioral science literature on the family as a basic unit in health and medical care discusses studies of family activities and family involvement with illness, care-seeking, and "becoming a patient," but does not reveal the existence of any appreciable body of research on the family as a determinant of health behavior. Other reviews of the literature (e.g., Baranowski & Nader, 1985; Campbell, 1978; Gochman, 1985) repeatedly affirm that little has been done on how family structure, process, or child-rearing practices affect children's overt health behaviors or their beliefs relevant to health and illness. Although there has been considerable research (e.g., Geertsen *et al.*, 1975; Suchman, 1965/1972) on how social integration operates through family values and beliefs to affect health behaviors such as utilization of professional services, family structure and process were not the primary focal points of such studies and were not examined systematically. One exception to this is Umberson's study (1987) demonstrating that specific family relationships such as marriage and parenting act as controls upon, or deterrents to, negative or risk-taking behaviors such as drinking and driving, and substance abuse.

Furthermore, where "familism," i.e., the presumed inclination to rely excessively on the family and to distrust the social world beyond the family, has been studied, its impact on health behaviors is not clear or consistent (e.g., Hoppe & Heller, 1975).

For convenience, research on family determinants can be discussed under three headings: children's health behaviors, adult health behaviors, and the family as a unit.

CHILDREN'S HEALTH BEHAVIORS

Among the few studies of how family factors determine children's health behaviors, Campbell (1975) showed that while mothers and children use the same signs and symptoms as a basis for attributing illness, there is no specific linkage within individual mother–child pairs, i.e., an individual mother's tendency to attribute illness did not predict her child's tendency to attribute illness. Campbell also observed (1978) that maternal valuing of self-direction in children is linked to children being more inclined to communicate to parents that they are sick, whereas maternal valuing of self-assertiveness (in contrast to being attentive to others) reduces this.

Dielman, Leech, Becker, Rosenstock, and Horvath (1982) did not find strong relationships between parental health beliefs and children's health beliefs. Blaxter and Paterson's examination (1982) of three generations of Scottish families—children, mothers, and grandmothers—found that while some of the grandmothers' advice on health-related child care influenced the mothers' behavior, there was less such influence than might have been expected; that contraception patterns between the two older generations were different; and that there was little intergenerational similarity in attitudes toward health and health services. Methodological problems precluded generalizations about family influences on use of health services.

Among the very few systematic studies using large numbers of variables, Bush, Iannotti, and Davidson's (1985) analyses showed that mothers' use of medicines was an important determinant of childrens' autonomous use of medicines.

In a different direction, Carandang, Folkins, Hines, and Steward (1979) presented interesting evidence, within a Piagetian framework, that the stresses associated with the presence of a child with diabetes in a family have a negative effect on their sibling's ability to conceptualize the causes and treatment of illness.

ADULT HEALTH BEHAVIORS

Little work has been done, moreover, on the family as a determinant of adult health beliefs and health behaviors. Nader *et al.* (1982) demonstrated the potential role of adolescents as gatekeepers of health information, which raises important questions about the multidirectionality of the determinants of health behavior within the family.

Horwitz (1978) showed that characteristics of the husband–wife dyadic relationship are related to informal help-seeking behaviors, i.e., use of relatives and friends. Persons whose marital relationships were characterized as conflicted were more likely to engage in active informal help-seeking for emotional problems among relatives and friends, than were those whose marital relationships were supportive and sympathetic.

THE FAMILY AS A UNIT: THE "ENERGIZED" FAMILY

A major obstacle to research lies in the failure to conceptualize the family *qua* family. Often, reports that contain *family* in their title use a characteristic of one of the parents, such as mother's education, as a major variable, but do not consider the family as a total unit. While such studies can have considerable value in broadening understanding of health behavior, they do not shed light on how the family *as a unit* acts as a determinant.

Pratt's seminal work on the "energized" family (1976) has been the most important effort in conceptualizing the family as a social system, and in relating variables derived from this conceptualization to health behavior. Members of Pratt's "energized" family demonstrate regular interaction with one another, maintain contacts with the community to advance their interests, and attempt to cope and to master their lives. Such families show fluidity in internal organization, a sharing of power, flexibility in role relationships, and concern for and support of the growth of family members (Pratt, 1976, pp. 3–4). Pratt provides evidence that "energized" families can promote sound health practices (1976), and that "developmental" child-rearing practices, i.e., those that demonstrate use of reasons, rewards, and the granting of autonomy, are more likely to lead to appropriate health behaviors in children than are methods that are based on punishment and discipline (1973).

Sallis and Nader's chapter reviews the literature on family determinants of behaviors that are related to health risks: smoking, eating, and physical activity. The chapter introduces the methodological concept of "aggregation," which facilitates identifying family influences, and then, more importantly, it presents a much-needed conceptual model, derived from well-established, basic theories of learning, to provide a mechanism for explaining the acquisition and maintenance of these and other health and safety-related behaviors.

REFERENCES

Baranowski, T., & Nader, P. R. (1985). Family health behavior. In D. C. Turk & R. D. Kerns (Eds.), *Health, illness, and families: A life-span perspective*. New York: Wiley.

Blaxter, M., & Paterson, E. (1982). *Mothers and daughters: A three-generational study of health attitudes and behaviour*. London: Heinemann.

Bush, P. J., Iannotti, R. J., & Davidson, F. R. (1985). A longitudinal study of children and medicines. In D. D. Breimer & P. Speiser (Eds.), *Topics in pharmaceutical sciences 1985*. Amsterdam: Elsevier.

Campbell, J. D. (1975). Attribution of illness: Another double standard. *Journal of Health and Social Behavior, 16,* 114–126.

Campbell, J. D. (1978). The child in the sick-role: Contributions of age, sex, parental status, and parental values. *Journal of Health and Social Behavior, 19,* 35–51.

Carandang, M. L. A., Folkins, C. H., Hines, P. A., & Steward, M. S. (1979). The role of cognitive level and sibling illness in children's conceptualization of illness. *American Journal of Orthopsychiatry, 49,* 474–481.

Dielman, T. E., Leech, S. L., Becker, M. H., Rosenstock, I. M., & Horvath, W. J. (1982). Parental and child health beliefs and behavior. In D. S. Gochman & G. S. Parcel (Eds.), Children's health beliefs and health behaviors [Special issue]. *Health Education Quarterly, 9,* 60–77.

Geertsen, R., Klauber, M. R., Rindflesh, M., Kane, R. L., & Gray, R. (1975). A re-examination of Suchman's views on social factors in health care utilization. *Journal of Health and Social Behavior, 16,* 226–237.

Gochman, D. S. (1985). Family determinants of children's concepts of health and illness. In D. C. Turk & R. D. Kerns (Eds.), *Health, illness, and families: A life-span perspective*. New York: Wiley.

Hoppe, S. K., & Heller, P. L. (1975). Alienation, familism and the utilization of health services by Mexican Americans. *Journal of Health and Social Behavior, 16,* 304–314.

Horwitz, A. (1978). Family, kin, and friend networks in psychiatric help-seeking. *Social Science and Medicine, 12,* 297–304.

Litman, T. J. (1974). The family as a basic unit in health and medical care: A social-behavioral overview. *Social Science and Medicine, 8,* 495–519.

Nader, P. R., Perry, C., Maccoby, N., Solomon, D., Killen, J., Telch, M., & Alexander, J. K. (1982). Adolescent perceptions of family health behavior: A tenth grade educational activity to increase family awareness of a community cardiovascular risk reduction program. *Journal of School Health, 52,* 372–377.

Pratt, L. (1973). Child rearing methods and children's health behavior. *Journal of Health and Social Behavior, 14,* 61–69.

Pratt, L. (1976). *Family structure and effective health behavior: The energized family*. Boston: Houghton Mifflin.

Suchman, E. A. (1972). Social patterns of illness and medical care. In E. G. Jaco (Ed.), *Patients, physicians and illness*. New York: Free Press. (Reprinted from *Journal of Health and Human Behavior,* 1965, *6,* 2–16).

Umberson, D. (1987). Family status and health behaviors: Social control as a dimension of social integration. *Journal of Health and Social Behavior, 28,* 306–319.

CHAPTER 6

Family Determinants of Health Behaviors

James F. Sallis and Philip R. Nader

The strong evidence linking behavior and health outcomes has led to the realization that truly healthy people, and truly healthy societies in these times, are distinguished by both a lack of physiological pathology and a pattern of behaviors that reduces one's risk of developing the major chronic diseases (Hamburg, Elliott, & Parron, 1982; Matarazzo, 1982). A small number of behaviors, namely smoking, diet, and exercise, have been shown to be related to the leading causes of morbidity and mortality in industrialized countries. Smoking is a major causative factor in several cancers (Levy, 1985), cardiovascular diseases (USPHS, 1979), and chronic pulmonary diseases (Brashear, 1980). Dietary habits, particularly intake of fats and saturated fats, have been linked to development of cancers (Levy, 1985), cardiovascular diseases (Glueck & Connor, 1978), and diabetes mellitus (Arky, Wylie-Rosett, & El-Beheri, 1982). Physical inactivity appears to play a role in cardiovascular diseases (Paffenbarger & Hyde, 1984) and diabetes mellitus (Rauramaa, 1984).

The observation that these behaviors are related to numerous prevalent diseases suggests that widespread adoption of "salutogenic" behaviors would decrease risk of several diseases. It is well understood that behaviors in adulthood are associated with increased risk of disease, but there is indirect evidence that similar behaviors in children have health consequences. There are relationships between dietary fats and serum cholesterol in children (Glueck *et al.,* 1982) and evidence that dietary therapy reduces cholesterol levels in hypercholesterolemic children (Glueck, Tsang, Fallat, & Mellies, 1977). Physically fit and active children appear to have lower levels of blood pressure (Fraser, Phillips, & Harris, 1983), serum cholesterol (Gilliam & Burke, 1978), and obesity (Bullen, Reed, & Mayer, 1964) than their more sedentary peers. It seems prudent to be concerned with both behavioral and physiological risks in children, because blood pressure and serum lipoproteins in children predict extent of atherosclerotic lesions several years later (Newman *et al.,* 1986). It is expected that children's health habits will be especially subject to family influences.

The purpose of this chapter is to review the role of the family in the development and alteration of health-related smoking, dietary, and exercise behaviors. Though the family is the major social institution in most societies, and its influence on seeking health services has been explored extensively (Crawford, 1971), family determinants of behaviors related to the prevention of major chronic diseases have received limited attention. For clarity,

JAMES F. SALLIS and PHILIP R. NADER • Department of Pediatrics, University of California at San Diego, La Jolla, California 92093.

discussion will be confined to smoking, dietary, and exercise behaviors, with emphasis on their relationships to cardiovascular diseases (CVD). It will be demonstrated that physiological risk is clustered within families, and that there is evidence of both genetic and environmental influences. A conceptual model of family influences on preventive health behaviors will be developed. The empirical data on family determinants of health behavior will be reviewed, and the implications for family-centered health promotion programs will be discussed.

THE CHANGING NATURE OF FAMILIES

The family plays a critical role in the socialization of children, but that role is becoming increasingly difficult to characterize. A report from the Select Committee on Children, Youth, and Families (1983) revealed some important trends. In 1982, 22% of children lived with only one parent and an additional 10% lived with one biological parent and one stepparent. These rates have been increasing dramatically, especially among blacks. Between 1970 and 1982 there was a 68% increase in the number of children living in female-headed households. There have also been large increases in the number of working mothers whose children are in day-care facilities. All of these structural changes would appear to have profound impacts on the influence of the family on health habits of members, but there has been little study related to preventive health issues (Loveland-Cherry, 1986).

These and other changes make it difficult both to define and to discuss "the family." In some parts of the United States, fewer than 50% of children live with both biological parents, so studies of families must consider single-parent families and blended families. In addition, many married couples are childless and other couples with children are not legally married.

The Bureau of the Census defines a "family" broadly as a group of two or more persons residing together and related by birth, marriage, or adoption. A "household" consists of all persons who occupy a housing unit. Even this definition of family would exclude some groupings which others would consider to be a family. Our aim is not to develop "the" definition of family, but to suggest that each investigator must develop explicit criteria for inclusion of families that are consistent with the objectives of the study.

FAMILY AGGREGATION OF CVD RISK FACTORS

The most consistent and dramatic evidence of family influences on CVD is family aggregation of physiological risk factors. "Family aggregation" refers to similarities in health variables among family members that are greater than similarities among nonfamily members. Although aggregation is frequently cited as an indication of genetic family influences, it can also be seen as a rationale for carefully investigating family influences on health risk and for identifying and intervening on high-risk families.

In several studies the parent–child and sibling–sibling correlations of blood pressure are approximately .24 (Feinleib, Garrison, & Havlik, 1980; Patterson, Kaplan, Sallis, & Nader, 1987) and the spouse–spouse correlations tend to be lower but significant (Sackett, 1975; Suarez, Criqui, & Barrett-Connor, 1983). Genetic determination of blood pressure is strong, but does not explain all of the variance (Sackett, 1975; Feinleib *et al.*, 1980).

A similar pattern is found with serum cholesterol and lipoproteins. Spouse–spouse correlations are generally low (Barrett-Connor, Suarez, & Criqui, 1982), but parent–child and sibling–sibling correlations for total cholesterol, HDL, and LDL are usually significant and range from .15 to .40 (Shear, Frerichs, Weinberg, & Berenson, 1978; Karlin *et al.*,

1982). Again, there is some evidence than genetic factors are more important than environmental factors (Greenberg, Green, Roggenkamp, & Barrett-Connor, 1984).

A study of 40,000 people revealed significant family aggregation of obesity (Garn & Clark, 1976). The parent–child correlation for body fat was approximately .25, and children of obese parents were fatter than children of thin parents at all ages. Sibling–sibling correlations were higher; approximately .38. With obesity, there is evidence that genetic factors are less important. For example, in the Garn and Clark study, spouse–spouse correlations of body fat were nearly .25, and this could not be accounted for by genetic relatedness. Similar parent–child body fat correlations with both natural and adopted parents suggest that shared environments are important in determining obesity (Garn, Cole, & Bailey, 1976). Although there is some disagreement among studies, the evidence indicates that physiological risk factors are aggregated within families, but the relative contributions of genetic and environmental influences are not clear. The remainder of this chapter consists of discussions of the environmental family influences on health behavior and risk for CVD.

FAMILY INFLUENCES ON PREVENTIVE HEALTH BEHAVIORS

In this section the empirical literature on family influences on smoking, dietary, and exercise behaviors is reviewed. A representative, rather than exhaustive, review is presented, with an emphasis on synthesizing research findings. Previous reviews provide other perspectives (Baranowski & Nader, 1985; Venters, 1986).

Smoking Behavior

There is a very large literature on determinants of smoking initiation in children, and most reviewers conclude that pressure from peers is the single most important influence (Flay, d'Avernas, Best, Kersell, & Ryan, 1983; Evans & Raines, 1982; NIE, 1979). Family influences are typically the second most important determinant. A national survey determined that about 14% of the children of smoking parents smoke, but only about 6% of the children of nonsmoking parents (NIE, 1979). This general pattern of family aggregation of smoking habits has been observed in many studies (Borland & Rudolph, 1975; Hunter, Baugh, Webber, Sklov, & Berenson, 1982; Biglan & Lichtenstein, 1984). Although most smoking parents do not approve of their children smoking (Evans & Raines, 1982), about 5% of adolescent smokers have their first cigarette with their parents (Biglan, Severson, McConnell, & Baury, 1983).

The influence of siblings who smoke also appears to be strong. In families with nonsmoking parents, approximately 17% of children with older siblings who smoke, do so. In families where neither parents nor older siblings smoke, the rate of smoking is 4% or less (NIE, 1979). The effect of sibling smoking has been observed rather consistently (Speilberger, Jacobs, Crane, & Russell, 1983; Biglan & Lichtenstein, 1984).

There is evidence of concordance in smoking habits among spouses (Venters, Jacobs, Luepker, Maiman, & Gillum, 1984; Sackett, Anderson, Milner, Feinleib, & Kannel, 1975), with one study finding a concordance rate 11% above chance expectations (Venters *et al.*, 1984). There was little evidence that concordance increased with years of marriage (Venters *et al.*, 1984; Sackett *et al.*, 1975), and one study did not find spouse concordance (Kolonel & Lee, 1981). For those smokers desiring to quit, spouse support appears to be helpful (Mermelstein, Cohen, Lichtenstein, Baer, & Kamarck, 1986), and spouses tend to quit smoking in tandem (Venters *et al.*, 1984).

In summary, there is a great deal of evidence that the smoking habits of parents and older siblings influence children, but it may be possible for children to be effective in assisting their parents in quitting (Flay, Hansen, Johnson, & Sobel, 1983). Spouse concordance in smoking may be related to selective marriage, but this effect is enhanced by similar cigarette consumption rates and dates of quitting (Venters *et al.,* 1984).

Risk-Related Dietary Behaviors

Many dietary factors are, or may be, related to chronic diseases, but total calories, fat, and sodium intake will be emphasized in this section. A number of studies have examined the family aggregation of dietary behaviors. Two studies reveal significant spouse concordance in intake of fat, but their results regarding calories and specific food items are discrepant (Eastwood, Brydon, Smith, & Smith, 1982; Lee & Kolonel, 1982). A large study noted similarity between spouses in use of discretionary salt (Venters *et al.,* 1984). Relationships of dietary habit similarities between parents and children have also been examined. Laskarzewski and colleagues (Laskarzewski *et al.,* 1980) found significant correlations ranging from about .15 to .30 for intake of fat and calories. Using urinary sodium and potassium as indicators of intake, two studies found evidence of moderate degrees of parent–child similarity (Connor, Connor, Henry, Sexton, & Keenan, 1984; Staessen *et al.,* 1985).

In a sample of San Diego families (Patterson, Rupp, Sallis, Atkins, & Nader, in press) intrafamily correlations tended to be higher in Mexican-American families than in Anglo families. Intakes of fat, sodium, and calories were significantly correlated between spouses, and in some parent–child pairs. Sibling correlations were significant more often in Mexican-American families.

A number of studies have documented the effects of specific family factors or parent behaviors on childhood eating behaviors, and these are reviewed by Hertzler (1983). Few of these studies specifically studied cardiovascular risk-related dietary habits, but some findings have implications for present purposes. Parental modeling seems to be an important determinant of child food preferences. Children's preferences are related to fathers' preferences (Bryan & Lowenberg, 1958), but there is an even higher similarity (76% agreement) in food dislikes with older siblings (McCarthy, 1935). Familiarity with foods, which is largely controlled by the family, has been shown to be a determinant of child eating patterns (Phillips & Kolasa, 1980).

Food is commonly used in families as a reward or punishment (Eppright *et al.,* 1969), and use of food in this manner, or even giving foods in a social context, can alter children's preferences for foods (Birch *et al.,* 1980). A number of family variables, including number of siblings, mother's work status, and mother's marital status, were found to be related to nutritional status, as measured by physical examination (Jacoby *et al.,* 1975). A measure of family functioning was related to food and nutrient intake in one study (Kintner *et al.,* 1981). More methodologically rigorous studies are needed to explore the complex relationships between family structure, family functioning, and dietary habits.

Family interaction patterns and their influence on diet have been studied. Klesges *et al.* (1983) found that parental encouragements to eat were highly related to child obesity status. Measures of family social support for diet were more highly correlated with a dietary index than rated social support from friends (Sallis, Grossman, Pinski, Patterson, & Nader, 1987).

In summary, there is strong evidence from several studies that health-related dietary habits are aggregated within families. A number of intrafamily processes appear to mediate these relationships. The processes include modeling, reward and punishment practices, family structure, family functioning, and social support. Much of the research has not been conducted with a high degree of methodological rigor, and problems of measuring diet introduce error, so the findings must be viewed as merely suggestive at this time.

Physical Activity Behaviors

Less research on family aggregation of health-related physical activity has been conducted than on smoking and diet. The type of physical activity of interest is primarily endurance or "aerobic" exercise that involves rhythmic movement of large muscle groups with adequate intensity, duration, and frequency (Haskell, Montoye, & Orenstein, 1985). However, in many studies physical activity is characterized very grossly. Venters *et al.* (1984) found significant concordance in physical activity between spouses, and in two multivariate studies parental factors were the strongest correlates of child physical activity (Gottlieb & Chen, 1985; Butcher, 1983). In a study of San Diego families, there were moderate parent–child correlations in physical activity, but less evidence of spouse and sibling pair similarities (Sallis, Patterson, Buono, Atkins, & Nader, 1988). Children with obese parents were less physically active than were children with nonobese parents (Griffiths & Payne, 1976).

Parents seem to be powerful agents of influence regarding their children's sports and exercise participation (Livingood, Goldwater, & Kurz, 1981), and parental encouragements are related to physical activity levels in young children (Klesges *et al.*, 1984). Parents' exercise attitudes were related to their children's attitudes (Dowell, 1973), and physically active adolescents were more likely than their sedentary classmates to believe that their parents wanted them to exercise (Godin & Shephard, 1984). Parental attitudes about exercise discriminated between physically active and inactive children, and active adults reported participating in more activities with their families (Harris, 1979). In addition to parental influences on children, there are a number of means by which children can alter their parents' participation in physical activity and sports (Snyder & Purdy, 1982).

Support from family members may be an important determinant of physical activity. Exercisers, especially coronary patients, are more likely to continue exercise if they have supportive spouses (Martin & Dubbert, 1982; Dishman, Sallis, & Orenstein, 1985). Ratings of family support were more highly correlated with exercise habits than were ratings of friend support (Sallis, Grossman, *et al.*, 1987).

In summary, there is limited but suggestive documentation that physical activity habits are aggregated within families. There are some indications that families influence children's attitudes toward physical activity, but both the quality and quantity of these studies are generally inadequate.

There are data suggesting that family determinants of smoking, dietary, and physical activity behaviors are important, but few conclusions can be confidently drawn from this diverse literature because of the ubiquitous methodological deficiencies. Specifically, most of the studies have been conducted on small numbers of families that were neither carefully selected nor adequately described in terms of family structure and basic demographic variables. Most studies investigated only one type of influence, so comparative strengths and interactions among determinants are unknown. There are few examples of investigators who have pursued a line of research devoted to increasing understanding of family influences on health behaviors, and it is likely that serious commitment to this area will be required to make significant advances.

MECHANISMS OF FAMILY INFLUENCE

The research on family determinants of preventive health behaviors is the product of a number of theoretical and nontheoretical approaches. It is the aim of this section to

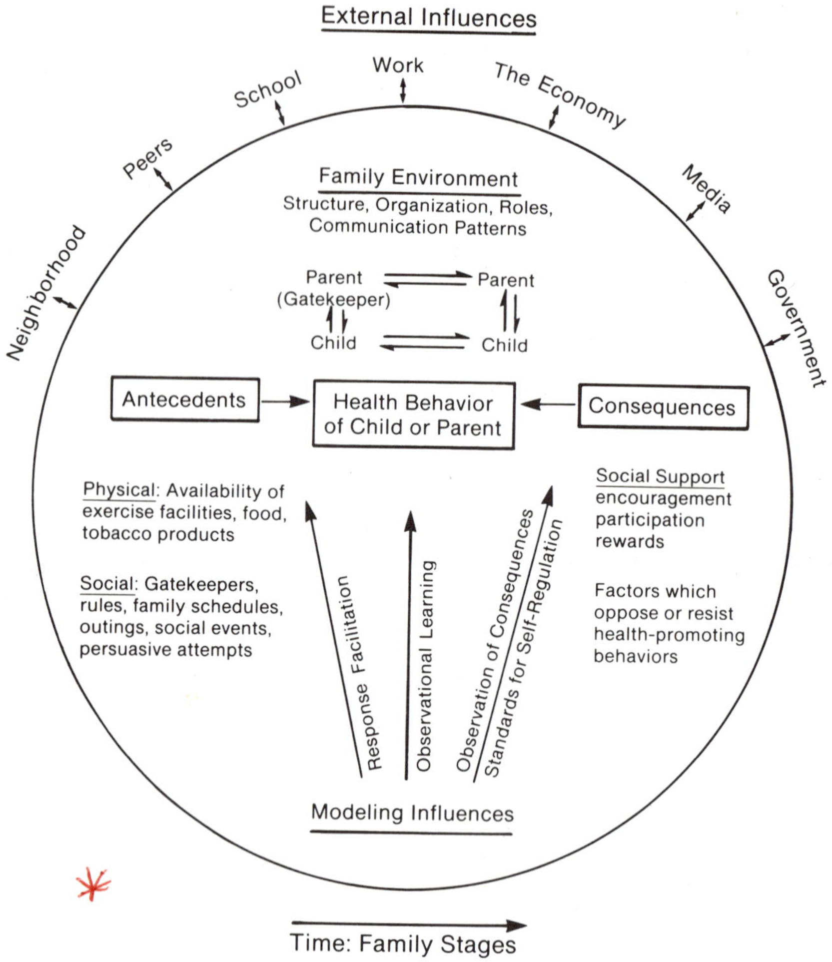

FIGURE 1. A model of family influences on health behavior.

present a single conceptual model that describes the mechanisms of influence suggested by previous research as well as points the way toward some additional areas of investigation. The model is an elaboration of cognitive–social learning theory (Bandura, 1977) and Skinnerian learning principles (Skinner, 1953). Social learning theory is a comprehensive theory of human behavior, based upon interrelationships among behavioral, cognitive, and emotional processing within the individual, and the surrounding physical and social environments. Skinnerian principles emphasize the influence of antecedent and consequent environmental events on behavior. These theories have been extremely effective in facilitating understanding and control of a wide range of human behaviors (Bellack, Hersen, & Kazdin, 1982). The major components of a social learning model of family influences are shown in Figure 1. While the model focuses on mechanisms of influence within the family, there are, of course, many additional influences, external to the family. These include social, organizational, and psychological factors that are the subjects of other chapters in this volume.

In the previous section it was demonstrated that family influences on health behaviors are consistently found. This is not surprising given the nature of family interactions. What is surprising is that these influences have not been documented more carefully and that their mechanisms have not been described. Family relationships are the most intensive, in terms of both quality and quantity, in the lives of most people. There are strong emotional bonds, and interactions among family members influence virtually every aspect of human life. Family members spend great amounts of time together, especially during child-rearing years, and the relationships typically endure for several decades, if not throughout life. There are so many opportunities for family influences on health habits that only a few potentially major factors can be singled out for discussion.

Family Environment

All of the social learning influences can be observed within the context of the family environment. There are many types of family structures in modern society. Although these structures undoubtedly have many implications for interactional dynamics, the impact on preventive health behaviors has seldom been addressed (Loveland-Cherry, 1986). Families are conceived of as complex systems with many dynamic properties (Watzlawick, Beavin, & Jackson, 1967). The different styles of interaction, dominance patterns, and role structures have been the object of investigation (Olson, Russell, & Sprenkle, 1983). However, the operationalization of these concepts is difficult and ideally involves direct observation of families with coding of verbal and nonverbal interactions. At least three commonly used self-report measures show promise as indices of family functioning that are practical for use in health research. The Family Environment Scale (Moos & Moos, 1981) consists of 10 subscales in three categories: relationships, personal growth, and system maintenance. Three of the subscales have been used as an index of quality of social support in the family (Holahan & Moos, 1983). The Family Adaptability and Cohesion Evaluation Scale (FACES; Olson, McCubbin, & Barnes, 1985) and the McMaster Family Assessment Device (Miller, Epstein, Bishop, & Keitner, 1985) are based on specific models of family functioning. While research on the relationship between these measures of family functioning and health habits is needed, more conceptual work is required to identify dimensions of family functioning that should be relevant to the development and alteration of health behaviors. Instead of merely borrowing concepts from the mental health field, specific theories should be developed for family preventive health.

It is important to keep in mind, when considering the social learning model of family determinants of health behavior, that influence among family members is multidirectional. Parent-to-child influences are most frequently discussed and may be the most powerful. However, when there are two parents, one parent will usually have the role of food gatekeeper, and this parent's effect on the dietary behavior of all family members may be especially important. Spouse-to-spouse influences are likely to be strong, and these have been discussed previously (Venters, 1986). While it has been argued that child-to-parent influences can be significant (Baranowski, 1978; Snyder & Purdy, 1982), they have been insufficiently studied. However, sibling-to-sibling influences have been demonstrated in regard to smoking and are expected to be important in other behavioral domains as well. These complex intrafamily patterns of influence indicate that any family member may model behavior and provide antecedents and consequences that influence the behavior of any other family members. Thus, researchers should consider all potential directions of influence in studies of mechanisms of family influence.

The Operant Core

It is well established that behavior is determined by the environmental stimuli that precede and follow it (Bandura, 1969; Skinner, 1953). The model depicted in Figure 1 is based on the assumption that family influences on antecedent and consequent events will be effective in shaping health behavior. Operant influences are the core of this model of family determinants because families control so many of the important environmental stimuli that shape behavior very strongly. Specific types of influences are tied to this simple, basic operant framework.

Modeling

Modeling is a core concept in social learning theory, and the influence of modeling (i.e., demonstration) of a wide variety of behaviors is strong and well understood (Rosenthal & Bandura, 1979). The influence of modeling is not simple because it serves a number of functions and is mediated by several factors. Rosenthal and Bandura (1979) identified four functions of modeling. First, the "observational learning effect" states that people learn to do things by watching others. As family members have so many opportunities to watch one another, this effect is pervasive. For example, children learn how to open a pack of cigarettes by observing their parents. Second, observing the positive or negative consequences of a model's actions serves to "disinhibit or inhibit" performance of a similar behavior. Thus, observing a sibling being chided for requesting ice cream will tend to discourage similar requests. Third, "response facilitation effect" means that modeling can be an antecedent event. One child asking father to go out and play basketball may stimulate other siblings to propose similar activities. This function is distinguished from observational learning in that no new behaviors are learned; only the timing or frequency of performance is affected. Fourth, modeling sets "cognitive standards for self-regulation." By observing the actions of others, one learns to set certain standards or expectations by which to judge oneself in similar situations. For example, if a child observes adults who spend most weekends sitting in front of the television, the observer will expect to act similarly when he or she becomes an adult. If two spouses are attempting to alter their eating habits and one spouse makes a point of being consistent in sticking to the goals, then the other spouse will tend to adopt similar standards.

The most important attributes of a model are relevance and credibility. Relevant models compel attention, and their behavior affords plausible standards to guide one's own conduct. If a model appears to deserve trust, then credibility is enhanced. For children, parents are models of profound relevance and credibility. Considering the frequency and duration of contact with parental and sibling models, it is expected that children will be influenced in very important ways by modeling of family members.

It should be noted in Figure 1 that modeling can act as an antecedent, can teach the actual behavior, and can influence consequences, so that this is a powerful and complex mechanism for family influence.

Antecedents

Antecedents are events that cue behaviors. Our environments are full of cues such as signs, reminders, and rules. The household is particularly rich with health-related cues, and families provide health-related antecedent social stimuli both in and out of the home.

Physical cues in the home environment are powerful determinants of behaviors. Presence or absence of cigarettes or various types of food at home exerts significant control over consumptive behavior. Even preschool children who had cigarettes in their home were more likely to report they would smoke in the future than children without such cues (Shute, St. Pierre, & Lubell, 1981). The most salient eating cues involve the foods that are served in the home. It is probable that access to physical activity-related equipment (e.g., bicycles, soccer ball) and resources (e.g., open space) is a determinant of level of physical activity. The family controls these potential antecedents in the home, but family habits also affect exposure to cues outside of the home. For example, frequent family trips to fast-food restaurants that do not offer salads produce eating-related cues that are very different from those in restaurants that feature salad bars. Choice of place of residence influences ease of access to playgrounds, sports facilities, and team sports opportunities. These are just a few of the many antecedents in the physical environment to which the family controls access. Systematic study to identify these variables and estimate their strength is recommended.

Social cues are probably even more influential, and the family provides a wide range of cues for health-related behavior. These cues tend to be provided frequently and over long periods of time by family members with whom there are strong emotional bonds. Though it is not possible to identify all of these social cues, a few general categories will be mentioned. Family members' smoking, dietary, and exercise habits are powerful antecedent stimuli, especially for children (see previous section on modeling). Regarding food, it is usually possible to identify a "gatekeeper" in each family. This person is primarily responsible for menu-planning, shopping, and cooking. There is often verbal persuasion and teaching about food that accompanies this role. In addition, food preferences may be a frequent topic of family conversation, with all members stating their own preferences and even attempting persuasion to their point of view. All of these food-related interactions can be construed as social antecedents. In some families there may be a similar gatekeeping role regarding physical activity or other recreational activities. Conversation and persuasion related to physical activity and use of leisure time also act as social cues to behavior.

Families may develop formal or informal rules to govern health-related habits. There may be proscriptions against tobacco use, or the family rule could be that one may smoke beginning at a certain age. Families can have rules pertaining to timing of snacks, type of snacks allowed, child's choice of meals, and child's input into shopping. These rules and practices will influence the eating habits of family members. In a similar way, family rules can affect the level of physical activity. Rules regarding TV viewing and parental recommendations on participation in team sports or other athletic endeavors will have significant impacts on children's physical activity habits. While the influence of family-controlled antecedents would appear to be strong, there is very little research to document these effects. However, Klesges and colleagues (Klesges *et al.*, 1983, 1984; Klesges, Malott, Boschee, & Weber, 1986) have conducted a number of studies documenting the influence of parental prompts on the dietary and physical activity habits of children. Interviews with adults changing their dietary and exercise habits revealed that family participation in these change efforts was both common and powerful. Exercising with a family member or assisting them in the preparation of a low-fat meal seemed to be effective methods of support (Sallis, Grossman, *et al.*, 1987).

Consequences

Some of the social antecedents discussed above can be considered to be social support; specifically, participation, encouragements, and reminders. Social support can also be helpful as a consequence.

Family members can support one another emotionally, materially, or with information (Caplan, 1982). There is evidence that families can be both supportive and nonsupportive; that is, they can sabotage attempts to alter health habits (Sallis, Grossman, *et al.*, 1987). Family members provide support by complimenting healthy eating, commenting upon missed exercise sessions, or setting up a reward program for quitting smoking. Negative support or opposition can take the form of complaining about the time spent exercising, complaining about an ex-smoker being too irritable, or refusing to eat healthy meals. Some parents systematically use food as rewards, and children tend to develop preferences for these foods (Birch *et al.*, 1980). This practice is relevant, since the most frequent "reward foods" tend to be high in fat and calories, such as pastries and other baked goods. Spouses continue this practice with one another, especially on special occasions. On the other hand, exercise may be occasionally used as punishment by some parents, as it is by coaches and drill sergeants. Thus, family members not only reward and punish certain health-related behaviors by word and action, but the act of rewarding or punishing may also contain lessons that may influence health habits.

The Time Dimension: Family Stages

Just as the developmental progression of individuals has been described (Erikson, 1963), families also have lives that evolve from one stage to another. It would seem that these life stages have the potential to influence family determinants of preventive health behaviors. The concept of family life cycle seems most relevant to families with children, though couples' relationships also change over time. One might expect families in the early stages of development, and especially those with young children, to be in a period of instability. Many life patterns are changing as the needs of other family members are assimilated, so health habits may be highly subject to modifying factors at this stage. With young children, parents exert almost total control over dietary habits and development of preferences, except when the child is with other caretakers.

In the middle stages of family life, for example when children are of school age, it is expected that dietary habits will become fairly stable, and the tendency will be for family members to continue with the customary dietary habits unless unusual forces for change are brought to bear from within the family or from outside. In contrast, attitudes and preferences regarding physical activity are just developing in elementary age children, and parents share influence over this development with external persons and institutions, such as peers and schools. Couples may become closer as they support one another in child-rearing, or they may not feel they have enough energy left over for their relationship.

In the later stages of family life, as children become more independent and eventually move away, and as the couples' relationships mature or, as often happens, dissolve, family influences decrease. As children spend more time with peers, they spend less time with parents and look to them for guidance less often. At the same time, children's influence over their parents' health habits may increase in many families as children develop divergent attitudes and habits regarding smoking, diet, or physical activity. The direction of couples' relationships would seem to be varied. They could move closer together as children leave home, or they could follow more independent paths. The diversity of patterns of spouse relationships may be related to the failure to find links between length of marriage and spousal similarity in health habits and risk factors (Greenberg *et al.*, 1984).

Summary

This model, based on social learning theory, suggests that families are powerful and lasting determinants of preventive health behaviors. Moreover, there are many mechanisms of influence; some of which are direct and some of which are subtle. Explicit identification of potentially important family variables can encourage researchers to develop appropriate measures so that the family determinants can be better understood.

IMPLICATIONS FOR INTERVENTION

One important benefit of increased understanding of family determinants is to influence the design of family-based health promotion programs. Family-based approaches seem particularly relevant to reduction of risk for CVD, because the underlying disease process continues for decades before it is clinically manifested. The family's potential impact is unique, because family influence is at its peak when dietary preferences are developed that eventually lead to overconsumption patterns that are associated with CVD. The family continues to influence dietary, smoking, and exercise habits for many years. Because of the long-term impact, and because the family is a dynamic system (Watzlawick *et al.,* 1967), it is hypothesized that health habit changes made in the *entire* family will be relatively stable and well maintained. This hypothesis is supported by intriguing data from a 5-year follow-up of child weight loss programs. The results suggest that the most important benefits of family-based programs are the long-term effects (Epstein, Wing, Koeske, & Valoski, 1987).

Representative studies exploring the role of family-based interventions on health habit changes are briefly reviewed.

The benefits of spouse involvement in adult weight loss programs have been studied, but the results are not clear. The first controlled study revealed a strong effect for spouse involvement (Brownell, Heckerman, Westlake, Hayes, & Monti, 1978) that persisted for 3 years (Heckerman & Zitter, 1979). However, these same investigators have been unable to replicate this finding (Wilson & Brownell, 1978; Brownell & Stunkard, 1981). Subsequently, several variations on this theme have been examined, with different methods of spouse involvement. In some studies spouse involvement was beneficial (Pearce, LeBow, & Orchard, 1981; Saccone & Israel, 1978), but in other studies there was no apparent effect (Dubbert & Wilson, 1984; Black & Lantz, 1984). In one study there was a significant effect for spouse involvement at 2 years, but not at the 4-year follow-up (Murphy, Bruce, & Williamson, 1985).

Another active area of investigation related to diet and exercise modification is parent involvement in child weight loss. In general, the results indicate that parent involvement in child weight control programs facilitates weight loss in children (Israel, Stolmaker, & Andrian, 1985; Epstein, Wing, Koeske, Andrasik, & Ossip, 1981; Epstein *et al.,* 1985; Wheeler & Hess, 1976) and in parents (Epstein *et al.,* 1981; Epstein, Wing, Steranchak, Dickson, & Michaelson, 1980; Israel *et al.,* 1985; Kingsley & Shapiro, 1977).

In several studies parent and child weight loss was correlated, at least during the initial treatment (Epstein & Wing, 1983). Moreover, children from larger families lost less weight (Epstein, Koeske, Wing, & Valoski, 1986). For overweight adolescents there is no evidence that conjoint parent–child interventions are beneficial (Coates, Killen, & Slinkard, 1982; Brownell, Kelman, & Stunkard, 1983). However, with preadolescents, the studies to date seem to indicate that family-based interventions are more effective with both children and adults, and there is evidence of substantial long-term maintenance (Epstein *et al.,* 1987).

A few studies of family-based programs to alter CVD risk-related behaviors have been reported. A family-based program to reduce sodium consumption in children with high blood pressure produced significant reductions when compared to a control group (Gillum, Elmer, Prineas, & Surbey, 1981). A very short-term program demonstrated changes in reported fat intake of families receiving the intervention (Witschi, Singer, Wulee, & Store, 1978), and another program with preschoolers produced changes in reported eating habits (Leonard, D'Augelli, & Smicklas-Wright, 1984). A combined school and family-based pilot program for children with high blood pressure increased knowledge and lowered urinary sodium values in participating children (Farris, Frank, Webber, & Berenson, 1985). A pilot study of 24 families revealed that a behavioral family-based intervention produced large reductions in dietary fat and salt intake, but no increases in aerobic exercise (Nader, Baranowski, Vanderpool, Dworkin, & Dunn, 1983). Other large studies of family-based programs to alter CVD-related dietary and exercise behaviors are ongoing (Nader *et al.,* 1986; Hollis, Connor, & Matarazzo, 1982). The studies conducted to date indicate the promise of harnessing family interactions for health promotion, but they also have demonstrated logistic difficulties such as low attendance at sessions. The ongoing studies will provide data on the feasibility and effectiveness of family health promotion on a large scale.

Despite the considerable influence of the family on smoking behavior, few studies have addressed family-based smoking cessation. One study suggested that children may be able to influence their parents to quit smoking (Flay, Hansen, *et al.*, 1983), and a series of case reports suggested that spouses who quit smoking at the same time may be able to support one another effectively (Lichstein & Stalgaitis, 1980). Perceived spouse support for quitting predicted short-term abstinence (Mermelstein *et al.*, 1986), but an experimental study did not demonstrate a significant impact of spouse training on cessation (McIntyre-Kingsolver, Lichtenstein, & Mermelstein, 1986). It appears that spouse influences on smoking cessation are complex.

Several major issues are unresolved. Although several methods of parent involvement in child weight loss programs have been investigated, there is no clear demonstration that one approach should be preferred over the others. While there appears to be no benefit for parent involvement in adolescent weight control programs, the reasons for this age-related finding have not been identified. The generalizability of family-based interventions such as those used with child weight loss, to other health behaviors is unknown.

SUMMARY AND CONCLUSIONS

The relatively meager quantity of research belies the importance of family determinants of CVD-related health behaviors. Though there are clearly genetic factors involved in the family aggregation of blood pressure, serum cholesterol and lipoproteins, and obesity, the family environment is responsible for the apparent aggregation of dietary habits, physical activity patterns, and smoking. It is largely through family influences over the physical and social environments that children gain their attitudes, knowledge, and early health practices, and those influences continue for many years at a reduced level.

The mechanisms through which family influences operate are obscure, and both theoretical and empirical work are required to provide an adequate understanding. A simple model, based on social learning theory, was presented to stimulate conceptualization of family determinants. The model emphasizes that family members influence one another's health behaviors in many ways, with high frequency, and over a long period of time.

The theoretical importance of family determinants has been partially documented by research, and several investigators are developing family-based interventions that attempt to alter existing patterns of family communication to support the goals of health promotion. The research to date generally supports the benefits of family-based behavioral programs that involve parents and children. However, many questions and problems remain to be addressed by future investigation.

It is critical to improve understanding of family determinants of preventive health behavior so that these powerful influences can be used to shape health-promoting habits in children. Working with the children holds potential for benefiting the adults in the family as well. Family-based interventions are essential for adopting a proactive health promotion strategy, i.e., health promotion should begin with socialization of infants and toddlers so that preferences are developed early for low-calorie foods and for an active rather than a sedentary life-style. Interventions targeting the entire family are the only way to achieve this goal of very early primary prevention. Interventions for families with very young children are the only way to reduce reliance on the current health promotion strategy of attempting to reverse already established and refractory health habits.

Research on the current state of knowledge of family determinants of health habits has suggested that family influences are important. However, many questions are left unanswered. Because family determinants have not been systematically studied or guided by models or theories, it is likely that many important determinants have not been identified. Of those that have, their relative power has not been estimated. Of those that appear to be powerful, measurement instruments are typically inadequate, and the mechanisms of influence and relationships to other determinants have not been studied. For most determinants, evidence of cause and effect is lacking, so that the need for well-conceptualized research programs on the family determinants of health behavior is great.

Acknowledgment

The authors thank Irma Valdez for her valuable assistance in the preparation of this chapter.

REFERENCES

Arky, R. A., Wylie-Rosett, J., and El-Beheri, B. (1982). Examination of current dietary recommendations for individuals with diabetes mellitus. *Diabetes Care, 5,* 59–63.

Bandura, A. (1969). *Principles of behavior modification.* New York: Holt, Rinehart, & Winston.

Bandura, A. (1977). *Social learning theory.* Englewood Cliffs, NJ: Prentice–Hall.

Baranowski, M. (1978). Adolescents attempted influence on parental behaviors. *Adolescence, 13,* 585–604.

Baranowski, T., & Nader, P. R. (1985). Family health behavior. In D. C. Turk & R. D. Kerns (Eds.), *Health, illness, and families: A life-span perspective* (pp. 51–80). New York: Wiley.

Barrett-Connor, E., Suarez, L., & Criqui, M. H. (1982). Spouse concordance of plasma cholesterol and triglyceride. *Journal of Chronic Diseases, 35,* 333–340.

Bellack, A. S., Hersen, M., & Kazdin, A. E. (Eds.). (1982). *International handbook of behavior modification and therapy.* New York: Plenum Press.

Biglan, A., & Lichtenstein, E. (1984). A behavior-analytic approach to smoking acquisition: Some recent findings. *Journal of Applied Social Psychology, 14,* 207–223.

Biglan, A., Severson, H. H., McConnell, S., & Baury, J. (1983). Social influence and adolescent smoking: A first look behind the barn. *Health Education,* 14–18.

Birch, L. L., Zimmerman, S. I., & Hind, H. (1980). The influence of social-affective context on the formation of children's food preferences. *Child Development, 51,* 856–861.

Black, D. R., & Lantz, C. E. (1984). Spouse involvement and a possible long-term follow-up trap in weight loss. *Behaviour Research and Therapy, 22,* 557–562.

Borland, B. L., & Rudolph, J. P. (1975). Relative effects of low socio-economic status, parental smoking and poor scholastic performance on smoking among high school students. *Social Science and Medicine, 9,* 27–30.

Brashear, R. E. (1980). Chronic obstructive pulmonary disease. In D. H. Simmons (Ed.), *Current pulmonology* (Vol. 2, pp. 1–39). Boston: Houghton Mifflin.

Brownell, K. D., Heckerman, C. L., Westlake, R. J., Hayes, S. C., & Monti, P. M. (1978). The effect of couples training and partner cooperativeness in the behavioral treatment of obesity. *Behaviour Research and Therapy, 16,* 323–333.

Brownell, K. D., Kelman, J. H., & Stunkard, A. J. (1983). Treatment of obese children with and without their mothers: Changes in weight and blood pressure. *Pediatrics, 71,* 515–523.

Brownell, K. D., & Stunkard, A. J. (1981). Couples training, pharmacotherapy, and behavior therapy in the treatment of obesity. *Archives of General Psychiatry, 38,* 1224–1229.

Bryan, M. S., & Lowenberg, M. E. (1958). The father's influence on young children's food preferences. *Journal of the American Dietetic Association, 34,* 30–34.

Bullen, B. A., Reed, R. B., & Mayer, J. (1964). Physical activity of obese and nonobese adolescent girls appraised by motion picture sampling. *American Journal of Clinical Nutrition, 14,* 211–223.

Butcher, J. (1983). Socialization of adolescent girls into physical activity. *Adolescence, 18,* 753–766.

Caplan, G. (1982). The family as a support system. In H. I. McCubbin, A. E. Cauble, & J. M. Patterson (Eds.), *Family stress, coping, and social support* (pp. 200–220). Springfield, IL: Thomas.

Coates, T. J., Killen, J. D., & Slinkard, L. A. (1982). Parent participation in a treatment program for overweight adolescents. *International Journal of Eating Disorders, 1,* 37–48.

Connor, S. L., Connor, W. E., Henry, H., Sexton, G., & Keenan, E. J. (1984). The effects of familial relationships, age, body weight, and diet on blood pressure and the 24-hour excretion of sodium, potassium, and creatinine in men, women, and children of randomly selected families. *Circulation, 70,* 76–85.

Crawford, C. O. (1971). *Health and the family: A medical sociological analysis.* New York: Macmillan Co.

Dishman, R. K., Sallis, J. F., & Orenstein, D. R. (1985). The determinants of physical activity and exercise. *Public Health Reports, 100,* 158–171.

Dowell, L. J. (1973). A study of physical and psychological variables related to attitudes toward physical activity. *International Journal of Sport Psychology, 4,* 39–47.

Dubbert, P. M., & Wilson, G. T. (1984). Goal-setting and spouse involvement in the treatment of obesity. *Behaviour Research and Therapy, 3,* 227–242.

Eastwood, M. A., Brydon, W. G., Smith, D. M., & Smith, J. H. (1982). A study of diet, serum lipids, and fecal constituents in spouses. *American Journal of Clinical Nutrition, 36,* 290–293.

Eppright, E. S., Fox, H. M., Fryer, B. A., Lamkin, G. H., & Vivian, V. M. (1969). Eating behavior of preschool children. *Journal of Nutrition Education, 1,* 16–19.

Epstein, L. H., Koeske, R., Wing, R. R., & Valoski, A. (1986). The effect of family variables on child weight change. *Health Psychology, 5,* 1–12.

Epstein, L. H., & Wing, R. R. (1983). Reanalysis of weight changes in behavior modification and nutrition education for childhood obesity. *Journal of Pediatric Psychology, 8,* 97–100.

Epstein, L. H., Wing, R. R., Koeske, R., Andrasik, F., & Ossip, D. J. (1981). Child and parent weight loss in family-based behavior modification programs. *Journal of Consulting and Clinical Psychology, 49,* 674–685.

Epstein, L. H., Wing, R. R., Koeske, R., & Valoski, A. (1987). Long-term effects of family-based treatment of childhood obesity. *Journal of Consulting and Clinical Psychology, 55,* 91–95.

Epstein, L. H., Wing, R. R., Steranchak, L., Dickson, B., & Michaelson, J. (1980). Comparison of family based behavior modification and nutrition education for childhood obesity. *Journal of Pediatric Psychology, 5,* 25–36.

Epstein, L. H., Wing, R. R., Woodall, K., Penner, B. C., Kress, M. J., & Koeske, R. (1985). Effects of family-based behavioral treatment on obese 5-to-8-year-old children. *Behavior Therapy, 16,* 205–212.

Erikson, E. H. (1963). *Childhood and society.* New York: Norton.

Evans, R. I., & Raines, B. E. (1982). Control and prevention of smoking in adolescents: A psychosocial perspective. In T. J. Coates, A. C. Petersen, & C. Perry (Eds.), *Promoting adolescent health: A dialog on research and practice* (pp. 101–136). New York: Academic Press.

Farris, R. P., Frank, G. C., Webber, L. S., & Berenson, G. S. (1985). A nutrition curriculum for families with high blood pressure. *Journal of School Health, 55,* 110–112.

Feinleib, M., Garrison, R. J., & Havlik, R. J. (1980). Environmental and genetic factors affecting the distribution of blood pressure in children. In R. M. Lauer & R. B. Shekelle (Eds.), *Childhood prevention of atherosclerosis and hypertension* (pp. 271–279). New York: Raven Press.

Flay, B. R., d'Avernas, J. R., Best, J. A., Kersell, M. W., & Ryan, K. B. (1983). Cigarette smoking: Why young people do it and ways of preventing it. In P. J. McGrath & P. Firestone (Eds.), *Pediatric and adolescent behavioral medicine: Issues in treatment* (pp. 132–183). Berlin: Springer.

Flay, B. R., Hansen, W. B., Johnson, C. A., & Sobel, J. C. (1983). *Involvement of children in motivating smoking parents to quit with a television program.* Paper presented at the American Psychological Association, Anaheim, CA.

Fraser, G. E., Phillips, R. L., & Harris, R. (1983). Physical fitness and blood pressure in school children. *Circulation, 67,* 405–412.

Garn, S. M., & Clark, D. C. (1976). Trends in fatness and the origins of obesity. *Pediatrics, 57,* 443–456.

Garn, S. M., Cole, P. E., & Bailey, J. M. (1976). Effect of parental fatness on the fatness of biological and adoptive children. *Ecology of Food and Nutrition, 6,* 1–3.

Gilliam, T., & Burke, M. B. (1978). Effects of exercise on serum lipids and lipoproteins in girls, ages 8 to 10 years. *Artery, 4,* 203.

Gillum, R. F., Elmer, P. S., Prineas, R. J., & Surbey, D. (1981). Changing sodium intake in children: The Minneapolis Children's Blood Pressure Study. *Hypertension, 3,* 698–703.

Glueck, C. J., & Connor, W. E. (1978). Diet–coronary heart disease relationships reconnoitered. *American Journal of Clinical Nutrition, 31,* 727–737.

Glueck, C. J., Tsang, R. C., Fallat, R. W., & Mellies, M. J. (1977). Diet in children heterozygous for familial hypercholesterolemia. *American Journal of Diseases of Children, 131,* 162–166.

Glueck, C. J., Waldman, G., McClish, D. K., Morrison, J. A., Khoury, P., Larsen, R., Salz, K., Rifkind, B. M., & Mattson, F. H. (1982). Relationships of nutrient intake to lipids and lipoproteins in 1234 white children. *Arteriosclerosis, 2,* 523–536.

Godin, G., & Shephard, R. J. (1984). Normative beliefs of school children concerning regular exercise. *Journal of School Health, 54,* 443–445.

Gottlieb, N. H., & Chen, M. S. (1985). Sociocultural correlates of childhood sporting activities: Their implications for heart health. *Social Science and Medicine, 5,* 533–539.

Greenberg, R. A., Green, P. P., Roggenkamp, K. J., & Barrett-Connor, E. (1984). The constancy of parent–offspring similarity of total cholesterol throughout childhood and early life. *Journal of Chronic Diseases, 37,* 833–838.

Griffiths, M., & Payne, P. R. (1976). Energy expenditure in small children of obese and non-obese parents. *Nature, 260,* 698–700.

Hamburg, D. A., Elliott, G. R., & Parron, D. L. (1982). *Health and behavior: Frontiers of research in the biobehavioral sciences.* Washington, DC: National Academy Press.

Harris, L. (1979). *Fitness in America: The Perrier Study.* Washington, DC: National Center for Health Statistics.

Haskell, W. L., Montoye, H. J., & Orenstein, O. (1985). Physical activity and exercise to achieve health-related physical fitness components. *Public Health Reports, 100,* 202–212.

Heckerman, C. L., & Zitter, R. E. (1979). *Spouse monitoring and reinforcement in the treatment of obesity.* Paper presented at the Association for the Advancement of Behavior Therapy, San Francisco.

Hertzler, A. A. (1983). Children's food patterns—a review: II. Family and group behavior. *Journal of the American Dietetic Association, 83,* 555–560.

Holahan, C. J., & Moos, R. H. (1983). The quality of social support: Measures of family and work relationships. *Journal of Clinical Psychology, 22,* 157–162.

Hollis, J. F., Connor, W. E., & Matarazzo, J. D. (1982). Lifestyle, behavioral health, and heart disease. In R. J. Gatchel, A. Baum, & J. E. Singer (Eds.), *Handbook of psychology and health* (Vol. 1, pp. 465–502). Hillsdale, NJ: Erlbaum.

Hunter, S. M., Baugh, J. G., Webber, S., Sklov, M. C., & Berenson, G. S. (1982). Social learning effects on trial and adoption of cigarette smoking in children: The Bogalusa Heart Study. *Preventive Medicine, 11,* 29–42.

Israel, A. C., Stolmaker, L., & Andrian, C. A. G. (1985). The effects of training parents in general child management skills on a behavioral weight loss program for children. *Behavior Therapy, 16,* 169–180.

Jacoby, A., Altman, D. G., Cook, J., Holland, W. W., & Elliott, A. (1975). Influence of some social and environmental factors on the nutrient intake and nutritional status of school children. *British Journal of Preventive and Social Medicine, 29,* 116–120.

Karlin, S., Williams, P. T., Farquhar, J. W., Barrett-Connor, E., Hoover, I., Wahl, P. W., Haskell, W. L., Bergelin, R. O., & Suarez, L. (1982). Association arrays for the study of familial height, weight, lipid, and lipoprotein similarity in three west coast populations. *American Journal of Epidemiology, 116,* 1001–1021.

Kingsley, R. G., & Shapiro, J. (1977). A comparison of three behavioral programs for the control of obesity in children. *Behavior Therapy, 8,* 30–36.

Kintner, M., Boss, P. G., & Johnson, N. (1981). The relationship between dysfunctional family environments and family member food intake. *Journal of Marriage and the Family, 43,* 633–641.

Klesges, R. C., Coates, T. J., Brown, G., Sturgeon-Tillish, J., Moldenhauer-Klesges, L. M., Holzer, B., Woolfrey, J., & Vollmer, J. (1983). Parental influences on children's eating behavior and relative weight. *Journal of Applied Behavior Analysis, 16,* 371–378.

Klesges, R. C., Coates, T. J., Moldenhauer-Klesges, L. M., Holzer, B., Gustavson, J., & Barnes, J. (1984). The FATS: An observational system for assessing physical activity in children and associated parent behavior. *Behavior Assessment, 6,* 333–345.

Klesges, R. C., Malott, J. M., Boschee, P. F., & Weber, J. M. (1986). The effects of parental influences on children's food intake, physical activity, and relative weight. *International Journal of Obesity, 5,* 335–346.

Kolonel, L. N., & Lee, J. (1981). Husband–wife correspondence in smoking, drinking, and dietary habits. *American Journal of Clinical Nutrition, 34,* 99–104.

Laskarzewski, P., Morrison, J. A., Khoury, K., Glatfelter, L., Larsen, R., & Glueck, C. J. (1980). Parent–child nutrient intake relationships in school children ages 6 to 19: The Princeton School District Study. *American Journal of Clinical Nutrition, 33,* 3250–3255.

Lee, J., & Kolonel, L. N. (1982). Nutrient intakes of husbands and wives: Implications for epidemiologic research. *American Journal of Epidemiology, 115,* 515–525.

Leonard, C. P., D'Augelli, A. R., & Smicklas-Wright, H. (1984). Effects of a weight-control program on parents' response to family eating situations. *Journal of the American Dietetic Association, 84,* 424–427.

Levy, S. M. (1985). *Behavior and cancer.* San Francisco: Jossey–Bass.

Lichstein, K. L., & Stalgaitis, S. J. (1980). Treatment of cigarette smoking in couples by reciprocal aversion. *Behavior Therapy, 11,* 104–108.

Livingood, A. B., Goldwater, C., & Kurz, R. B. (1981). Psychological aspects of sports participation in young children. *Advances in Behavioral Pediatrics, 2,* 141–169.

Loveland-Cherry, C. J. (1986). Personal health practices in single parent and two parent families. *Family Relations, 35,* 133–139.

Martin, J. E., & Dubbert, P. (1982). Exercise applications and promotion in behavioral medicine: Current status and future directions. *Journal of Consulting and Clinical Psychology, 50,* 1004–1017.

Matarazzo, J. D. (1982). Behavioral health's challenge to academic, scientific, and professional psychology. *American Psychologist, 37,* 1–14.

McCarthy, D. (1935). Children's feeding problems in relation to the food aversions in the family. *Child Development, 6,* 277–283.

McIntyre-Kingsolver, K., Lichtenstein, E., & Mermelstein, R. J. (1986). Spouse training in a multicomponent smoking program. *Behavior Therapy, 17,* 67–74.

Mermelstein, R., Cohen, S., Lichtenstein, E., Baer, J. S., & Kamarck, T. (1986). Social support, smoking cessation and maintenance. *Journal of Consulting and Clinical Psychology, 54,* 447–453.

Miller, I. W., Epstein, N. B., Bishop, D. S., & Keitner, G. I. (1985). The McMaster family assessment device: Reliability and validity. *Journal of Marital and Family Therapy, 11,* 345–356.

Moos, R. H., & Moos, B. S. (1981). *Family Environment Scale manual.* Palo Alto, CA: Consulting Psychologists Press.

Murphy, J. K., Bruce, B. K., & Williamson, D. A. (1985). A comparison of measured and self-reported weights in a 4-year follow-up of spouse involvement in obesity treatment. *Behavior Therapy, 16,* 524–530.

Nader, P. R., Baranowski, T., Vanderpool, N., Dworkin, R. J., & Dunn, K. (1983). The Family Health Project: Cardiovascular risk reduction education for children and parents. *Developmental and Behavioral Pediatrics, 4,* 3–10.

Nader, P. R., Sallis, J. F., Rupp, J., Atkins, C., Patterson, T., & Abramson, I. (1986). The San Diego Family Health Project: Reaching families through the schools. *Journal of School Health, 56,* 227–231.

National Institute of Education. (1979). *Teenage smoking: Immediate and long-term patterns.* Washington, DC: U.S. Government Printing Office.

Newman, W. P., Freedman, D., Voors, A. W., Gard, P. D., Srinivasan, S. R., Cresanta, J. L., Williamson, G. D., Webber, L. S., & Berenson, G. S. (1986). Relation of serum lipoprotein levels and systolic blood pressure to early atherosclerosis. *New England Journal of Medicine, 314,* 138–144.

Olson, D., McCubbin, H., & Barnes, H. (Eds.). (1985). *Families: What makes them work.* Beverly Hills: Sage.

Olson, D. H., Russell, C., & Sprenkle, D. (1983). Circumplex model of marital and family systems VI: Theoretical update. *Family Process, 22,* 69–83.

Paffenbarger, R. S., & Hyde, R. T. (1984). Exercise in the prevention of coronary heart disease. *Preventive Medicine, 13,* 3–22.

Patterson, T. L., Kaplan, R. M., Sallis, J. F., & Nader, P. R. (1987). Aggregation of blood pressure in Anglo American and Mexican American families. *Preventive Medicine, 16,* 616–625.

Patterson, T. L., Rupp, J. W., Sallis, J. F., Atkins, C. J., & Nader, P. R. (in press). Aggregation of dietary calories, fats, and sodium in Mexican-American and Anglo families. *American Journal of Preventive Medicine.*

Pearce, J. W., LeBow, M. D., & Orchard, J. (1981). Role of spouse involvement in the behavioral treatment of overweight women. *Journal of Consulting and Clinical Psychology, 49,* 236–244.

Phillips, B. K., & Kolasa, K. K. (1980). Vegetable preferences of preschoolers in daycare. *Journal of Nutrition Education, 12,* 192–196.

Rauramaa, R. (1984). Relationship of physical activity, glucose tolerance, and weight management. *Preventive Medicine, 13,* 37–46.

Rosenthal, T. L., & Bandura, A. (1979). Psychological modeling: Theory and practice. In S. L. Garfield & A. E. Bergin (Eds.), *Handbook of psychotherapy and behavior change* (2nd ed., pp. 621–658). New York: Wiley.

Saccone, A. J., & Israel, A. C. (1978). Effects of experimenter versus significant other-controlled reinforcement and choice of target behavior on weight loss. *Behavior Therapy, 9,* 271–278.

Sackett, D. L. (1975). Studies of blood pressure in spouses. In O. Paul (Ed.), *Epidemiology and control of hypertension* (pp. 21–35). Miami: Symposium Specialists.

Sackett, D. L., Anderson, G. D., Milner, R., Feinleib, M., & Kannel, W. B. (1975). Concordance for coronary risk factors among spouses. *Circulation, 52,* 589–595.

Sallis, J. F., Grossman, R. M., Pinski, R. B., Patterson, T. L., & Nader, P. R. (1987). The development of scales to measure social support for diet and exercise behaviors. *Preventive Medicine, 16,* 825–836.

Sallis, J. F., Patterson, T. L., Buono, M. J., Atkins, C. J., & Nader, P. R. (1988). Aggregation of physical activity habits in Mexican-American and Anglo families. *Journal of Behavioral Medicine, 11,* 31–41.

Select Committee on Children, Youth, and Families. (1983). *U.S. children and their families: Current conditions and recent trends.* Washington, DC: U.S. House of Representatives.

Shear, C. L., Frerichs, R. R., Weinberg, R., & Berenson, G. S. (1978). Childhood sibling aggregation of coronary artery disease risk factor variables in a biracial community. *American Journal of Epidemiology, 107,* 522–528.

Shute, R. E., St. Pierre, R.W., & Lubell, E. G. (1981). Smoking awareness and practices of urban pre-school and first grade children. *Journal of School Health, 51,* 347–351.

Skinner, B. F. (1953). *Science and human behavior.* New York: Macmillan Co.

Snyder, E. E., & Purdy, D. A. (1982). Socialization into sport: Parent and child reverse and reciprocal effects. *Research Quarterly for Exercise and Sport, 53,* 263–266.

Speilberger, C. D., Jacobs, G. A., Crane, R. S., & Russell, S. F. (1983). On the relation between family smoking habits and the smoking behavior of college students. *International Review of Applied Psychology, 32,* 53–69.

Staessen, J., Bulpitt, C. J., Fagard, R., Joosens, J. V., Lijnen, P., & Amery, A. (1985). Familial aggregation of blood pressure, anthropometric characteristics and urinary excretion of sodium and potassium—A population study in two Belgian towns. *Journal of Chronic Diseases, 38,* 397–407.

Suarez, L., Criqui, M. H., & Barrett-Connor, E. (1983). Spouse concordance for systolic and diastolic blood pressure. *American Journal of Epidemiology, 118,* 343–351.

U.S. Public Health Service. (1979). *Smoking and health: 1979. A report of the Surgeon General* (DHEW (PHS) Publication No. 79-50066). Washington, DC: U.S. Government Printing Office.

Venters, M. H. (1986). Family life and cardiovascular risk: Implications for the prevention of chronic disease. *Social Science and Medicine, 22,* 1067–1074.

Venters, M. H., Jacobs, D. R., Luepker, R. V., Maiman, L. A., & Gillum, R. F. (1984). Spouse concordance of smoking patterns: The Minnesota Heart Survey. *American Journal of Epidemiology, 120,* 608–616.

Watzlawick, P., Beavin, J. H., & Jackson, D. C. (1967). *Pragmatics of human communication: A study of interactional patterns, pathologies, and paradoxes.* New York: Norton.

Wheeler, M. E., & Hess, K. W. (1976). Treatment of juvenile obesity by successive approximation control of eating. *Journal of Behavior Therapy and Experimental Psychiatry, 7,* 235–241.

Wilson, G. T., & Brownell, K. (1978). Behavior therapy for obesity: Including family members in the treatment process. *Behavior Therapy, 9,* 943–945.

Witschi, J. C., Singer, M., Wulee, M., & Store, F. (1978). Family cooperation and effectiveness in a cholesterol-lowering diet. *Journal of the American Dietetic Association, 12,* 384–389.

Social Determinants

Social Structure and Networks

An appreciable literature exists relating social factors to mortality, to incidence and prevalence (morbidity) of diseases, to accessibility and availability of care, and so on (e.g., Mechanic, 1978, Chapters 5–7; Syme & Berkman, 1986; Wolinsky, 1988, Chapter 1). In contrast, rigorous research on the social determinants of health behavior reflecting clear conceptualizations of the social factors is less abundant. Much research that has been labeled, indexed, or "keyworded" as "social," "sociocultural," or "sociopsychological" has dealt with demographic attributes of the person, i.e., age, gender, race, and so on, rather than with variables that are essentially social. However, a truly "social" literature is emerging. Research on the social determinants of health behavior is discussed in two sections: the first deals with characteristics of social structure; the second, with social roles.

Research related to the social structure determinants of health behavior can be considered under two headings: group characteristics, including research on group membership, group norms, social status or stratification; and network characteristics, including research on the characteristics of social ties or linkages.

GROUP CHARACTERISTICS

Suchman's (1965/1972) investigation of the dimension of social group organization and the utilization of health services has had a pronounced heuristic impact on medical sociology as well as on health behavior research. Suchman's work integrated demography, family structure, and social status in an attempt to use group characteristics to predict utilization of services as well as attitudes toward scientific medicine. He concluded that degree of "parochialism" or "cosmopolitanism" of family backgrounds influenced patterns of beliefs about illness and medical care, and ultimately affected patterns of utilization. Suchman's studies have generated both considerable research and an appreciable amount of controversy.

Subsequent investigations have shown the need to revise Suchman's conclusions. Geertsen's chapter presents both a précis and an assessment of Suchman's model, and a reexamination of its validity in the face of new data. Geertsen suggests an alternate model that takes into account the content of specific social and subcultural beliefs and values relevant to health and modern medicine.

In a complementary approach to group characteristics, Greenley and Mechanic's (1976) examination of reference groups in relation to seeking care for personal problems revealed that college students who sought counseling from members of the clergy were more oriented to the traditional student culture, while those who used outpatient psychiatric facilities for those problems were more oriented to the student "counterculture."

SOCIAL STRATIFICATION

The stratification patterns of American and other societies have become the bases for numerous investigations of health behavior. Koos's large-scale study of health and illness in "Regionville" (1954) is an early analysis of how social status is related to the interpretation of signs of illness. However, the definition of social class, or socioeconomic status, has been the subject of much debate. To define class or status solely in terms of income, money, and/or property would make it a "personal" rather than a "social" characteristic. Among the earliest systematic investigators of stratification in American society, Warner (e.g., 1949) demonstrated that class or status was multifaceted, that it reflected education, occupation, life-style, and mobility in addition to income and property, and that it reflected not only objective measures of these factors but also social appraisals or evaluations. Yet many attempts to relate socioeconomic position to health behaviors have employed overly simplistic measures that reflect individual income, educational, occupational levels in some additive fashion. Most studies, if well-conceived and properly conducted, have revealed little if any relationship between income and health behaviors (e.g., Rundall & Wheeler, 1979). Neighbors (1984) urged a thoughtful reconsideration of how income is used in analyses of health behavior research data. Moreover, Allen (1970) cautioned against making inappropriate assumptions about the true beliefs and values of poor persons, and about overgeneralizing from "the culture of poverty."

In contrast to a simplistic approach, Coburn and Pope (1974), using a measure of socioeconomic status reflecting income, occupation, and education, together with measures of six variables such as social participation, work self-direction, and powerless/planfulness, thought to reflect "life-style" factors that would go beyond personal attributes and that would help account for the effects of socioeconomic status, found that education, income, and social participation were positively related to making preventive dental visits and vaccinations for polio. Moreover, the relationship between socioeconomic status and having routine preventive physical examinations was curvilinear, with those lowest and highest in socioeconomic status making more such visits than those in the middle socioeconomic ranges. The research raised questions about the overall predictive value of socioeconomic status; social participation was considered to be the most predictive of the explanatory variables.

Questions about the value of socioeconomic status as determinants of health beliefs also arise in the work of Moody and Gray (1972) who observed that it was less valuable a predictor of preventive behavior than was social integration; and in the work of Suchman (1965/1972) and Gochman (1975).

Cockerham, Lueschen, Kunz, and Spaeth (1986) employ a concept of group status which is related to the "esteem a person is accorded by other people" (p. 4) and which thus represents a social appraisal. Persons who have low group status perceived a greater number of symptoms as requiring medical care, and were more likely to have made physician's visits for those symptoms, than persons who have higher group status. But more important was the finding that group status did not otherwise appreciably relate to healthy life-styles. Cockerham and his associates advance the concept of "culture of medicine" to replace the "culture of poverty" concept as a way of looking at those few social group differences that were observed.

Among other studies of social stratification, social status, or social class, Britt (1975) observed that social class and sick-role incumbency have a reciprocal relationship, mediated by the stresses arising from the poor housing, crowding, and inadequate social conditions associated with low incomes. Miller (1973) observed that upper and middle class persons were more likely to consult only with a spouse before seeking professional care for cancer symptoms, but that there were no class differences in informal consultations with medically knowledgeable persons. Moreover, socioeconomic status was found to be inversely related to taking lay advice. Osborn (1973) found that social ranking was directly related to positive self-evaluations of health status, but that the influence of rank on these evaluations was greatest among those with no reported chronic conditions.

Pflanz, Basler, and Schwoon (1977) reported that among adult German males (but not among females) there was a greater use of tranquilizing drugs among those in the upper and upper middle classes than in the lower class. However, this difference could not be accounted for by social participation or any other of several social characteristics. In an Indian study, Ramachandran and Shastri (1983) were unable to relate occupational status to choice of source of medical care. Verbrugge (1978) was unable to find that socioeconomic status was related to being among the "early accepters" or "new users" of contraceptive methods for family planning.

SOCIAL NETWORKS

In both the Ramachandran and Shastri (1983) and Verbrugge (1978) studies, the absence of socioeconomic status effects was complemented by observations of the importance of social networks and informal social contacts. Ramachandran and Shastri, for example, observed that decisions to seek medical care at specific sites were often influenced by the location of relatives near such sites. Verbrugge noted the importance of certain communicator characteristics of the "early accepters" as effective transmitters of information, advice, and influence throughout informal networks of their relatives, friends, and neighbors. It is the interactions among such informal social contacts—the degree to which persons participate in a variety of social interaction processes—that comprise the essence of research on social networks.

Moody and Gray (1972), using Suchman's model, provided one of the earliest demonstrations of the important role played by social interaction in contrast to socioeconomic status, in predictions of mothers' having their children participate in oral polio immunization. Mothers who had higher levels of social integration, i.e., higher rates of participating in community activities, and lower levels of alienation were more likely to have their children participate in the immunization program than were mothers who had lower levels of social integration and higher levels of alienation. These relationships were found, in general, to be independent of socioeconomic status.

Pilisuk and Froland (1978) indicated how circles of "intimates" have replaced families in urbanized and mobile societies, pointed out the value of such social support networks in the area of health and illness, and outlined a model of network analysis. Wallston, Alagna, DeVellis, and DeVellis (1983), in the context of reviewing the literature on social support and physical health, identified how social supports are related to adherence to medication regimens and to self-management programs. Levy's review of the literature on social support and compliance (1983) clearly identifies some major problems in the definition and description of social support in research studies. Hammer (1983) examined the relationships among social networks, health status, buffering of stresses, and health behaviors, and concluded that although social networks may mediate health status through their effects on health behaviors, their impact on health status cannot be accounted for solely through this mediation. Jacobson (1986) called attention to the need to examine the timing of support, in addition to increasing specificity about the type of support. Neighbors and Jackson (1984) identified patterns of illness behavior in the black community in relation to differential use of informal networks and professional help. Women were more likely to use informal networks than were men; and persons with physical problems were less likely to use *only* informal networks than were persons with emotional problems, and use of these informal networks for physical problems was likely to result in decisions to seek professional care.

Ritter's chapter distinguishes between social support and social networks; calls attention to the need for greater precision and conceptual clarity in dealing with these concepts; relates social networks and social support to health beliefs, utilization of services, and health-promoting behaviors; and presents a model to account for the influence of social networks.

The importance of social integration is also evidenced in Langlie's analysis (1977) of health belief model variables and preventive behaviors. Langlie dealt not only with social group characteristics, but also with patterns of family and social interaction as well, and made an important conceptual and empirical distinction between "indirect risk" and "direct risk" preventive health behaviors. Other ways in which the breadth of social networks and support systems influence health behaviors are observed in Finlayson's (1976) observations that women whose husbands had more successful recoveries from heart attacks had wider social contacts than those whose husbands had less successful recoveries; in Baranowski and colleagues' (1983) observations of the differential influence on breastfeeding of specific members of a mother's network, depending on ethnicity; in Calnan's (1983) observations in Britain that in the case of sudden illnesses or accidents away from home, decisions to seek medical care are made more quickly when others are consulted than when no one is consulted; in Frankel and Nuttall's (1984) findings in a Canadian sample that social support becomes a significant predictor of use of physician services for persons experiencing high distress; in Furstenberg and Davis's (1984) case history observations showing how conversations among older persons which either sought or transmitted information, or which led to help with daily tasks, also led to social support that reinforced health actions and use of health services.

REFERENCES

Allen, V. (1970). Theoretical issues in poverty research. *Journal of Social Issues, 26,* 149–167.

Baranowski, T., Bee, D. E., Rassin, D. K., Richardson, C. J., Brown, J. P., Guenther, N., & Nader, P. R. (1983). Social support, social influence, ethnicity and the breastfeeding decision. *Social Science and Medicine, 21,* 1599–1611.

Britt, D. W. (1975). Social class and the sick role: Examining the issue of mutual influence. *Journal of Health and Social Behavior, 16,* 178–182.

Calnan, M. (1983). Social networks and patterns of help-seeking behaviour. *Social Science and Medicine, 17,* 25–28.

Coburn, D., & Pope, C. R. (1974). Socioeconomic status and preventive health behaviour. *Journal of Health and Social Behavior, 15,* 67–78.

Cockerham, W. C., Lueschen, G., Kunz, G., & Spaeth, J. L. (1986). Social stratification and self-management of health. *Journal of Health and Social Behavior, 27,* 1–14.

Finlayson, A. (1976). Social networks as coping resources. *Social Science and Medicine, 10,* 97–103.

Frankel, B. G., & Nuttall, S. (1984). Illness behaviour: An exploration of determinants. *Social Science and Medicine, 19,* 147–155.

Furstenberg, A. L., & Davis, L. J. (1984). Lay consultation of older people. *Social Science and Medicine, 18,* 827–837.

Gochman, D. S. (1975). The measurement and development of dentally relevant motives. *Journal of Public Health Dentistry, 35,* 160–164.

Greenley, J. R., & Mechanic, D. (1976). Social selection in seeking help for psychological problems. *Journal of Health and Social Behavior, 17,* 249–262.

Hammer, M. (1983). 'Core' and 'extended' social networks in relation to health and illness. *Social Science and Medicine, 17,* 405–411.

Jacobson, D. E. (1986). Types and timing of social support. *Journal of Health and Social Behavior, 27,* 250–264.

Koos, E. L. (1954). *The health of Regionville: What the people thought and did about it.* New York: Columbia University Press.

Langlie, J. K. (1977). Social networks, health beliefs, and preventive health behavior. *Journal of Health and Social Behavior, 18,* 244–260.

Levy, R. L. (1983). Social support and compliance: A selective review and critique of treatment integrity and outcome measurement. *Social Science and Medicine, 18,* 1329–1338.

Mechanic, D. (1978). *Medical sociology: A comprehensive text* (2nd ed.). New York: Free Press.

Miller, M. H. (1973). Seeking advice for cancer symptoms. *American Journal of Public Health, 63,* 955–961.

Moody, P. M., & Gray, R. M. (1972). Social class, social integration, and the use of preventive health services. In E. G. Jaco (Ed.), *Patients, physicians and illness: A sourcebook in behavioral science and health* (2nd ed.). New York: Free Press.

Neighbors, H. W. (1984). Professional help use among Black Americans: Implications for unmet need. *American Journal of Community Psychology, 12,* 551–566.

Neighbors, H. W., & Jackson, J. J. (1984). The use of informal and formal help: Four patterns of illness behavior in the Black community. *American Journal of Community Psychology, 12,* 629–644.

Osborn, R. W. (1973). Social rank and self-health evaluation of older urban males. *Social Science and Medicine, 7,* 209–218.

Pflanz, M., Basler, H.-D., & Schwoon, D. (1977). Use of tranquilizing drugs by a middle-aged population in a West German city. *Journal of Health and Social Behavior, 18,* 194–205.

Pilisuk, M., & Froland, C. (1978). Kinship, social networks, social support and health. *Social Science and Medicine, 12B,* 273–280.

Ramachandran, H., & Shastri, G. S. (1983). Movement for medical treatment: A study in contact patterns of a rural population. *Social Science and Medicine, 17,* 177–187.

Rundall, T. G., & Wheeler, J. R. C. (1979). The effect of income on use of preventive care: An evaluation of alternative explanations. *Journal of Health and Social Behavior, 20,* 397–406.

Suchman, E. A. (1972). Social patterns of illness and medical care. In E. G. Jaco (Ed.), *Patients, physicians and illness: A sourcebook in behavioral science and health* (2nd ed.). New York: Free Press. (Reprinted from *Journal of Health and Human Behavior,* 1965, *6,* 2–16).

Syme, S. L., & Berkman, L. F. (1986). Social class, susceptibility, and sickness. In P. Conrad & R. Kern (Eds.), *The sociology of health and illness* (2nd ed.). New York: St. Martin's.

Verbrugge, L. M. (1978). Peers as recruiters: Family planning communications of West Malaysian acceptors. *Journal of Health and Social Behavior, 19,* 51–68.

Wallston, B. S., Alagna, S. W., DeVellis, B. M., & DeVellis, R. F. (1983). Social support and physical health. *Health Psychology, 2,* 367–391.

Warner, W. L. (1949). *Democracy in Jonesville: A study of quality and inequality.* New York: Harper Brothers.

Wolinsky, F. D. (1988). *The sociology of health: Principles, practitioners, and issues* (2nd ed.). Belmont, CA: Wadsworth.

CHAPTER 7

Social Group Characteristics and Health Behavior

Reed Geertsen

How does the organization of social relationships affect human responses to potentially disruptive situations like illness or the possibility of illness? After several decades of speculation and research, much has been learned, although most of what we know in this area continues to be challenged and reinterpreted through ongoing research. In the field of sociology, these challenges have taken several different directions. New and more sophisticated methodologies continue to be applied to earlier data sets in an effort to substantiate, refute, or modify previous research findings. Once-popular theories and modes of explanation like systems theory and functionalism have given way to alternative approaches like network theory. Replications of research using diverse population groups have helped to clarify and, in many cases, correct previous conclusions of how key variables combine to influence behavior.

EARLY CONTRIBUTIONS

No contribution to medical sociology has stimulated more interest or received more criticism than Parsons's (1951) conception of the sick role. His model showing how illness can be influenced by social relationships and how sickness constitutes a social role has had a major impact on medical care research. Basically, Parsons argued that, under normal circumstances, the preillness relationships and responsibilities of sick persons subjected them to certain rights and contingent obligations called the "sick role," which helped to regulate illness behavior and facilitate a return to normal functioning as soon as possible. Attempts to untangle how all of this worked empirically for various types of illness and disease raised numerous methodological, theoretical, and population-specific questions. For example, subsequent research uncovered a lack of uniformity across different ages and cultural groups and revealed variations which did not apply equally well to acute and chronic diseases. Furthermore, a middle class bias in the initial model was detected as it was applied to different socioeconomic segments of the population. With these and other findings have come clarifications and elaborations of the sick role which have helped to advance the field of medical sociology (Cockerham, 1986, pp. 137–142).

REED GEERTSEN • Department of Sociology, Utah State University, Logan, Utah 84322.

Other early contributions to medical sociology have gone through this same cycle of questioning, testing, and elaboration through several decades of research. Zborowski's (1952) research on ethnic groups and the clinical reporting of pain raised questions about the variability of such differences and provided explanations that are still being wrestled with today. Zborowski examined 146 male patients drawn from four different ethnic backgrounds in the New York City borough of The Bronx. Jewish and Italian patients were found to be much more emotional in describing pain and were more likely to exaggerate their pain experience than were Irish or several-generation American patients. Although similar in their responses to pain, Italian and Jewish patients had very different attitudes toward this experience. Italians were mainly concerned with the immediacy of the pain, wanted quick relief, and tended to express a confident attitude toward the doctor. Jewish patients focused instead on the symptomatic meaning of pain, wanted diagnosis rather than quick relief, tended to be skeptical of the doctor's actions, and were concerned about the future implications of the pain experience. Zola (1966) later expanded this research by emphasizing the cultural context of symptoms among patients at the Massachusetts General Hospital in Boston. Italians, unlike the Irish, were found to spread and generalize their complaints. As a result they reported significantly more symptoms in more bodily locations and noted a greater variety of dysfunctions. They also tended to emphasize the effects of symptoms on interpersonal behavior. Zola linked these tendencies to underlying Italian cultural traits like expressiveness and dramatization. Opposite tendencies among the Irish were identified with other cultural traits. To date, the different responses to pain in over 29 ethnic groups have been examined following Zborowski's lead (Lipton & Marbach, 1984).

Although many researchers have investigated the possible link between social group characteristics and health behavior, none have had greater impact on medical sociology than Suchman. His research (Suchman, 1964, 1965) on various ethnic groups in the Washington Heights section of New York City was the first comprehensive attempt to explore the possible interrelationships between individual medical orientations, medical behaviors, and social group structures. This work has become an important landmark for theory and research on social networks in medical sociology. Like Parsons and Zborowski, Suchman's work has been reexamined, criticized, replicated, and challenged by others. This chapter will examine his influence on a growing body of research on social networks which has helped to clarify how group structures are related to medical behavior.

SUCHMAN'S MODEL

Suchman's model of medical behavior was developed during a time when "social system" thinking, emphasizing the mutual dependence and interrelatedness of social processes, structures, and behaviors, dominated the field of sociology. During this time, attempts to link different dimensions of personality to various aspects of social structure were appearing in the literature. Parsons and Shils's (1962) portrayal of institutionalization and Kanter's (1968) analysis of commitment in utopian communities illustrate this interest in the linkage between social arrangements and personality. At the same time there was a growing concern over ethnic and socioeconomic variations in health care. Koos's (1954) work revealed sharp social class differences in awareness and interpretation of symptoms requiring medical attention. King (1962) and Brown (1964) also stressed the importance of ethnic, cultural, and socioeconomic factors in medical care.

During this time, Freidson (1960) drew attention to the possible discrepancies between professional beliefs and lay practices. He focused on "social networks" and was one of the earliest writers to emphasize the importance of social group ties in medical behavior.

This "lay referral system" represented a potential source of influence in the seeking of medical care. In his words,

> Indeed, the whole process of seeking help involves a network of potential consultants, from the intimate and informal confines of the nuclear family through successively more select, distant, and authoritative laymen, until the "professional" is reached. This network of consultants, which is part of the structure of the local lay community and which imposes form on the seeking of help, might be called the "lay referral structure." Taken together with the cultural understandings involved in the process, we may speak of it as the "lay referral system." (p. 377)

Freidson's emphasis on both social relationships and cultural themes helped shape Suchman's thinking and research. At about the same time, Bloom's (1963) analysis of doctor–patient interaction placed the patient in the middle of successive circles of influence. Closest to the individual was the family. Encompassing both the individual and the family was the sociocultural context. Suchman's work brought together many of these concepts within a systematic empirical framework. The basic assumption underlying his research was that group structures influence individual attitudes which in turn influence health and medical behavior.

The main problem addressed by Suchman (1965) was the lack of agreement in expectations and orientations between medical professionals and patients that was often observed in the delivery of medical care. To Suchman these differences had two important implications for patient behavior. First, patients with orientations which contradicted those of medical professionals were not likely to seek professional medical care on a regular basis. Second, when they did seek such care, they were less likely to cooperate in treatment programs. Suchman's aim was to explain lay persons' orientations toward modern medicine by relating them to social group structures. He took the position that skepticism and distrust of modern medicine were an outward expression of an underlying set of social relationships characterized by restricted participation in society. This hypothesis that attitudes and information are acquired through structured ties in social relationships was later to become a major postulate of modern network theory (Wellman, 1983, p. 165).

Group Structures and Medical Orientation

Empirical investigation required definition and measurement of social group structure, medical orientation, and medical behavior. Conceptually, group structure was broken down into family, friend, and community components. These were defined as the three basic levels of social influence on the individual. Because Suchman was interested in the degree to which restrictive group structures influenced attitudes, he developed a series of questions to measure this aspect of social involvement empirically at these three important levels. To represent the family level, he developed an index called "family authority." Questions were asked about the authority of the household head and about the family's emphasis on custom and tradition. At the social group level, he produced a measure called "friendship solidarity." By this he meant close friendships of long duration. Respondents were asked if their close friends were also friends with each other, if they had the same religious background, and if their families knew each other well. At the community level, he measured "ethnic exclusivity" by asking if parents and the parents of friends came from the same country, and if respondents preferred to shop where clerks shared a common cultural background. Collectively, individuals with social ties characterized by high family authority, friendship solidarity, and ethnic exclusivity were considered to have ingroup tendencies or "parochial" group structures. Social ties characterized by the opposite attributes were called "cosmopolitan" group structures.

Individual medical orientations were measured through questions designed to tap how people thought (cognitive), felt (affective), and behaved (behavioral) with respect to illness and medical care. The cognitive dimension of the medical orientation was defined as "knowledge of disease" and was measured by responses to 13 questions about common diseases. The affective dimension was defined as "skepticism of medical care" and was captured by questions about doubts and misgivings about medical professionals. The behavioral dimension was defined as "dependency during illness" and was measured in terms of whether persons found it hard to give up the special care received as they began to recover from illness. Medical behavior was limited to health status and usual source of care. Usual source of care was assessed as the respondent's first point of contact with the health care system and dichotomized as either private (e.g., private physician) or public (e.g., outpatient clinics). Suchman assumed that persons with parochial group ties would tend to use a private physician rather than impersonal outpatient facilities as the point of first contact in those instances where medical visits were made.

Testing the Model

Using the foregoing empirical measures, Suchman designed a study to see if individuals in ethnically exclusive community groups, highly cohesive friendship groups, and authority-, tradition-oriented families would have less knowledge of disease, more skepticism, and greater dependency than those with cosmopolitan group ties. For a study population, he chose the Washington Heights section of New York City. This area's large mix of nonwhite and foreign-born whites provided considerable ethnic and socioeconomic variation. It also contained a wide range of medical facilities. Such a population was felt to be necessary to provide sufficient variation in the social group variables to allow testing of the hypothesis. His study was limited to adult members of households over 21 years of age. Data were obtained through personal interviews conducted in homes.

The data revealed three basic findings (Suchman, 1964, 1965). First, the three measures of social group organization were all found to be significantly interrelated. Persons whose social relationships demonstrated high ethnic exclusivity were typically found to show high friendship solidarity and high family authority and vice versa. From this, he concluded that the three variables could be combined to form a single index ranging from "parochial" to "cosmopolitan" group structures. Second, the individual medical orientation variables were also found to be highly interrelated. Persons with low knowledge of disease were usually found to be skeptical toward medical care and to have a high dependency in illness. Consequently, these three variables were combined to form an index called "scientific" versus "popular" health orientation with "popular" representing low knowledge, high skepticism, and high dependency.

A third basic finding was an apparent strong connection between group structures and medical orientations. High ethnic exclusivity was found to be associated with significantly lower knowledge about disease, higher skepticism of medical care, and higher dependency in illness. Likewise, high friendship solidarity, as well as a family orientation toward tradition and authority, were found to be associated with low knowledge of disease, high skepticism, and high dependency. The importance of these findings was underscored by the fact that ethnic group variations within the population were found to correspond to the social group variables (Suchman, 1964). Puerto Ricans who were found as a group to be the most parochial were also found to have the fewest individuals reporting a scientific orientation. On the other hand, Protestant and Jewish respondents typically reported both cosmopolitan rather than parochial group structures and scientific rather than popular health orientations. Variations within each ethnic group were also found to be consistent with Suchman's predictions. That is, Puerto Ricans reporting more cosmopolitan group structures were found to be more scientific in their health orientations than Puerto Ricans reporting parochial group structures. These findings were consistent across all ethnic groups examined. From this he assumed support for the basic idea that group structures influence medical orientations.

One significant shortcoming in this research was the limited measurement of medical behavior. Although usual sources of care (defined as private or public at time of first contact) and health status were examined, no data were collected on the frequency of use of medical services. This created a problem for the model because the hypothesized connection of the social group and medical orientation variables with source of care proved to be inconsistent, and was probably influenced more by socioeconomic status than by the study variables.

REACTIONS TO THE SUCHMAN MODEL

The potential implications of Suchman's research for the delivery of medical care soon drew attention to his work. Although his findings were frequently cited in the literature and usually accepted at face value, efforts to substantiate and at least partially replicate them were not published until 1973. One such study was conducted in Los Angeles, California (Reeder & Berkanovic, 1973). Although less diverse ethnically than Washington Heights, the study population did have a significant number of blacks and Mexican-Americans; however, unlike Suchman's study group, very few of these were foreign-born. The Los Angeles data collected in 1970 failed to support Suchman's data collected in 1960. As indicated by the researchers (Reeder & Berkanovic, 1973, p. 142): "where Suchman's parochials represented the least informed segments of the community, the parochials in our study may be the most knowledgeable about medical matters and, by virtue of living in ethnically exclusive enclaves, be the least skeptical about the medical care available to them."

Unfortunately, the findings are not as easily interpreted as the investigators suggest. Although Suchman's medical orientation variables were measured in identical fashion, the social group structures were not. Instead, they were assessed using questions that only partially resemble the questions used by Suchman (Reeder & Berkanovic, 1973, p. 137). The concept of "preferential parochialism" was substituted for family authority and tradition, and was measured by questions on the extent to which respondents preferred community members to be alike, opposed school desegregation, and resisted new ways of doing things. Exclusivity was defined as "behavioral parochialism," and was measured as participation in voluntary organizations within their local community and by engaging in shopping, visiting, and other activities within the community, but with no emphasis on ethnicity. Measures of friendship solidarity (rephrased as "perceptual parochialism") were likewise different and were based on questions about whether people in the community were similar to the respondent and whether the respondent thought of the community as a real home.

In the same year, McKinlay (1973) used Suchman's concepts of social group structure to examine help-seeking behavior. Although the study did not include measures of individual medical orientations, it did provide additional information on kinship and friendship networks as they relate to the utilization of health and welfare services. In this study the underutilizers were found to rely on a readily available network of friends and relatives as lay consultants before using the service. On the other hand, utilizers appeared to differentiate more between friends and relatives, and to be more independent of both in their decision to seek help. Although informative, these findings were not easily interpreted relative to Suchman's work.

AN ALTERNATIVE MODEL

The incomplete attempts at replicating Suchman's work, along with the diverse findings resulting from using substitute measures, raised questions as to its applicability in other populations. To reduce some of the growing confusion, an exact replication of the Suchman study was undertaken by researchers in Salt Lake City, Utah (Geertsen, Klauber, Rindflesh, Kane, & Gray, 1975). The Utah culture presented some interesting possibilities with respect to Suchman's proposed model due to the emphasis on both modern medicine and strong families. The Utah Mormons have always been told to abstain from tobacco and hard drinks and to use good health practices. Church-operated hospitals using modern medical technology were once widespread in Utah. Continued contacts with relatives and strong family ties facilitated through family reunions and genealogy records and frequent association with church members are promoted through various church programs and organizations such as neighborhood "wards" (O'Dea, 1964). Parochial group structures supporting rather than opposing modern medicine appeared to be a strong possibility in Utah. This population seemed well suited either to support Suchman's model or to provide further clarification of the suggested relationships. Interviews very similar to those used in New York were collected in 1969 from 535 randomly selected male and female heads of households in Salt Lake City. Suchman's exact questions for measuring the basic variables were used. Some new questions were added dealing with the actual use of health services, such as number of visits to a physician or outpatient clinic, number of visits to a dentist, and number of visits to other medical facilities during the previous year.

A comparison of the Salt Lake City and Washington Heights samples showed only slight variation in age and sex. Socioeconomic data revealed a higher overall social class standing for the Salt Lake sample, some of which was attributed to the later date at which the data were collected. As expected, sharp differences were observed in the ethnic and religious composition of the two samples. Whereas the Washington Heights sample consisted of 25% blacks, 27% Jews, 20% Catholics, and 9% Puerto Ricans many of whom (except for the blacks) were foreign-born, in Salt Lake City the sample was made up primarily of white nonethnics, whose families had lived in America for several generations, 70% of whom belonged to the Mormon religious faith. These differences were anticipated and considered to be useful in further testing the Suchman model (Geertsen *et al.*, 1975, p. 229).

Empirical Inconsistencies

An examination of the Utah data began to reveal discrepancies in how the variables were related in the two populations. Family authority was found to coincide with friendship solidarity but not with ethnic exclusivity. For medical orientations, individuals who scored low on knowledge of disease were not found to be more skeptical of medical care or to have a higher dependency in illness. However, the relationship between skepticism of medical care and dependency in illness was similar to that found by Suchman. Persons high on skepticism were also high on dependency. Further differences were uncovered when cross-tabulating social group variables with medical orientations. Whereas Suchman found that high family authority and strong friendship solidarity were related to low knowledge of disease, just the opposite was found in the Salt Lake City study. Likewise, family authority and friendship solidarity were found to be associated with low rather than high skepticism.

One modification in the Utah study was the substitution of actual utilization of health services for source of care. Only two of the six variables—family authority and knowledge of disease—were found to be associated with utilization regardless of the socioeconomic status of respondents. Friendship solidarity was found to be associated with utilization, but only among respondents of lower socioeconomic status.

The Utah study raised some concerns about Suchman's work. First, it questioned the validity of combining different levels of social group structure and different dimensions of medical orientation into summary measures of cosmopolitan–parochialism and scientific–popular health orientation. Second, the Utah data revealed that close and exclusive social ties could be associated with supportive orientations toward medical care.

Cultural Orientations

The comparative findings from the two studies produced an alternative explanation to that provided by Suchman. Cultural orientations were singled out as underlying factors in the use of medical services, with social group ties acting as intervening variables in this more basic relationship. Persons belonging to close and exclusive groups, especially tradition- and authority-oriented families, were considered to be (1) more likely to respond to a medical problem by seeking medical care if this was consistent with their culture beliefs and practices, or (2) less likely to seek medical care where cultural beliefs and practices emphasized skepticism and distrust. Using this alternative explanation and the apparent differences in the two studies, a new model of health care was proposed.

A simplified version of the Utah model is diagrammed in Figure 1. As indicated, the variables in the model are activated by the presence of some health condition or symptom(s) of possible illness. Subcultural orientations may have different influences depending on the nature of group ties. If group ties interlock as Suchman found, these ties will tend to strengthen the subcultural response. If group ties are weak or contain competing subcultural orientations, then the subcultural response will be weakened. Family authority, knowledge of disease, and friendship solidarity are singled out as the main intervening variables of those identified by Suchman. They influence medical behavior by helping to determine whether or not a health condition is interpreted as a health problem and by helping to identify appropriate forms of response to the problem. Yet these factors probably only have strong influences when they interlock with each other as well as with other social ties, and when all social relations support a particular cultural orientation.

OTHER POPULATION GROUPS

Gypsies

The Utah study raised questions concerning other population groups. The possibility of parochial group structures supporting rather than opposing the use of medical services was found to be true of Gypsies in Boston. Contrary to popular beliefs about Gypsies, Salloway (1973) found them to be very knowledgeable in finding their way through the hospital system. Most of this knowledgeability was traced to an extensive set of social ties with other Gypsies. Visits to health practitioners were found to be socially supported, with other Gypsies knowing what the suspected health problem was, how it was being treated, and how the affected family felt about the treatment received. In this regard the Gypsy culture emphasizes family authority and tradition and places severe restriction on relations with the *gadge* or outsiders who are considered to be *marime* or defiled (Kephart, 1987). This results in a strong ethnic identity corresponding to what Suchman calls ethnic exclusivity with a strong degree of ingroup solidarity. Yet these ties support the use of medical services.

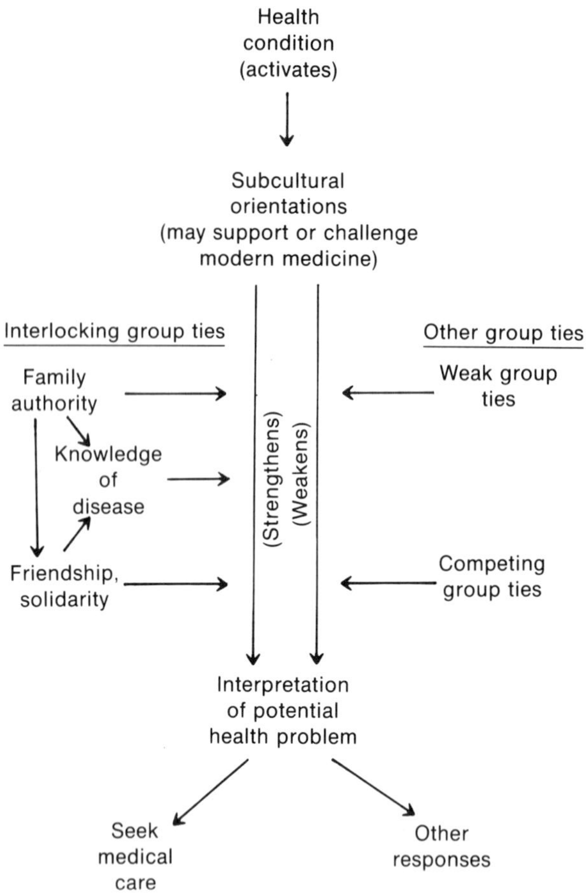

FIGURE 1. Simplified version of the Utah model.

Mexican-Americans

Farge (1978) examined the Suchman variables using identical measures among Hispanic-Americans in Houston. Positive associations were found among all three social group variables, consistent with the New York and Salt Lake City studies. But the link between family authority and friendship solidarity was weak. In Utah the weakest link was between family authority and ethnic exclusivity. For the medical orientation variables, the Houston results were closer to the Utah than the New York findings. Consistent with Utah, no relationship was found between knowledge of disease and dependency in illness. In Houston the association between knowledge and skepticism was opposite to that found in New York, whereas no association was found in Utah. The relationship between skepticism of care and dependency in illness was found to be even stronger in Houston than in the other two studies. Suchman's distinction between scientific and popular medical orientations clearly does not fit either of the other two populations. Unfortunately, due to the small sample size, the moderate relationships observed between several variables were not found to be statistically significant, and by focusing only on statistically significant relationships (which reflect sample size) rather than on the degree of observed association, Farge misinterpreted some of her findings relative to the Salt Lake City and New York populations.

The most important finding from the Houston study was the connection between social group structures and medical orientations. The findings again are opposite to those observed by Suchman. As in Utah, high family authority was found to be associated with more accurate knowledge of disease and lower skepticism of medical care. Similar though less pronounced associations were observed between friendship solidarity and these two variables. Although less clear, the relationships of ethnic exclusivity with knowledge and skepticism were found to come closer to the Utah findings than the New York findings. Unlike both the Utah and New York studies, dependency in illness was not found to be associated with family authority, friendship solidarity, or ethnic exclusivity.

Overall the Houston results reaffirm the underlying premise of the Utah model which maintains that close and exclusive group relationships can support, as well as inhibit, positive medical orientations. Unfortunately, no data on health service utilization were reported in the Houston study.

Early Conceptions. The greater knowledge and lower skepticism found among those with strong family ties raise questions about early conceptions of health care among Hispanics. Typically, early investigators (e.g., Saunders, 1954) wrote about the negative influences of Hispanic culture on the seeking and acceptance of modern medical care. Folk beliefs emphasizing magic and herbs, "nonscientific" healers such as curanderos and medicas with alternative treatments, and various rituals and attitudes of fatalism and skepticism were cited as obvious hindrances to modern medical care.

Nall and Speilberg (1967) were among the first to examine empirically the view that Mexican-American culture interfered with modern medicine. Folk beliefs, religious rituals, and use of folk curers were not found to be significantly related to acceptance or rejection of treatment for tuberculosis. Poor participation in the treatment regimen was associated more with family factors like being married and having relatives in the home, and with other factors like seeking advice from associates. On the other hand, the socially alienated were the most likely to accept treatment. All of the 53 subjects (a small sample size) in their study were residents of McAllen, Texas (rural, mostly unskilled). Others writing at about the same time reaffirmed the importance of the extended family in the delay or "last resort" orientation of Mexican-Americans toward Anglo medicine (Madsen, 1964; Rubel, 1966).

In the 1970s studies began to show contradictory findings on the relationship between family ties and use of medical services among Mexican-Americans. Some researchers (Hoppe & Heller, 1975; Quesada & Heller, 1977) reported better access to care where family ties were strong. Others (Welch, Comer, & Steinman, 1973) found no relationship between low utilization and integration within the ethnic subcommunity.

Changing Views. More recent data from general population surveys with greater urban representation, show utilization rates for Mexican-Americans to be very similar to those found in other population groups. One study (Andersen, Lewis, Giachello, Aday, & Chiu, 1981), using 1976 national survey data for the Southwest, found lower use of physician services among Mexican-Americans before making statistical adjustments for need and socioeconomic status. After adjustments, the differences nearly disappeared. The adjusted figures showed that 73% of the Hispanics saw a physician during the previous year compared with 76% of the total U.S. population. According to the authors, much of the difference in utilization was explained by younger age (need), lower income (SES), and lower insurance coverage, rather than by negative cultural orientations. A three-generation study in Texas conducted in 1985 (Markides, Levin, & Ray, 1985) confirms that Mexican-Americans do not underutilize physician services. This was found to hold for all three generations of family members residing in a 50-mile area.

The inconsistency in these findings seems to reflect the time period, research methods, and population characteristics of the groups studied. Earlier Hispanic studies focused on rural, homogeneous populations, used nonprobability samples, and were conducted prior to the full impact of Medicare and Medicaid.

Blacks

Sharp, Ross, and Cockerham's (1983) more recent study of blacks suggests that the attitudes of the economically disadvantaged have changed since the 1960s. Illinois health survey data for 1980 revealed an absence of skepticism toward the medical profession and a strong awareness of symptom seriousness among blacks. As Sharp *et al.* (1983) have indicated:

> We find a comparative lack of skepticism among Blacks and the less educated about visiting the doctor. In fact, the reverse seems true; these groups held attitudes and evaluated symptoms in such a way that would predispose them to use physician services when ill. These data support our original hypothesis that attitudes and beliefs among the less privileged no longer serve as barriers to utilization.

But this has not always been the case. Earlier studies document the lower rates of utilization and more negative attitudes toward physicians characteristic of blacks in the 1960s and early 1970s (Hines, 1972; Dutton, 1978).

Implications from Other Groups

Research on other population groups suggests that the parochial group influence detected by Suchman might change as cultural assimilation takes place. The immigrant and migrant composition of his study population accentuates the possible time element in the findings. Over one-third of the white ethnics were foreign-born. Many of the blacks were immigrants from the South (Lendt, 1960). Research on assimilation shows a general distrust of the dominant society and its institutions among recent immigrants from contrasting cultural backgrounds. The ingroup tendencies have also been observed as ways of easing the adjustment process as members find security through familiar customs and social support (Gordon, 1964). Suchman's data may thus be time bound and reflect the immigration and socioeconomic barriers to medical care that were still prevalent in the 1960s.

NETWORK APPROACHES TO SOCIAL GROUP STRUCTURE

Two questions always arise when examining earlier research. First, are the findings unique to the groups studied or do they apply generally to other population groups? Second, have the variables been measured properly or can they be better measured in some other way? Studies generated by Suchman's work have moved in both directions. The Utah and Houston studies addressed the first question but not the second; no answers were provided as to whether variables like family authority and tradition (1) were adequately measured or (2) represented the most important family variables in the utilization of health services.

Several other studies that were reactions to Suchman's work have, however, focused on the second question. These studies show the expanding influence of network analysis in sociology. As Wellman (1983) pointed out, network analysts "concentrate on studying how the pattern of ties in a network provides significant opportunities and constraints because it affects the access of people and institutions to such resources as information, wealth, and power." By using expanded measures of social group structure, these studies too have helped to redirect thinking and to open up new possibilities concerning the possible links among social groups, medical attitudes, and health behavior. Instead of focusing on certain limited aspects of family, friends, and ethnicity, attention has been broadened to include a variety of new dimensions in the study of social networks.

Measuring Social Networks

A recent example of this approach (Horwitz, Morgenstern, & Berkman, 1985) provides support for the basic contention of the Utah model. In a follow-up investigation of more than 500 children participating in a Yale pediatric study, the authors say: "These results are compatible with the conclusion of Geertsen *et al.* (Utah study) that extensive, tightly knit social groups are more likely to insure that the network members adopt the group's health norms." Their measurements of group structure, however, are different from those used by Suchman. Rather than looking at social group structure in terms of ethnic exclusivity, friendship solidarity, and family authority, they examined instead the size, density, intimacy, durability, geographic dispersion, and homogeneity of social contacts. For example, network size was measured by asking how many close friends and relatives each respondent had. They also asked how far away different network members lived. Several of their social network measures like size and geographical proximity were found to be positively correlated with yearly utilization rates. In seeking to explain these findings, the authors singled out the health beliefs of social networks, although they were unable to test this possibility fully due to insufficient information about the health beliefs of network members.

The network measures used by Horwitz *et al.* were derived from earlier research by Salloway and Dillon (1973) and McKinlay (1973). Salloway and Dillon measured social networks by asking respondents in a suburb of Boston about frequency of contact with friends and relatives (including telephone calls), and about expected support in the form of grocery shopping, house cleaning, and lending money. In this research, family networks were analyzed separately from friendship networks. The investigators hypothesized that family networks were more likely to be closed and close-knit with many interlocking ties, and would thus provide many alternatives to seeking outside help. Conversely, friendship networks were more likely to be open, with less mutual contact and sharing of ideas, and thus less likely to keep the individual from seeking outside help. In Suchman's terms, family networks were hypothesized to be more parochial and friendship networks more cosmopolitan. Though not conclusive, the findings of Horwitz *et al.* showed that friend and family networks might operate in opposite ways in terms of delay in the use of health services (friends less delay, family more delay). The differences, however, were very small.

A similar approach was used by McKinlay (1973), but his sample was confined to lower class families. He measured kinship networks using proximity of relatives, frequency of interaction, places of usual visits, and ages of relatives. Friendship networks were examined in a similar way, except that duration of friendship was substituted for places of usual visits. The expanded measures allowed greater precision in the examination of network composition. In this lower class sample, delay and underutilization of prenatal care were found to be most common among those with strong, undifferentiated network ties among relatives and friends. In other words, for this group friends tended to be family friends, and the family and friendship networks tended to be strong and to interlock. On the other hand, utilizers tended to have weaker family ties, and where friendships were strong, they tended to have no independent linkages to family members other than through the respondent. Even more important was McKinlay's analysis of advice seeking. He asked respondents about which persons they consulted on problems like sickness, pregnancy, and finances. The persons who utilized services were found to seek advice less, and when they did it was from friends and husbands. In contrast, persons who underutilized services consulted more and used a wider variety of readily available friends and relatives, especially mothers. Other research (Birkel & Reppucci, 1983) on network ties, but not dealing specifically with health problems, confirms the network influence among lower class respondents. Overall network density, measured by the extent to which network members maintained contacts with one another independently of the respondent, was negatively correlated (−.49) with child-rearing consultations. Of special interest is their finding that self-competence, measured by self-ratings, can modify network influences. Women with low competence in high-density networks sought consultation the most, whereas women with low competence in low-density networks sought consultation the least.

Longitudinal Dimension of Social Networks

In the 1980s more advanced statistical and methodological procedures have been applied using even broader measures of social networks. Efforts have been made to overcome the limitations of using single-point data collection based on respondent recall since this makes causal analysis very difficult. This is particularly true with behavior like visiting a physician which is not likely to be influenced by attitudes or group structures in the absence of some specific illness episode or persistent health problem. This difficulty is reaffirmed by Mechanic's (1979) observation that attitudes *alone* do not greatly influence utilization.

One way to overcome these limitations is to examine multiple factors within a panel design using regression techniques. A series of such studies was undertaken by Berkanovic and others in Los Angeles (Berkanovic, Telesky, & Reeder, 1981). In these studies 1210 individuals were contacted and reinterviewed every 6 weeks over a 12-month period. Of that number 769 reported some health problem during the year. With such periodic contacts, the investigators were able to determine which persons sought medical help in response to actual symptoms. Multiple indicators of need, sociodemographics, access to care, social networks, and health orientations were examined using regression techniques to sort out the relative influences of different variables on seeking medical care. Of special interest are the two different types of network measurements used in the studies. First, a factor analysis was performed on information obtained at the beginning of the study on general network ties. This revealed three clusters: contact or physical closeness, consultation with others on health matters, and support from others in various situations of need. Second, information was obtained concerning the actual use of social networks during the year when real symptoms were experienced. No factor analysis was performed on the second type of information. Medical orientations were also obtained in both ways; that is, one set of measures was obtained during the first interview dealing with general orientations, and another set of symptom-specific measures was gathered as illness episodes were uncovered through repeated interviews.

In the first of these studies (Berkanovic *et al.*, 1981), all of the variables were combined in a regression model which was able to account for 57% of the variance in the initial decision to seek medical help. Of this amount, need factors accounted for 12%. General network contact and general network support added small though statistically significant amounts to the variance explained. Respondents with frequent general contact and consultation with network members were *less* likely to see a doctor than those with less frequent contact and consultation. However, those reporting high general network support were *more* likely to see a doctor than those with low support. Most important, however, was the finding that over 40% of the variance was accounted for by symptom-specific network contacts and medical orientations. Network advice about seeing a doctor, perceived seriousness of symptoms, and especially perceived efficacy of care (Suchman's skepticism measured in the opposite direction) were found to be key predictor variables in the decision to seek help. It should be noted that the dependent variable involved only the initial decision to see a doctor and did not include follow-up visits.

The findings of this first study reveal inconsistent and relatively weak influences of general network factors such as contact and support on the seeking of medical care. Yet, they show that network advice is very influential when it concerns specific symptoms of possible illness. Likewise, attitude-specific responses to actual symptoms are much more influential than general orientations such as Suchman's knowledge of disease. These findings, emphasizing the importance of medical need and the interaction between symptoms and attitudes, are reaffirmed in other studies. A review of the utilization literature by Hulka and Wheat (1985, p. 455) emphasizes that "health status is the most important determinant of utilization." Sharp *et al.* (1983) also concluded that general attitudes alone do not predict utilization, but the combination of having symptoms and evaluating them as serious does have a substantial effect on utilization behavior. These findings are consistent with the Utah model emphasis on a health problem as the most specific and direct influence on utilization behavior.

Network Advice

The second in the series of studies by Berkanovic and Telesky (1982) added a new dimension to the attitude–network question. Cases were examined where specific network advice to see a doctor was either congruent or incongruent with personal beliefs about the seriousness of symptoms. It should be noted, however, that none of their respondents reported being advised *not* to see a doctor, so networks operated either by withholding advice or by giving positive advice to seek help. They found that persons who considered the symptom to be serious were much more likely to see a doctor (85.6%) if network members also advised this action than if no advice was received (65.2%). Where symptoms were not considered to be serious, those receiving network advice to see a doctor were much more likely to visit the doctor (49.3%) than where no such advice was received (13.4%). However, of special interest is their finding that "when the network advises seeking care but beliefs do not support this behavior, fewer individuals actually seek care than in the other incongruent condition" (p. 1026). The other incongruent condition consisted of no network advice to seek care but beliefs that supported care. Unlike the first study, general network characteristics (contact, consulting, support) were found to have a noticeable influence in situations where network advice contradicted what the individual personally believed. This finding pointed to the possible contingent nature of network influences. In this case the more general and enduring network factors seemed to exert their greatest influence when informational conflicts were present in the immediate situation. This raised the possibility that the direction of network influences might also be contingent on the sociocultural backgrounds of individuals and networks as suggested in the Utah model. Because the sociocultural dimension was ignored in the first two studies, a third study was undertaken.

Sociocultural Variables

In the third of their studies, Berkanovic and Telesky (1985) tried to correct their oversight of sociocultural factors by reexamining their findings among subgroups of blacks, Mexican-Americans, and whites. Again it should be noted that negative cultural orientations resulting in advice not to seek professional care were missing in the study population. Although small subsample sizes hampered their analysis (193 for Mexican-Americans and 100 for blacks), ethnicity was still found to be potentially important through its interactions with networks and cognitive orientations. For example, general health orientations were found to be influential in the decision of blacks to seek medical care but not in the decision of whites or Mexican-Americans to do so. Likewise, network advice was more influential in the decision to seek care among whites and Mexican-Americans than among blacks, while having a regular source of care was much more important in this decision for blacks than for whites and Mexican-Americans. These and other differences emphasize the potential importance of cultural differences. According to Berkanovic and Telesky (1985):

> The present analysis suggests that the failure of the social networks and health orientations to contribute to the variance explained in the main effects analysis was due, in part, to heterogeneity among the Whites in the sample. As was suggested at the outset of this paper, the Whites are drawn from many diverse ethnic groups. Hence, contradictory tendencies among them would be expected. However, the present analysis also indicates that ethnicity plays a role in determining responses to illnesses through its interaction with networks and cognitive orientations. Thus, Black-Americans and Mexican-Americans, the two distinguishable ethnic groups in this analysis, differ both from each other and from the Whites with respect to the variables that predict the reporting of illnesses, disability and the decision to seek medical care.

In other words, social network ties may have very different influences on individual behavior depending on the particular sociocultural background and the extent to which it is shared by other network members.

It is becoming increasingly apparent that subcultural variations exist within particular network configurations. Furthermore, the direction of the network influence can shift as sociocultural change takes place. As this is gaining wider recognition, Suchman's concepts continue to be applied to a wider variety of related problems. Fox and Storms (1981) tried to untangle some of the inconsistencies in research on health care satisfaction by using Suchman's approach to health orientations. Others have been using his concepts to better understand seeking help from public authorities (Nelson, 1980), health care in developing countries (Kroeger, 1983), and consumer health self-care (Green, Werlin, Schauffler, & Avery, 1977).

PROBLEMS AND IMPLICATIONS

Social Networks

The investigation of how the organization of social relationships and group ties affects medical attitudes and behavior continues to be an active question in the field of medical sociology. From Freidson's "lay referral system" and Suchman's "cosmopolitan–parochial" group structures, research has grown to include a variety of other dimensions in the analysis of social networks. However, the influence of social networks is more diverse and complicated than originally recognized. First, network structures do influence health behavior. But contrary to Suchman's prediction, this influence can support as well as inhibit the seeking of help, depending on the sociocultural background shared by the individual and other network members. One major shortcoming in research has been a lack of specific measurements of the beliefs and orientations of network members.

Second, network influences are stronger when direct advice is sought from network members rather than generally implied through past contacts, but the influence of network structure in this process is still unclear. It is apparent that network advice is more likely to result in a specific response to seeking or avoiding care when it relates to an individual's immediate symptom experience.

Third, the influence of social networks may vary according to individual cognitions. Of particular interest is the increased importance of general network structures when personal belief and network advice are incongruent. This observation raises questions regarding possible network influences under other forms of incongruence within Suchman's model, such as high knowledge of disease combined with skepticism of care. Also, increased sensitivity to networks among persons with a low sense of competence introduces the dimension of self-concept in a way that helps to broaden our understanding of potential network influences.

Fourth, social networks are multidimensional and appear to contain contradicting influences in the seeking of help. For example, there is evidence in the research cited that family networks and friendship networks may influence individuals in different ways depending on their relative density, autonomy, and frequency of use. Large network size and frequent contact do not necessarily mean network support. These two types of network variables seem to influence behavior in opposite directions. To complicate things further, additional research (Schaefer, Coyne, & Lazarus, 1981) suggests that social support is not a unitary concept. Clearly Suchman's social group measures only partially tap the complexities associated with social networks and the potential implications of group ties. The network literature offers many other dimensions that have yet to be examined in relation to social ties and how they might influence health behavior (Pilisuk & Froland, 1978). Within specific networks, other dimensions such as symmetry, intensity, and intimacy need to be added to the dimensions such as frequency, proximity, and duration of ties that have typically been examined. In terms of overall network structure, clustering, dispersion, homogeneity, and density deserve further attention. Although Suchman's measures imply some of these dimensions, they lack precision and specificity.

Finally, a neglected area in the network and health behavior research is the person's location within these networks. Persons occupying central positions within large, dense, closed networks are more likely to be influenced by network values and norms and to experience greater demands for their continued performance than less involved members on the fringe. Yet larger network size increases the likelihood of role substitutes who can take over in time of need, thus reducing pressures to perform. These and other cross pressures related to a person's network location deserve attention.

Research Problems

Several weaknesses in research methods are apparent from the studies examined. One concerns sample selection and the measurement of cultural orientations. Most studies have attributed certain cultural orientations to particular ethnic and religious groups. Recent studies showing new attitudes and cultural outlooks among Mexican-Americans and blacks question the validity of such global indicators. The problem is particularly troublesome in large cross-sectional studies where persons are treated as being culturally similar due to ethnicity or race, without adequate empirical verification. Better indicators of cultural background are needed.

A second problem comes from the potential unreliability of self-reported data. Nearly all of the research has measured variables through respondent recall after the utilization behaviors have taken place. The possibility of behavior influencing recall through increased sensitivity cannot be dismissed. The panel design used by Berkanovic *et al.* (1981) reduces part of the problem by shortening the time span in recall but potential biases still remain. There is always the danger of responses reflecting justifications for action rather than actual circumstances. Where possible, independent sources of verification are needed. For example, a respondent's estimates of network contact need to be compared with estimates of such contact made by other network members.

The variability in utilization behavior and its contingency on medical need is also problematic. People visit doctors for a wide variety of reasons. Some visits are initiated in response to acute episodes while others are made as part of the management of chronic, long-term conditions. In either case, individuals may appear to be high users of health services, yet the frequency of their visits may fall short of what doctors expect. Some individuals may dislike going to the doctor and still be frequent utilizers due to the severity of their health conditions. Those visiting the doctor frequently may also be poor compliers in treatment programs. Still others may visit doctors for preventive measures or for a variety of other reasons such as family or personal stress. This variability is reflected in the studies which have closely examined Suchman's work. Part of the inconsistency in the findings emerging from network research is no doubt attributable to the diverse outcome measures employed. Utilization has been defined and measured in terms of source of care, total number of visits, acute episode visits, delay in seeking care, and participation in specific treatment programs. Some studies have ignored utilization completely and looked only at attitudes. Network influences may be stronger for some types of utilization than for others, but this is hard to untangle due to wide variations in study samples and measurements used.

REFERENCES

Andersen, R., Lewis, S. Z., Giachello, A. L., Aday, L. A., & Chiu, G. (1981). Access to medical care among the Hispanic population of the southwestern United States. *Journal of Health and Social Behavior, 22,* 78–89.

Berkanovic, E., & Telesky, C. (1982). Social networks, beliefs, and the decision to seek medical care: An analysis of congruent and incongruent patterns. *Medical Care, 20,* 1018–1026.

Berkanovic, E., & Telesky, C. (1985). Mexican-American, Black-American and White-American differences in reporting illnesses, disability and physician visits for illness. *Social Science and Medicine, 20,* 567–577.

Berkanovic, E., Telesky, C., & Reeder, S. (1981). Structural and social psychological factors in the decision to seek medical care for symptoms. *Medical Care, 19,* 693–709.

Birkel, R. C., & Reppucci, N. D. (1983). Social networks, information seeking, and the utilization of services. *American Journal of Community Psychology, 11,* 185–205.

Bloom, S. W. (1963). *The doctor and his patient.* New York: Free Press.

Brown, E. L. (1964). *Newer dimensions of patient care. Part 3: Patients as people.* New York: Russell Sage Foundation.

Cockerham, W. C. (1986). *Medical sociology.* Englewood Cliffs, NJ: Prentice–Hall.

Dutton, D. B. (1978). Explaining the low use of health services by the poor: Costs, attitudes, or delivery systems. *American Sociological Review, 43,* 348–368.

Farge, E. J. (1978). Medical orientation among a Mexican-American population: An old and a new model reviewed. *Social Science and Medicine, 12,* 277–282.

Fox, J. G., & Storms, D. M. (1981). A different approach to sociodemographic predictors of satisfaction with health care. *Social Science and Medicine, 15A,* 557–564.

Freidson, E. (1960). Client control of medical practice. *American Journal of Sociology, 65,* 374–382.

Geertsen, R., Klauber, M. R., Rindflesh, M., Kane, R. L., & Gray, R. (1975). A re-examination of Suchman's views on social factors in health care utilization. *Journal of Health and Social Behavior, 16,* 226–237.

Gordon, M. M. (1964). *Assimilation in American life.* London: Oxford University Press.

Green, L. W., Werlin, S. H., Schauffler, H. H., & Avery, C. H. (1977). Research and demonstration issues in self-care. *Health Education Monographs, 5,* 161–189.

Hines, R. (1972). The health status of black Americans: Changing perspectives. In E. Jaco (Ed.), *Patients, physicians and illness* (pp. 40–50). New York: Free Press.

Hoppe, S. K., & Heller, P. L. (1975). Alienation, familism, and the utilization of health services by Mexican Americans. *Journal of Health and Social Behavior, 16,* 304–314.

Horwitz, S. M., Morgenstern, H., & Berkman, L. F. (1985). The impact of social stressors and social networks on pediatric medical care use. *Medical Care, 23,* 946–959.

Hulka, B. S., & Wheat, J. R. (1985). Patterns of utilization: The patient perspective. *Medical Care, 23,* 438–460.

Kanter, R. M. (1968). Commitment and social organization: A study of commitment mechanisms in utopian communities. *American Sociological Review, 33,* 499–517.

Kephart, W. M. (1987). *Extraordinary groups.* New York: St. Martin's Press.

King, S. H. (1962). *Perceptions of illness and medical practice.* New York: Russell Sage Foundation.

Koos, E. (1954). *The health of Regionville.* New York: Columbia University Press.

Kroeger, A. (1983). Anthropological and socio-medical health care in developing countries. *Social Science and Medicine, 17,* 147–161.

Lendt, L. A. (1960). *A social history of Washington Heights, New York City.* New York: Columbia–Washington Heights Community Mental Health Project.

Lipton, J. A., & Marbach, J. J. (1984). Ethnicity and the pain experience. *Social Science and Medicine, 19,* 1279–1298.

Madsen, W. (1964). *Mexican Americans of south Texas.* Chicago: Holt, Rinehart & Winston.

Markides, K. S., Levin, J. S., & Ray, L. A. (1985). Determinants of physician utilization among Mexican Americans: A three generation study. *Medical Care, 23,* 236–246.

McKinlay, J. B. (1973). Social networks, lay consultation and help-seeking behavior. *Social Forces, 51,* 275–292.

Mechanic, D. (1979). Correlates of physician utilization: Why do major multivariate studies of physician utilization find trivial psychosocial and organizational effects. *Journal of Health and Social Behavior, 20,* 387–396.

Nall, F. C., & Speilberg, J. (1967). Social and cultural factors in the responses of Mexican-Americans to medical treatment. *Journal of Health and Social Behavior, 8,* 299–308.

Nelson, B. J. (1980). Help-seeking from public authorities: Who arrives at the agency door? *Policy Sciences, 12,* 175–192.

O'Dea, T. F. (1964). *The Mormons.* Chicago: University of Chicago Press.

Parsons, T. (1951). *The social system.* Glencoe, IL: Free Press.

Parsons, T., & Shils, E. A. (Eds.). (1962). *Toward a general theory of action.* New York: Harper & Row.

Pilisuk, M., & Froland, C. (1978). Kinship, social networks, social support and health. *Social Science and Medicine, 12B,* 273–280.

Quesada, G. M., & Heller, P. L. (1977). Sociocultural barriers to medical care among Mexican Americans in Texas. *Medical Care, 15* (Suppl.), 93–101.

Reeder, L. G., & Berkanovic, E. (1973). Sociological concomitants of health orientations: A partial replication of Suchman. *Journal of Health and Social Behavior, 14,* 134–143.

Rubel, A. J. (1966). *Across the tracks: Mexican Americans in a Texas city.* Austin: University of Texas Press.

Salloway, J. (1973). Medical utilization among urban gypsies. *Urban Anthropology, 2,* 113–126.

Salloway, J. C., & Dillon, P. B. (1973). A comparison of family networks and friend networks in health care utilization. *Journal of Comparative Family Studies, 4*(Special Issue), 131–142.

Saunders, L. (1954). *Cultural difference and medical care.* New York: Russell Sage Foundation.

Schaefer, C., Coyne, J. C., & Lazarus, R. S. (1981). The health-related functions of social support. *Journal of Behavioral Medicine, 4,* 381–405.

Sharp, K., Ross, C. E., & Cockerham, W. C. (1983). Symptoms, beliefs, and the use of physician services among the disadvantaged. *Journal of Health and Social Behavior, 24,* 255–263.

Suchman, E. A. (1964). Sociomedical variations among ethnic groups. *American Journal of Sociology, 70,* 319–331.

Suchman, E. A. (1965). Social patterns of illness and medical care. *Journal of Health and Human Behavior, 6,* 2–16.

Welch, S., Comer, J., & Steinman, M. (1973). Some social and attitudinal correlates of health care among Mexican Americans. *Journal of Health and Social Behavior, 14,* 205–213.

Wellman, B. (1983). Network analysis: Some basic principles. In R. Collins (ed.), *Sociological theory* (pp. 155–179). San Francisco: Jossey–Bass.
Zborowski, M. (1952). Cultural components in response to pain. *Journal of Social Issues, 8,* 16–30.
Zola, I. (1966). Culture and symptoms—An analysis of patients' presenting complaints. *American Sociological Review, 31,* 615–630.

CHAPTER 8

Social Supports, Social Networks, and Health Behaviors

Christian Ritter

INTRODUCTION

The purpose of this chapter is to examine some of the recent work that has bearing on the relationship between social supports, social networks, and health behavior. It is not intended to provide an exhaustive review of the literature in any of these areas. Nor is the purpose to propose a conceptual model that can then be applied to a variety of health behaviors. Instead, this chapter will identify methodological problems and conceptual concerns that have not been adequately dealt with in the area of health behavior research, and draw from the larger literature on social supports and social networks in an attempt to add clarity to this area of research. A major goal of the chapter then is to provide a research agenda for better understanding the nature of the relationship between social ties and health behaviors.

This goal will be achieved by beginning with a general review of the literature on social supports and social networks and their relationship to health status, followed by a discussion of the differences between social supports and social networks and the implications of such differences. After this, specific research efforts assessing the relationship between social ties and health behaviors will be critically reviewed. The chapter then considers the mechanisms proposed to explain these relationship differences in health behavior and health status. Finally, future directions for the field will be considered in the light of the evidence reviewed.

The basic premise of this chapter is that in order to understand specific behaviors such as health-promoting behaviors, it is essential to situate the behavior conceptually within the larger processes in which it is embedded. It is for this reason the chapter begins with a discussion of the more general question of how social ties are linked to health status. Once this issue is examined along with questions related to the theoretical and methodological advantages of concept clarification and precision of measurement, any insights can then be applied to the more specific area of health behavior.

In the sections which follow, research will be reviewed with an eye toward what can be gleaned from prior conceptualization of social networks and their effects on health. The

CHRISTIAN RITTER • Department of Sociology and Anthropology, Kent State University, Kent, Ohio 44242-0001.

purpose is to provide a basis from which greater clarity of issues can be achieved in order to propose ways in which social networks research can specifically be applied to health behaviors.

SOCIAL SUPPORTS, SOCIAL NETWORKS, AND HEALTH STATUS

The positive effects of social supports have been widely researched. As Berkman (1984) stated, no other risk factor has recently gained so much continued attention so rapidly. There is much evidence to support the notion that social supports are related to good health and well-being. Early work indicated that social supports have a direct positive effect on health status as well as an indirect effect through moderating the impact of stress on mental and physical health (Broadhead *et al.*, 1983; Cassel, 1976; Cobb, 1976; Kaplan, Cassel, & Gore, 1977).

Studies have demonstrated that social supports are directly related to psychiatric symptomatology (Andrews, Tennant, Hewson, & Vaillant, 1978; Berkman & Syme, 1979; Billings & Moos, 1981; Goldberg, Van Natta, & Comstock, 1985; Henderson, Duncan-Jones, McAuley, & Ritchie, 1978; Lin, Ensel, Simeone, & Kuo, 1979; Thoits, 1982). A direct relationship has also been documented for physical health (Gore, 1978) and mortality (Berkman & Syme, 1979; Blazer, 1982; Gottlieb, 1981).

As buffers, social supports have been shown to moderate the relationship between life events and health. This type of relationship has been documented for psychological distress (Brown & Harris, 1978; Eaton, 1978; Turner, 1981; Winefield, 1979) and serum cholesterol levels (Gore, 1978).

However, beyond the evidence that persons with social supports are healthier than those without social supports, the relationship remains unclear. Some reasons for this lack of greater understanding have to do with how social support and social networks have been conceptualized (House & Kahn, 1984); other reasons have to do with how they are measured (cf. Wortman, 1984; Berkman, 1986).

Lack of Conceptual Clarity

The literature on social supports in health demonstrates a lack of clarity about what the term *social support* means. It has been used to designate a variety of different ways in which an individual is linked to others. This poses a problem in drawing general conclusions from comparisons of studies in which the term has been used in different ways.

For example, some approaches consider social support in terms of demographic or family-related factors such as marriage and living arrangements (Eaton, 1978). Others look at the general availability of social supports in terms of network involvement or social ties (i.e., Berkman & Syme, 1979). Neither of these approaches examines the specific source of the support. Yet it is important to know where the support is coming from within the context of interpersonal relationships, as well as to identify the different types of support that are available (Hirsch, 1981; Weiss, 1974).

Hirsch (1981) made the argument that social supports and social networks are best seen in conjunction with one another. He views social networks in terms of their relationship to coping activities. Behaviors related to coping take place within what Hirsch terms personal communities that support critical social identities. This perspective suggests that social supports and social networks may have distinct yet interrelated effects on health behaviors. Health behaviors may be affected most by certain individuals within the network who are providing specific types of support, and not by the network characteristics or by the role performance of that individual within the network. However, before such possibilities are considered, it is essential that the potential dimensions of social supports be further clarified.

The careful delineation of different types of network characteristics that are related to support is especially important as social supports and social networks have been shown to have different effects on morbidity and mortality (Berkman, 1984). By looking at supports and networks as separate concepts, one is able to determine their relative effects on health and health behaviors.

A primary reason for lack of clarity in findings related to the impact of networks on health is that social networks also tend to be too inaccurately conceptualized to allow for clear examination of all of the relevant processes (Hammer, 1983). Networks have been variously conceptualized as the number of contacts with friends and relatives (Henderson, Byrne, Duncan-Jones, Scott, & Adcock, 1980), perceived support from others (Lin *et al.*, 1979), or the availability of a confidant (Lowenthal & Haven, 1968). When attempts are made to look at the multiple dimensions of support, these are usually post hoc and include only a few imprecisely measured dimensions.

Social Supports, Social Networks, Social Ties: Conceptual Distinctions

The term *social supports* is often used to refer to general group characteristics: network size, network involvement, social ties, and supportive interpersonal relationships. This usage is misleading because it implies that all network characteristics are potentially supportive. Individuals with larger networks are assumed to have more social supports than those with smaller networks. Similarly, individuals who are married or who are living with another person are assumed to have more supports than single individuals or those who live alone. While social support is likely to be related to these network characteristics, it is equally likely that these network characteristics are independent of one another.

As awareness of the necessity of considering various dimensions of social supports and social networks grows, more care is being taken in the use of these concepts. Definitions are becoming increasingly precise and specific functions of each term are being more carefully delineated.

Social Ties. Social ties, or social linkages, is used to represent the general degree of, and nature of interpersonal contact and interaction. Social ties include both social networks and social supports.

A number of theories have been advanced about the functions of social ties (Brim, 1974; Caplan, 1974; Mitchell & Trickett, 1980; Weiss, 1969). Weiss, for example, identified six functions of social ties: intimacy, integration or belonging, opportunities for nurturant behavior, reassurance of worth, assistance and guidance, and advice. Berkman (1984) suggested that many of these theories overlap and asserted that the six major functions proposed by Weiss encompass the most important functions listed by the others. Walker, MacBride, and Vachon (1977) additionally suggested access to new contacts and diverse information.

Social Supports. Social supports are thus a part of social ties, but have a more precise and limited meaning. Social supports refer to interpersonal relationships that protect people from the negatives of stress (Kessler, Price, & Wortman, 1985). Although this is a useful definition of the concept, the nature, meaning, and measurement of social supports are widely debated in the literature.

Social supports can be classified according to whether they relate to *structural* or *functional* aspects of the relationship. Structural aspects of the relationship include: living arrangements, frequency of contact, participation in social activities, and involvement in social networks. Functional aspects include: emotional support, encouraging expression of feelings, provision of advice or information, provision of material aid (Kessler *et al.*, 1985).

House (1981) classified supportive behavior from others in terms of four general classes: emotional, appraisal, informational, and instrumental. Emotional support refers to feedback and affirmation. Informational support includes suggestions, advice, and information that one gets from others only. Instrumental support has to do with labor, money, and time that one can obtain from those with whom one affiliates.

In order to understand health behaviors and health status, it is necessary to look beyond social supports and to consider the broader social networks in which supports may or may not take place. The network approach provides a number of advantages including the delineation of social interactions in terms of a number of network characteristics. This would allow for more precise assessment of the context of interpersonal ties, as well as the number and frequency of interactions (Israel, 1982, 1985).

Social Networks. Mitchell (1969) defined social networks as having three dimensions: the structural, the interactional, and the functional. The structural dimension refers to the size, density, and interconnectiveness of specific linkages between individuals. The interactional dimension is more concerned with the nature of the relationship, the quality of interactions, and the degree of reciprocity of relationships to others. The functional dimension is, by definition, concerned with functions provided by various network numbers. These would include affective and instrumental functions, among them the development of new contacts and the maintenance of identity.

This view of networks describes and categorizes social relationships independently of whether they provide social support. The advantage of this approach over a "pure" support approach is that all linkages between one person and another are taken into account. This allows for categorizing all reported contacts and the associated web of social ties that surround an individual (Mitchell, 1969).

Wellman (1981) suggested that the network approach allows examination of the structure of relationships and how this influences the flow of resources through specific ties. The specific structural dimensions considered by Wellman include density and complexity, size, symmetry, reciprocity, geographic proximity or dispersion, homogeneity, and accessibility (Granovetter, 1973; Wellman, 1979, 1981). These structural aspects are examined along with the interaction dimensions of frequency, strength, intensity, and durability over time. Each of these properties can then be applied to a particular kind of network—such as family, friends, co-workers, and/or neighbors (Berkman, 1984).

Support and Networks Contrasted. Although there is certainly some overlap between social networks and social supports, social support is a distinct concept and should be treated as such. Social support refers to emotional, instrumental, and financial aid that is obtained from one's social network (House, 1981). It is, in effect, an exchange that actually takes place (Berkman, 1984). Thoits's (1982) refinement of Kaplan and colleagues' (1977) definition holds that support is the degree to which a person's basic social needs are gratified through interaction with others. Given these definitions, it is clear the social networks may or may not be supportive. In order to study situations under which individuals do and/or do not get support, it is necessary that we distinguish between these two concepts.

The distinction between social networks and social supports centers on the difference between the actual provision of and the potential availability of such aid. Research has shown that even within the area of social supports the perception of support does not have the same effects as the actual support received (Wethington & Kessler, 1986).

Social Supports, Social Networks, and Utilization

Health behavior research has systematically not examined the role of social supports *per se*. Instead, it has examined various aspects of social organization as they are related to help-seeking and the utilization of services.

Social networks have been found to influence a variety of health behaviors. Since Suchman's (1965) work, the influence of other persons and of social groups or networks on the decision to seek medical care has received research attention (Mitchell, 1969; Freidson, 1970; Geertsen, Klauber, Rindflesh, Kane, & Gray, 1975; Kadushin, 1969; McKinlay, 1973; Horwitz, 1978). Whether it be the positive effects of the role of family and friendship networks (McKinlay, 1973), the influence of lay referral systems (Freidson, 1970), the role of friends in providing connections to formal institutions (Kadushin, 1969), the general use of informal social networks (Horwitz, 1978), or the facilitating effect of friendship solidarity and strong family ties (Geertsen *et al.*, 1975), the utilization of services has consistently been shown to be affected by the health attitudes and norms of the network within which the individual is embedded.

Although there is consistent evidence that this relationship exists, very little is known about its specific nature or about the mechanism that links social networks to health behaviors. Relatively little effort has been made to address the nature of this relationship. Much of the earlier literature points to general cultural or subcultural influences of the groups in which the individual actor is embedded. Although groups are thereby shown to have influence on the behavior of the individuals, the nature of this influence and the associated networks of relationships are not made explicit.

The reasons for this lack of knowledge are conceptual and methodological. Lack of complete and precise conceptualization of the nature of the relationship between social networks and health behaviors has resulted in insufficient data gathering, and thus relatively little progress in defining the precise role played by network embeddedness in the use of health services.

Gottlieb (1981) and others have made progress in linking informal support structures with the utilization of formal services, areas which are usually looked at separately. His basic premise is that lay resources, as represented by social networks, provide informal, alternative structures of support (Gottlieb, 1981; Cassel, 1976; Caplan, 1974). Gottlieb suggests that various types of support are provided through informal groups. He argues that what has been previously conceptualized under the general category of "natural" support groups (as opposed to formal, public services) includes a variety of mutual help groups that are not always natural in that they are actively maintained and often deliberately planned and created by some layperson. These mutual help groups include neighborhood-based associations, as well as kin networks and primary group ties. Gottlieb posits that it is necessary to clarify what is meant by informal support structures and to develop terms that are more precise than natural support systems. Through this clarification of terminology we can then assess ways in which types of informal social supports differentially affect health and the utilization of formal services. Furthermore, we can assess how alternatives to formal services are organized through the initiation of informal mutual help groups.

Gottlieb's clarification suggests that the concept of social support needs to be considered in terms of three dimensions: social integration and participation, interaction in social networks that have particular structural properties, and access to a set of resources present in intimate peer relationships. These three dimensions of support, representing a range of levels of analysis from the "microprocesses" of intimacy to the macro-level phenomena of social integration, can then be examined in terms of their differential impact on the utilization of formal services.

Moreover, with this multidimensional framework of informal support systems, one can better understand the nature of the relationship between informal and formal support systems. Gottlieb suggests that this link is especially important in terms of the potential role of informal helpers in the delivery of services, whereby informal networks are used by health care practitioners to affect changes in the behavior of clients in regard to health maintenance.

For example, participation in cancer screening programs has been shown to be influenced by obtaining information from others (Sanson, Wakefield, & Pinnok, 1971; Howe, 1981; Gravell, Zapka, & Mamon, 1985). Partner support has also specifically been shown to have an effect upon cessation of smoking (Coppatelli & Orleans, 1985). The evidence suggests that the transmission of positive values toward medical care and the sharing of health-related knowledge is accomplished through social network interaction. In this sense social networks provide specific linkages that are used to interpret an individual's behavior and to provide cues to preventive behavior. Under the assumption that the social network is therefore the place to start in attempts to influence the health-promoting behavior of individuals, it has been suggested that interventions might well take the form of providing key network members with pertinent health-promoting information in an effort to stimulate informed discussion within social networks, thereby increasing the probability of preventive health behaviors (Gravell *et al.,* 1985).

SOCIAL TIES AND HEALTH STATUS

Although there is evidence to suggest that extensiveness and strength of social ties is related to positive mental and physical health, the specific mechanism for this relationship is unclear. This section of the chapter further discusses some of the explanations of why individuals who have relatively stronger or more extended social ties tend to be healthier than those who have relatively weaker or more constricted social ties. These explanations will then be considered in terms of their implications for the study of health behaviors.

Cohen and Syme (1985) suggested that social integration may have a direct effect on health status by encouraging health-promoting changes in behavior which in turn affect health status. They also suggest an alternative conceptualization in which social networks buffer the relationship between stress and health. Thoits (1983) argued that a variety of role involvements produce a sense of multiple identities (the consequence of enacting numerous role relationships) which gives greater purpose and meaning to one's life and thus reduces distress. Drawing from this position, Cohen and Syme suggested that healthful behaviors are facilitated by positive feedback from others. It is this positive feedback that leads to the adoption of both "appropriate" roles and healthful behaviors (Cassel, 1976; Hammer, 1983; Hirsch, 1981; Thoits, 1983).

Horwitz, Morgenstern, and Berkman (1985) provided some clarity about how social networks influence health behaviors. Drawing from the literature on the effects of stress on health, they proposed two alternative conceptualizations which can be empirically assessed. The first alternative considers the specific role of social networks as support systems that buffer against the potential harm of life changes, as sources of information, as resources, as shapers of beliefs and values, and so on (Cassel, 1976; Cobb, 1976; Gore, 1978; Kaplan *et al.,* 1977; Nuckolls, Cassel, & Kaplan, 1972). The second alternative considers social networks generally, or social supports specifically, in terms of their direct positive effect on health (Mueller, 1980; Berkman & Syme, 1979; Thoits, 1982).

Mechanisms of Influence

As Horwitz *et al.* (1985) stated, very little is known about which network characteristics affect health beliefs; nor about whether social networks are related to utilization through network beliefs, or through the level of adequacy of network support, or by the moderating network effect on health status, or some other determinant. Testing alternative conceptual models derived from more precisely defined and measured network characteristics and geared to specific types of health behaviors, or specific types of utilization, will certainly lead to progress in the field.

There is evidence that support systems serve to buffer against the potential harm of stress by affecting health beliefs. Horwitz *et al.* find that extensive, tightly knit social groups are more likely to ensure that network members adopt the group health norms. Once these health beliefs are shared, the individual members are more likely to use preventive health services because they have acquired the group's promedical health care beliefs, or less likely to use their services because they have acquired the group's antimedical health care beliefs. Although these results are similar to the conclusions reached by Geertsen *et al.* (1975), and certainly add clarity to the issues at hand, we are still left wondering how this transmission occurs. These findings are particularly troublesome because there is no specific information about what beliefs are held by the network members. As is often the case with other research in this area, it is assumed that extensive tightly knit networks have normative beliefs about health care, and that these beliefs are somehow transmitted to the individual network members.

In a more detailed review of potential resolutions to methodological and conceptual uncertainties, Berkman (1985) stated that we need to know how social networks "enter" the body to influence disease processes. In order to make progress in the field, we need to begin to sort out the specific role of social supports in their effect on health. Berkman suggested that to accomplish this goal it is necessary to (1) separate social networks from social supports, (2) sort out whether lack of social networks is a source of stress or serves to moderate the relationship between stress and health, (3) clarify the role of cultural expectations, and (4) sort out the pathway(s) between social support and health status.

Berkman suggested that social support probably affects health status by the advice and direct aid that it provides, by decreasing susceptibility to disease, and through health-promoting or health-hindering group influence. Specifically, she suggested that peer pressure may be an important factor determining whether one engages in health-promoting behaviors.

The focus on peer pressure makes explicit what has been implicitly suggested in prior research. Berkman and Syme (1979) observed some social networks to be associated with poor health practices: smoking, drinking, bad eating habits, obesity; as well as with the use of health services. Although these relationships were shown to exist, they have not been disentangled or really explained. As Hammer (1983) argued, there is little evidence for how the process works, nor does the evidence account for all of the effects of networks on health. It has also been suggested that social feedback processes should also be incorporated in any model in which people's health habits are predicted to be reinforced by others (Cassel, 1976).

Berkman proposed a number of ways in which social networks and social supports may be linked to disease and/or physical health in general. The first explanation is that social ties may provide advice, services, and access to new social contacts (cf. Gottlieb, 1981; Horwitz *et al.*, 1985). Individuals with particular network ties are more likely to be "successful" in obtaining medical care than are others who lack such ties. The transmission of promedical care values and knowledge also varies as a function of the social network to which one is tied. This explanation is similar to the hypothesis implicit in the early work on utilization of services by various ethnic groups (i.e., Suchman, 1965; Geertsen *et al.*, 1975)—that cues to action and the type of medical care sought are, in part, a function of the "cultural" beliefs of one's network; and furthermore that the knowledge of how to obtain formal medical services is related to the subsequent access to and the utilization of those services. It is the utilization of these services as a consequence of this knowledge that is related to better health care and better health.

The second explanation of how networks "enter" the process in improving physical health focuses on the specific health practices of the networks in which individuals are embedded. Some networks can be considered to be "healthier" than others. They are made up of persons who are in better health and who take better care of one another than are found in other networks. This care is provided either directly through the provision of instrumental aid, or through the provision of economic assistance which would allow one to achieve better physical health. In this model, the social network is considered the source of specific benefits that serve to improve health. Here the potential provision of health-enhancing services increases as a function of network size and density.

A third explanation advanced by Berkman (1984) looks specifically at the role that social integration plays in influencing behavior from a normative perspective. Instead of conceiving of network involvement as a source of information and promedical values or of a source of specific aid (economic and otherwise), Berkman suggested that social networks may also serve as a mechanism of social control whereby individuals are influenced by peer pressure. According to this alternative, individuals are influenced by social networks in that they often feel constrained to behave like the other members of their network. This perspective allows one to go beyond what is often an ephemeral "cultural" influence to a more specific conceptualization in terms of the influence that others exert through the norms of the group. Here the key research issue is to focus on the specific process whereby individual behavior is affected by the behavior of one's social networks or reference groups. This perspective is best suited for specifically assessing the role of health behaviors in the relationship between social network characteristics and health, and for sorting out the mechanism by which normative behaviors and associated group norms are transmitted to the individual and thereby influence the individual's health protective behaviors. These behaviors take a number of forms and are likely to have different origins within the general category of networks. Furthermore, these origins are likely to vary throughout the life course.

For example, health behaviors such as cigarette smoking, excessive use of alcohol, drug use, lack of physical activity, poor eating habits, lack of sleep, and excessive sleep are learned patterns that begin at various points in one's life and are differentially influenced by various members of the social groups to which one belongs. Throughout life, friends, family, neighbors, and co-workers have varying salience in terms of their influence on behaviors. Progress in understanding the relative effects of various group members on health behaviors is therefore in part related to when in the life cycle the health behaviors are studied, and how long the behaviors have been enacted. This is critical in order to help distinguish initiation from continuation, resumption, and discontinuation of various health behaviors.

The fourth possibility that Berkman put forward is that social networks may in fact alter biological risk factors such as blood pressure and serum cholesterol. Berkman argued that lack of ties may itself be a source of stress, created by not having sufficient social ties to provide for intimacy, or a sense of belonging, and the opportunity to provide as well as to receive nurturance. This possibility suggests that social networks directly affect susceptibility to illness (Antonovsky, 1972, 1974; Berkman & Syme, 1979; Cassel, 1976). Another possibility is that social networks may affect the course of many diseases through multiple physiological mechanisms, although these are not specified (Berkman, 1984). Regardless of the specific physiological mechanism that links social networks and health, this conceptualization has some relevance for the study of health behaviors. This approach directly suggests that life events that are related to a loss of social supports or a reduction in the number of social supports available would increase susceptibility to disease. It is also reasonable to suspect that individuals with larger and less restricted social networks would be less affected by such a loss and would therefore be less likely to be negatively affected by the loss because the total network configuration would be less at risk for being altered by the event.

It is equally possible that health behaviors themselves are affected by network losses. It is also possible that individuals who engage in protective health behaviors may be less vulnerable to the increased susceptibility resulting from either the ongoing lack of support from social ties or the loss of social supports.

FUTURE DIRECTIONS

In order to understand the mechanisms that link social supports, social networks, health behaviors, and health status, it is clear from this discussion that we must move beyond previous attempts to look only at component parts of these processes. Studies should consider changes in health behavior over time and include precise measures of supports and network characteristics and health status as they also change over time.

In addition, the influence of specific network members should be more carefully assessed. As has been discussed, advice from or influence of others may produce either positive or negative changes in health behaviors. For example, an individual may initiate health-risk behaviors, such as smoking, because the behavior is enacted by a significant other. However, the mechanisms by which others influence health behaviors are unclear.

In order to clarify the nature of the influence, specific aspects of potential influence must be considered. Models of decision making and attitude theory can help in specifying the influence of others in changing health behaviors. Most prominent of these models is the Fishbein and Ajzen model of behavioral intentions.

This model of behavior intentions (Fishbein & Ajzen, 1975; Ajzen & Fishbein, 1977) and revisions of the model have been applied to a number of behaviors that have health consequences. According to the model, behavior is the function of an individual's intention to perform the specific behavior. Intentions are in turn a function of attitudes toward the behavior and the subjective norm regarding the behavior. Attitudes or affective evaluations reflect beliefs about the consequences of behavior weighted by the subjective evaluation of the consequences. Subjective norms, or perceived general social norms concerning the behavior, are thought to reflect beliefs about the behavioral expectations of significant others, weighted by the motivation to conform to them, summed over all significant others (Liska, 1984). All other predictors of behavior operate indirectly through intentions to behave, either by affecting subjective norms or attitudes toward the behavior.

This model has been applied to a number of health behaviors (Oliver & Berger, 1979; Montano, 1986, Bentler & Speckart, 1981). Oliver and Berger (1979) and Montano (1986) applied the model to vaccinations; Bentler and Speckart considered its application to exercise, and to alcohol and drug use (Bentler & Speckart, 1979; Lacy, 1981). Although the results of these studies indicate that the original model developed by Fishbein and Ajzen does not always fit the data as well as alternative formulations, in each case subjective norms as measured by perceived normative expectations of significant others are shown to have a strong effect on the behaviors in question.

The advantage of this approach to the measure of group influence is that it can be applied to specific others in the individual's network or to groups of individuals such as friends or neighbors. Social influence is measured by the perception of whether others want an individual to behave in certain ways, and the individual's motivation to comply with these expectations. Although concepts such as peer pressure and partner support have been found to have significant effects on behavior in terms of smoking and alcohol use (i.e., Gottlieb & Baker, 1986; Coppatelli & Orleans, 1985), this conceptualization of the influence of others as providing subjective norms for behavior provides a clearer understanding of how individuals are affected by others. To conceive of others' influence as a perception of what is normative, and to measure these perceptions for specific target individuals or groups of individuals (i.e., friends, parents, neighbors), provides a well-defined link between group beliefs and values and individual behavior: individuals are in large part influenced by others to the degree that they are aware of the values and subsequent behavioral expectations held by others.

This approach would then allow for a specific assessment of which group or individual subjective norms have the greatest impact on specific health behaviors. The relative impact of peer versus family normative expectations on health-related behaviors is likely to vary over the life span with peer influence having greater salience during adolescence and the family having greater influence during childhood and adulthood. Additionally, certain health behaviors are probably more influenced by normative expectations than are others. Further, it is reasonable to expect that the effects of subjective norms would vary according to whether we are interested in predicting the initiation, discontinuation, or resumption of health-related behaviors. There is currently some indirect evidence to suggest that these processes are not equally predicted by the same factors. For example, Bentler and Speckart (1981) and Montano (1986) found that the effects of each of the components of the model are reduced when prior behavior or habit are included in the model predicting intentions to behave and subsequent behavior. These findings imply that it is essential to distinguish unique behaviors from ongoing behaviors that are resumed and discontinued over a period of months or years. It is not enough merely to control for prior behavior. Models must be developed that attempt to account for these diverse behavioral patterns.

The behavioral intention model can also be incorporated into more comprehensive models tailored to specific behaviors for subpopulations. Such subgroup analysis would clarify the relative influences of components of the models for types of health behaviors within various populations at risk. An important aspect of such specification would be to determine under which conditions social support and types of social ties have the greatest influence, and alternatively under which conditions they have little or no effect on health behaviors of interest.

Other future research might determine whether the relationship between social ties and health-promoting behaviors is linear. Although prior research has for the most part been carried out with the implicit assumption that good health and the probability of engaging in health-promoting behavior increases linearly as a function of increased social ties, larger social networks, and more social support, it is not clear that this is the case. It would be useful to identify at what point, if any, additional support does not add to positive health status and whether there is a point at which too much support is related to negative health status by producing a "smothering" effect.

Finally, future research should look at the effect of role transitions (i.e., marriage, employment, retirement, divorces) as they produce changes in social networks and supports, and ultimately changes in health behaviors and health status. Role transitions that affect network configuration and are related to a loss of support may well increase psychological distress which then leads to a change in health behaviors which is subsequently related to changes in health status. At present we can only speculate as to the nature and strength of these relationships.

In addition to the need for increased conceptual clarification, research addressing social ties and health behaviors and health status would benefit from, as has been suggested here and elsewhere, increased methodological precision and rigor. Advances in this area would include: more sophisticated measures of social networks and social supports (cf. Marsden, 1987; Burt & Minor, 1983); behavioral measures of social support (House & Kahn, 1984; Kessler *et al.*, 1985); the use of heterogeneous populations with regard to key variables from high- and low-risk categories; adjustment for physical health to sort out the direction of the relationship between social ties and morbidity (Berkman, 1986); and the use of longitudinal data with measures at multiple points in time.

Incorporating these data requirements in prospective studies of numerous specific health behaviors, and collecting data that are clearly derived from theory, will hasten progress in increasing understanding of the relationship between social ties and health behaviors. Failure to incorporate theoretical clarity and methodological refinements in future studies of these processes will only serve to reify many dubious assumptions about these relationships.

REFERENCES

Ajzen, T., & Fishbein, M. (1977). Attitude–behavior relations: A theoretical analysis and review of empirical research. *Psychological Bulletin, 84,* 888–918.

Andrews, G., Tennant, C., Hewson, D. M., & Vaillant, G. E. (1978). Life event stress, social support, coping style, and risk of psychological impairment. *Journal of Nervous and Mental Diseases, 116,* 307–316.

Antonovsky, A. (1972). Breakdown: A needed fourth step in the conceptual armamentarium of modern medicine. *Social Science and Medicine, 6,* 537–544.

Antonovsky, A. (1974). Conceptual, methodological problems in the study of resistance resources and stressful life events. In B. S. Dohrenwend & B. P. Dohrenwend (Eds.), *Stressful life events: Their nature and effects* (pp. 245–259). New York: Wiley.

Bentler, P. M., & Speckart, G. (1979). Models of attitude–behavior relations. *Psychological Review, 86,* 452–464.

Bentler, P. M., & Speckart, G. (1981). Attitudes cause behavior: A structural equation analysis. *Journal of Personality and Social Psychology, 40,* 226–238.

Berkman, L. F. (1984). Assessing the physical health effects of social networks and social support. *Annual Review of Public Health, 5,* 413–432.

Berkman, L. F. (1986). Social networks, support, and health: Taking the next step forward. *American Journal of Epidemiology, 123,* 559–562.

Berkman, L. F., & Syme, S. L. (1979). Social networks, host resistance and mortality: A nine year follow-up study of Alameda County residents. *American Journal of Epidemiology, 109,* 186–204.

Billings, A. G., & Moos, R. H. (1981). The role of coping responses and social responses in attenuating the impact of stressful life events. *Journal of Behavioral Medicine, 4,* 139–157.

Blazer, D. G. (1982). Social support and mortality in an elderly community population. *American Journal of Epidemiology, 115,* 684–694.

Brim, J. (1974). Social network correlates of avowed happiness. *Journal of Nervous and Mental Diseases, 158,* 432–439.

Broadhead, W. E., Kaplan, B. H., James, S. A., Wagner, E. H., Schoenbach, V. J., Grimson, R., Heyden, S., Tibblin, G., & Gehlback, S. H. (1983). The epidemiological evidence for a relationship between social support and health. *American Journal of Epidemiology, 117,* 521–537.

Brown, G. W., & Harris, T. O. (1978). *Social origins of depression: A study of psychiatric disorder in women.* New York: Free Press.

Burt, R. S., & Minor, M. S. (1983). *Applied network analysis.* Beverly Hills: Sage.

Caplan, G. (1974). *Social systems and community mental health.* New York: Behavioral Publishers.

Cassel, J. (1976). The contribution of social environment to host resistance. *American Journal of Epidemiology, 104,* 107–123.

Cobb, S. (1976). Social support as a moderator of life stress. *Psychosomatic Medicine, 15* (5, Suppl.), 47–57.

Cohen, C., & Syme, S. L. (1985). *Social support and health*. New York: Academic Press.
Coppatelli, H. C., & Orleans, C. T. (1985). Partner support and other determinants of smoking cessation maintenance among women. *Journal of Consulting and Clinical Psychology, 53,* 455–460.
Eaton, W. W. (1978). Life events, social supports and psychiatric symptoms: A reanalysis of the New Haven data. *Journal of Health and Social Behavior, 19,* 230–234.
Fishbein, M., and Ajzen, I. (1975). *Beliefs, attitudes, intentions and behavior: An introduction to theory and research*. Reading, MA: Addison–Wesley.
Freidson, E. (1970). *Profession of medicine*. New York: Dodd, Mead.
Geertsen, R., Klauber, M. R., Rindflesh, M., Kane, R. L., & Gray, R. (1975). A re-examination of Suchman's views on social factors in health care utilization. *Journal of Health and Social Behavior, 16,* 226–237.
Goldberg, E. L., Van Natta, P., & Comstock, G. W. (1985). Depressive symptoms, social networks and social support of elderly women. *American Journal of Epidemiology, 121,* 448–456.
Gottlieb, B. H. (1981). Social networks and social support in community mental health. In B. H. Gottlieb (Ed.), *Social networks and social support* (pp. 11–42). Beverly Hills: Sage.
Gottlieb, N. H., & Baker, J. A. (1986). The relative influence of health beliefs, parental and peer behaviors and exercise program participation on smoking, alcohol use and physical activity. *Social Science and Medicine, 22,* 915–927.
Gore, S. (1978). The effect of social support in moderating the health consequences of unemployment. *Journal of Health and Social Behavior, 17,* 157–165.
Granovetter, M. (1973). The strength of weak ties. *American Journal of Sociology, 78,* 1360–1380.
Gravell, J., Zapka, J. G., & Mamon, J. A. (1985). Impact of breast self-examination planned educational messages on social network communications: An exploratory study. *Health Education Quarterly, 12,* 51–64.
Hammer, M. (1983). Core and extended social networks in relation to health and illness. *Social Science and Medicine, 17,* 405–411.
Henderson, S., Byrne, D. G., Duncan-Jones, P., Scott, R., & Adcock, S. (1980). Social relationships, adversity, and neurosis: A study of associations in a general population sample. *British Journal of Psychiatry, 136,* 574–583.
Henderson, S., Duncan-Jones, P., McAuley, M., & Ritchie, K. (1978). The patient's primary group. *British Journal of Psychiatry, 132,* 74–86.
Hirsch, B. J. (1981). Social network and the coping process: Creating personal communities. In B. H. Gottlieb (Ed.), *Social networks and social support* (pp. 149–170). Beverly Hills: Sage.
Horwitz, A. (1978). Family, kin, and friend networks in psychiatric help-seeking. *Social Science and Medicine, 12,* 297–304.
Horwitz, S. M., Morgenstern, H., & Berkman, L. F. (1985). The impact of social stressors and social networks on pediatric medical care use. *Medical Care, 23,* 946–959.
House, J. S. (1981). *Work, stress and social support*. Reading, MA: Addison–Wesley.
House, J. S., & Kahn, R. (1984). Measuring social support. In S. Cohen & L. Syme (Eds.), *Social support and health* (pp. 83–108). New York: Academic Press.
Howe, H. L. (1981). Social factors associated with breast self-examination among high risk women. *American Journal of Public Health, 71,* 251–255.
Israel, B. A. (1982). Social networks and health status: Linking theory, research and practice. *Patient Counseling and Health Education, 4,* 65–79.
Israel, B. A. (1985). Social networks and social support: Implications for natural helper and community level interventions. *Health Education Quarterly, 12,* 65–80.
Kadushin, C. (1969). *Why people go to psychiatrists*. New York: Atherton.
Kaplan, B. H., Cassel, J. C., & Gore, S. (1977). Social support and health. *Medical Care, 15* (Suppl.), 47–58.
Kessler, R. C., Price, R. H., & Wortman, C. B. (1985). Social factors in psychopathology: Stress, social support, and coping processes. *Annual Review of Psychology, 36,* 531–572.
Lacy, W. B. (1981). The influence of attitudes and current friends on drug use intentions. *Journal of Social Psychology, 113,* 65–76.
Lin, N., Ensel, W. M., Simeone, R. S., & Kuo, W. (1979). Social support, stressful life events, and illness: A model and an empirical test. *Journal of Health and Social Behavior, 20,* 108–119.

Liska, A. E. (1984). A critical examination of the causal structure of the Fishbein/Ajzen attitude–behavior model. *Social Psychology Quarterly, 47,* 61–74.

Lowenthal, M. F., & Haven, C. (1968). Interaction and adaptation: Intimacy as a criterion variable. *American Sociological Review, 33,* 20–30.

Marsden, P. V. (1987). Core discussion networks of Americans. *American Sociological Review, 52,* 122–131.

McKinlay, J. (1973). Social networks, lay consultation, and help seeking behavior. *Social Forces, 51,* 275.

Mitchell, J. C. (1969). The concept and use of social network. In J. C. Mitchell (Ed.), *Social networks in urban situations* (pp. 1–50). Manchester: University Press.

Mitchell, R. E., & Trickett, E. J. (1980). Task force report: Social networks as mediators of social support—An analysis of the effects and determinants of social networks. *Community Mental Health Journal, 16,* 27–44.

Montano, D. E. (1986). Predicting and understanding influenza vaccination behavior. *Medical Care, 24,* 438–453.

Mueller, D. P. (1980). Social networks: A promising direction for research on the relationship of the social environment to psychiatric disorder. *Social Science and Medicine, 14A,* 147–161.

Nuckolls, K. B., Cassel, J., & Kaplan, B. H. (1972). Psychosocial assets, life crisis and the prognosis of pregnancy. *American Journal of Epidemiology, 95,* 431–441.

Oliver, R. L., & Berger, P. K. (1979). A pathanalysis of preventive health care decision models. *Journal of Consumer Research, 6,* 13–121.

Sanson, C. D., Wakefield, J., & Pinnok, K. M. (1971). Choice or change? How women come to have a cytotest done by their family doctor. *International Journal of Health Education, 14,* 127–138.

Suchman, E. (1965). Social patterns of illness and medical care. *Journal of Health and Human Behavior, 6,* 2–16.

Thoits, P. A. (1982). Conceptual, methodological, and theoretical problems in studying social support as a buffer against stress. *Journal of Health and Social Behavior, 23,* 145–159.

Thoits, P. A. (1983). Multiple identities and psychological well-being. *American Sociological Review, 48,* 174–187.

Turner, R. J. (1981). Social support as a contingency in psychological well-being. *Journal of Health and Social Behavior, 22,* 357–367.

Walker, K., MacBride, A., & Vachon, M. (1977). Social support networks and the crisis of bereavement. *Social Science and Medicine, 11,* 35–41.

Weiss, R. (1969). The fund of sociability. *Transition, 1,* 36–43.

Weiss, R. (1974). The provisions of social relationships. In Z. Rubin (Ed.), *Doing unto others* (pp. 17–26). Englewood Cliffs, NJ: Prentice–Hall.

Wellman, B. (1979). The community question. *American Journal of Sociology, 84,* 1201–1231.

Wellman, B. (1981). Applying network analyses to the study of support. In B. H. Gottlieb (Ed.), *Social networks and social support* (pp. 171–200). Beverly Hills: Sage.

Wethington, E., & Kessler, R. C. (1986). Perceived support, received support, and adjustment to stressful life events. *Journal of Health and Social Behavior, 27,* 78–89.

Winefield, H. B. (1979). Social support and social environment of depressed and normal women. *Australian and New Zealand Journal of Psychiatry, 13,* 335–339.

Wortman, C. B. (1984). Social support and the cancer patient: Conceptual and methodological issues. *Cancer, 53,* 2339–2360.

Social Determinants

Social Roles

The concept of "role" provides a way of integrating the individual and society; of relating personal behavior to group or societal norms; of examining individual performances within the context of social expectations about those performances. Research on health behavior makes use of two critical role concepts: the sick role and gender-based roles.

SICK ROLE

Parsons's (e.g., 1951, 1972) conception of the sick role has provided an important framework for understanding the behavior of sick persons in terms of role and role relationships in the context of the social system, particularly in relation to American values such as achievement, autonomy, and productivity. By virtue of accepting the role, and by performing it appropriately, the incumbent in the sick role is temporarily allowed to demonstrate dependency and is relieved of performing other roles and tasks, i.e., is allowed to behave in ways that are contrary to the society's dominant values. Within the Parsonian framework, the "sick role" is only conditionally legitimate.

Twaddle's elaboration (1979) of the concept of sick role treats health and illnesses as statuses, with health having a higher value than illness. Health and illness are thus seen as the bases for social evaluations and consequently for social stratification. Twaddle further considered health as a norm and illness as deviance from this norm.

In a lively debate, Gallagher (1976/1979) systematically critiqued parts of Parsons's position, to which Parsons himself (1975) developed a rejoinder. Arluke, Kennedy, and Kessler's (1979) literature review of research on the sick role showed that although little association exists within individual beliefs about the four major sick-role dimensions, and although some economic and social factors are related to individual sick-role dimensions, there is nonetheless consensus in the way people conceptualize the sick role. Segall (1976) also raised questions about the "coherence" of the role's several components and about its universality. Despite both conceptual and empirical criticisms, the construct of "sick role" has been unquestionably heuristic and has generated research linking personal health behavior to the demands, expectations, status, and value systems of the social world.

Social class and/or socioeconomic status have been important variables in research related to the sick role. Britt (1975) provided insight into the reciprocal relationships between sick role and social class, i.e., occupying the sick role tends to reduce income and income-generating opportunities. These reductions, in turn, increase both stress and certain behaviors that may additionally decrease employability (e.g., reduction of job seeking) and thus increase the likelihood that sick-role occupation will be continued. Campbell (1978) provided insight into how components of parental social class are related to children's sick-role behavior.

Arluke's chapter provides a critical examination of the current status of the sick-role concept.

Physicians are traditionally considered to be the legitimate gatekeepers of entry into the sick role. Field (1961/1972) described economic and political factors that affect physicians' behavior in relation to granting the sick role, i.e., to the certification or legitimization of illness. Dodier (1985) reported on how French physicians may vary in their moral evaluations of workers, and how these evaluations affect their allowing workers to occupy the sick role.

The physician's power to legitimate the sick role thus increases in importance as society becomes overmedicalized. The overmedicalizing of American society (e.g., Fox, 1977) is reflected in the medicalization of deviance, i.e., the selective labeling of nonnormative behaviors, such as alcoholism and other behavioral problems, as illnesses. How certain behavior problems have been labeled as illnesses, and how professionals employ sick-role concepts in dealing with them, can be demonstrated in the research of Chalfant and Kurtz (1971) and Kurtz and Giacopassi (1975). Wolinsky's chapter discusses the issue of sick-role legitimization in light of changing social and economic conditions.

Brown and Rawlinson's (1977) analysis of sick-role incumbency after recovery from cardiac surgery showed that males more readily relinquish the sick role than do females, and thus points to the issue of gender and its relationship to health behavior.

GENDER-BASED ROLES

Gender has historically been an important basis for role differentiation within social systems, whether these be as small as the family, or as large as a culture, although anthropologists have shown that little or no biological determinism accounts for this (e.g., Mead, 1950). Nathanson (1975) and Harrison (1978) both provided critical analyses of the linkages between gender-based roles and health status. Nathanson noted higher morbidity rates among women as well as their higher rates of utilization of health services—independent of reproduction-related conditions—and identified hypotheses to provide a conceptual frame of reference for understanding the relationship between illness and the female role. In complementary fashion, Harrison's literature review indicated that there were health dangers inherent in the male role.

Harrison's work is anomalous. Generally, research into gender differences has focused on women—on their allegedly poorer health status relative to men, and on their increased use of health services. The problem itself is often unknowingly stated in sexist terms, of the woman behaving inappropriately through *over*use, rather than in terms of the inappropriate *under*use of health services by men, or of the seeming reluctance of men to enter the sick role when doing so is appropriate.

The linkages between gender and health status are mediated in large measure by health behaviors, such as perceptions of health status, accepting the sick role, and utilizing appropriate health services. Horwitz (1977) identified gender differences in discussing problems with others: women are more inclined to do so than men.

A literature is accumulating that looks critically at dimensions of gender roles to determine whether some common assumptions or hypotheses about these linkages are warranted. Verbrugge's critical review (1985) of such gender differences also provides an integration of different approaches to accounting for them, e.g., gender differences in biological risks, acquired risks, psychosocial aspects of symptoms and care, health reporting behavior, and history of health care.

Multiple-Role, Fixed-Role, Nurturant-Role Hypotheses

In the decade between 1975 and 1985, the literature on gender-based differences in health behavior has moved rapidly from the well-considered conceptualizations of Nathanson and Harrison, to the testing of specific role-related hypotheses. The most prominent models advanced as ways of explaining some of the gender differences in psychosocial aspects of symptoms and care are the multiple-role, fixed-role, and nurturant-role hypotheses. Verbrugge (1983) systematically explored the multiple-role hypothesis and showed that the combination of roles in which a person is involved (i.e., employee, spouse, parent) does not have any *special* effect on health or health behavior. Although individual roles do have an impact on health and health behaviors, no additional interactive impact is observed for combinations of roles. Thus, data showing women's greater utilization of health services and drugs cannot be explained in terms of their engaging in fewer rather than in multiple roles. Furthermore, when age and number of roles were controlled, gender differences in health diminished. Verbrugge reasoned, however, that ability to occupy roles such as that of spouse or parent, or to perform successfully as an employee, may itself require at least some minimal level of health status.

Marcus and Siegel's (1982) exploration of the fixed-role hypothesis that women typically have fewer "fixed" role obligations to others (e.g., to employers) that prevent them from seeking services, revealed no gender differences in utilization of care for acute conditions, and that the gender differences in utilization observed for chronic conditions disappeared when role obligations were controlled. Other related research (Marcus, Seeman, & Telesky, 1983) showed that fixed-role obligations were related to remaining in the sick role but not likely to explain adoption of the sick role. Moreover, they pointed out that deciding to adopt the sick role may itself be congruent with commitments to fulfilling a number of other role obligations in the long run.

Gove (1984a) proposed the nurturant-role hypothesis as an alternative to the fixed-role hypothesis to account for women's higher rates of illness. According to this hypothesis, women's role as nurturer places them in a position where they have greater responsibilities for meeting the needs and demands made by others, that these demands are likely to draw attention to their own troubles, and that the lack of structure of the nurturant role gives women more time to dwell upon their troubles. Marcus, Seeman, and Telesky (1984) and Gove (1984b) debated the relative merits of their hypotheses.

Hibbard and Pope (1983) showed that although females are more likely than males to report experiences of symptoms, there were no observable gender differences in acceptance of the sick role when ill. They further observed that women with greater role responsibilities used medical services more than did women with fewer such responsibilities. Moreover, Hibbard and Pope reasoned from their data that the perceptual and behavioral aspects of illness operate differently in males and females; that the greatest gender differences occur in relation to perception of symptoms rather than in utilization behavior; and that role responsibilities may be related to differences in paying attention to and/or interpreting ambiguous—as opposed to powerful or obvious—symptoms. The complexity of their analyses enabled them to show, for example, that increased reports of symptoms were inversely related to adoption of the sick role among females.

Hibbard and Pope clearly pointed out how difficult it is to compare males and females on role responsibilities; that it is difficult to control for the amount of time and attention that the genders give to any particular role.

Waldron's chapter systematically explores gender differences in a number of health behaviors, and relates these differences to social and cultural role patterns. Waldron notes that in some non-Western cultures, the gender differences in utilization of services are reversed: males use health services more frequently than do females!

REFERENCES

Arluke, A., Kennedy, L., & Kessler, R. C. (1979). Reexamining the sick-role concept: An empirical assessment. *Journal of Health and Social Behavior, 20,* 30–36.

Britt, D. W. (1975). Social class and the sick role: Examining the issue of mutual influence. *Journal of Health and Social Behavior, 16,* 178–182.

Brown, J. S., & Rawlinson, M. E. (1977). Sex differences in sick role rejection and in work performance following cardiac surgery. *Journal of Health and Social Behavior, 18,* 276–292.

Campbell, J. D. (1978). The child in the sick role: Contributions of age, sex, parental status, and parental values. *Journal of Health and Social Behavior, 19,* 35–51.

Chalfant, H. P., & Kurtz, R. A. (1971). Alcoholics and the sick role: Assessments by social workers. *Journal of Health and Social Behavior, 12,* 66–72.

Dodier, N. (1985). Social uses of illness at the workplace: Sick leave and moral evaluation. *Social Science and Medicine, 20,* 123–128.

Field, M. G. (1972). The doctor–patient relationship in the perspective of "fee-for-service" and "third-party" medicine. In E. G. Jaco (Ed.), *Patients, physicians and illness: A sourcebook in behavioral science and health* (2nd ed.). New York: Free Press. (Reprinted from *Journal of Health and Human Behavior,* 1961, *2,* 252–262).

Fox, R. C. (1977). The medicalization and demedicalization of American society. In J. H. Knowles (Ed.), *Doing better and feeling worse: Health in the United States.* New York: Norton.

Gallagher, E. B. (1979). Lines of reconstruction and extension in the Parsonian sociology of illness. In E. G. Jaco (Ed.), *Patients, physicians and illness* (3rd ed.). New York: Free Press. (Reprinted from *Social Science and Medicine,* 1976, *10,* 207–218).

Gove, W. R. (1984a). Gender differences in mental and physical illness: The effects of fixed roles and nurturant roles. *Social Science and Medicine, 19,* 77–84.

Gove, W. R. (1984b). On understanding illness, illness behavior and reading what has been written: A reply to Marcus, Seeman and Telesky. *Social Science and Medicine, 19,* 88–91.

Harrison, J. (1978). Warning: The male sex role may be dangerous to your health. *Journal of Social Issues, 34,* 65–86.

Hibbard, J. H., & Pope, C. R. (1983). Gender roles, illness orientation and use of medical services. *Social Science and Medicine, 17,* 129–137.

Horwitz, A. (1977). The pathways into psychiatric treatment: Some differences between men and women. *Journal of Health and Social Behavior, 18,* 169–178.

Kurtz, R. A., & Giacopassi, D. J. (1975). Medical and social work students' perceptions of deviant conditions and sick role incumbency. *Social Science and Medicine, 9,* 249–255.

Marcus, A. C., Seeman, T. E., & Telesky, C. W. (1983). Sex differences in reports of illness and disability: A further test of the fixed role hypothesis. *Social Science and Medicine, 17,* 993–1002.

Marcus, A. C., Seeman, T. E., & Telesky, C. W. (1984). Teetering on the horns of a dilemma: Professor Gove's latest paper on sex differences in illness behavior. *Social Science and Medicine, 19,* 84–88.

Marcus, A. C., & Siegel, J. M. (1982). Sex differences in the use of physician services: A preliminary test of the fixed role hypothesis. *Journal of Health and Social Behavior, 23,* 186–197.

Mead, M. (1950). *Sex and temperament in three primitive societies.* New York: Mentor.

Nathanson, C. A. (1975). Illness and the feminine role: A theoretical review. *Social Science and Medicine, 9,* 57–62.

Parsons, T. (1951). *The social system.* Glencoe, IL: Free Press.

Parsons, T. (1972). Definitions of health and illness in the light of American values and social structure. In E. G. Jaco (Ed.), *Patients, physicians and illness: A sourcebook in behavioral science and health* (2nd ed.). New York: Free Press.

Parsons, T. (1975). The sick role and the role of the physician reconsidered. *Milbank Memorial Fund Quarterly, 53,* 257–278.

Segall, A. (1976). The sick role concept: Understanding illness behavior. *Journal of Health and Social Behavior, 17,* 163–170.

Twaddle, A. C. (1979). *Sickness behavior and the sick role*. Boston: Schenkman.

Verbrugge, L. M. (1983). Multiple roles and physical health of women and men. *Journal of Health and Social Behavior, 24,* 16–30.

Verbrugge, L. M. (1985). Gender and health: An update on hypotheses and evidence. *Journal of Health and Social Behavior, 26,* 156–182.

CHAPTER 9

The Sick-Role Concept

Arnold Arluke

THE MODEL

Structural–Functional Approach

Over three decades ago, Parsons elaborated a model of how societies operate and continue to exist. His structural–functional approach is concerned with how different parts of society relate to each other and contribute to a state of equilibrium. Although the approach focuses on the maintenance of social systems, the individual is not entirely excluded from his analysis. Through a process of socialization, individuals learn to share similar normative expectations for behavior in a variety of different social positions or roles. The social system, which is a network of roles, functions smoothly only insofar as persons perform their roles adequately. Deviation from the normal performance of these roles can become a threat to the stability of society. Given the potential negative consequences of role deviance, social control mechanisms arise to minimize its occurrence.

According to Parsons, illness represents one such form of deviance because of its impact on society. If people fail to meet their normal role obligations, occupationally or familially, for example, they create a problem for society and for the people around them. Even though this failure is due to disease, it is deviant because the person is not behaving as expected.

Sick-Role Expectations

In order to minimize the potentially destabilizing effects of illness on the social system, Parsons posits the ideal-type concept of the sick role. He argues, without empirical validation, that institutionally determined expectations exist in all illness situations in American society, and that these expectations are internalized by Americans and ensure the "minimization of illness" (Parsons, 1951). Two rights and two duties make up this "conditionally legitimate deviant role." More specifically, the sick person has: (1) a right to be exempt from normal social roles, (2) a right not to be held responsible for the condition, (3) a duty to try and get well, and (4) a duty to seek and cooperate with technically competent help.

The first expectation in the Parsonian model is that the sick person has the right to

ARNOLD ARLUKE • Department of Sociology and Anthropology, Northeastern University, Boston, Massachusetts 02115.

be exempt temporarily from normal social responsibilities. The extent of role exemption depends on the nature and severity of the illness. Greater exemption is permitted with more severe illness; less exemption with less severe illnesses. This incapacity to perform one's social roles is what makes sickness a deviant role. The sick person also has the right to be exempt from responsibility for the incapacity. The individual is not considered to be culpable for the condition, and therefore for the inability to perform normal roles, because sickness is not thought to be willfully chosen. Nor is sickness willfully overcome by the patient alone. The ability to heal oneself is not seen as a matter of individual motivation or desire.

These two rights, however, are granted to the sick person only if certain conditions are met. Two sick-role duties ensure that the privileges of sickness are only temporary and that the sick person will once again participate in the social system in the same fashion as he or she did prior to illness.

Thus, the sick person has an obligation to define illness as an inherently undesirable state, and because it is so undesirable, to recover completely and resume normal social roles as soon as possible. This sick-role duty is what, for Parsons, makes sickness a legitimate deviant role. The sick person also has an obligation to seek and cooperate with competent help because not all illnesses are minor and self-limiting. In American society, physicians are generally considered to be competent medical help. By seeking a physician, the sick person enters the role of the patient and is thereby expected to facilitate recovery by cooperating with medical advice. This includes willingness to submit to the techniques and therapies of medical science, to the care of nonphysician personnel, and to hospitalization if necessary.

These duties, Parsons observes, are compatible with key American values. Activism, for instance, calls on the individual to master one's environment rather than to adjust to the inevitable. This value is conspicuous in America where sickness is seen as a challenge to be met by seeking appropriate medical care. A second value, instrumentalism, emphasizes the achievement of specific goals. It is believed that through hard work progress can be made toward the attainment of goals and that success is possible. Sickness is approached instrumentally by "working" at getting better; reassuming one's normal productive roles is the goal (Parsons, 1964).

Secondary Gains

The rights and privileges of the sick role may be jeopardized if these values are not embodied in the sick person's behavior. Sick-role occupancy will probably be seen as illegitimate if the person fails to seek competent medical care, follow the physician's orders, and openly want to get better. Under such circumstances, the person risks being seen as a malingerer, feigning sickness in order to acquire privileges accorded the sick, or what Parsons calls "secondary gains."

A variety of interactional or social psychological features affect whether people will seek out the secondary gains of the sick role. Personal experience with and exposure to persons who have benefited from being sick may influence others who then try to gain role exemptions when the opportunity occurs. Leigh and Reiser (1980) cited the example of a person who goes to a physician with "exaggerated lingering symptoms of a minor injury" after seeing a friend receive a generous financial award from an industrial accident. Conversely, the stigma associated with particular illnesses such as venereal disease may reduce motivation to adopt the sick role.

Abuse of the sick role may also occur when people need a temporary excuse for not performing up to some standard. Aronowitz (1973) provided an example of this in his study of auto assembly-line workers who shirked their duties by calling in sick. The sick role may provide a more permanent excuse for people in a dependent state. Empirical studies support the idea that individuals may use the sick role as a "substitute status" (Cockerham, Lueschen, Kunz, & Spaeth, 1986, p. 11). Cole and Lejeune (1972), for example, found that welfare mothers used sickness to justify nonperformance.

People may also seek the secondary gains of the sick role if they need help in coping. Studies by Arluke, Kennedy, and Kessler (1979) and Nuttbrock (1986) suggested that the sick role may provide the elderly with social support for dependent behavior. In addition, among persons unable to care for themselves, the sick role may justify other people assuming a caretaking function, or in more extreme cases, hospitalization or institutionalization. Nursing home placement of the elderly, for example, sometimes occurs because of a failure to cope socially; the sick role becomes a method or vehicle to justify institutionalization.

The sick role can help people cope in yet another way. Illness can be used to acquire rewards. Shuval, Antonovsky, and Davies (1973) observed that in Israel illness is sometimes used as an "allocative tool." Scarce rewards such as lighter work loads, improved housing, tax relief, and so on, can be gained through the sick role, as illness is one of the criteria used for the distribution of resources in Israel.

Social Control

Parsons considers the attractiveness of the secondary gains of the sick role to be a potentially serious problem for the social system because the wish for exemption from the pressures of everyday life is continually present and inherent in the division of labor and in the very nature of American society. If large numbers of people sought to engage in such deviant behavior as the sick role, the social system would be undermined. Therefore, society controls the number of people claiming to be sick by using physicians to regulate entry into the sick role. The model requires that people go to physicians to ensure the absence of malingering and to restore people to their normal roles. As a form of social control, then, the sick role allows the medical treatment of sick people while it discourages imaginary illness. The sick-role duties promote getting well and reduce the incentive to falsify illness. The sick person is also isolated from most healthy people, making it difficult for the sick person to become a model for others who might be tempted into such deviancy.

The social control aspect of the sick-role concept has influenced the writings of many sociologists. In particular, analysis has focused on how physicians become agents of social control whose duty it is to certify illness and either permit or restrict sick-role adoption. One example can be seen in Field's (1967) study of the application of the sick role in the Soviet Union during its rapid industrialization in the 1930s. Physicians were allowed to authorize fewer sick leaves for people who worked in industries judged essential to the survival of Stalinist Russia than for those in less critical industries. Indeed, in unusual situations such as wartime where the demand for performance of normal responsibilities is high (e.g., combat), illness may be viewed by physicians as malingering even when not feigned. Schneider's (1947) participant observation study of sick call in World War II reported that military physicians were so suspicious of soldiers using illness as a way of escaping duty that real illness was sometimes seen as malingering and soldiers were often blamed for getting sick as in the case of venereal disease which was treated as a disciplinary offense.

Waitzkin (1971) also found that the sick role serves a social control function in American institutions. He noted that the sick role can reduce conflict and help maintain social order. In so doing, the sick role can provide secondary gains for both institutions and individuals. For institutions, sick-role adoption can mitigate disruptive strains by stabilizing role relationships. For individuals, the sick role can satisfy needs for attention or nurturance. One example he offered is based on a 4-month field study of sick call in a large urban penal institution. Waitzkin argued that the range of behavior seen as appropriate for adopting the sick role in prison will be wide compared to other institutions because the sick role provides prisoners a legitimate outlet for deviant behavior which, if released, could threaten the prison institution. In addition to the latent stabilizing functions of the sick role for the prison, there are secondary gains for individual prisoners. Sick-role adoption can provide for the inmate's personal and psychological needs. For example, if sick, the inmate can be excused from prison labor or sheer confinement. In addition, while in the infirmary, the inmate can communicate with other prisoners or have homosexual contacts. Also, nurturance and support may be had from the medical encounter itself, in addition to medications which can be used in nonmedical ways. Howe, Froom, Culpepper, and Mangone (1977) provided experimental confirmation of Waitzkin's theory that the sick role serves many purposes in prisons. When lower levels of care were made available for prisoners, total sick-role enactment remained constant although the desire for physicians' care decreased.

For Parsons, therefore, medical practice is a mechanism by which society tries to control deviance. The sick role becomes a vehicle by which new forms of deviance can be brought under the medical profession's domain, treated medically, and redefined morally and socially. Conrad's (1975) study of hyperactivity, for instance, showed how a social problem such as classroom disruption was relabeled as a medical problem. Such medicalization extends the medical profession's jurisdiction and increases its role as an agent of social control.

The trend toward medicalizing social problems led Arluke and Peterson (1981) to theorize that the sick role has been applied to groups not considered deviant. They pointed out that the aging process itself has come to be viewed as an illness and that the elderly, by the fact of their age, are treated as though they occupy the sick role even in the absence of physical illness. That is, they are expected to reduce their normal social and occupational responsibilities and assume more dependent roles.

An experimental study by Fisher, Arluke, and Levin (1984–85) offered some empirical support for the suggestion that old age is being medicalized. Subjects were randomly given vignettes of people with identical illness characteristics and background information, but different ages and employment statuses. Subjects were more likely to expect an old, rather than a middle-aged, man not to recover. However, subjects were also more likely to expect reduction in role obligations when the man was retired than when he was employed, regardless of age. At least regarding old age, medicalization does not appear to be complete; some of the sick-role expectations, such as role reduction, are not ascribed solely on the basis of age.

A similar ambivalence regarding the ascription of sick-role expectations was detected by Kurtz and Giacopassi (1975) in their study of 399 medical and social work students. They found their subjects were much more willing to award sick-role incumbency to physical ailments, such as heart disorders, than to mental or addictive disorders. It seems, then, that the general trend toward medicalization may, in the case of particular social problems, be incomplete; only some of the sick-role expectations may be applicable to these problems and those that are may only be applied with some hesitancy.

CRITICISMS

The Parsonian model has proven to be remarkably controversial as well as provocative. At least four basic lines of criticism of the sick-role concept have been made; namely, that the Parsonian sick role is (1) limited to acute disorders, (2) iatrogenic, (3) medicocentric, and (4) culture-bound and class-bound.

Limited to Acute Disorders

Critics of Parsons maintain that the sick-role model is accurate when applied to acute and episodic illness, but fails to describe the experiences of patients with chronic or terminal illnesses (Callahan, Carroll, Revier, Gilhooly, & Dunn, 1966; Cogswell & Weir, 1964; Gustafson, 1972; Kassebaum & Baumann, 1965), mental disorders (Cockerham, 1981; Denzin & Spitzer, 1966; Sobel & Ingalls, 1964; Waxler & Mishler, 1963), and physical disabilities (Davis, 1961; Kojima, 1977; Litman, 1962; Thomas, 1966). If we take the example of the chronically ill patient, the validity of this criticism will be apparent.

It may be difficult to be excused from everyday role responsibilities if one has a chronic problem precisely because of the potentially long-term nature of such role reductions. Some chronically ill people may resist such indulgence because they may not want to be seen as "special cases." Such patients feel an imperative to cover-up their conditions and keep-up their routines so their relationships generally remain normal (Wiener, 1975). Others may resist the reduction of everyday responsibilities because these activities may be important to their self-esteem or to the structuring of their lives (Rosengren, 1980). Employers, friends, and family may themselves not always be willing to make special accommodations and reduce their expectations of the chronically ill. In one study (Honig-Parnass, 1981) of 430 females associated with Israel's largest health care organization, it was found that the chronically ill were allowed less dependency than the acutely ill.

Also, the issue of culpability for becoming sick may be an issue for some people with chronic illness. The patient may do a lot of soul-searching in order to understand the reasons for being struck by a permanent and sometimes disabling problem. In some cases, this may entail self-blame. Arthritis patients, for instance, often blame themselves for getting the disease (Elder, 1973). Some feel they are being punished by God for prior immoral behavior, whereas others cite their life-style as the cause of the problem.

Nor can the patient with chronic illness expect to get better. Of course, there may be remissions and the effects of the illness may be minimized, but there is no absolute recovery in the strict sense of the Parsonian sick role. Moreover, the duty to get well as a dominant motive may be an "unpleasant encumbrance" (Rosengren, 1980, p. 284) if it means that the rest of one's life must be organized with recovery as a central interest.

Lastly, the chronically ill patient does not as a rule fully cooperate with the medical advice of physicians. Research indicates that such patients are likely to act autonomously and take over management of their medical problems. In one study of people with multiple sclerosis (Stewart & Sullivan, 1982), the behavior of patients ran contrary to what one would predict from the model of the sick role in acute illness. Social consensus and definitional clarity were not found to exist between doctor and patient. Instead, the doctor–patient relationship was a process of social negotiation rather than normative restraint. Patients refused to accept their physicians' judgments regarding their symptoms and advanced their own definition of their condition.

The values, beliefs, and resources of chronically ill patients, as well as their social and environmental situation, influence how they cooperate with the medical care provided by physicians. In one study (Arluke, 1980), the beliefs of rheumatoid arthritis patients were found to have a potentially enormous impact on whether the advice of physicians was followed. These patients generated their own lay definition of what constituted an effective drug and made assessments of efficacy using various personal methods. The net result was that some patients modified or abandoned their therapies, and did so without consulting their physicians.

Parsons (1975) responded to this critique. He maintained that even if complete recovery is impossible, chronic disease often can be managed so the patient can return to a normal range of function. Thus, while chronic diseases cannot be cured, they should not be thought of as so different from acute diseases. Despite the attempt by Parsons to modify his thinking, the sick-role expectations can still not be applied to a variety of chronic situations without substantial modification of his model. In addition, he did not address the fact that the process of sick-role adoption in chronic illness seems marked by dissensus and conflict rather than harmony and cooperation characteristic of physician–patient relationships in cases of acute disorders.

Iatrogenesis

Criticism of the Parsonian model also focuses on the iatrogenic consequences of sick-role adoption. Carlson (1975) and Illich (1976) argued that dependence on physicians and medications, and willingness to adopt the sick role, induces illness and reduces ability to cope. Research on the iatrogenic consequences of the sick role generally supports this notion (e.g., Lowrey, 1963; McLamb & Huntley, 1967). Myles (1978), for one, notes that the "institutional organization of being ill tends to reinforce patterns of illness behavior among clients by constraining the individual increasingly to adopt attitudes and behavior consistent with the assumption of the sick role" (p. 508). Once institutionalized, sick persons may inevitably come to believe that they are sick and behave accordingly. To test this idea, Myles examined whether institutionalized elderly patients were more likely to incorporate the sick role into their self-concept than were noninstitutionalized elderly. Contrary to this expectation, Myles found that the institutionalized elderly were less likely to incorporate the sick role into their definition of self than were the noninstitutionalized elderly. However, the author noted that this finding may only reflect the general situation of the elderly within the larger society; that is, the living environments of noninstitutionalized elderly may be more problematic than those of institutionalized elderly.

The sick role may also be iatrogenic when the patient is suffering from alcoholism, mental illness, or drug addiction. A number of researchers (e.g., Lesser, 1974; Roman & Trice, 1968; Stuart, 1970) suggest that with illnesses such as these, the sick role may prevent patients from being seen as responsible for their behavior, and therefore less likely to do anything to change their behavior. In addition, if these patients are hospitalized, the behavior expected of them may not be consistent with what is expected of them in everyday life. There may also be iatrogenic effects with conditions that are viewed as desirable, but that are being medicalized. For instance, Rosengren (1962) and McKinlay (1972) both commented on the dangers of treating pregnancy as an illness.

Medicocentrism

A third criticism is that the sick-role model is conceptually problematic because it is based on an idealized view of the American medical profession. Parsonian norms regarding medical practice and values in America represent the way the medical profession has defined itself (Landy, 1977). This official view of the health care process portrays physicians as parentlike, strong figures who are permissive, supportive, objective, and ethical. Patients in this scheme become what Parsons calls "desocialized," and act as relatively weak, dependent, childlike figures.

This view, claims Gallagher (1976), is medicocentric; that is, it places physicians at the center of the health-care process, thereby overestimating their therapeutic impact and underestimating the socioclinical significance of other health-care practitioners, nonmedical professionals, and lay support systems. Patently, Parsons focused too narrowly on only the physician as the legitimizer and gatekeeper to the sick role. Nonmedical professionals may also be instrumental in deciding whether the sick role is awarded. Chalfant and Kurtz (1971), for instance, in their study of 224 social workers in welfare agencies, discovered that many social workers of alcoholics saw drinking as motivated behavior, and alcoholics therefore as culpable actors not entitled to the right to be exempt from normal responsibilities. Lay people, especially in chronic disease situations, may also occupy a significant position in the successful awarding of the sick role. Suchman (1965) observed that sick people first seek provisional validation of the sick role from family and friends. If awarded, they gain temporary exemption from routine tasks and obligations. Indeed, the lay support system has been shown to have a great influence on entry and performance in, as well as exit from, the sick role with the chronically ill (e.g., Markson, 1971), the disabled (e.g., Litman, 1962), and mentally ill (Greenley, 1972).

Medicocentrism may also lead to an overestimation of the moral authority of the physician. Parsons's characterization of the acutely ill patient as passive and dependent may no longer be accurate given changes in American values and the organization of health care. Some maintain that the authority of physicians has waned in recent years and that patients are now more likely to adopt a consumer stance toward medical care (Haug, 1976). Wolinsky and Wolinsky (1981) support this notion. Their data indicate that younger people, not socialized to traditional norms of obedience to physicians, are less likely to expect sick-role legitimation than older people.

McCormack (1981) also questioned the assumption by Parsons that the doctor–patient relationship must be hierarchical because the patient lacks knowledge and objectivity to serve as an equal partner. The trusting dependency relationship which results from this inequality is subject to abuse "if the professional is not sufficiently self-disciplined by a moral code" (p. 41). As long as the physician occupies a "fiduciary trusteeship" with patients, "there is no hope of democratizing the relationship between professional and patient, of developing a more horizontal partnership of equals. . . ."

Culture-Bound and Class-Bound

Finally, the Parsonian model is based on an ideal type of American middle-class family, and is therefore culture-bound and class-bound. Medical anthropologists note that the specific features of the Parsonian sick-role model are far from being universal (e.g., Fabrega, 1974). Although many non-Western societies also have patterned expectations about the rights and obligations of the sick, the particular expectations outlined by Parsons seem applicable mainly to the industrial capitalist societies of America and Western Europe. One extreme example of the inapplicability of the Parsonian scheme to other cultures is discussed in Lebra's (1972) study of the sick role in a Japanese religious sect. Members of this sect believe that sickness is caused by the neglect of religious duties, and that people should therefore be held responsible for their diseases. Recovery involves self-healing through prayers by sick people themselves. They also believe sickness is not an occasion for dependence. In short, there is no sick role among members of this Japanese subculture.

Even within the United States, it is difficult to apply the Parsonian model to the behavior of people. The behavior that one would predict on the basis of the sick-role expectations is not what one finds across different segments of the population. In fact, relatively few people seek medical attention, despite the widespread presence of clinically serious signs in the population (Zola, 1966). What does have a profound influence on sick-role behavior is a person's sociocultural position. Ethnic and social status affects the interpretation of symptoms, physician utilization, responsibility for health and sickness, and cooperation with medical advice (e.g., Calnan, 1983; Frankel & Nuttall, 1984; Hammer, 1983; Meile, 1986; Segall, 1976a; Zborowski, 1952).

The sick-role model is also class-bound in that it is built upon the values of the American middle class (Landy, 1977). Cockerham (1982) maintained that the sick role's emphasis on individual responsibility and the desirability of good health is anchored in middle-class values which encourage rational problem-solving, hard work to overcome adversity, and deferred gratification. Lower-class culture, on the other hand, may lead people to feel they have little control over their lives and that success is difficult to attain. They may also deny the sick role and its secondary gains because they may have to continue working, despite how they feel, in order to survive economically.

A number of empirical studies support the argument that the sick-role model is class-bound (e.g., Petroni, 1969; Pill & Stott, 1982). Ossenberg (1962), for instance, reported that the meaning of illness as a form of deviance varies by social class. In this study, hospitalized middle-class patients were more likely to feel legitimately excused from role performance than were hospitalized lower-class patients, who were more likely to experience their illness as deviance.

Although sick-role behavior is often studied, frequently with results critical of the Parsonian model, the normative basis of the sick-role concept is rarely subjected to empirical assessment. The few studies that have done this research tend to find a significant amount of public consensus regarding the sick-role expectations, thereby lending support to the normative component of the model.

For example, Twaddle (1969) examined the extent to which 29 late-middle-age, married people agreed with all four expectations in Parsons's sick-role model. Although only a minority of subjects agreed with all four, the model did describe the modal response of subjects when the expectations were analyzed separately. Similarly, Segall (1976b) studied the sick-role expectations of 70 Jewish and Protestant housewives. A majority of subjects agreed with individual sick-role expectations and few disagreed completely with all four.

Despite the normative acceptance reported in these studies, their findings suggest some religious variation in the expectations held by their subjects. Yet two much larger studies document a great deal of acceptance of individual sick-role expectations across a variety of sociocultural groups. Gordon (1966), for instance, studied 808 New York City residents and found that once a person is defined as sick, all SES groups share similar sick-role expectations. Other equally plausible bases of variation, such as race or ethnicity, were examined in the study by Arluke *et al.* (1979), which concludes that when the expectations are considered discretely, the Parsonian model is fairly accurate. In other words, although few people accept all four expectations, there is widespread public acceptance of individual sick-role expectations.

The fact that there seems to be a great deal of normative acceptance of the sick role is very important in making an overall assessment of the validity of the Parsonian model. Many critics forget that the core of the model describes the general tendency of the population at large to share certain beliefs about illness. This general tendency, or normative ideal type, is important to the social-structural level of explanation used by Parsons to explain the functioning of the social system (Berkanovic, 1972). But people have incorrectly assumed that the sick-role concept should be valid at the level of individual behavior regardless of sociocultural background. Thus, it must be concluded that, although some criticisms of the model are appropriate, the normative basis of the sick-role model may be quite valid. Of course, as only a handful of studies have tried empirically to verify this aspect of the model, future research should concentrate on this goal, along with other lines of research specified below.

FUTURE RESEARCH POSSIBILITIES

Although the sick role has generated a considerable literature, a number of questions still need answering to further our understanding of the illness experience. Perhaps the most urgent question is provoked by the limitations of conceiving of illness as a social role. When approached as a social role, analysis is restricted to public identity or interpersonal expectations for behavior. This is of course what Parsons intended, and is the very strength of his contribution. Yet the intrapersonal side of disease is ignored. We know little about the psychological basis of sick-role behavior or the psychological consequences of sick-role adoption.

Psychological Basis of Sick-Role Behavior

To what extent, if at all, do the psychological attributes of individuals influence sick-role behavior? Shuval *et al.* (1973) suggested that willingness to enter the sick role, and to be comfortable in it, will be influenced by one's "orientation toward life." People with active orientations may find it difficult if not guilt-producing to be in the sick role. This is because the sick role entails two kinds of passivity—abrogation of responsibilities and submissiveness to authority. For people with an active orientation toward life, the sick role may be incompatible with their outlook. On the other hand, people with a passive orientation toward life may find that the sick role complements their general orientation.

Moving beyond Shuval and colleagues' hypothesis, studies have only recently begun to examine how psychological attributes are linked both to social demographic characteristics and to patterned differences in sick-role expectations. Arluke *et al.* (1979) found that persons with lower SES are most likely to believe that people should not be held responsible for their illnesses. They suggested that this belief may stem from broader class differences in the imputation of responsibility and control. Research on locus of control is consistent with this notion; lower-class people tend to have a more passive orientation toward life and are less willing to take responsibility for problems in their lives. A recent study by Cockerham *et al.* (1986) provided additional support for the link between social class, beliefs about control, and sick-role behavior. They argued that the culture of poverty influences the emergence of psychological traits such as fatalism, dependence, and devaluation of health. They found that the poor tend "to invest responsibility for their own health in the health care delivery system than in themselves" (p. 10). For instance, the more affluent, in their study, were more likely to treat themselves whereas the poor adopted a more dependent stance toward physicians.

Psychological Consequences of Sick-Role Adoption

Conversely, we also need to study how the sick role, once entered, influences the individual's experience of illness. For many people, a central component of illness is the loss of a sense of personal invulnerability. Sickness can challenge our conception of the body as indestructible and provide an alternative—although perhaps temporary—view of human frailty. But to what extent, if at all, do sick-role expectations engender the view of oneself as vulnerable? Sick people often lose the feeling that events and their causes can be understood and controlled. As members of a modern Western society, many individuals may rely on the dominant rational explanation of illness provided by their culture. But magical, moral, and religious explanations may also exist to explain sickness when transformations of one's body are beyond the person's rational understanding. For example, some illnesses may elicit a deep emotional reaction in patients, such that they search for some personal and moral responsibility for causing their condition. Fox (1968, p. 91) noted the example of seriously ill hospital patients "grappling with the 'whys' of their illness in moral, religious, and cosmic" ways. But to what extent is the loss of confidence in one's ability to explain and control external events also rooted in the sick role itself?

In short, the sick role may be even more powerful than previously thought in terms of influencing the human experience of disease. The role may have just as much patterned influence over our public selves as it has over our private lives, thoughts, and feelings. It is time to articulate the nature and extent of such a relationship.

REFERENCES

Arluke, A. (1980). Judging drugs: Patients' conceptions of therapeutic efficacy in the treatment of arthritis. *Human Organization, 39,* 84–88.

Arluke, A., Kennedy, L., & Kessler, R. (1979). Reexamining the sick-role concept: An empirical assessment. *Journal of Health and Social Behavior, 20,* 30–36.

Arluke, A., & Peterson, J. (1981). Accidental medicalization of old age and its social control implications. In C. Fry (Ed.), *Dimensions: Aging, culture and health* (pp. 271–284). New York: J. F. Bergin.

Aronowitz, S. (1973). *False promises: The shaping of American working class consciousness.* New York: McGraw–Hill.

Berkanovic, E. (1972). Lay conceptions of the sick role. *Social Forces, 51,* 53–64.

Callahan, E. M., Carroll, S., Revier, Sister P., Gilhooly, E., & Dunn, D. (1966). The "sick role" in chronic illness: Some reactions. *Journal of Chronic Disease, 19,* 883–897.

Calnan, M. (1983). Social networks and patterns of help-seeking behaviour. *Social Science and Medicine, 17,* 25–28.

Carlson, R. (1975). *The end of medicine.* New York: Wiley.

Chalfant, H. P., & Kurtz, R. (1971). Alcoholics and the sick role: Assessments by social workers. *Journal of Health and Social Behavior, 12,* 66–72.

Cockerham, W. C. (1981). *Sociology of mental disorder.* Englewood Cliffs, NJ: Prentice–Hall.

Cockerham, W. C. (1982). *Medical sociology.* Englewood Cliffs, NJ: Prentice–Hall.

Cockerham, W. C., Lueschen, G., Kunz, G., & Spaeth, J. L. (1986). Social stratification and self-management of health. *Journal of Health and Social Behavior, 27,* 1–14.

Cogswell, B. E., & Weir, D. D. (1964). A role in process: The development of medical professionals' role in long-term care of chronically diseased patients. *Journal of Health and Social Behavior, 5,* 95–103.

Cole, S., & Lejeune, R. (1972). Illness and the legitimation of failure. *American Sociological Review, 37,* 347–356.

Conrad, P. (1975). The discovery of hyperkinesis: Notes on the medicalization of deviant behavior. *Social Problems, 23,* 12–21.

Davis, F. (1961). Deviance disavowal: The management of strained interaction by the visibly handicapped. *Social Problems, 9,* 121–132.

Denzin, N. K., & Spitzer, S. P. (1966). Paths to the mental hospital and staff predictions of patient role behavior. *Journal of Health and Human Behavior, 7,* 265–271.

Elder, R. G. (1973). Social class and lay explanations of the etiology of arthritis. *Journal of Health and Social Behavior, 14,* 28–38.

Fabrega, H. (1974). *Disease and social behavior.* Cambridge, MA: MIT Press.

Field, M. (1967). *Soviet socialized medicine: An introduction.* New York: Free Press.

Fisher, W., Arluke, A., & Levin, J. (1984–85). The elderly sick role: An experimental analysis. *International Journal of Aging and Human Development, 20,* 161–165.

Fox, R. (1968). Illness. In *International encyclopedia of the social sciences* (pp. 90–97). New York: Macmillan Co. and Free Press.

Frankel, B. G., & Nuttall, S. (1984). Illness behaviour: An exploration of determinants. *Social Science and Medicine, 19,* 147–155.

Gallagher, E. B. (1976). Lines of reconstruction and extension in the Parsonian sociology of illness. *Social Science and Medicine, 10,* 207–218.

Gordon, G. (1966). *Role theory and illness: A sociological perspective.* New Haven, CT: College University Press.

Greenley, J. R. (1972). The psychiatric patient's family and length of hospitalization. *Journal of Health and Social Behavior, 13,* 25–37.

Gustafson, E. (1972). Dying: The career of the nursing home patient. *Journal of Health and Social Behavior, 13,* 226–235.
Hammer, M. (1983). 'Core' and 'extended' social networks in relation to health and illness. *Social Science and Medicine, 17,* 405–411.
Haug, M. R. (1972). The erosion of professional authority: A cross-cultural inquiry in the case of the physician. *Milbank Memorial Fund Quarterly, 54,* 83–106.
Honig-Parnass, T. (1981). Lay concepts of the sick role: An examination of the professionalist bias in Parsons' model. *Social Science and Medicine, 15A,* 615–623.
Howe, B., Froom, J., Culpepper, L., & Mangone, D. (1977). Adoption of the sick role by prisoners: Report on a multi-functional experiment. *Social Science and Medicine, 11,* 507–510.
Illich, I. (1976). *Medical nemesis.* New York: Bantam.
Kassebaum, G. G., & Baumann, B. O. (1965). Dimensions of the sick role in chronic illness. *Journal of Health and Human Behavior, 6,* 16–27.
Kojima, Y. (1977). Disabled individuals in Japanese society. *Rehabilitation World, 3,* 18–25.
Kurtz, R. D., & Giacopassi, D. J. (1975). Medical and social work students' perceptions of deviant conditions and sick role encumbency. *Social Science and Medicine, 9,* 249–255.
Landy, D. (1977). *Culture, disease, and healing.* New York: Macmillan Co.
Lebra, T. S. (1972). Religious conversion and elimination of the sick role. In W. Lebra (Ed.), *Transcultural research in mental health* (pp. 282–292). Hawaii: University of Hawaii Press.
Leigh, H., & Reiser, M. F. (1980). *The patient.* New York: Plenum Press.
Lesser, M. E. (1974). Perceptions of illness at a therapeutic community for ex-drug addicts: "Legitimate deviance" or escape? *Social Science and Medicine, 8,* 575–583.
Litman, T. J. (1962). The influence of self-conception and life orientation factors in the rehabilitation of the orthopedically disabled. *Journal of Health and Social Behavior, 3,* 249–257.
Lowrey, G. (1963). The problem of hospital accidents to children. *Pediatrics, 32,* 1064–1068.
Markson, E. W. (1971). Patient semeiology of a chronic disease—Rheumatoid arthritis. *Social Science and Medicine, 5,* 159–167.
McCormack, T. (1981). The new criticism and the sick role. *Canadian Review of Sociology, 18,* 30–47.
McKinlay, J. B. (1972). The sick role—Illness and pregnancy. *Social Science and Medicine, 6,* 561–572.
McLamb, J. T., & Huntley, R. R. (1967). The hazards of hospitalization. *Southern Medical Journal, 60,* 469–472.
Meile, R. L. (1986). Pathways to patienthood: Sick role and labeling perspectives. *Social Science and Medicine, 22,* 35–40.
Myles, J. (1978). Institutionalization and sick-role identification among the elderly. *American Sociological Review, 43,* 508–521.
Nuttbrock, L. (1986). The management of illness among physically impaired older people: An interactionist interpretation. *Social Psychology Quarterly, 49,* 180–191.
Ossenberg, R. J. (1962). The experience of deviance in the patient role: A study of class differences. *Journal of Health and Social Behavior, 3,* 277–282.
Parsons, T. (1951). *The social system.* Glencoe, IL: Free Press.
Parsons, T. (1964). *Social structure and personality* (pp. 257–291). New York: Free Press.
Parsons, T. (1975). The sick role and the role of the physician reconsidered. *Milbank Memorial Fund Quarterly, 53,* 257–278.
Petroni, F. A. (1969). Social class, family size, and the sick role. *Journal of Marriage and the Family, 31,* 728–735.
Pill, R., & Stott, N. C. H. (1982). Concepts of illness causation and responsibility: Some preliminary data from a sample of working class mothers. *Social Science and Medicine, 16,* 43–52.
Roman, P. M., & Trice, H. M. (1968). The sick role, labelling theory and the deviant drinker. *International Journal of Social Psychiatry, 14,* 245–251.
Rosengren, W. (1962). The sick role during pregnancy: A note on research in progress. *Journal of Health and Social Behavior, 3,* 213–218.
Rosengren, W. (1980). *Sociology of medicine: Diversity, conflict, and change.* New York: Harper & Row.

Schneider, D. M. (1947). The social dynamics of physical disability in army basic training. *Psychiatry, 10,* 323–333.
Segall, A. (1976a). The sick role concept: Understanding illness behavior. *Journal of Health and Social Behavior, 17,* 163–170.
Segall, A. (1976b). Sociocultural variation in sick role behavioural expectations. *Social Science and Medicine, 10,* 47–51.
Shuval, J., Antonovsky, A., & Davies, A. M. (1973). Illness: A mechanism for coping with failure. *Social Science and Medicine, 7,* 259–265.
Sobel, R., & Ingalls, A. (1964). Resistance to treatment: Explorations of the patient's sick role. *American Journal of Psychotherapy, 18,* 562–573.
Stewart, D. C., & Sullivan, T. J. (1982). Illness behavior and the sick role in chronic disease. *Social Science and Medicine, 16,* 1397–1404.
Stuart, R. (1970). *Trick or treatment.* Champaign, IL: Research Press.
Suchman, E. (1965). Stages of illness and medical care. *Journal of Health and Social Behavior, 6,* 114–128.
Thomas, E. J. (1966). Problems of disability from the perspective of role theory. *Journal of Health and Human Behavior, 7,* 2–14.
Twaddle, A. C. (1969). Health decisions and sick role variations: An exploration. *Journal of Health and Social Behavior, 10,* 105–115.
Waitzkin, H. (1971). Latent functions of the sick role in various institutional settings. *Social Science and Medicine, 5,* 45–75.
Waxler, N. E., & Mishler, E. G. (1963). Hospitalization of psychiatric patients: Physician-centered and family-centered influence patterns. *Journal of Health and Human Behavior, 4,* 250–257.
Wiener, C. L. (1975). The burden of rheumatoid arthritis. In A. L. Strauss (Ed.), *Chronic illness and the quality of life* (pp. 71–80). St. Louis: Mosby.
Wolinsky, F. D., & Wolinsky, S. R. (1981). Expecting sick-role legitimation and getting it. *Journal of Health and Social Behavior, 22,* 229–242.
Zborowski, M. (1952). Cultural components in response to pain. *Journal of Social Issues, 8,* 16–30.
Zola, I. (1966). Culture and symptoms—An analysis of patients' presenting complaints. *American Sociological Review, 31,* 615–630.

CHAPTER 10

Sick-Role Legitimization

Fredric D. Wolinsky

The purpose of this chapter is to consider in detail the issue of sick-role legitimization. There are three major sections to the chapter. The first provides a brief review of the sick role in light of American values and social structure, including a description of the traditional Parsonian scheme and the changes in it that have been necessitated by modifications in the health care delivery system. This section also considers the emergence of sick-role legitimization as a crucial contemporary issue in health behavior, focusing on its use as a coping response, as an avoidance mechanism, and as a justification for failure. The second section focuses on the prevalence of sick-role legitimization, including the taking of sick leave, and the receipt of medications and other visible badges of courage. In the final section we consider the major implications of sick-role legitimization: the increasing demand for it in the face of the coming physician surplus, and its effect on the stability of structural role interdependencies in highly differentiated societies.

INTRODUCTION

The Sick Role in Light of American Values and Social Structure

Parsons's (1951; see also Parsons & Fox, 1952; Parsons, 1958, 1975) idea of the sick role is perhaps the single most important sociological concept in health behavior (see Fox, 1979, 1985; Levine & Kozloff, 1978; Wolinsky, 1988). Nearly all subsequent theoretical or conceptual frameworks in sociological approaches to health behavior have emerged as the result of attempts to refute or to extend the sick-role concept. It tells us what type of behavior we should be able to expect from and associate with the sick person. The four basic aspects of the Parsonian sick role include: (1) the nonresponsibility of the individual for the condition, (2) the exemption of the sick individual from normal task and role obligations, (3) the recognition that being sick is undesirable and that one should want to and try to get well, and (4) the obligation to seek out competent help.

The first aspect of the sick role is that the sick individual is not to be held responsible for the condition. The sick individual's incapacity to perform social roles and tasks is recognized as being beyond the individual's power to overcome by merely deciding to get well. Therefore, for the individual to become well some therapeutic process is necessary.

FREDRIC D. WOLINSKY • Department of Sociology, Texas A & M University, College Station, Texas 77843-4351.

From a theoretical standpoint it does not matter whether the recovery process is spontaneous or aided by other factors (e.g., physicians and medications). The point is that the sick individual is not capable of being healed merely by a personal desire or motivation to get well.

Because of the incapacity to perform social roles and tasks, the individual is defined as being sick. This incapacity to perform one's social roles and tasks becomes the basis for the legitimate social exemption from such performance, with the extent and duration of that legitimate exemption depending on the nature and severity of the illness. The more severe the illness, the greater is the exemption; the less severe the illness, the lesser the exemption. This legitimate exemption, however, is only partial and conditional; its continuation depends on the performance of the other aspects of the sick role.

The basic condition for the temporary exemption of the sick individual from task and role obligations is rooted in the recognition that being sick is a socially undesirable state of affairs. Because it is so undesirable, the individual must want to get well (which also serves as a proscription against malingering), and is obligated to try to get well. To get well, the sick individual must cooperate with others because recovery is not possible through the individual's efforts alone. Thus, although the sick person may enjoy the temporary but legitimate exemption from normal task and role obligations, there is the new obligation to try to get well as soon as possible.

It is the nature of most illnesses that spontaneous cures or recoveries cannot be expected to occur very often, to occur very fast, or to occur completely. The sick individual, however, is expected to recover completely and as soon as possible. Consequently, the sick individual (and anyone responsible for his or her welfare) is saddled with a second obligation. He or she must seek out competent help and cooperate in a concerted effort to recover from the incapacitating illness. Traditionally, the competent helper who is sought and whose instructions are to be followed is the physician.

In order for others to recognize and respect an individual's adoption of the sick role, one of two processes must take place. In the first, *provisional validation* of the petition for sick-role status is granted by the individual's lay referral system (see Freidson, 1970; Suchman, 1965a,b). This occurs early in the illness behavior career when the individual makes the decision that what is being experienced is an illness which needs medical care. The ill individual begins to seek alleviation of the symptoms through self-treatment and home remedies, seeking out information and advice concerning the symptoms from family and friends. In so doing, provisional validation of the sick role is requested. If granted, it results in the temporary exemption from some normal task and role obligations. In essence, the ill individual turns to the lay referral system by discussing the condition and future behavior with the appropriate significant others.

Although provisional validation from the lay referral system permits the sick role to be adopted on a temporary basis, the ill individual does not become a bona fide occupant of the sick role until patient status has been *legitimized by the physician*. This legitimization requires more than mere contact with the physician. The physician must also indicate that the patient is indeed sick. One way to do this is with the simple verbal statement, "yes, you are sick." There are two principal reasons why this straightforward method of conferring sick-role legitimization may not be acceptable to the patient. The first is that simply telling the patient this may be insufficient to meet the patient's emotional needs. Because being sick is considered to be such an undesirable state, the patient will generally expect a more rigorous response (see Parsons, 1951, 1958). Some form of explicit intervention will be required, even if it involves merely the reaffirmation of the patient's self-treatment regimen. Otherwise, the patient will be left to face the emotional strain of being sick without the support of knowing that a positive course of action has been set in motion by the appropriate social control agent (the physician).

The second reason why simply telling the patient may not be acceptable involves its lack of effect on others. Inasmuch as most patient–practitioner encounters (especially those occurring in ambulatory settings) remain private backstage affairs, such unsubstantiated conferrals of sick-role legitimization carry little currency beyond the examining room (see Wolinsky & Wolinsky, 1981). At issue here is the verification of privileged communications. Unless the physician provides some observable sign of having conferred the sick role on the patient, the patient will have difficulty in obtaining the benefits of the sick role from important reference groups. The most drastic observable sign, of course, would be hospitalization. Less severe, yet still effective methods include written communications authorizing the extension of sick-role benefits (missing school for children, sick leave for adults), calling in the appropriate significant others (family, teachers, employers) for a more extended discussion of the illness and the treatment regimen, and issuing prescribed medications (an obtrusive badge of courage, the extent of which is fundamentally up to the patient). Any of these signs should permit the patient to gain access to the benefits of the sick role, as long as the obligations associated with them are met.

There are, of course, a number of necessary modifications in the traditional Parsonian sick role that have been brought about by changes in the health care delivery system (for extended reviews of these issues see Levine & Kozloff, 1978; Wolinsky, 1988). Of principal relevance for the current discussion of sick-role legitimization is the increasing negotiation that occurs between patient and practitioner. This reflects a general decline in the asymmetry of their relationship. For example, Hayes-Bautista (1976a,b) described the process of treatment modification in which patients use convincing and/or countering tactics to obtain what they consider to be more appropriate regimens from their physicians. One aspect of the treatment process that was particularly susceptible to negotiation was drug therapy. Similarly, Haug and Lavin (1983) examined the rise of consumerism in medicine, and noted the existence of a cohort phenomenon. Among patients they found that it was the younger, more knowledgeable ones who were more likely to exhibit consumerist attitudes and behaviors. Among physicians they found that it was the younger practitioners who took a more antiauthority stance who were more likely to accommodate consumerist patients. In a related study, West (1984) used conversational analysis of actual medical encounters to assess the asymmetry of the patient–practitioner relationship. Her findings were somewhat mixed. Although physicians retained and exercised more power than their patients, in the end their interaction was more of an unfolding drama that the two negotiated with much improvisation.

Two factors that mark the beginning of a new era in health care lie at the root of these changes in the traditional patient–practitioner relationship. The first is the general trend toward consumerist behavior in American society. As consumers, patients are better informed and more discriminating than ever before (McKinlay, 1975). Many are no longer willing to take the physician's authority for granted (Haug & Lavin, 1981). They are willing to assert their rights, and want to share in making decisions about their treatment (see Haug & Lavin, 1983). The second factor involves the changing nature of the health care delivery system (see Starr, 1982; Anderson, 1985). By the end of this decade there will be a surplus of some 60,000 physicians in the United States (GMENAC, 1982). Hospital occupancy rates are at their lowest levels in years (AHA, 1986). Nonetheless, health care costs continue on their unending upward spiral (DHHS, 1987). The resulting increase in competition for patients has made both individual physicians and institutional providers (e.g., hospitals and health maintenance organizations) far more sensitive to meeting the needs, especially the nonmedical needs, of their patients (see Light, 1986; McKinlay, 1986). Indeed, although "guest services" (i.e., hotel-like amenities) are a relatively recent approach in health care management, they have become critically important for survival.

These factors suggest that ever-increasing pressure will be placed on physicians' gatekeeping function as the legitimizers of the sick role.

Sick-Role Legitimization as a Contemporary Issue

There is yet another aspect of contemporary life that enhances the salience of sick-role legitimization as an issue worthy of discussion. It involves using the sick role as a coping device, as an avoidance mechanism, or as a justification for failure. In all three uses, sick-role legitimization is sought and employed as a method of dealing with the social pressures of task and role performance expectations. What distinguishes these methods from each other is both their degree of permanence, and the individual's degree of conscious reliance on them. At one extreme, using the sick role as a coping response is likely to be a temporary and unconscious method of adapting to stressful situations and life events. At the other extreme, using the sick role to justify failure permanently is more likely to involve a conscious rationalization process. Relying on the sick role to avoid certain task and role obligations represents the middle range; it may or may not be a conscious and/or permanent method. Let us briefly consider these three uses of the sick role, all of which fall outside of the traditional bounds of appropriateness.

Using the sick role as a coping mechanism follows directly from Parsons's (1951) structural functionalist perspective which emphasizes the integrative functions of medicine in contemporary American society. When traditional linkages between individuals and the social fabric are torn (e.g., the death of a spouse, the loss of a job, or marital dissolution), some alternative means for social integration is necessary. Without it, individuals with fewer links and/or those who have their links taken away are more likely to experience pathological health and illness behavior than their counterparts (i.e., higher rates of psychological distress, suicide, and so forth; see Durkheim, 1897, 1903). It has recently been argued that a decline or loss of integrative links in one area may be partially or fully offset by an increase in other existing integrative links, or by the establishment of new ones (see Coe, Wolinsky, Miller, & Prendergast, 1984; Wan, 1985). Accordingly, it seems plausible that when faced with a decline or loss of integrative links in other functional areas, individuals may attempt to increase their integrative links or develop new ones with health care providers in order to maintain a homeostatic state of integration.

Research supporting this line of conceptual development has developed in two areas. In the first the focus has been on the effects of latent social needs on physician utilization. Shuval (1970) used this perspective to explain why, after adjusting for medical need, more recent immigrants to Israel had higher health services utilization rates than did their earlier arriving counterparts. Her research suggested that the need for catharsis (i.e., emotional support) had a direct effect on the use of health services during the earlier years of the new immigrants' tenure in Israel, and that as they became more integrated their health services utilization became more similar to that of their older immigrant and native Israeli counterparts. A recent replication of that study found that while the cathartic need still persisted among these immigrants, it had become a poor predictor of their current physician utilization. That is, with the passage of time the former immigrants seemed to have abandoned their previous method of turning to physicians to gratify their cathartic needs (Honig-Parnass, 1982).

The second set of studies that have employed this perspective are typified by those of Mechanic and his colleagues (Mechanic, 1978, 1979, 1980, 1983; Tessler & Mechanic, 1978; Tessler, Mechanic, & Dimond, 1976). In these studies the focus is not on the event that reduces or eliminates the integrative link, but on the inference that psychological distress results from such diminishment or removal. In particular, Mechanic and his colleagues have examined the impact of psychological distress on the use of physician services. In retrospective and prospective studies, they have shown that psychological distress is one of the most important predictors of physician utilization, whether the population under study is part of a health maintenance organization, inmates of a state penitentiary, or the noninstitutionalized community.

Although these two sets of studies may seem quite different, they stem from the same theoretical tradition. Both focus on the use of physician services as a method of coping with problems that are not strictly medical. In both cases the principal motivation for seeing the doctor is the satisfaction of the psychological distress induced by significant life events (see Holmes & Rahe, 1967) regardless of whether those life events are part of the immigration process or the routine stressors of daily living. As both the incidence and prevalence of routine stressors increase in contemporary society, it seems reasonable to anticipate an increase in physician utilization as a coping response.

Using the sick role as a justification for failure represents the other extreme of the continuum. Parsons's (1951) initial description of the sick role noted that the sick may be unconsciously motivated to remain so in order to retain the privileges and temporary exemptions associated with being sick (i.e., to extend the benefits of secondary gain). Subsequently, Parsons (1958) expressed a concern that the increasingly high achievement levels associated with contemporary American life might accentuate that motivation. At about the same time, Merton (1957) and others (see especially Blau & Duncan, 1967) had already clearly identified the strong cultural values in American society which stress the importance of moving up in the social hierarchy.

Building on these insights, Cole and Lejeune (1972) suggested that illness may be used to justify a failure to fulfill socially prescribed roles. By adopting the sick role the individual who has failed to meet task and role obligations avoids being blamed because being sick is believed to be beyond individual control. Thus, Cole and Lejeune hypothesized that "wherever there are high rates of self-defined failure there will be high rates of self-defined poor health." In a more general sense, one would expect to find physicians' services overutilized (relative to need) among those who have not been able to perform their task and role assignments.

Similarly, this situation might also apply to those who, although they have been able to perform their current task and role assignments, have not been able to move up in the social hierarchy in the traditionally expected manner. In contemporary American society this scenario has become increasingly likely due to two factors. First, the traditional population pyramid that facilitated normative intergenerational occupational advancement patterns during the first two-thirds of this century can be relied upon no longer. This change was brought about by the combination of decreased mortality rates, decreased fertility rates, and a marked delay in the onset of child-bearing (see Rice & Feldman, 1983; Myers, 1985). Second, the rapid economic expansion experienced during the post-World War II boom has not survived the 1980s. Indeed, the cycle between recessions seems to have shortened, and the annual growth of the gross national product has been relatively inconsequential. Coupled with the changing demographic structure, these poorer economic conditions have resulted in fewer new opportunities for advancement and a marked reduction in the recycling of existing advancement opportunities. Therefore, intergenerational occupational advancement will be considerably less likely for future cohorts, perhaps motivating an increase in the pursuit of sick-role legitimization as a justification for not getting ahead.

Somewhere between the use of sick-role legitimization as a coping device and as a justification for failure lies its possible use as an avoidance mechanism. Perhaps the best example here would be the use of the sick role to defend a less than aggressive pursuit of normatively desired goals, such as upward mobility. Consider the case of the departmental administrator who does not wish to compete for (or receive) a line administrator's position.

Or consider the individual in the clerical pool who does not wish to compete for an office managership. These individuals may rely on sick-role legitimization as a means to avoid advancement to positions for which the pressures of task and role performance would be greater than they are willing to tolerate.

In a similar vein, but less directly related to occupational mobility, would be the use of sick-role legitimization to avoid the assignment of the more stressful tasks and roles within one's present status configuration. For example, in selecting (or vying) for assignments among a pool of co-workers, an individual may use his or her health status as a means of avoiding the more challenging endeavors in order to obtain the more mundane, routine, and otherwise less-threatening assignments. In this way the potential for failing to perform task and role assignments successfully is reduced, making life "safer" and more successful (albeit at a lower "degree of difficulty") for the individual.

What all three of these uses of sick-role legitimization (as a coping device, as a justification for failure, or as an avoidance mechanism) have in common is that they represent an encroachment on the normative expectation of the undesirability of being sick. In a sense, this suggests a voluntary medicalization of life that appears to contrast rather markedly with the *in*voluntary expropriation described by Illich (1976) and Conrad (1975; Conrad & Schneider, 1980). Those scholars argued that medicine was changing the traditional way in which pain, suffering, and deviance were viewed as part of the human condition. The uses of sick-role legitimization described above, however, suggest that individuals themselves are implicitly and explicitly using medicine temporarily and permanently to shield themselves from their daily hassles, lack of commitment to traditional goals, and failure to get ahead. This represents a significant departure from traditional sick-role behavior, and has important implications for the future of the health care delivery system.

THE PREVALENCE OF SICK-ROLE LEGITIMIZATION

As indicated, measuring sick-role legitimization is not an easy task (see also Wolinsky & Wolinsky, 1981). This is primarily due to the fact that what occurs in most patient–practitioner encounters in ambulatory settings is a private, backstage affair. Indeed, even when an obtrusive indicator of sick-role legitimization has been provided (such as prescribed medications, or proscriptions against certain activities), the patient has the opportunity to manage the visibility of that indicator. Thus, charting the prevalence of sick-role legitimization is necessarily an indirect process. There are, however, two plausible initial steps. The first focuses more on the provisional validation of the sick role by charting the distribution of sick leave. The second addresses sick-role legitimization more directly by focusing on the receipt of prescription medications in the ambulatory setting.

The Taking of Sick Leave

Sick leave is available to most employed persons in the United States, although the terms and conditions under which it may be taken vary considerably. This makes the use of sick leave data somewhat tenuous. Moreover, there is no uniform mechanism for the reporting and registration of sick leave. Thus, official data on sick leave at the national level are hard to come by and difficult to interpret. An alternative is to rely on self-reported restricted activity, bed-disability, or work or school days lost due to health problems. Questions about these have traditionally been included in the annual national Health Interview Survey (HIS), which typically involves detailed face-to-face interviews with a probability sample of about 110,000 individuals residing in some 40,000 households.

Four such indirect measures can be tracked between 1971 and 1983 (the broadest time period available at present). These include: (1) the number of days lost from work for currently employed persons aged 18 years or more; (2) the number of school days missed by youths aged 5–17 years; (3) the number of days spent in bed (which may overlap with item 1 or 2); and (4) the number of other days on which a person cuts down on his or her usual activity level due to a health problem. The health problems underlying all four indicators include illness, injury, or impairment, and they may be of either an acute or a chronic nature. They are expressed here as rates per person per year (DHHS, 1986a).

The number of work and school days lost due to health reasons has declined over this 13-year period. The change in lost work days (from 5.1 to 4.2), although not quite one day per person, nonetheless represents almost a 20% decline. The change in lost school days (from 5.5 to 5.0) is more modest; it represents about a 10% decline. These indicators suggest that the provisional validation of the sick role was somewhat less frequent in 1983 than in 1971. The data on the number of bed days, however, contradict this. They show a little more than a half day per person (or approximately 10%) increase (from 6.1 to 6.7). Finally, the number of restricted activity days has declined (from 15.7 to 14.5) by a little over one day per person per year, or about 6%. Overall, then, three of the four indicators suggest a general decline in the prevalence of taking sick leave.

That interpretation, however, may not be accurate. Although these data are self-reports of requests for the provisional validation of the sick role, they are not normed to the existence of actual health conditions. Unfortunately, the HIS data provide no opportunity for directly adjusting the taking of sick leave for the need to take it. It is possible, however, to arrive at an approximation for that adjustment process by calculating the ratio of the number of acute conditions reported in 1983 to that reported in 1971. This ratio is 174.7/218.5 or 0.80. Thus, although the prevalence of acute conditions had by 1983 declined to 80% of its 1971 level, there was not a comparable decline in the taking of sick leave. Indeed, only the relative rate of lost work days remained the same. Accordingly, these data provide some support for the hypothesis that sick-role legitimization is relatively more pervasive today, at least as measured by these indirect indicators.

The Receipt of Prescription Medications

Data on the prevalence of prescription medications can be derived from the National Ambulatory Medical Care Survey (NAMCS), conducted by the National Center for Health Statistics. NAMCS involves a national probability sample of 89,447 patient visits to 3676 office-based physicians. Unfortunately, the data on prescribed drug therapy are presently available only for the years 1980 and 1981. Thus, changes in prescribed drug-taking behavior cannot be charted in the same way that changes in the taking of sick leave could. Detailed data, however, are available for the patients of general and family practitioners (who happen to prescribe drugs more often than their fellow practitioners, accounting for two-thirds of all prescriptions), and for antimicrobial drugs (which may be more likely to be dispensed in order to satisfy patient requests for sick-role legitimization). In any event, the data (DHHS, 1983, 1986b) are staggering.

During 1980 and 1981, office-based general or family practitioners prescribed or administered some form of drug therapy to 74% of their office patients. Moreover, the average number of drugs mentioned per visit was 1.39 (1.89 among those with at least one drug mentioned). This underscores the general proclivity toward drug therapy in ambulatory care. Focusing specifically on the domain of antimicrobial drug therapy (defined as the use of penicillins, cephalosporins, macrolides and lincosamides, tetracyclines, sulfonamides and trimethoprim, and miscellaneous antimicrobials) reveals similar results. At least one antimicrobial drug was prescribed in 188.8 million office visits, or one out of every six that took place. In addition, an average of 0.9 other drugs were prescribed to supplement the antimicrobials.

What these data fail to indicate is whether or not these drugs were justly prescribed. By the physicians' own admissions, however, 2.4% of all the antimicrobial drugs prescribed involved situations where the reason for the visit was *not* for illness care (DHHS, 1986b). Moreover, data from the 1977 and 1978 NAMCS (DHHS, 1982) indicate physicians believed that the reasons for nearly 4.9 million office visits were to counsel patients about their social problems. Thus, it would seem that the prevalence of drug therapy exceeds the medical need it. This can be taken as an indirect indication of patients' pressures for sick-role legitimization. What cannot be determined from these data is whether the pressure for sick-role legitimization, in the form of prescribed medications, has been increasing over time.

IMPLICATIONS FOR HEALTH CARE DELIVERY AND THE SOCIAL SYSTEM

As already indicated, there are theoretical reasons to expect increased pressure from patients for sick-role legitimization in the ambulatory care setting. Principal among these are the increasing levels of social stress and the decreasing opportunities for occupational attainment being faced by younger cohorts in contemporary American society. The three behavioral variants discussed involve having the physician as the gatekeeper legitimize the sick role so that the petitioner can (1) use the temporary exemption from some task and role obligations to cope with the daily stressors of life, (2) use the more permanent but less complete exemption from some task and role obligations to avoid pursuing goals or assignments that may be self-defined as out of reach, and (3) use the permanent and complete exemption from task and role obligations to justify failure in general. The first situation is likely to involve only an initial visit to the doctor for an acute episode, the second is likely to include a series of follow-up visits for a relatively mild chronic ailment, and the third is likely to involve a prolonged series of follow-up visits for a serious chronic complaint. We now turn to the implications of the expected increase in the demand for sick-role legitimization on the health care delivery system, and on the social system.

Implications for the Health Care Delivery System

The effect of the potential increase in the demand for sick-role legitimization on the health care delivery system may best be discussed in tandem with the coming physician surplus. The Graduate Medical Education National Advisory Committee (1981) has projected a physician surplus of some 60,000 by 1990. Light (1986) considered this estimate to be quite conservative and expects the surplus to be closer to 90,000 physicians. Thus, although the size of the surplus is subject to debate, there is general agreement that the supply of physicians will exceed the demand for their services (estimated on the basis of need).

If the demand for sick-role legitimization as a coping response, an avoidance mechanism, or a justification for failure increases as expected, however, the surplus physician supply may be substantially reduced. Moreover, McKinlay (1986) has argued (and Haug and Lavin's [1983] earlier work suggests) that the physician surplus will bring about an era in which physicians are more tolerant of and receptive to their patients' needs and wants. Indeed, I suggest that it may herald a much-needed shift in conceptual focus from "doctor-shopping" to "doctor-manipulation."

The increased competition among physicians harnessed with the increased demand for sick-role legitimization among patients may result in a considerable expansion of the ambulatory care market, especially with regard to the use of prescribed drug therapy. Therefore, in the future we may expect to see the annual rate of physician visits per person increase, especially among 25- to 55-year-olds, because they are most likely to bear the brunt of the increased stress that results from the reduced opportunities for intergenerational advancement. Associated with this increase in ambulatory physician utilization (and the concomitant prescribed drug therapy), of course, will be additional upward pressures on per capita health care costs.

This suggests that much more research is needed on *why* people go to see the doctor. Although an extensive literature on health services utilization already exists, most of it focuses on who uses what health services, when, where, and how. The "why" question has escaped most health services researchers if for no other reason than it is quite difficult to answer (see Wolinsky, 1988). Nonetheless, what is needed now is more ground-breaking research patterned after Mechanic's (1978, 1979, 1980, 1983) longitudinal studies on how psychological distress *causes* the use of health services. In particular, it is imperative that future studies pay exacting detail to determining the degree to which physician visits are used for medical reasons or for inappropriate sick-role legitimization (i.e., for coping, avoidance, or justification). This further will require the development of far more specific longitudinal protocols which focus on the psychosocial factors (conscious and unconscious) that trigger patients to seek out their doctors (especially their general or family practitioners).

Implications for the Social System

There are at least three implications of the expanding use of sick-role legitimization on the social system that warrant attention. All three stem from the fact that the use of sick-role legitimization as a coping response, as an avoidance mechanism, or as a justification for failure represents an encroachment on the undesirability of being sick. This has serious implications for both the sick-role concept and the broader social system of which it is an integral part.

The first implication is a change in the basic moral fabric of society. As Illich (1976) and Conrad (1975; Conrad & Schneider, 1980) have suggested, the domain of medicine has been expropriating to its jurisdiction a sizeable portion of the pain, suffering, and deviance that had traditionally been considered to be part of the human condition. Individuals' use of sick-role legitimization to cope with, justify, or avoid their failures represents a further and voluntary shift away from individual responsibility for and commitment to the traditional American work ethic. Indeed, it may herald the end of an era characterized by its achievement orientation, and the emergence of a more hedonistic period in which a "me" outlook and "entitlement" attitudes prevail. To be sure, it indicates weakened obligations to the traditional social order.

This reduced commitment to the social order suggests the second implication. If individuals in highly structurally differentiated societies exhibit less commitment to performing their task and role obligations (as evidenced in their use of sick-role legitimization for coping with, avoiding, or justifying their failures), then the institutions in which they operate must respond by decreasing the potential disruption that may occur from that declining commitment. One approach would be to increase the redundancy of workers. This could be achieved either by employing backup workers for each sensitive position, or by reducing the specificity of each worker's tasks. Either method, however, involves retreating from the advantages of structural role interdependencies in highly differentiated societies.

The third implication of the use of sick-role legitimization for coping, avoidance, or justification purposes is that the sick-role concept itself may be in need of a major theoretical overhaul. In the Parsonian (1951, 1958, 1975) scheme, physicians are recognized as the legitimate social control agents for any deviance that occurs because the individual cannot perform assigned tasks and roles. The three circumstances discussed in this chapter, however, seriously strain that interpretation (i.e., the individuals are able, but not willing to carry out their expected assignments). Indeed, if physicians succumb to such requests for sick-role legitimization, then their ability to serve as social control agents will have been substantially diminished. This focuses not on the individual, but on the structural integrity of physicians to serve in such a crucial role. Therefore, modifications of the Parsonian scheme (including the sick role, the physician's role, and the patient–practitioner relationship) are necessary if this structural–functional approach to maintaining the social order in highly differentiated societies is to remain applicable.

REFERENCES

American Hospital Association. (1986). *Hospital statistics* (1985 ed.). Chicago: American Hospital Association.

Anderson, O. W. (1985). *Health services in the United States: A growth industry since 1875*. Ann Arbor: Health Administration Press.

Blau, P. M., & Duncan, O. D. (1967). *The American occupational structure*. Chicago: University of Chicago Press.

Coe, R. M., Wolinsky, F. D., Miller, D. K., & Prendergast, J. M. (1984). Complementary and compensatory functions in social network relationships among the elderly. *The Gerontologist, 24,* 396–400.

Cole, S., & Lejeune, R. (1972). Illness and the legitimation of failure. *American Sociological Review, 37,* 347–356.

Conrad, P. (1975). The discovery of hyperkinesis: Notes on the medicalization of deviant behavior. *Social Problems, 23,* 12–21.

Conrad, P., & Scheider, J. W. (1980). *Deviance and medicalization*. St. Louis: Mosby.

Department of Health, Education, and Welfare. (1975). *Current estimates from the Health Interview Survey, United States, 1973* (DHEW Publication No. 75–1522). Washington, DC: U.S. Government Printing Office.

Department of Health and Human Services. (1982). *Patients' reasons for visiting physicians: National Ambulatory Medical Care Survey, United States, 1977–1978* (DHHS Publication No. 82-1717). Washington, DC: U.S. Government Printing Office.

Department of Health and Human Services. (1983). *Patterns of ambulatory care in general and family practice: The National Ambulatory Medical Care Survey, United States, January 1980–December 1981* (DHHS Publication No. 83–1734). Washington, DC: U.S. Government Printing Office.

Department of Health and Human Services. (1986a). *Current estimates from the National Health Interview Survey, United States, 1983* (DHHS Publication No. 86-1582). Washington, DC: U.S. Government Printing Office.

Department of Health and Human Services. (1986b). *Use of antimicrobial drugs in office-based practice, United States, 1980–81* (DHHS Publication No. 86-1746). Washington, DC: U.S. Government Printing Office.

Department of Health and Human Services. (1987). *Health, United States, 1986* (DHHS Publication No. 87-1232). Washington, DC: U.S. Government Printing Office.

Durkheim, E. (1897; translated 1951). *Suicide: A study in sociology*. New York: Free Press.

Durkheim, E. (1903; translated 1961). *Moral education: A study in the theory and application of the sociology of education*. New York: Free Press.

Fox, R. C. (1979). *Essays in medical sociology*. New York: Wiley.

Fox, R. C. (1985). Reflections and opportunities in the sociology of medicine. *Journal of Health and Social Behavior, 26,* 6–14.

Freidson, E. (1970). *The profession of medicine: A study in the sociology of applied knowledge*. New York: Harper & Row.
Graduate Medical Education National Advisory Committee. (1981). *Summary report of the Graduate Medical Education National Advisory Committee* (DHHS Publication No. 81-651). Washington, DC: U.S. Government Printing Office.
Haug, M., & Lavin, B. (1981). Practitioner or patient: Who's in charge? *Journal of Health and Social Behavior, 22,* 219–229.
Haug, M., & Lavin, B. (1983). *Consumerism in medicine: Challenging physician authority*. Beverly Hills: Sage.
Hayes-Bautista, D. (1976a). Termination of the patient–practitioner relationship: Divorce, patient style. *Journal of Health and Social Behavior, 17,* 12–22.
Hayes-Bautista, D. (1976b). Modifying the treatment: Patient compliance, patient control, and medical care. *Social Science and Medicine, 10,* 233–238.
Holmes, T. H., & Rahe, R. H. (1967). The social readjustment rating scale. *Journal of Psychosomatic Research, 11,* 213–218.
Honig-Parnass, T. (1982). The effects of latent social needs on physician utilization by immigrants: A replication study. *Social Science and Medicine, 16,* 505–514.
Illich, I. (1976). *Medical nemesis*. New York: Pantheon.
Levine, S., & Kozloff, M. (1978). The sick role: Assessment and overview. *Annual Review of Sociology, 4,* 317–343.
Light, D. (1986). *Organizational consequences of a physician surplus: An overview*. Paper presented at the annual meeting of the American Sociological Association.
McKinlay, J. (1975). Who is really ignorant: Patient or practitioner? *Journal of Health and Social Behavior, 16,* 136–145.
McKinlay, J. (1986). *Proletarianization and the social transformation of doctoring*. Paper presented at the annual meeting of the American Sociological Association.
Mechanic, D. (1978). *Medical sociology: A comprehensive text* (2nd ed.). New York: Free Press.
Mechanic, D. (1979). Development of psychological distress among young adults. *Archives of General Psychiatry, 36,* 1233–1239.
Mechanic, D. (1980). The experience and reporting of common physical complaints. *Journal of Health and Social Behavior, 21,* 146–155.
Mechanic, D. (1983). The experience and expression of distress: The study of illness behavior and medical utilization. In D. Mechanic (Ed.), *Handbook of health, health care, and the health professions*. New York: Free Press.
Merton, R. K. (1957). *Social theory and social structure*. New York: Free Press.
Myers, G. (1985). Aging and world-wide population change. In R. Binstock & E. Shanas (Eds.), *Handbook of aging and the social sciences* (2nd ed.). Princeton, NJ: Van Nostrand–Reinhold.
Parsons, T. (1951). *The social system*. New York: Free Press.
Parsons, T. (1958). Definitions of health and illness in light of American values and social structure. In E. G. Jaco (Ed.), *Patients, physicians, and illness*. New York: Free Press.
Parsons, T. (1975). The sick role and the role of the physician reconsidered. *Milbank Memorial Fund Quarterly, 53,* 257–278.
Parsons, T., & Fox, R. C. (1952). Illness, therapy, and the modern urban American family. *Journal of Social Issues, 8,* 31–44.
Rice, D. P., & Feldman, J. (1983). Living longer in the United States: Changes and health needs of the elderly. *Milbank Memorial Fund Quarterly, 61,* 362–396.
Shuval, J. T. (1970). *The social functions of medical practice*. San Francisco: Jossey–Bass.
Starr, P. (1982). *The social transformation of American medicine: The rise of a sovereign profession and the making of a vast industry*. New York: Basic Books.
Suchman, E. (1965a). Social patterns of illness and medical care. *Journal of Health and Human Behavior, 6,* 2–16.
Suchman, E. (1965b). Stages of illness and medical care. *Journal of Health and Human Behavior, 6,* 114–128.
Tessler, R., & Mechanic, D. (1978). Psychological distress and perceived health status. *Journal of Health and Social Behavior, 19,* 254–262.

Tessler, R., Mechanic, D., & Dimond, M. (1976). The effect of psychological distress on physician utilization: A prospective study. *Journal of Health and Social Behavior, 17,* 353–364.
Wan, T. T. H. (1985). *Gerontological health and role loss in the later years*. Lexington: Lexington Books.
West, C. (1984). *Routine complications: Troubles with talk between doctors and patients*. Bloomington: Indiana University Press.
Wolinsky, F. D. (1988). *The sociology of health: Principles, practitioners, and issues* (2nd ed.). Belmont: Wadsworth.
Wolinsky, F. D., & Wolinsky, S. R. (1981). Expecting sick-role legitimation and getting it. *Journal of Health and Social Behavior, 23,* 229–242.

CHAPTER 11

Gender and Health-Related Behavior

Ingrid Waldron

INTRODUCTION

For this review, health-related behavior has been defined broadly to include any behavior that has a significant effect on health or is generally believed to have such an effect. Health-related behavior can be subdivided into risky behavior, preventive behavior, and treatment-seeking or self-treatment. The following paragraphs briefly summarize gender differences in each of these categories of health-related behavior.

In Western countries, males tend to engage in more risky behavior than do females, particularly for risky behavior that involves physical daring or illegal behavior (Waldron, 1983a, 1986a). Males more often than females use guns, take physical risks in recreation, drive unsafely, drink heavily, use illicit drugs, and work at physically hazardous jobs. Males also smoke more, except among teenagers and young adults in some countries (U.S. Department of Health and Human Services, 1980; Waldron, 1983b, 1988). Similar patterns are observed in non-Western countries. For example, males have more accidents in non-Western as well as Western countries (Waldron, 1986a). In many non-Western societies, more men than women smoke and drink, although in some groups women are as likely as men to smoke or to drink (Child, Barry, & Bacon, 1965; Waldron, Bratelli, Carriker, Sung, Vogeli, & Waldman, 1988). Although many types of risky behavior are more common among males, there are some types that are more common among females. For example, in contemporary Western societies females are much more likely to engage in the severe food intake restriction characteristic of anorexia nervosa (Garfinkel & Garner, 1982).

Gender differences in preventive behavior are highly variable. In the United States, women more often than men take vitamins, brush their teeth, and use dental floss or a waterpick, but men get as much or more vigorous physical exercise than do women (National Center for Health Statistics, 1986a,b; Waldron, 1983a). No consistent gender differences have been found in the proportion of adults who use seat belts or in the proportion who obtain immunizations (Kohn & White, 1976; Waldron, 1983a). In the United States and Canada, women visit a physician for a general checkup more often than do men, but in several European countries men obtained checkups more often.

Gender differences in treatment-seeking and self-treatment are also quite variable. In Western countries it appears that women are more likely to respond to many types of

INGRID WALDRON • Department of Biology, University of Pennsylvania, Philadelphia, Pennsylvania 19104-6018.

symptoms by seeking medical care and/or self-medication, but for symptoms of certain types of serious illness there do not appear to be gender differences in obtaining medical care (Dean, Holst, & Wagner, 1983; Kohn & White, 1976; Verbrugge, 1982; Waldron, 1983a). In some non-Western societies, females obtained less medical care than did males (Waldron, 1983a).

Thus, gender differences in health-related behavior vary depending on the type of behavior and the cultural context. This variability suggests that gender differences in health-related behavior are not due primarily to a single variable, such as gender differences in the degree of concern with health. Evidence presented in subsequent sections of this chapter supports the conclusion that concerns with the health effects of behavior have little or no influence on gender differences in many types of health-related behavior. This conclusion is compatible with previous evidence that concerns with health effects have only a minor influence on the adoption of many types of health-related behavior (Cahalan, Cisin, & Crossley, 1969; Garfinkel & Garner, 1982; US DHHS, 1980). Because concerns with health effects have little influence on the adoption of many types of behavior that affect health, I have chosen to use the term *health-related behavior* rather than *health behavior*.

The observation that gender differences in health-related behavior vary depending on the type of behavior and the cultural context suggests that the causes of these gender differences also vary for different types of behavior and in different cultural contexts. Therefore, my analysis of the causes of gender differences in health-related behavior will focus on several specific types of health-related behavior, with attention to cultural variation where data are available. The following three sections present analyses of the causes of gender differences in smoking, drinking, and accidents, each of which is an important cause of men's higher mortality in Western countries (Waldron, 1986a,b). The subsequent section analyzes reasons why females more often diet in order to lose weight and why females more often develop the eating disorders, anorexia nervosa and bulimia. Next I analyze gender differences in physician visits. General conclusions derived from these analyses are presented in the final section. One important conclusion is that, for many types of health-related behavior, gender differences are determined in large part by the compatibility of the specific type of health-related behavior with general male and female roles and expectations concerning appropriate male and female behavior.

Most of the available evidence concerning health-related behavior is derived from studies in the United States and other Western countries, so the conclusions and generalizations presented apply primarily to these countries. In this chapter the evidence presented is for Western countries unless explicitly designated as evidence for non-Western countries.

Due to limitations of space, this review is necessarily selective rather than comprehensive. Additional information concerning the patterns and causes of gender differences in health-related behavior and additional references to the original literature can be found in the reviews cited herein.

SMOKING

Historical data for Western countries indicate that, in general, more men than women used tobacco, although in a few historical situations tobacco use was nearly universal for both men and women (Waldron, 1988). At the beginning of the 20th century in the United States and Great Britain, pipe and cigar smoking and tobacco chewing were much more common among men than among women. As cigarette smoking became popular, this new tobacco habit was also adopted primarily by men. By the end of World War I cigarette smoking was common among men and rare among women (US DHHS, 1980; Waldron, 1988). Women took up cigarette smoking several decades later than men, and by World War II gender differences in smoking prevalence were decreasing. This decrease has been particularly striking for teenagers and young adults; in this age range females have been as likely or more likely than males to be smokers in many Western countries in recent years (Hill & Gray, 1984; Johnston, O'Malley, & Bachman, 1986; US DHHS, 1980; Waldron, 1986a, 1988).

Data for non-Western societies also show that smoking has been more common among men than among women in almost all cases studied (Finau, Stanhope, & Prior, 1982; Joly, 1975; Mougne, MacLennan, & Atsana, 1982; Waldron, 1983a, 1986a; Waldron *et al.*, 1988). However, there has been considerable variation in the magnitude of gender differences, and in a few cases smoking has been about equally common for women and men. I have not found evidence of any group in which smoking has been substantially more prevalent among women.

In addition to the gender differences in the prevalence of smoking, there are gender differences in smoking habits among smokers. For example, in both Western and non-Western societies, men generally smoke more per day and inhale more deeply (Finau *et al.*, 1982; Joly, 1975; US DHHS, 1980; Waldron, 1986a, 1988; Waldron *et al.*, 1988).

It appears that the most important single factor contributing to gender differences in smoking has been widespread social disapproval of women's smoking. Such disapproval has been reported from regions as diverse as Japan, India, Sri Lanka, Ethiopia, and Kenya in recent decades and the United States and Great Britain in the early 20th century (Waldron, 1986a, 1988; Waldron *et al.*, 1988). Social disapproval of women's smoking has decreased considerably in Western countries during this century, and this has been an important reason for the decrease in gender differences in smoking prevalence.

Survey data provide additional evidence for the importance of social disapproval of women's smoking, at least in some cultural conditions. For nonsmokers in the United States in the mid-1960s, women much more frequently than men reported that the reason they had not taken up cigarette smoking was that smoking was not socially acceptable (U.S. Department of Health, Education and Welfare, 1969; Waldron, 1988). In addition, women more often than men reported family members' objections as a reason for having never smoked. In Latin American cities in 1971–72, a third of female nonsmokers reported that they had never smoked because smoking was unfeminine, and a quarter of male smokers reported that they had begun to smoke because it gave them an increased sense of masculinity (Joly, 1975; Waldron *et al.*, 1988). These attitudes appear to have made a major contribution to the gender differences in smoking.

The reasons for the widespread social disapproval of women's smoking have not been clearly identified, but disapproval of women's smoking appears to be related to several aspects of traditional sex roles (Waldron *et al.*, 1988). For example, in many societies men have had greater power and freedom of behavior, and social proscriptions against women's smoking appear to have been related to more general restrictions on women's behavior. In some cultures, women who smoke have been considered promiscuous or prostitutes, and the social pressures against women's smoking have been linked to the restrictions on women's sexual behavior. These attitudes have been reported from cultures as diverse as the United States and Great Britain in the early 20th century, Japan in the mid-20th century, and several African cultures in recent decades (Fass, 1977; Waldron, 1988; Waldron *et al.*, 1988).

There appear to be other links between traditional sex roles and gender differences in smoking. For example, in Western countries cigarette smoking has been encouraged in the military and discouraged by some religions. Thus, men's greater involvement in the military and women's greater involvement with religion appear to have contributed to gender differences in smoking, although these effects appear to have been small in magnitude in recent decades (US DHEW, 1969; Waldron, 1988). Rebelliousness and rejection of adult authority have been tolerated more in boys, and boys' greater rebelliousness appears to have contributed to their higher rates of teenage smoking in earlier periods (Bachman, Johnston, & O'Malley, 1981; Waldron, 1988).

Gender differences in roles have decreased during the 20th century in Western societies, and it appears that this has been an important underlying cause of the decrease in gender differences in smoking. One specific hypothesis is that increases in women's employment have contributed to increases in women's smoking, because employed women have been exposed more to the world of men's opinions and habits, employed women have been less subject to conventional constraints on women's behavior, and employed women have had more access to the money with which to buy cigarettes. This hypothesis is not supported by the available data.

In earlier data for the United States, employed women were slightly more likely than housewives to be smokers, but this difference is not observed in recent data for young and middle-aged women (US DHHS, 1986; Waldron, 1988). Smoking rates vary by occupation, with women in managerial and administrative occupations more likely than housewives to be smokers and women in professional and technical occupations less likely than housewives to be smokers. In Latin American cities in 1971–72, smoking was equally common for housewives and women in blue-collar and clerical occupations, but women in administrative and professional occupations were more likely to smoke (Joly, 1975). In these Latin American cities, women with more education were more likely to smoke, and the effects of education may account for the higher smoking rates among women in administrative and professional occupations. In international data, women's labor force participation rates are not related to either the prevalence of smoking among women or gender differences in the prevalence of smoking (Waldron, 1988).

These data suggest that, on the average, a woman's employment has little *direct* effect on whether she becomes a smoker. However, it appears that there has been an indirect link between women's employment and smoking. The increases in women's employment during this century have contributed to increasing equality between women and men and general liberalization of norms concerning women's behavior. One aspect of these general social trends has been increasing social acceptance of women's smoking, and this increasing acceptance appears to have been a major cause of the increases in women's smoking.

A link between general attitudes toward women's rights and women's smoking is indicated by the observation that, in the 1920s in the United States, young women who smoked explicitly asserted their right to smoke as part of their general equal rights with men (Fass, 1977). However, recent data do not support an association between support of feminism and smoking (Waldron, 1988).

One aspect of sex roles may have contributed to increased smoking by women in recent decades. Appearance and physical attractiveness have been particularly important for girls and women and recently, at least in the United States, there has been increasing emphasis on a slim figure as a crucial aspect of attractiveness for women (Garfinkel & Garner, 1982; Rodin, Silberstein, & Striegel-Moore, 1985). Smoking appears to help prevent weight gain. Thus, it is not surprising that women more often report the belief that smoking prevents weight gain as a reason for smoking (Hill & Gray, 1984; US DHHS, 1980; Waldron, 1988).

A final hypothesized link between sex roles and smoking is that women are more involved in health care for other family members and are more concerned with their own health and, consequently, might be expected to avoid a health-damaging behavior such as smoking. Conversely, males are encouraged to take more physical risks and males more often engage in a variety of risky behaviors, and thus might be expected to be less concerned with the health-damaging effects of smoking. However, a variety of evidence indicates that concerns with the health consequences of smoking have not had a greater influence on women's smoking than on men's smoking and health-related motivations have not made a substantial contribution to gender differences in smoking.

Surveys in Western countries typically find little gender difference in knowledge or beliefs concerning the health-damaging effects of smoking and, when gender differences are observed, greater knowledge or concern is shown as frequently by men as by women (Hill & Gray, 1984; NCHS, 1986b; US DHEW, 1969; Waldron, 1988). Similarly, surveys of reasons for never having smoked or reasons for having quit smoking have shown that men were at least as likely as women to mention health reasons (Joly, 1975; US DHEW, 1969). In addition, current evidence indicates that programs to publicize the health effects of smoking have had at least as great an effect on men's smoking as on women's (Waldron, 1988).

The patterns of gender differences in specific types of tobacco use also suggest that concern about health effects has not been an important cause of women's lower rates of tobacco use, and the relative social acceptability of various types of tobacco use for men and women has played a more important role. Gender differences are modest in magnitude for cigarette smoking, the riskiest type of tobacco use, but the most socially acceptable for women. In contrast, gender differences are large for pipe and cigar smoking and tobacco chewing, which are relatively safer, but much less socially acceptable for women (Jarvis, 1984; US DHEW, 1969; Waldron, 1988). Men who quit smoking cigarettes have often switched to cigar smoking, while women have rarely done so. This appears to be a major reason why men have been more likely than women to quit cigarette smoking in some periods in the United States and Great Britain (Jarvis, 1984).

In addition to the social influences on gender differences in smoking, biological influences have been hypothesized. There is some evidence that females may metabolize nicotine more slowly than do males and consequently girls may be more likely than boys to experience nicotine overdose and feel sick when they smoke their first cigarette (Waldron, 1983b, 1988). As a result, girls might be less likely to become cigarette smokers, particularly if low-nicotine cigarettes are not available. However, evidence from the United States in the mid-1960s suggests that gender differences in feeling sick after smoking a first cigarette probably made only a minor contribution to gender differences in smoking adoption (Palmer, 1970; Waldron, 1988). One reason why gender differences in the response to a first cigarette were relatively unimportant was that many girls and women never smoked even a single cigarette, and this in itself was a major reason for gender differences in smoking in this period (Palmer, 1970; US DHEW, 1969). Thus, available evidence suggests that sex differences in nicotine metabolism and the tendency to experience nicotine overdose have not been a major cause of gender differences in the prevalence of smoking.

Another hypothesis has been that smoking cessation may result in more withdrawal symptoms for women than for men and this might contribute to lower smoking cessation rates for women (US DHHS, 1980). However, recent studies of both objectively and subjectively assessed withdrawal symptoms do not show the hypothesized gender differences, at least within the first few days after smoking cessation (Svikis, Hatsukami, Hughes, Carroll, & Pickens, 1986; Waldron, 1988). In addition, there has been considerable historical and cross-cultural variation in gender differences in smoking cessation rates, with higher cessation rates for women than for men in many non-Western countries (Finau *et al.*, 1982; Waldron, 1988; Waldron *et al.*, 1988). This variability indicates that inherent sex differences in withdrawal symptoms have not been the primary determinant of gender differences in smoking cessation rates.

In summary, smoking has been more common among men in almost all available cross-cultural and historical data. However, this gender difference has varied in magnitude, and in a few cases females have been as likely or slightly more likely to be smokers. Social disapproval of women's smoking has been a major cause of gender differences in smoking, and growing social acceptance of women's smoking appears to have been an important reason for the decline in gender differences in smoking in Western countries in the 20th century. Increases in women's employment have contributed to increasing general equality between the sexes, and this in turn has contributed to increasing acceptance of women's smoking. However, it appears that, on the average, a woman's employment has little direct effect on her smoking habits. A variety of additional factors have influenced gender differences in smoking. For example, boys' greater rebelliousness has tended to increase males' smoking rates, while females' greater concern with weight control tends to increase females' smoking rates. Thus, available evidence indicates that several aspects of sex roles and expectations concerning gender-appropriate behavior have influenced gender differences in smoking. Several other hypotheses were not supported by available evidence. For example, there appears to have been little gender difference in concern with the health effects of smoking, and health-related motivations appear to have made little or no contribution to gender differences in smoking.

ALCOHOL CONSUMPTION

In Western societies in the 20th century, boys and men have consumed more alcohol than girls and women (Clark & Midanik, 1982; Ferrence, 1980; Johnston *et al.,* 1986; NCHS, 1986a,b). In the present-day United States and Canada, gender differences are large for daily drinking, heavy drinking, and problem drinking, each of which is roughly three times more common among men. Gender differences are generally smaller if infrequent users of alcohol are included. Indeed, among teenagers in the United States and Canada today, there is little or no gender difference in the proportion who drink at least occasionally.

Trends in gender differences in alcohol consumption are somewhat controversial due to limited data and the complexity of the observed patterns. For adults in the United States and Canada it appears that in recent decades there has been relatively little convergence in the drinking habits of men and women (Clark & Midanik, 1982; Ferrence, 1980; Wilsnack, Wilsnack, & Klassen, 1986). For adolescents there appears to have been a decrease in gender differences in alcohol use during the 1970s (Ferrence, 1980; Johnston *et al.,* 1986). In contrast, for college students gender differences have increased recently for one measure of heavy drinking: the frequency of consuming five or more drinks in a row has increased for college men but not for college women (Johnston *et al.,* 1986).

Gender differences in alcohol consumption vary considerably cross-culturally. In a third of nonindustrial societies studied, men and women consumed alcohol equally (Child *et al.,* 1965). In all cases in which a gender difference was observed, men drank more than women. More recent data for non-Western countries also indicate that more men drink, but in some cases this difference is quite small (Finau *et al.,* 1982; Mougne *et al.,* 1982).

The patterns of gender differences in alcohol consumption show many similarities to the patterns of gender differences in cigarette smoking, but there are also important differences. For example, in the present-day United States men drink and smoke more, but gender differences are larger for drinking than for smoking (NCHS, 1986a). The causes of gender differences in alcohol consumption show many similarities to the causes of gender differences in smoking, but there are also significant differences. The evidence to be presented concerning causes of gender differences in drinking is based primarily on data for the United States.

A major cause of gender differences in alcohol consumption has been social acceptance, even approval, of men's drinking and social disapproval of women's drinking, particularly heavy drinking (Gomberg, 1982; Lemle, 1984, cited in Biener, 1987). The gender differences in the social acceptability of drinking are observed even among contemporary teenagers. For example, among high school seniors, girls are substantially more likely than boys to report that their close friends disapprove or would disapprove of them drinking daily or heavily (Johnston, Bachman, & O'Malley, 1984).

It has been hypothesized that many traditional societies developed social proscriptions against heavy drinking by women because even occasional drunkenness interfered with adequate care of babies and young children, whereas occasional drunkenness may have been compatible with the usual responsibilities of men in nonindustrial societies (Child *et al.*, 1965). Another hypothesized reason for the greater social disapproval of heavy drinking by women is that drunkenness in women is thought to be associated with sexual availability, promiscuity, and prostitution; this link is thought to be stronger and much less socially acceptable for women than for men (Gomberg, 1982). Thus, social disapproval of heavy drinking by women appears to be linked to traditional sex roles and expectations concerning gender-appropriate behavior.

There are additional links between gender differences in alcohol consumption and general gender differences in roles and behavior. Frequent church attendance or strong religious commitment is associated with lower alcohol use, so females' greater involvement with religion has contributed to their lower alcohol consumption (Bachman *et al.*, 1981; Cahalan *et al.*, 1969; Liban & Smart, 1980). Boys' greater rebelliousness and involvement in antisocial behavior appear to contribute to their greater alcohol consumption (Bachman *et al.*, 1981; Thompson & Wilsnack, 1984).

Another possible link between contemporary sex roles and alcohol consumption is suggested by the finding in several studies that employed women are more likely than housewives to be problem drinkers or heavy drinkers, at least among young women (Ferrence, 1980; Johnson, 1982; Liban & Smart, 1980). However, no evidence for this association was found in two other studies (Welch & Booth, 1977; Wilsnack, Wilsnack, & Klassen, 1984). Another study found that employed women were more likely than housewives to use alcohol when they were tense and worried (Timmer, Veroff, & Colten, 1985). Evidence from another study indicates that women with more egalitarian sex role attitudes consumed more alcohol (Celentano & McQueen, 1984). Although these findings suggest that employed women or women with egalitarian sex role attitudes may drink more, these hypothesized relationships would appear to be in conflict with the evidence that during the recent period of rapidly increasing women's employment and increasingly egalitarian sex role attitudes, there appears to have been little or no increase in the prevalence of heavy drinking or problem drinking among women (Clark & Midanik, 1982; Ferrence, 1980; Wilsnack *et al.*, 1984, 1986).

It is unclear whether there are gender differences in concerns about the health effects of drinking that might contribute to gender differences in drinking. A recent survey indicates that women are somewhat more aware of the health effects of heavy drinking (NCHS, 1986b), but an earlier survey found men at least as likely as women to give health-related reasons for abstaining or drinking less than formerly (Cahalan *et al.*, 1969). Females rate alcohol consumption as more harmful or risky than do males, both among contemporary teenagers and among adults in the 1960s (Cahalan *et al.*, 1969; Johnston *et al.*, 1984; Pascale, Trucksis, & Sylvester, 1985). It is unclear whether this gender difference in perceived risk reflects greater female concern with health problems and/or with psychosocial problems that can be caused by drinking.

An additional reason why women drink less than men may be that alternative responses to stress may be more socially acceptable for women. In response to stress, women more often use psychotropic medications, pray, or talk with friends or relatives, whereas men more often drink alcohol (Cahalan *et al.*, 1969; Clark & Midanik, 1982; Timmer *et al.*, 1985; Waldron, 1983a).

It has been hypothesized that an X-linked recessive gene may be responsible for higher rates of alcoholism among men than among women, but several lines of evidence indicate that this hypothesis is probably incorrect (Waldron, 1983b).

In summary, there appear to be many similarities between the causes of gender differences in drinking and the causes of gender differences in smoking. Factors that contribute to gender differences in drinking and smoking include social disapproval of these behaviors for girls and women, girls' and women's greater involvement in religion, and lesser rebelliousness of girls than boys. In addition to these similarities, there are important differences in the patterns and causes of gender differences in drinking and smoking. For example, gender differences in alcohol consumption are larger than gender differences in smoking in the present-day United States. One important reason appears to be the continuing strong social disapproval of heavy drinking by women, possibly related to the loss of control following heavy alcohol consumption and the increase in vulnerability to seduction or rape of women who are drunk. In addition, other factors, such as women's greater use of cigarette smoking to regulate body weight, may contribute to smaller gender differences in smoking than in alcohol consumption.

ACCIDENTS

Males have more accidents than do females, and this gender difference is substantial in magnitude and widespread cross-culturally (Verbrugge, 1985; Waldron, 1986a; World Health Organization, 1981). Accidental death rates are higher for males for almost all types of accidents for almost all age groups in many different countries throughout the world.

The evidence to be reviewed indicates that males' higher accident rates are due primarily to a variety of behaviors that have been more expected or accepted for males. Most of this evidence is derived from data for the United States, with scattered supporting evidence from other countries.

Male drivers have substantially higher rates of fatal motor vehicle accidents than do female drivers, because males drive more and because males have more fatal accidents per mile driven (Veevers, 1982; Waldron, 1986a). Observational studies show that males tend to drive faster and less cautiously and more often violate traffic regulations. Male drivers are considerably more likely to have high blood alcohol levels (Ferrence, 1980; Waldron, 1986a). Thus, major causes of males' higher rates of fatal motor vehicle accidents are males' less safe driving habits and their higher frequency of driving after drinking.

Men's higher rates of accidents on the job are another major cause of their higher accidental death rates (Waldron, 1986a). Men have more work accidents because more men are employed and because employed men are more likely than employed women to have physically hazardous jobs.

Other types of accidents that show particularly large gender differences are gun accidents and drownings. Fatalities due to gun accidents and accidental drownings are over five times as high for males as for females in the United States (Waldron, 1986a).

Boys play in more risky ways than do girls and this contributes substantially to their higher rates of accidents (Waldron, 1983a). Gender differences in play may be due in part to the effects of male sex hormones which may contribute to boys' higher levels of physical activity (Waldron, 1983b). Differences in the socialization of girls and boys also contribute to boys' higher levels of physical activity and risk-taking (Waldron, 1986a).

In conclusion, many of the behaviors that contribute to males' higher rates of accidents have been more socially accepted or expected for males than for females. Drinking alcohol, taking risks physically, working at hazardous jobs, and gun use have all been more expected of males than of females in Western societies as well as in many non-Western societies. Differential socialization of boys and girls with regard to these behaviors has been widespread cross-culturally, reflecting the widespread differences in men's and women's roles (Waldron, 1986a). Thus, sex roles and the associated cultural influences on gender differences in behavior appear to makes a major contribution to males' higher rates of accidents.

DIETING AND EATING DISORDERS

The relationship between dieting and health is complex, with possible beneficial effects due to the reduction of obesity and possible harmful effects due to the inadequate nutrition that can result from some weight loss diets, the health-damaging effects of some drugs used to suppress appetite, and the possible deleterious effects of repeated weight loss and weight gain. The extreme restriction of food intake and substantial weight loss that are characteristic of anorexia nervosa undoubtedly harm health and can be fatal (Garfinkel & Garner, 1982). Binging and subsequent purging (e.g., self-induced vomiting) is characteristic of bulimia. Bulimia is rarely fatal, but frequently leads to health problems as well as psychological problems.

In the present-day United States, women are twice as likely as men to report that they are dieting in order to lose weight (Stephenson, Levy, Sass, & McGarvey, 1987). In contemporary Western countries, adolescent girls and young women are roughly ten times as likely as adolescent boys and young men to develop anorexia or bulimia (Garfinkel & Garner, 1982; Striegel-Moore, Silberstein, & Rodin, 1986).

The major reason why dieting, anorexia, and bulimia are so much more common among females appears to be related to one aspect of sex roles, the greater emphasis on females' appearance (Rodin *et al.,* 1985; Striegel-Moore *et al.,* 1986). Being attractive leads to a wide variety of social and psychological advantages, especially for females, and the contemporary beauty ideal for females emphasizes a very slim figure (Garfinkel & Garner, 1982; Rodin *et al.,* 1985). In contrast, female bodies inherently tend to store more fat than do male bodies, particularly during puberty and pregnancy. The discrepancy between a very slim ideal body form for females and a heavier ''natural'' body weight leads to women's frequent preoccupation with weight control and dieting. In extreme cases this preoccupation with weight control and dieting can be manifested as anorexia nervosa. Dieting may also predispose women to the binging characteristic of bulimia (Polivy & Herman, 1985). Thus, the primary reasons for girls' and womens' higher rates of dieting, and disordered eating behaviors appear to be the cultural emphasis on slimness as a very important desirable attribute for girls and women, in combination with the inherent tendency of adolescent and postadolescent female bodies to deposit fat.

PHYSICIAN VISITS

In Western countries women generally make more physician visits than do men (Verbrugge, 1985; Waldron, 1983a). In contrast, in some non-Western societies, for example, in Japan in the 1950s, men have had as high or higher rates of physician visits than women (Waldron, 1983a).

Women's more complex and demanding reproductive functions are a major reason for women's higher rates of physician visits, especially among young and middle-aged adults (Nathanson & Lorenz, 1982; Verbrugge, 1985; Waldron, 1983a). In the United States, pregnancy accounts for about one-third of the gender difference in physician visits in the 15- to 44-year-old age range, and other reproduction-related and sex-specific diagnoses account for roughly an additional quarter of the gender difference in physician visits. It should be noted that the inherent sex differences in reproductive biology have varying effects on gender differences in physician visits depending on the cultural context. In many poor countries, such as India and Egypt, many women obtain little or no obstetric and gynecological medical care (Lopez & Ruzicka, 1983).

In Western countries, another reason for women's higher rates of physician visits is that women have more self-reported symptoms and poorer self-rated health (Waldron, 1983a). It is at present unclear why women report more symptoms and poorer health than do men. It has been hypothesized that, for a given physiological condition, women are more likely than men to report symptoms and rate their health as poor. Tests of this hypothesis have yielded mixed results (Waldron, 1983a). Comparisons between symptom reports and medical indicators of an illness have not shown consistent gender differences in symptom reporting. Comparisons of self-ratings and physicians' ratings of general health suggest that women's self-ratings of general health are more pessimistic than are men's. These findings suggest that both gender differences in somatic condition and gender differences in perception may contribute to women's higher rates of symptoms and poorer self-perceived health, and these in turn contribute to women's higher rates of physician visits.

In addition, it appears that, for a given level of self-perceived health, women may be more likely to make a physician visit (Waldron, 1983a). Gender differences in the likelihood of visiting a physician vary depending on the type of symptom. It appears that for less serious conditions, such as overweight and mild chronic conditions, women are more likely to make physician visits. In contrast, for symptoms of several types of serious somatic illness, men are as likely as women to seek treatment. For example, for most types of cancer, no gender differences have been found in the lag time from first noticing symptoms to seeking medical care and no gender differences have been found in the stage of cancer at diagnosis. Similarly, for myocardial infarctions, the lag time from first symptoms to seeking medical care is as long or longer for women as for men. Also, the proportion of myocardial infarctions that are not diagnosed or treated at the time of occurrence appears to be as high for women as for men.

These data indicate that women are not more likely to obtain treatment for several types of major illness. In contrast, for another potentially serious condition, hypertension, women are more likely to obtain treatment. Among hypertensives, more women than men are aware of their condition, and among hypertensives who are aware of their condition, more women have obtained treatment (Apostolides *et al.*, 1980; Hartel, Keil, & Cairns, 1985). Hypertension is generally asymptomatic, but is easily diagnosed in a medical visit, so women's more frequent physician visits can account for women's greater awareness of their hypertension. Women's higher rates of treatment seeking for hypertension may reflect gender differences in general attitudes (Waldron, 1983a). It appears that untreated hypertensives have greater need for autonomy and less need for sympathy, help, and being taken care of than treated hypertensives, and thus women's greater expressed need for sympathy, help, and care may contribute to their higher rates of treatment for hypertension.

Survey data for the United States indicate other gender differences in attitudes that appear to contribute to gender differences in physician visits. Males more often report that they can and do ignore pain (Mechanic, 1964; Verbrugge, 1982), and this may contribute to their lower rates of physician visits. Also, women rate the importance of health somewhat higher than do men (Cahalan *et al.*, 1969; US DHEW, 1969, 1976; Verbrugge, 1982). Gender differences in attitudes toward health care are suggested by the observations that women more often have a personal physician or regular source of health care and men more often report not needing a doctor as their reason for not having a regular source of medical care (Cleary, Mechanic, & Greenley, 1982; NCHS, 1986b).

In the United States, women may have greater faith in the value of preventive medical care and this may contribute to their higher rates of physician visits for preventive care (Cleary *et al.*, 1982; Waldron, 1983a). Gender differences in physician visits for preventive care vary cross-culturally. In several European countries, men make more visits for physical examinations in the absence of illness, even after exclusion of physical examinations for administrative reasons such as job requirements (Kohn & White, 1976).

Another hypothesis has been that men have more "fixed role" obligations such as employment and the inflexible time demands of these fixed role obligations may make it difficult for men to arrange time for a physician visit. One study found evidence that employment may make a modest contribution to gender differences in physician visits for chronic illnesses (Marcus & Siegel, 1982). However, comparisons of employed women and housewives have shown no consistent difference in their propensity to visit a physician when ill (Cleary *et al.*, 1982; Nathanson & Lorenz, 1982). Also, women are as likely as men to report inconvenience in arranging time for physician visits (Verbrugge, 1982; Waldron, 1983a). This suggests that there may be a balance between men's greater role obligations due to employment and women's greater role obligations due to responsibility for care of children and other family members. Thus, it appears that, overall, gender differences in employment and other role obligations are not a major cause of gender differences in physician visits.

Another hypothesis has been that physicians may treat men and women differently, and this may contribute to women's higher rates of physician visits. There is some evidence that physicians' advice may tend to elevate women's utilization of medical care, for example, in recommendations of follow-up care for back pain or dizziness or in recommendations for gynecological surgery in the United States (Verbrugge & Steiner, 1981; Waldron, 1982). However, most of the available evidence suggests little gender difference in physicians' recommendations of medical care for a given condition (Verbrugge, 1985; Verbrugge & Steiner, 1981; Waldron, 1982).

In contrast to the pattern observed in Western countries, in some non-Western countries it appears that men are more likely than women to obtain medical care. For example, in Bangladesh men were more likely to obtain care for diarrheal infections, and in Japan men obtained medical care for bladder cancer at earlier stages than did women (Lopez & Ruzicka, 1983; Waldron, 1983a). Men's greater likelihood of obtaining medical care in these situations reflects several aspects of general sex roles and expectations concerning gender-appropriate behavior. For example, in some non-Western societies, restrictions on women's traveling and norms concerning modesty for women limit women's access to medical care. In addition, in quite a few societies, males' higher status and the perception that males are more valuable result in discrimination against females and greater male access to scarce resources such as medical care (Waldron, 1983a, 1986a).

In conclusion, gender differences in physician visits reflect both biological and cultural causes. In Western countries, sex differences in reproductive biology are a major reason for women's higher rates of physician visits. It appears that gender differences in the perception of health and the propensity to seek medical care also contribute to women's higher rates of physician visits. Gender differences in the propensity to visit physicians are only observed for certain types of conditions; men are as likely as women to seek medical care for many types of major, symptomatic illness. In some non-Western societies, females obtain less adequate medical care, reflecting sex discrimination and other factors associated with general sex roles in these societies.

CONCLUSIONS

The analyses presented of the causes of gender differences in smoking, drinking, accidents, dieting, eating disorders, and physician visits illustrate that many different factors influence gender differences in health-related behavior. The specific causal factors of importance vary depending on the particular type of behavior. As a result of this variation in causal factors, the magnitude and direction of gender differences in health-related behavior vary depending on the particular type of health-related behavior. Cultural influences have a major impact on gender differences in health-related behavior and, consequently, gender differences in health-related behavior have varied cross-culturally and historically.

One important generalization that applies to many of the diverse patterns observed is that gender differences in specific types of health-related behavior are strongly influenced by the compatibility of the behavior with general sex roles and expectations concerning appropriate male and female behavior. For example, expectations that males more than females will use guns, take physical risks in recreation, and have certain types of physically risky jobs contribute significantly to males' higher rates of accidents. A major reason for gender differences in drinking has been widespread social disapproval of women's drinking, particularly heavy drinking, and this appears to have been due, at least in part, to concerns that heavy drinking could interfere with women's responsibility for the care of young children and concerns that heavy drinking could contribute to promiscuity among women.

Other aspects of sex roles and expectations concerning gender-appropriate behavior have also influenced gender differences in health-related behavior. Greater tolerance of rebelliousness in males and males' lesser involvement in religion have contributed to males' higher rates of drinking and smoking, at least in 20th century United States. Emphasis on appearance and slimness for females contributes to their higher rates of dieting, anorexia nervosa, and bulimia and may also tend to increase their smoking rates in contemporary Western societies. Greater acceptability of concern with pain and care-seeking for females may contribute to their higher rates of physician visits in the United States and other Western societies. In contrast, in some non-Western societies, discrimination against females has prevented them from obtaining as much medical care as males, and this type of discrimination has been linked to gender differences in roles and power.

These examples illustrate that sex roles and general expectations concerning gender-appropriate behavior have influenced gender differences in health-related behavior in many different ways. Cross-cultural and historical variation in sex roles and expectations concerning gender-appropriate behavior has also contributed to variation in gender differences in health-related behavior.

One interesting question is whether the increasing employment of women in Western countries in the 20th century has contributed to decreases in gender differences in health-related behavior. For the types of behavior analyzed in this review, little evidence was found for a direct effect of employment on women's health-related behavior, although, among young women in the United States, employed women may be more likely than housewives to be problem drinkers. Women's employment may have had more important indirect effects on gender differences in health-related behavior. Increasing employment of women contributed to general cultural changes such as increasing equality for women and liberalization of norms concerning women's behavior, including increased social acceptance of smoking. The increased social acceptability of women's smoking has been one important reason for the decreasing gender differences in smoking.

Although sex roles have varied cross-culturally and historically, certain aspects of sex roles have been widespread cross-culturally and these common features of sex roles have contributed to certain widespread gender differences in health-related behavior. For example, because of inherent sex differences in reproductive biology, women have been more involved in the care of babies and young children in all or almost all cultures, while men have generally had greater responsibility for certain types of physically risky activities that are incompatible with child care (Waldron, 1983b). These gender differences in roles and related differences in the socialization of males and females appear to have contributed to the widespread gender differences in accident rates, alcohol consumption, and possibly some other types of health-related behavior. Thus, sex differences in reproductive biology have resulted in the cultural evolution of certain aspects of male and female roles that are widespread cross-culturally, and these in turn have contributed to certain widespread gender differences in health-related behavior.

There are also more direct effects of sex differences in biology on gender differences in health-related behavior. For example, effects of male hormones may contribute to males' higher levels of physical activity, and this may be one reason why males have higher accident rates in many different countries throughout the world. Similarly, women's more complex and demanding reproductive functions have been a major cause of women's higher rates of physician visits in Western countries. Despite the inherent sex differences in reproductive biology, women have had lower rates of physician visits than men in some poor societies where inadequate medical resources and discrimination against females have prevented many women from obtaining adequate medical care. Thus, inherent sex differences may interact with cultural factors to produce culturally variable patterns of gender differences in health-related behavior.

One final point is that concerns about the health effects of behavior have had little or no impact on gender differences in many types of health-related behavior. Data for the United States indicate that women place a somewhat greater importance on health than do men, and this apparently contributes to women's higher rates of physician visits. However, despite women's greater expressed concern with health, men are as likely or more likely to engage in some types of preventive behavior, such as seat belt use and vigorous physical exercise, and females are much more likely to engage in the risky behaviors associated with anorexia or bulimia. Also, gender differences in health concerns appear to have made little or no contribution to gender differences in smoking, despite the major health effects of smoking. Thus, women's greater concern with health is not a major determinant of gender differences in many types of health-related behavior. This is not surprising given that gender differences in the valuation of health are modest in magnitude and many types of health-related behavior are much more strongly influenced by a variety of other factors than by health-related motivations. The evidence reviewed in this chapter suggests that gender differences in many types of health-related behavior have been influenced less by gender differences in health-related motivations and more by the compatibility or incompatibility of the specific type of health-related behavior with male and female roles.

Acknowledgments

This research has been supported in part by a grant from the MacArthur Foundation Network on the Determinants and Consequences of Health-Damaging and Health-Promoting Behavior. I am grateful to Christine Vogeli for her excellent assistance in preparing this review.

REFERENCES

Apostolides, A. Y., Cutter, G., Kraus, J. F., Oberman, A., Blaszlsowski, T., Borhami, N. O., & Entwisle, G. (1980). Impact of hypertension information on high blood pressure control between 1973 and 1978. *Hypertension, 2*(1), 8–13.

Bachman, J. G., Johnston, L. D., & O'Malley, P. M. (1981). Smoking, drinking, and drug use among American high school students: Correlates and trends, 1975–1979. *American Journal of Public Health, 71,* 59–69.

Biener, L. (1987). Gender differences in the use of substances for coping. In R. C. Barnett, L. Biener, & G. K. Baruch (Eds.), *Gender and stress.* New York: Free Press.

Cahalan, D., Cisin, I., & Crossley, H. (1969). *A national study of drinking behavior and attitudes.* New Haven: College & University Press.

Celentano, D. D., & McQueen, D. V. (1984). Alcohol consumption patterns among women in Baltimore. *Journal of Studies on Alcohol, 45,* 355–358.

Child, I. L., Barry, H., III, & Bacon, M. K. (1965). A cross-culture study of drinking. III. Sex differences. *Quarterly Journal of Studies on Alcohol, 3* (Suppl.), 49–61.

Clark, W., & Midanik, L. (1982). Alcohol use and alcohol problems among U.S. adults. In National Institute on Alcohol Abuse and Alcoholism, *Alcohol and health,* Monograph No. 1, pp. 3–53.

Cleary, P. D., Mechanic, D., & Greenley, J. R. (1982). Sex differences in medical care utilization: An empirical investigation. *Journal of Health and Social Behavior, 23,* 106–119.

Dean, K. J., Holst, E., & Wagner, M. G. (1983). Self-care of common illnesses in Denmark. *Medical Care, 21,* 1012–1032.

Fass, P. S. (1977). *The damned and the beautiful American youth in the 1920's.* London: Oxford University Press.

Ferrence, R. G. (1980). Sex differences in the prevalence of problem drinking. *Research Advances in Alcohol and Drug Problems, 5,* 69–124.

Finau, S. A., Stanhope, J. M., & Prior, I. A. M. (1982). Kava, alcohol and tobacco consumption among Tongans with urbanization. *Social Science and Medicine, 16,* 35–41.

Garfinkel, P. E., & Garner, D. M. (1982). *Anorexia nervosa—A multidimensional perspective.* New York: Brunner/Mazel.

Gomberg, E. S. L. (1982). Historical and political perspective: Women and drug use. *Journal of Social Issues, 38,* 9–23.

Hartel, U., Keil, U., & Cairns, V. (1985). Medical care utilization and self-reported health of hypertensives—Results of the Munich Blood Pressure Study. In R. Kaplan & M. Criqui (Eds.), *Behavioral epidemiology and disease prevention* (pp. 201–215). New York: Plenum Press.

Hill, D., & Gray, N. (1984). Australian patterns of tobacco smoking and related health beliefs in 1983. *Community Health Studies, 8*(3), 307–316.

Jarvis, M. (1984). Gender and smoking: Do women really find it harder to give up? *British Journal of Addiction, 79,* 383–387.

Johnson, P. B. (1982). Sex differences, women's roles and alcohol use: Preliminary national data. *Journal of Social Issues, 38,* 93–116.

Johnston, L. D., Bachman, J. G., & O'Malley, P. M. (1984). *Monitoring the future—Questionnaire responses from the nations' high school seniors, 1983.* Ann Arbor: Institute for Social Research, University of Michigan.

Johnston, L. D., O'Malley, P. M., & Bachman, J. G. (1986). *Drug use among American high school students, college students, and other young adults.* Rockville, MD: National Institute on Drug Abuse, U.S. Department of Health and Human Services.

Joly, D. J. (1975). Cigarette smoking in Latin America—A survey of eight cities. *Bulletin of the Pan American Health Organization, 9,* 329–344.

Kohn, R., & White, I. (Eds.). (1976). *Health care—An international study: Report of the World Health Organization/International Collaborative Study of Medical Care Utilization.* London: Oxford University Press.

Liban, C., & Smart, R. G. (1980). Generational and other differences between males and females in problem drinking and its treatment. *Drug and Alcohol Dependence, 5,* 207–221.

Lopez, A., & Ruzicka, C. T. (Eds.). (1983). *Sex differentials in mortality.* Canberra: Australian National University, Demography Department.

Marcus, A. C., & Siegel, J. M. (1982). Sex differences in the use of physician services: A preliminary test of the fixed role hypothesis. *Journal of Health and Social Behavior, 23,* 186–197.

Mechanic, D. (1964). The influence of mothers on their children's health attitudes and behavior. *Pediatrics, 33,* 444–452.

Mougne, C., MacLennan, R., & Atsana, S. (1982). Smoking, chewing and drinking in Ban Pong, northern Thailand. *Social Science and Medicine, 16,* 99–106.

Nathanson, C. A., & Lorenz, G. (1982). Women and health: The social dimensions of biomedical data. In J. Z. Giele (Ed.), *Women in the middle years—Current knowledge and directions for research and policy* (pp. 37–87). New York: Wiley.

National Center for Health Statistics. (1986a). Trends in smoking, alcohol consumption, and other health practices among U. S. adults, 1977 and 1983. *Advance data from vital and health statistics,* No. 118. DHHS Publication No. (PHS) 86-1250 and unpublished tables.

National Center for Health Statistics. (1986b). Persons with and without a regular source of medical care: United States. *Vital and health statistics,* Ser. 10, No. 151. DHHS Publication No. (PHS) 85-1579.

Palmer, A. B. (1970). Some variables contributing to the onset of cigarette smoking among junior high school students. *Social Science and Medicine, 4,* 359–366.

Pascale, P. J., Trucksis, F. E., & Sylvester, J. (1985). Regional trends and sex differences of drug use and attitudes of high school students in northeast Ohio 1977–1983. *Journal of Drug Education, 15,* 241–251.

Polivy, J., & Herman, C. P. (1985). Dieting and binging—A causal analysis. *American Psychologist, 40,* 193–201.

Rodin, J., Silberstein, L., & Striegel-Moore, R. (1985). Women and weight: A normative discontent. In T. B. Sonderegger (Ed.), *Psychology and gender: Nebraska symposium on motivation* (pp. 267–307). Lincoln: University of Nebraska Press.

Stephenson, M. G., Levy, A. S., Sass, M. L., & McGarvey, W. E. (1987). 1985 NHIS findings: Nutrition knowledge and baseline data for the weight-loss objectives. *Public Health Report, 102,* 61–67.

Striegel-Moore, R. H., Silberstein, L. R., & Rodin, J. (1986). Toward an understanding of risk factors for bulimia. *American Psychologist, 41,* 246–263.

Svikis, D. S., Hatsukami, D. K., Hughes, J. R., Carroll, K. M., & Pickens, R. W. (1986). Sex-differences in tobacco withdrawal syndrome. *Addictive Behaviors, 11,* 459–462.

Thompson, K. M., & Wilsnack, R. W. (1984). Drinking and drinking problems among female adolescents: Patterns and influences. In S. C. Wilsnack & L. J. Bechman (Eds.), *Alcohol problems in women* (pp. 37–65). New York: Guilford Press.

Timmer, S. G., Veroff, J., & Colter, M. E. (1985). Life stress, helplessness and the use of alcohol and drugs to cope. In S. Shiffman & T. A. Wills (Eds.), *Coping and substance use* (pp. 171–198). New York: Academic Press.

U.S. Department of Health and Human Services. (1980). *The health consequences of smoking for women—A report of the surgeon general.* Rockville, MD: U.S. Department of Health and Human Services.

U.S. Department of Health and Human Services. (1986). *The health consequences of smoking—Cancer and chronic lung disease in the workplace—A report of the surgeon general—1985.* Rockville, MD: U.S. Department of Health and Human Services.

U.S. Department of Health, Education, and Welfare. (1969). *Use of tobacco: Practices, attitudes, knowledge, and beliefs, United States—Fall 1964 and Spring 1966.* National Clearinghouse for Smoking and Health.

U.S. Department of Health, Education, and Welfare. (1976). *Adult use of tobacco—1975.* National Clearinghouse for Smoking and Health.

Veevers, J. (1982). Women in the driver's seat: Trends in sex differences in driving and death. *Population Research and Policy Review, 1,* 171–182.

Verbrugge, L. M. (1982). Sex differences in legal drug use. *Journal of Social Issues, 38,* 59–76.

Verbrugge, L. M. (1985). Gender and health: An update on hypotheses and evidence. *Journal of Health and Social Behavior, 26,* 156–182.

Verbrugge, L. M., & Steiner, R. P. (1981). Physician treatment of men and women patients: Sex bias or appropriate care? *Medical Care, 19*(6), 609–632.

Waldron, I. (1982). An analysis of causes of sex differences in mortality and morbidity. In W. R. Gove & G. R. Carpenter (Eds.), *The fundamental connection between nature and nurture* (pp. 69–116). Lexington, MA: Lexington Books.

Waldron, I. (1983a). Sex differences in illness incidence, prognosis and mortality. *Social Science and Medicine, 17,* 1107–1123.
Waldron, I. (1983b). Sex differences in human mortality: The role of genetic factors. *Social Science and Medicine, 17,* 321–333.
Waldron, I. (1986a). What do we know about causes of sex differences in mortality? A review of the literature. *Population Bulletin of the United Nations,* No. 18-1985, 59–76.
Waldron, I. (1986b). The contribution of smoking to sex differences in mortality. *Public Health Reports, 101,* 163–173.
Waldron, I. (1988). *Patterns and causes of gender differences in smoking*. Submitted paper, available from author upon request, Department of Biology, University of Pennsylvania.
Waldron, I., Bratelli, G., Carriker, L., Sung, W. C., Vogeli, C., & Waldman, E. (1988). Gender differences in tobacco use in Asia, Africa, and Latin America. *Social Science and Medicine*, in press.
Welch, S., & Booth, A. (1977). Employment and health among married women with children. *Sex Roles, 3,* 385–397.
Wilsnack, R. W., Wilsnack, S. D., & Klassen, A. D. (1984). Women's drinking and drinking problems. *American Journal of Public Health, 74,* 1231–1238.
Wilsnack, R. W., Wilsnack, S. D., & Klassen, A. D. (1986). Antecedents and consequences of drinking and drinking problems in women. *Nebraska Symposium on Drinking* (pp. 85–158). Geneva: World Health Organization.
World Health Organization. (1981). *World health statistics annual*. Geneva: Author.

Institutional Determinants

Institutional determinants refer to factors associated with organizations (or bureaucracies, in the original meaning of the term), namely those social units which are deliberately planned in order to accomplish certain goals (e.g., Etzioni, 1964). Although relatively few systematic studies have been reported, health behavior is presumed to be affected by aspects of the institution in which it takes place; most often these institutions are clinics and hospitals, but they can also be schools and workplaces.

Institutions have both social, or organizational, dimensions, and environmental dimensions. The social or organizational dimensions broadly include goals and values; policies related to authority, decision-making, division of labor, and personnel; and managerial styles; as well as how these effect employee morale and productivity (e.g., Etzioni, 1964). The environmental dimensions broadly include location; building height; room size and shape; arrangements of space; color and texture; and acoustics, ventilation, and lighting.

The linkage between institutional characteristics and the health behaviors of clients, patients, or consumers, the satisfaction of whose needs is presumably a goal or value of health care institutions, and the morale of whom is a concern of workplace institutions, has seldom been systematically examined. Gish (1984), for example, proposed a framework for identifying health care institutions in terms of whether they are resource oriented, disease oriented, political decision-makers, or organized sellers and purchasers of health care, and analyzed how these exhibit different values related to health care from country to country, particularly in regard to whether health is considered to be a social objective or a market commodity, but this promising conceptual model has not yet been subject to much empirical testing in relation to health behavior. What research exists can be discussed under three headings: organizational characteristics, environmental characteristics, and system barriers.

ORGANIZATIONAL CHARACTERISTICS

Two important organizational characteristics that have been related to health behavior are policies and organization of tasks.

Policies

In an example of early research on institutional policies, Berkanovic, Reeder, Marcus, and Schwartz (1975) examined the differential effects of prepayment and nonprepaid, fee-for-service policies in relation to the financing of care, and found that prepayment did not lead to significantly greater difficulty in obtaining appointments or in seeing a physician without an appointment. However, under the nonprepaid arrangements, patients were somewhat more dubious about their physician's ability.

Wolinsky's analysis (1976) of attitudinal data related to health maintenance organizations (HMOs) indicated that the HMO policy of heavily emphasizing prevention, together with the HMO's appeal to persons who were already more interested in prevention would account for some of the apparent dissatisfaction with HMOs: potential users are already likely to be involved in preventive care. Thus, when these joined an HMO they would experience a "ceiling effect"; they could not increase such utilization by very much. Luft (1978), on the other hand, concluded from examination of the literature on HMO services that the greater use of preventive services by HMO enrollees was attributable to their being covered for it financially, rather than to the HMO's preventive ideology, as persons who were covered for preventive services under third-party fee-for-payment reimbursement policies did not differ from HMO enrollees in use of such services.

Institutions also differ in their policies on client participation in policy making. Glogow (1973) reviewed a variety of arguments both for and against increased community involvement and participation in developing and implementing policies for public health services, and reasons strongly for increased openness in such policy making. Eardley and colleagues' (1985) examination of attendance patterns at cervical screening clinics in Britain revealed that it was the clinic's policies related to inviting the women and to providing them with insufficient information, together with non-user-oriented policies such as those requiring the women to take the initiative in setting the appointment, that had negative impacts on use of screening.

Task Organization

Hoping to find that staff/patient ratios and degree of bureaucratization of work routines were related to nurses' encouraging of perinatal maternal behavior, i.e., behaviors such as touching, smiling at, and otherwise reacting to their infants, Moss (1984) observed few clear-cut effects attributable to formal properties of hospitals' organization. Moss found that the highest amount of maternal affectionate behavior occurred in a setting where there was fairly well-differentiated task organization, and where mothers had moderate control over their own activities, rather than where tasks were loosely organized and where mothers had higher degrees of control. Moss introduced intervening factors, such as strict task organization leading to nurses having more time at their disposal to work with mothers, and the differential impact of lack of structure on women of different social classes, to account for the absence of straightforward organizational effects.

One critical component of task organization is "role discretion." Greenley and Schoenherr (1981) observed that "role discretion," the ability to make autonomous work decisions, is the single attribute that has an impact on client satisfaction. Greenley and Davidson's chapter provides a further examination of the effects of role discretion, together with an analysis of other institutional characteristics, such as claimed and *de facto* "domains," and availability of resources, on care-seeking behavior and on patient satisfaction.

ENVIRONMENTAL CHARACTERISTICS

Taylor (1984) provided no empirical linkages, but exhorted that "things that are well designed for people tend to foster wellness . . . things that are ill designed tend to frustrate people and thereby foster illness" (p. 130). Three environmental characteristics that have been specifically related to health behavior are size, location, and space.

Size

Ross and Duff (1982) examined a variety of organizational factors in relation to experiences and satisfaction with patient care and observed that clients who had good experiences with quality care within a large, bureaucratic multispecialty prepaid clinic were more likely to make appropriate, need-based return visits than clients of smaller, fee-for-service practices. The size of the bureaucracy was apparently less of a barrier to care than the financial constraints of the fee-for-service arrangements. Size and impersonal treatment by themselves are not deterrents to care-seeking.

Mishler (1981), reviewing research findings related to institutional size, noted that increased size had a negative impact on health, that patients in larger institutions tended to be less open and less free in expressing their feelings. Larger institutions apparently place less emphasis on understanding patients' personal problems. While Mishler's observations reflected health status rather than health behavior, the findings point to some important directions for health behavior research: the effects of size on patient–physician interactions and on patient acceptance of regimens.

Location

Bohland (1984) analyzed use of emergency rooms for primary care in an urban Oklahoma county, and found that geographical proximity of the site was as important a determinant of its use as socioeconomic status. Davis and Kunitz (1978) reported that although the Navajo have distinctively different morbidity rates than does the larger United States population, reflecting both their poverty and their not-yet-completed transition from a population primarily at risk for acute infectious diseases to one primarily at risk for chronic diseases, the frequency with which they use hospital health services is more attributable to the proximity—and thus to the accessibility—of these services than to medical need.

Space

In a dramatically written analysis of how public places are experienced, Hiss (1987a,b) called attention to the important role that total perception of the environment plays in our feelings of comfort and well-being as well as in our behavior. Hiss suggested that the scale of the physical environment, its opportunities for viewing, and its richness must be considered in plans for buildings and neighborhoods.

Armstrong provided a cogent analysis of the implications of changes in the physical context of British primary care (1985), from practice conducted within the physician's own living quarters, through practice conducted within a separate part of the physician's home, to practice in clinics. The changes in the physical spatial arrangements are associated causally with changes in the characteristics of the physician–patient encounter, as well as in the meanings of medical practice and community health.

Moos and Schaefer (1985) discussed how physical and architectural factors of health care settings can influence how their staffs function and relate to patients, but their findings do not directly relate to health behaviors.

SYSTEM BARRIERS

In the context of their analysis of social, cultural, and demographic factors in utilization of health services, Berkanovic and Reeder (1974) extrapolated from available evidence and suggested that professional prejudices about clients' race, moral status, or responsibility for illness may serve as barriers to utilization of services. Furthermore, Rundall and Wheeler (1979) demonstrated that not having a regular source of care, problems in transportation to care sites, and long waiting times were all system barriers to utilization of preventive services.

Whitehead, Fusillo, and Kaplan's chapter on designing physical environments integrates some current conceptions of size, space, and other environmental characteristics and elaborates on ways in which they may be related to health behavior. As the literature, together with their chapter, makes clear, much research remains to be conducted to generate empirical knowledge beyond concepts and models.

REFERENCES

Armstrong, D. (1985). Space and time in British general practice. *Social Science and Medicine, 20,* 659–666.

Berkanovic, E., & Reeder, L. G. (1974). Can money buy the appropriate use of services? Some notes on the meaning of utilization data. *Journal of Health and Social Behavior, 15,* 93–99.

Berkanovic, E., Reeder, L. G., Marcus, A. C., & Schwartz, S. (1975). The effects of prepayment on access to medical care: The PACC experience. *Milbank Memorial Fund Quarterly, 53,* 241–253.

Bohland, J. (1984). Neighborhood variations in the use of hospital emergency rooms for primary care. *Social Science and Medicine, 19,* 1217–1226.

Davis, S., & Kunitz, S. J. (1978). Hospitalization utilization and elective surgery on the Navajo Indian reservation. *Social Science and Medicine, 12B,* 263–272.

Eardley, A., Elkind, A. K., Spencer, B., Hobbs, P., Pendleton, L. L., & Haran, D. (1985). Attendance for cervical screening—Whose problem? *Social Science and Medicine, 20,* 955–962.

Etzioni, A. (1964). *Modern organizations.* Englewood Cliffs, NJ: Prentice–Hall.

Gish, O. (1984). Values in health care. *Social Science and Medicine, 19,* 333–339.

Glogow, E. (1973). Community participation and sharing in control of public health services. *Health Services Reports, 88,* 442–448.

Greenley, J. R., & Schoenherr, R. A. (1981). Organization effects on client satisfaction with humaneness of service. *Journal of Health and Social Behavior, 22,* 2–18.

Hiss, T. (1987a, June 22). Experiencing places. *The New Yorker,* pp. 45–68.

Hiss, T. (1987b, June 29). Experiencing places. *The New Yorker,* pp. 73–86.

Luft, H. S. (1978). Why do HMOs seem to provide more health maintenance services? *Milbank Memorial Fund Quarterly, 56,* 140–165.

Mishler, E. G. (1981). Social contexts of health care. In E. G. Mishler, L. R. Amarasingham, S. D. Osherson, S. T. Hauser, N. E. Waxler, & R. Liem (Eds.), *Social contexts of health, illness, and patient care.* London: Cambridge University Press.

Moos, R. H., & Schaefer, J. A. (1985, August). *Evaluating health care work settings: A holistic conceptual framework.* Paper presented at the Veterans Administration Medical District 26 Conference on Evaluation Research, San Francisco.

Moss, N. (1984). Hospital units as social context: Effects on maternal behavior. *Social Science and Medicine, 19,* 515–522.

Ross, C. E., & Duff, R. S. (1982). Returning to the doctor: The effect of client characteristics, type of practice, and experiences with care. *Journal of Health and Social Behavior, 23,* 119–131.

Rundall, T. G., & Wheeler, J. R. C. (1979). The effect of income on use of preventive care: An evaluation of alternative explanations. *Journal of Health and Social Behavior, 20,* 397–406.

Taylor, C. W. (1984). Promoting health strengthening and wellness through environmental variables.

In J. D. Matarazzo, S. M. Weiss, J. A. Herd, N. E. Miller, & S. M. Weiss (Eds.), *Behavioral health: A handbook of health enhancement and disease prevention*. New York: Wiley.

Wolinsky, F. D. (1976). Health service utilization and attitudes toward health maintenance organizations: A theoretical and methodological discussion. *Journal of Health and Social Behavior, 17,* 221–236.

CHAPTER 12

Organizational Influences on Patient Health Behaviors

James R. Greenley and Robert E. Davidson

INTRODUCTION

Modern technological and scientific medicine is a relatively new phenomenon (Anderson, 1985). The modern profession of medicine has developed in the past 100 years. The delivery of medical care in formal organizations and bureaucratic settings has accelerated rapidly in the last few decades (Mechanic, 1976). Practitioners and health services researchers have come to increasingly appreciate the extent to which these organizational settings influence patient behaviors. These influences are difficult to study because they usually involve comparing different kinds of patients across a variety of organizations. Nevertheless, there has appeared a small but significant body of theory and research guiding our understanding of these organizational influences on patient health behaviors. This chapter will describe a particular theoretical perspective to explain organizational behaviors vis-à-vis patients and to interpret data about patient behavior in different organizational contexts.

Patient health behaviors are many and varied. Patients appraise their own bodily feelings, assess their prospects of getting well with and without professional services, decide whether to comply with treatment regimes, and so forth. No doubt all of these behaviors are influenced to some extent by the organizational structure of medical care. However, certain of these behaviors are much more directly affected by organizational forms than are others. This chapter will focus on certain behaviors we feel are most influenced by organizational structures: the decision whether to seek professional care, the choice of a particular service provider, the use of a certain volume of services, and the evaluation of the service provider. We feel these are most influenced by organizational structures because: (1) our theoretical perspective provides a closer link between these patient behaviors than many others, and (2) some data exist which show relationships between several of these patient behaviors and organizational structures and processes.

JAMES R. GREENLEY • Department of Sociology, University of Wisconsin, Madison, Wisconsin 53706. ROBERT E. DAVIDSON • Department of Social Science, Illinois Institute of Technology, Chicago, Illinois 60616.

THEORETICAL PERSPECTIVE

The structure of organizations both reflects and influences the behavior of organizational participants. It shapes and is shaped by the values and attitudes of those who work in them and those who receive services. Organizational structure shapes and reflects the expectations that staff and clients have of each other and may include policies for enforcing those expectations.

In this chapter we will set out a series of dimensions for the analysis of the ways in which organizations influence client behavior. These include organizational domain characteristics, patient selection mechanisms, and the interactional style of participants. These are some—but by no means all—of the ways in which organizations' struggle for resources and for autonomy from unwanted external constraints affect clients.

One of the most striking aspects of the health care system in the United States is its diversity and fragmentation. In contrast to health care systems in some other countries, such as Great Britain where most health care is provided in one large bureaucratic system, health care in the United States is provided through a variety of independent organizations (Cumming, 1967). These health care organizations arose like flora on a varied landscape, each one establishing itself in a particular niche where its unique characteristics enabled it to survive. Some were hospitals and others clinics; some were public and others private. They were set up by and for different professionals, such as physicians, dentists, sectarian healers, and nurses. There were prepaid and fee-for-service organizations, general medical and specialty mental health services, and many other specific types. Most were not linked to any larger administrative system or umbrella organization. Many public organizations, such as county and city hospitals, operated with a great deal of independence. This diversity and independence of organizations is reflected in problems common in our health care system: fragmentation, lack of coordination, poor continuity of care, truncated and segmented referral networks, duplication of equipment and services across organizations, and so forth (Black and Krause, 1963; Barth, 1963; Wilensky and Lebeaux, 1958).

Independent organizations have been found to strive for two major things: resources and autonomy (Thompson, 1962, 1967; Gouldner, 1959). Like other organizations, health provider organizations seek resources in order to grow and endure. They need resources in order to perform their functions, to reward people in the organizations for their efforts, and to have raw materials on which to work. The resources are of many types. Money is a rather flexible resource which can be used to pay staff, provide space and other facilities, and purchase equipment. Good will in the community is, for example, another resource without which most health care organizations could operate much less successfully. However, the most important resource to health care organizations is probably patients (Levine and White, 1961). Patients are the health care organization's avowed reason for existing. Patients are the source of other resources such as money (Greenley & Kirk, 1976; Rubington, 1965; Scott, 1969). Without patients, it would be difficult to attract health care professionals to work in the organization.

Like other organizations, health care organizations try to maintain autonomy, or the freedom to decide what they wish to do and how they will do it (Gouldner, 1959). Organizations that lose all of their autonomy cease to be independent entities. Organizations and their members fiercely guard their autonomy (Mott, 1968; Wilkie & Notkin, 1958). Elling (1963), for example, described how a community hospital withdrew from participation in a communitywide hospital improvement plan because the hospital's board of directors did not wish to sacrifice the hospital's identity and autonomy in a proposed merger with two other hospitals. Even subsections of large organizations, such as parts of public systems and private hospital chains, defend their own decision-making ability.

Organizations are continually interacting with their environment, accepting inputs and producing outputs (Gouldner, 1959; Thompson, 1967). An organization's environment influences its inputs and the nature of the tasks it performs. In this sense organizations are open systems (Thompson, 1962). The outputs of health care organizations include services provided for patients and the reactions of patients to this service. Its inputs include money, equipment, staff, and patients. A health care organization's environment includes other organizations, as well as governing bodies, the general public, specific client populations, professional organizations, and funding bodies. For purposes of this chapter, the most important part of its environment is the patient population it serves or may serve. These patients or potential patients are critical inputs and their experiences and behaviors are important outputs.

The value that a given organization places on autonomy, control of particular resources, and other matters reflects its identity or ideology. Organizational decisions are made by people behaving in a context of their experiences, their beliefs about the environment, and their beliefs about how organizations ought to be or act. These values and beliefs constitute an organizational culture. The conceptions of the actions that should be taken to achieve its goals constitute an organizational ideology. All organizations have an ideology and culture.

The behavior of health care organizations is often profoundly influenced by organizational ideologies and culture. Organizations may be committed to certain types of treatment (e.g., psychoanalysis or drug therapy for mental illness) or certain types of populations (care for specific patient populations defined by age, sex, disease, social class, or even religion).

Health care organizations, like other organizations, vary in structure and administrative process. An organizational chart captures several dimensions of organizational structure, such as horizontal and vertical differentiation, span of control, and patterns of hierarchies. Organizations differ by administrative processes of communication, coordination, formalization, and methods of control. Tasks may be differentially organized, standardized, or routinized. It is beyond the scope of this chapter to review the effects of these multiple factors on patient behaviors. We will concentrate on one salient factor, the role discretion of individual staff members.

ORGANIZATIONAL PROCESSES AND PATIENT BEHAVIORS

Choice of Service Provider

In our health care system, patients choose their health care provider from among many types of services and individual organizations and professionals. The process by which individuals choose to use a service and select particular providers is often referred to as the process of help-seeking. Help-seeking is influenced by individual characteristics of patients and by organizational characteristics (Greenley, 1980a,b).

Health care organizations adopt certain procedures and postures in order to attract or discourage patients from seeking help from them. The desirability of a patient to a particular organization depends on to what degree and in what ways patients might be a resource to the organization. Organizational behaviors toward patients as resources are very complex in large part because patients are complex resources. Patients can be assets because they fit with organizational ideologies of service, such as a commitment to help the poor. Certain patients can be valuable because they supply links to other organizations which are the sources of resources such as funds or space (Nagi, 1974). The same patients can be liabilities because they do not fit with other organizational ideologies, such as a preference for clients who will do well in psychotherapy. Some patients are relatively more costly than others because they bring in less money, as in the case of Hill–Burton patients treated free by hospitals. Others comprise more nonmonetary costs, such as lowered staff morale and higher staff turnover related to patients not improving, being uncooperative, and having inappropriate problems. Some of the complexities in the patterns that have been observed may result from patients being a resource in one respect and a liability in another.

In the broadest sense, organizations attract patients by making it known that they provide certain services. The claims they make about the types of clients served and services offered have been referred to as an organization's *claimed domain* (Levine & White, 1961; Greenley & Kirk, 1973). They make these claims through advertisements, and in many other ways. New organizations often offer a wide range of services (a large claimed domain) in order to attract much needed patients and establish themselves in the community (Rosengren, 1970). Organizations may redefine their eligibility requirements (claimed domain) when patients are in short supply in order to attract more, different kinds, and even previously unacceptable patients (Nagi, 1974; Sills, 1957). These claims seem to attract people to seek help at these organizations. For example, when general practitioners in England provided information about the services they offered, such as whether they would stitch a cut leg, patients of these physicians tended to have accurate knowledge about such services. When these patients were faced with deciding whether to take a particular problem to their doctor or to the hospital emergency service, they acted on their knowledge about what their physician would and would not do (Cartwright, 1967). Thus, claimed domains shape patient behaviors. Claimed domains are established because they are a major source of patients, and thus of autonomy and resources (Meyer, 1975).

While many help-seekers receive health care at the site where they initially apply for service, many if not most do not. One review of research on applicants for health and social services concluded that an average of 34% were rejected, 26% were referred, and 40% were served (Kirk & Greenley, 1974). Help-seekers often do not receive services because they are attracted to health care organizations by claimed domains that do not accurately reflect the service the organization actually provides.

The population actually served and the services rendered may be called the *de facto* domain (Greenley & Kirk, 1973). This *de facto* domain may not be congruent with an organization's claimed domain. Often the two domains do not cover the same problems, populations, and services (Stanton, 1970; Scott, 1969; Perrow, 1979). The difference between claimed domain and *de facto* domain is referred to as "domain discrepancy."

Domain discrepancy often accounts for help-seekers not receiving service in an organization that seems appropriate to their problems. Domain discrepancy occurs most often when *de facto* domains become smaller than claimed domains. Some health care organizations are unable to provide all promised or even mandated services due to insufficient resources or unavailable technologies. For example, state psychiatric hospitals that had limited resources were successfully sued for confining patients for the purpose of treatment but providing them only with custodial care (Brooks, 1974; Herr, Arons, & Wallace, 1983). Other organizations are established with unrealistically wide claimed domains for essentially political reasons (such as to shield themselves from criticism). For such reasons, Planned Parenthood organizations often offered fertility counseling services although they were primarily interested in preventing unwanted pregnancies (Kirk & Greenley, 1974). Certain organizations never fully planned to provide all services in claimed domains. In other circumstances, contracting organizational resources may force reduction of services, resulting in a shrunken *de facto* domain. *De facto* domains also contract as the result of organizations achieving a more secure resource base (Rosengren, 1970). This is because the organization with more resources can be more selective in the types of clients it chooses to serve. When domain discrepancy exists, potential patients may be attracted by a health care organization's claimed domain and will apply for services that the organization is not providing.

Alternatively, *de facto* domains may become larger than claimed domains. Providing service to a particular type of patient may be valuable to an organization, but acknowledging this service as part of the organization's claimed domain may not be. For example, a public mental health clinic funded to provide acute psychiatric care for the poor was observed to allow certain staff to provide long-term psychoanalytic psychotherapy to some persons with high income (Greenley, 1980b). This was allowed in order to improve recruitment possibilities and staff morale, even though recognition of this service in the organization's claimed domain would undermine its ability to get public funds. Because these higher income people were being served, there was less staff time for the poorer population, and some of these poor people thus had to be refused service.

When persons seeking help are not provided services, as a result of domain discrepancy, the health care organization staff usually provides reasons to explain this to the clients. This is called "active selection" and denotes that it is overt and occurs before service begins. Health care professionals often employ explanations and rationales that reflect their professional ideologies. Patients usually accept these explanations as legitimate because of the professional's status and implied expertise. In one multisite study, only 10% of patients identified by staff as having been rejected felt they had been rejected (Greenley & Schoenherr, 1981).

Sometimes, professional reasons for not serving clients are not readily available. In such cases, use of bureaucratic explanations centering on organizational rules and regulations is more common. In some organizations, staff have been observed to retreat into ritualistic "compulsive defending behavior" as a way of managing the pressures necessitated by obligatory selectivity (Wasserman, 1971). Ritualistic behavior refers here not only to a narrowly conceived deviant adaptation (Merton, 1968) but also to the broader tendency to focus on legalistic rules and regulations. Whether through expert pronouncements or ritualistic behavior, help-seekers find themselves being actively selected out. Domain discrepancy in its various forms, therefore, is thought to account for a large proportion of those patient experiences referred to as rejection, referral, dropping out of treatment, and so forth.

Volume of Services

Health care organizations appear to have a substantial amount of control over the volume of services provided. It has been estimated that approximately 80% of all service use is controlled by health care providers. In one study, less than 2% of 1628 hospital admissions were patient initiated. The remainder were physician initiated (Anderson & Sheatsley, 1959).

Health care organizations also have incentives to control the volume of service provided to any one patient. This is because patients very often are resources to the organization in relationship to the volume of services used. This is a very common situation in our health care system where fee-for-service payment is so pervasive. In a fee-for-service system, the organization can charge the patient directly for each unit of service. A contrasting example is the case of an HMO which may want more patients to choose them as a provider, but once chosen the patients are a greater resource if they consume fewer units of service. In a recent unpublished study (J.G.), one psychiatric clinic was observed providing fewer visits to prepaid patients within an HMO than to those funded through fee-for-service and insurance arrangements.

Staff in health care organizations may also provide fewer services to certain patients due to nonmonetary costs. Some patients are perceived as undesirable because they are ugly, incompetent, unreliable, uncooperative, or untreatable (Papper, 1970; Davidson & Factor, 1987). Health care organizations may have incentives to influence the volume of services used by patients for these nonmonetary reasons also.

An organization may want to limit services because it is forced to accept more patients than it can or wants to serve. Organizations with low "boundary control" often are in this situation. Boundary control refers to the ability of the organization to regulate the flow of inputs, including patients, into the organization. An organization with low boundary control over patients may be forced to accept patients who are inappropriate or unwanted. Public organizations may be placed in this position by law or regulations requiring them to serve certain populations. An extreme example is the public mental hospital which must take involuntarily committed patients even when such patients cannot be appropriately treated by the hospital's services. Commitment laws were passed in the 19th century precisely to force public mental hospitals to take patients who they did not want (Rothman, 1971, 1980). Similarly, the Community Mental Health Act of 1963 defined services by geographic "catchment area" to try to force mental health professionals to serve lower-class and minority chronically mentally ill citizens who were traditionally considered undesirable and were underserved (Lorber & Satow, 1977, 1978; Brown, 1985). The Veterans Administration Hospital faces similar restrictions and obligations to provide services to specified veteran populations (Thompson, 1981).

Rein (1980) observed that organizations that are forced to accept unwanted patients tend to be large public organizations with low boundary control and few resources. They are like the organizations in the immediately preceding examples (state mental hospitals, VA hospitals, and community mental health centers). They do not have the autonomy to control the type of patients they serve. They tend to get a large number of difficult patients, which taxes their resources. To reduce costs, they often implement bureaucratic procedures to routinize and standardize patient processing. In contrast to this type of organization, there are private organizations with sufficient autonomy to control their boundaries, with smaller, selected patient populations, and with more resources (Rein, 1980).

Organizations that feel that they must, or are legally obligated to, take patients have difficulty using active selection to deal with the flow of patients into their organization. They must usually try to adjust volume of services provided to these patients. They do this usually through passive selection techniques. In passive selection, patients are encouraged to decide to leave on their own. Common examples of passive selection are barriers to care used by some health care organizations to ration services. These include the establishment of a waiting list, long delays before one can get an appointment, shorter lengths of time with the doctor, and the provision of services in unpleasant physical surroundings (Schwartz, 1975). Inconveniences of location and hours, as well as the high cost of services can be passive barriers to care. These types of organizational situations and behaviors tend to discourage patients. At times patients may be counseled to request less care or seek care elsewhere, sometimes in the guise of treatment recommendations. In one situation observed by the author (J.G.), when prepaid HMO patients in a psychiatric clinic exceeded the number of visits budgeted into their prepayment, they were told that they did not need any more care. A review of literature revealed that in general those programs with the least stringent admission requirements (low boundary control) had the highest voluntary client dropout rate (Baekeland & Lundwall, 1975). Other organizations may have low boundary control because they are so resource poor that they feel they must take patients even when they are of small benefit in terms of resources. They may be forced by circumstances to take more undesirable patients and patients they do not know how to treat effectively (Lorber & Satow, 1977, 1978; Peyrot, 1982). For example, a struggling new group practice may not wish to turn away even relatively undesirable patients. Thus, organizations that value patients will be less likely to use passive selection techniques to reduce the number of patients. For example, Schwartz (1974) observed that "clients who bring the most profit to the server enjoy a competitive advantage; they wait the least, to the disadvantage of their lesser endowed brethren who can find no one to honor the value of their time."

Patients express dissatisfaction at passive selection techniques, such as long waiting times (Davie, Goldberg, & Rowe, 1974), and patient dissatisfaction is related to patient help-seeking and service utilization behaviors (Koos, 1954; Comstock & Sloan, 1973). Patients at a university general medical outpatient clinic expressed dissatisfaction due to the long waiting times and to the short time spent with physicians (Fisher, 1971).

Passive selection techniques are also directly related to patient behaviors. For example, patients who changed physicians voluntarily without referral reported reasons including the unwillingness of doctors to spend time talking to them, the high cost of services, and the inconvenience of location and hours. Of course, these passive selection factors may not always (or even often) be adopted consciously to reduce pressures of patient demands. At times they are probably unwittingly created and may not even be in the best interest of the organization. In general, however, they serve the organizational function of controlling and reducing patient demand.

In other instances, an organization may want to increase the volume of services provided patients. This may be particularly likely to occur when a larger volume of services provided to each patient can compensate for an insufficient number of patients. It also may occur where the cost of providing an additional unit of service to a current patient is less than the cost of providing a unit of service to a new patient. In such situations, organizations have incentives to provide a greater volume of services to certain patients.

These situations occur most often when funding depends on units of service provided, such as patient days in a hospital. A hospital can, for instance, compensate for having fewer patients by keeping patients longer. A recent study found that in order to maintain a daily census, administrators at a public psychiatric hospital advised staff not to discharge patients too quickly (Schulz, Greenley, & Peterson, 1984; Thompson, 1981). This pattern tended to occur in times of decreasing admissions due to deinstitutionalization campaigns. The tendency of these administrators to prolong length of stay was seen as compensating for the drop in new admissions (Brown, 1985; Connery, 1968). Similarly, VA hospitals are evaluated in part on the volume of service they deliver. Physicians and administrators feel the pressure to increase utilization, so there is a tendency to keep patients longer and to admit them more readily (Sapolsky, 1977). In outpatient general medical care, the request for a return visit also generates a greater volume of service from the same number of patients.

Patient Satisfaction

Patient reports about satisfaction with care are thought to reflect attitudes and opinions about care that may influence other patient behaviors, such as choice of provider, amount of services used, and compliance. In addition, patient satisfaction reports are behaviors in their own right.

Most research on patient satisfaction focuses on how patient characteristics are related to satisfaction reports. The few studies of organizational factors tend to show that these have a substantial impact on patient satisfaction, albeit a smaller impact than patient characteristics. For example, Greenley and Schoenherr (1981, p. 13) found that organizational characteristics accounted for 30% of the explained variance in patient satisfaction and patient characteristics accounted for 70%.

It has been well established that there are multiple dimensions of patient satisfaction (Ware, Snyder, & Wright, 1976). These include accessibility, humaneness, technical competence, and cost. There appears to be a halo effect in patient satisfaction reports, i.e., satisfaction in one area will tend to make a patient report higher satisfaction in others. Nevertheless, there are certain distinct organizational factors which influence each of these kinds of satisfaction.

Satisfaction with accessibility is known to be related to the patient's distance to the organization's facility and the hours the facility is open. More subtle organizational behaviors that provide passive barriers at the entry to service, such as long waiting times to get an appointment or to see a provider, are related to dissatisfaction with service (Schwartz, 1975). Dissatisfaction with access was the most common reason given by patients in one study for "doctor shopping," consulting more than one doctor without referral (Olsen, Kane, & Kasteler, 1976).

Satisfaction with the interpersonal aspects of care, such as concern, privacy, respect, and so forth, was related to the role discretion of the provider in a study of health and social service organizations (Greenley & Schoenherr, 1981). Role discretion is the ability of the provider to make decisions without checking with someone else first. Providers with little role discretion are probably seen as less concerned with patients as individuals, and less able to provide them privacy. The lack of role discretion is probably the reason that highly bureaucratic organizations are often disliked by clients. Becker, Drachman, and Kirscht (1974) reported that mothers who were randomly assigned to an experimental pediatric clinic in which staff felt more role discretion, had more flexibility in their jobs, and were able to do more of what they wanted, were more satisfied on most dimensions than were mothers assigned to another clinic.

Highly bureaucratic organizations are hierarchical, have written orders, have routinized procedures (deal with similar cases in the same way), and have specialized personnel (Weber, 1946). These characteristics might all lower the patient's perception of the role discretion of the provider. In more highly bureaucratic organizations, providers would more often be specialized and thus have to provide referrals or seek consultations about problems outside their area of expertise. They would have to ask permission from their superiors more often and would have to refer to written orders more often, and they would appear less flexible. All these could help explain why clients would be more dissatisfied with service in organizations where staff members have less role discretion.

Patients have been thought to be incapable of judging the technical competence of the health care they receive. Nevertheless, patients have strong opinions about the competence of doctors and the quality of care at different provider organizations (Robinson, 1971; Haug & Lavin, 1983). To some extent, patients generalize their satisfaction from dimensions such as humaneness to the competence dimension, an example of the halo effect. In this sense, the organizational determinants of satisfaction with competence would be similar to those for satisfaction with humaneness. Patients also assess competence directly through useful but imperfect indicators such as staff confusion, modernity of equipment and facilities, or the quality of data gathering or information giving to the patient. In one recent study, psychiatric patients' satisfaction was significantly positively related to other objective and subjective measures of the quality of hospital care (Schulz *et al.*, 1984). Also, patients treated in a general medical ward reported more satisfaction with the amount of information they were given when they knew more about medications prescribed for them, indicating that satisfaction was related to the adequacy of information given (Parkin, 1976).

Patient dissatisfaction is related to a variety of patient behaviors. In a sample of patients subsequently hospitalized, dislike or distrust of physicians was given as a reason for delaying between the time symptoms were first noticed and seeing a physician (Anderson & Sheatsley, 1959). In a Nova Scotia survey of three communities, more untreated symptoms were present in groups expressing low satisfaction with past medical care in general (Elliot, 1972). Among older patients at an outpatient clinic, those who expressed more discontent with the clinic's medical care had more untreated illnesses and more often sought medical care elsewhere (Hyman, 1970). Negative attitudes toward a student health service were positively related to the proportion of visits made to other (nonuniversity health services) physicians (Anderson & Bartkus, 1973). Auto workers in Detroit who were more satisfied with the union's prepaid health care plan had less out-of-plan utilization (Bashshur, Metzner, & Warden, 1967). A study of prepaid health plans in California found that approximately 90% of the voluntary disenrollment documents filed were the result of patient dissatisfaction (D'Onofrio & Mullen, 1977). Most of the sources of dissatisfaction were organizational or bureaucratic. "Doctor shopping," consulting another physician about the same problem without a referral, is related to patient dissatisfaction with a physician (Kasteler, Kane, Olsen, & Thetford, 1976). Thus, diverse studies show that patient satisfaction results in various patient health behaviors (see also Cahal, 1962; Gray & Cartwright, 1953).

Organizational behaviors and characteristics do not produce the same reaction in all patients. Satisfaction varies by what patients expect and value (Noyes, Levy, Chase, & Vory, 1974), and patients vary on what they expect and value. For example, one patient may dislike a large group practice because it is more bureaucratic, and another may like the same group practice because it is more efficient in processing insurance forms (Ross & Duff, 1982). Unmet expectations are a major source of dissatisfaction (Francis, Korscht, & Morris, 1969).

EFFECT OF NEW ORGANIZATIONAL FORMS

In recent years there has been a proliferation of new organizational forms of health care, largely promoted to improve control over costs. A major change has been in the area of prepayment for care, with the resultant growth of health maintenance organizations (HMOs) in their various forms. Another change has been a movement toward making the amount of payment contingent on the type of condition treated, as in the diagnostic-related groups (DRGs) scheme of the government and associated similar state plans. Both of these change the way in which patients are resources to organizations. These changes in how patients use resources have effects that are predictable from our theoretical perspective. A few of these effects on organizational behavior and client experiences will be mentioned in this section. It is beyond the scope of this chapter to review the growing literature on these topics.

The changes brought about by both HMOs and DRGs tend to make the patient's choice to use a provider financially rewarding for the provider. Under DRG plans, the hospital is paid a set fee for the admission of a patient with a particular disorder. Similarly, an HMO receives funds when a patient decides to get care from that HMO and pays the enrollment fee. Unlike the earlier fee-for-service model, in these cases the organization benefits from attracting the patient into care but not from actually providing the care. Thus, organizations under these conditions should be expected to make an effort to attract patients by advertising, favorable rates, and so forth. Promised packages of services should be expected to get larger, because claimed domains tend to expand for organizations with incentives to attract patients.

Yet once the patient is recruited, the organization has less incentive to provide services, as there is normally no additional payment for giving additional services. Provider organizations would have an incentive to have a larger claimed domain than *de facto* domain. They would be reluctant to use active selection, as this would mean a loss of patients and associated revenue. These organizations would use passive selection to limit the service provided. This could mean telling people they did not need the service, creating waiting lists and long waiting times, and giving generally less pleasant service.

The organizations *would* use active selection to prevent having to give care only to those patients expected to use more organizational resources than they would bring in, such as patients with more difficult and chronic disorders. HMOs and DRG hospitals would be expected to attempt to attract patients with less risk of having a difficult and chronic disorder, a process called "creaming." Conversely, hospitals and HMOs with established reputations for quality, such as those associated with research universities, attract patients who expect to need complex services, a process called "adverse selection."

One result of these organizational adjustments is that some patients seek care in different places than they did previously. Another result is increased dissatisfaction with care at HMO and DRG hospitals. The largest number of complaints about HMOs reflect unsatisfactory adjustment to the HMO model of delivering service, i.e., rotating staff, insufficient time per visit, and restricted access to physicians and once-standard tests. These are all good examples of passive selection.

RESPONSE OF MANAGERS, PRACTITIONERS, AND PATIENTS

The organization of health services has always influenced patient behaviors, but the organizational factors of interest have changed as health services have evolved. The solo medical practitioner of the last century influenced patients through ideology and practices as surely as the modern physician in a large prepaid health practice. However, the organization of the services is strikingly different, and as might be expected, the organizational factors influencing patient behaviors have changed. These changes continue to bring new challenges to the health services researcher who tries to understand how these new and evolving organizational forms influence patient health behaviors.

In the United States, the health delivery system has progressed from the era of the solo practitioner to increasingly bureaucratized corporate medicine. The corporate actors focus a significant portion of their efforts on regularizing the impact of the organization on patient behaviors, including use of services, enrollment in payment plans, and patient satisfaction. They also try to manage patient behavior by selective recruitment and by advertising that emphasizes patient satisfaction as well as clinical skill.

As corporate clinical organizations have grown, so has the influence of the nonclinician professional managers who run these organizations. Although they compensate for the managerial weaknesses of many clinician-administrators who lack administrative training, they have not been trained as health care professionals or socialized through years of clinical training and mentorship with experienced care-givers with strong patient care ideologies. Future research should inquire into how the values and beliefs of these corporate managers structure their attempt to mold patient behaviors in the interest of the organization. Corporate managers take no Hippocratic oath to behave in a patient's best interest.

For some time the organizational needs of large health care organizations have been in conflict with physicians' beliefs about professional standards. Increasingly, it seems, these organizational needs and standards have come to dominate the professional standards. We need to ask how this changes professional standards, influences the activities and sense of obligation of health care professionals, and, in turn, affects patient behaviors. How will these changing standards and practice settings influence medical education and the values and beliefs acquired by young practitioners in the course of their training?

Future research should focus also on the processes by which patients assess organizational forms and activities. Much of our current work draws on a picture of patients forming their opinions and behaviors through intense contact with a family physician, often someone they have known for some time. Though perhaps always exaggerated, fewer patients have such ongoing relationships with individual physicians today. Many more deal with bureaucratic organizations in which multiple faces and organizational rules influence their experiences. How are these experiences turned into assessments of organizational competence and caring? How do they affect compliance with treatment regimes and continued loyalty to the organization? Will patients employ a new calculus in assessing health care, as health care organizations have with regard to patients? Will patients lose trust in health care organizations and develop new ways to deal with them in a less personal and comforting era? Will patients increase their reliance on self-help groups and patterns of lay referral? Students of health behavior must adapt their research methods and questions to these new organizational patterns.

FUTURE RESEARCH DIRECTIONS

Factors such as organizational autonomy, quest for resources, domain, and staff role discretion shape patient behaviors and will continue to do so. Further research focusing on these concepts and relationships is needed because their impact is not widely understood. Good research in this area often involves comparative organizational studies which are difficult to do. Nevertheless, such research should be encouraged because it provides the clearest avenue to further insight.

Rapid changes in the structure of health services delivery will bring other patient behaviors and organizational factors into prominence in the coming years. New concepts and paradigms, new approaches to data gathering, and new organizational forms will test the ingenuity of researchers.

Many of the changes will come from the continuing bureaucratization and systematization of health care delivery organizations. These changes have been accompanied by—and in part brought about by—the introduction of large numbers of professional business-oriented managers without clinical training. These health care administration specialists have a mandate to make services more "rational" and run organizations in a more "businesslike" manner. We anticipate that the attitudes, values, and orientations of these managers will increasingly shape patients' reactions to health care organizations. Traditional health care professions, especially medicine, have resisted this orientation. Health care professionals are socialized to provide care in a certain manner and to believe that what they do is best for the patient. They find their values challenged by the more distant and financially driven concerns of professional managers. We believe that over time, nonclinical management perspectives will increasingly dominate health care organizations as traditional health care professionals adapt to new settings and as newly trained professionals are socialized in these new institutional climates. Of course the outcome of the conflict between the traditional professionals and the business-oriented managers will depend on the local market strength of each group, the support of leaders in the professional communities, and other political and economic factors. Nevertheless, both the process of conflict and its outcome will affect patient behavior.

For example, HMO patients and some staff have objected to management-imposed strict screening rules governing access to physicians and authorization of lab tests. Patients may come to distrust health care institutions' claims that they have the patient's best interest at heart. Organizations may respond with changes designed to make patients feel better about the organization but which are irrelevant to the quality of care.

The bureaucratization and systematization of health care organizations may also affect the professional socialization of new practitioners. Practitioners socialized to different values and practices may elicit new and different patient behaviors and reactions to service.

There is some evidence already that organizational forms may be changing socialization patterns of both doctors and nurses (Kindig & Lastiri, 1986). For example, nurses are being trained for the greater autonomy of HMO and other nontraditional jobs (Davidson & Factor, 1988). Researchers need to be sensitive to changes in patterns of socialization and resultant value orientations of practitioners. We need to study patient responses to differently socialized practitioners.

Another important area of future research concerns how patients individually and collectively try to make sense of their health problems and the health care system. Patient self-help groups have proliferated in the past decade to help patients and their families cope with the burden of severe or stigmatizing illnesses or medical conditions (Tessler, Killian, & Gubman, 1987; Gartner & Riessman, 1977; Lieberman, Borman, Bond, Antzer, & Levy, 1979). They have often grown into sophisticated national lobbies and fund-raisers for research into their disease, as well as networks of local advocacy groups. As they learn more about their disease, their attitudes toward the professional community often change from being suspicious and antagonistic to being cautiously accommodating. As advocates, they have developed both anecdotal and systematic knowledge of specific providers and forms of treatment to serve as a guide for members who are new to the treatment system. They are a whole new source of patient values and beliefs about treatment that providers will have to deal with (Davidson & McKee, 1986). Thus, we expect important future research to focus on increasingly organized and systematic lay referral systems which mirror the development of the health services. Research should track these processes, their impact in specific disease groups (e.g., multiple sclerosis and mental illness), membership characteristics associated with forms of professional contact (e.g., social class, race, insurance coverage), and other differentiating factors.

In sum, we expect the major research issues in future years to focus on factors in the organization of services and the organization of patient responses that follow from the current large changes in the bureaucratization and corporatization of medicine.

CONCLUSION

The basic processes that determine how health care organizations treat people will remain, even though the organizational forms and organizational environments will evolve. Patient behaviors will continue to be shaped by these organizational behaviors.

Our analysis is predicated on the notion that health care is provided through a fragmented system in which many organizational entities fight for their share of the resources. Could the adoption of a centralized system of care change this? We think not. Even within a centralized health system such as the English National Health Service, we have observed individual suborganizational units, such as district hospitals, work hard to avert centralized control and gain role discretion. The organizational subunits act like independent organizations, and the central administration often seems to have surprisingly little control. The organizational processes described here would exist even under a centralized health care delivery system, though the specific incentives may differ.

As health care organizations and systems evolve, continued attention should be paid to organizational effects on patient behavior. In this chapter we have only been able to focus on a very few organizational characteristics and processes, a select few key patient behaviors, and a specific theoretical perspective. A broad comparative organizational perspective is needed. Relevant interorganizational research is costly and difficult to do. Nevertheless, it should remain high on our health services research agenda.

REFERENCES

Anderson, J. G., & Bartkus, D. E. (1973). Choice of medical care: A behavioral model of health and illness behavior. *Journal of Health and Social Behavior, 14,* 348–362.

Anderson, O. (1985). *Health services in the United States.* Ann Arbor: Health Administration Press.

Anderson, O. W., & Sheatsley, P. B. (1959). *Comprehensive medical insurance—A study of costs, use, and attitude under two plans.* Chicago: Health Information Foundation, Research Service 9.

Baekeland, F., & Lundwall, L. (1975). Dropping out of treatment: A critical review. *Psychological Bulletin, 82*(5), 738–783.

Barth, E. A. (1963). The causes and consequences of interagency conflict. *Sociological Inquiry, 33,* 51–57.

Bashshur, R. L., Metzner, C. A., & Warden, C. (1967). Consumer satisfaction with group practice, the CHA case. *American Journal of Public Health, 57,* 1991–1999.

Becker, M., Drachman, R., & Kirscht, J. (1974). A field experiment to evaluate various outcomes of continuity of physician care. *American Journal of Public Health, 64,* 1062–1070.

Black, B. J., & Krause, H. M. (1963). Inter-agency cooperation in rehabilitation and mental health. *Social Service Review, 37,* 26–32.

Brooks, A. D. (1974). *Law, psychiatry, and the mental health system.* Boston: Little, Brown & Co.

Brown, P. (1985). *The transfer of care.* London: Routledge & Kegan Paul.

Cahal, M. F. (1962). What the public thinks of the family doctor: Folklore and facts. *General Practice, 25,* 146–157.

Cartwright, A. (1967). *Patients and their doctors: A study of general practice.* London: Routledge & Kegan Paul.

Comstock, L. N., & Sloan, D. (1973). A health survey of students. II. Satisfaction, attitudes, and knowledge. *Journal of the American College of Health Association, 22,* 156–159.

Connery, R. H. (1968). *The politics of mental health.* New York: Columbia University Press.

Cumming, E. (1967). Allocation of care to the mentally ill. In M. N. Zald (Ed.), *Organizing for community welfare* (pp. 109–159). Chicago: Quadrangle.

Davidson, R. E., & Factor, R. M. (1987). *Undesirable patients in psychiatry.* Unpublished manuscript, Department of Psychiatry, University of Wisconsin.

Davidson, R. E., & Factor, R. M. (1988). Psychiatric nursing roles in a community mental health center. *Community Mental Health Journal, 24,* 83–86.

Davidson, R. E., & McKee, D. (1986, August). *Ideology, expressed emotion, and the Alliance for the Mentally Ill.* Paper presented at the annual meeting of the Society for the Study of Social Problems, New York.

Davie, J. S., Goldberg, B., & Rowe, D. S. (1974). Consumer acceptance of Yale health plan. *Journal of the American College of Health Association, 22,* 325–331.

D'Onofrio, C. N., & Mullen, P. D. (1977). Consumer problems with prepaid health plans in California. *Public Health Reports, 92*(2), 121–134.

Elling, R. H. (1963). The hospital support game in urban centers. In E. Freidson (Ed.), *The hospital in modern society* (pp. 87–88). Glencoe, IL: Free Press.

Elliot, J. L. (1972). Cultural barriers to the utilization of health services. *Inquiry, 9*(4), 28–35.

Fisher, A. W. (1971). Patients' evaluation of outpatient medical care. *Journal of Medical Education, 46,* 238–244.

Francis, V., Korsch, B., & Morris, M. (1969). Gaps in doctor–patient communication: Patient response to medical advice. *New England Journal of Medicine, 10,* 535–540.

Gartner, A., & Riessman, F. (1977). *Self-help in the human services.* San Francisco: Jossey–Bass.

Gouldner, A. W. (1959). Organizational analysis. In R. K. Merton, L. Broom, & L. S. Cottrell, Jr. (Eds.), *Sociology today* (pp. 400–428). New York: Basic Books.

Gray, P. G., & Cartwright, A. (1953). Choosing and changing doctors. *Lancet, II,* 1308–1309.

Greenley, J. R. (1980a). Sociocultural and psychological aspects of the utilization of health services. In M. H. Brenner, A. Mooney, & T. J. Nagy (Eds.), *Assessing the contributions of the social sciences to health* (pp. 169–207). Boulder: Westview.

Greenley, J. R. (1980b). Organizational processes and client selectivity in social welfare services. In

D. Grunow & F. Hegner (Eds.), *Welfare or bureaucracy: Problems in matching welfare services to client needs* (pp. 79–92). Cambridge, MA: Oelgeschlager, Gunn, & Hain.

Greenley, J. R., & Kirk, S. (1973). Organizational characteristics of agencies and the distribution of services to applicants. *Journal of Health and Social Behavior, 14,* 70–79.

Greenley, J. R., & Kirk, S. (1976). Organizational influences on access to health care. *Social Science and Medicine, 10,* 317–322.

Greenley, J. R., & Schoenherr, R. (1981). Organization effects on client satisfaction with humaneness of service. *Journal of Health and Social Behavior, 22,* 2–18.

Haug, M., & Lavin, B. (1983). *Consumerism in medicine.* Beverly Hills: Sage.

Herr, S. S., Arons, S., & Wallace, R. E. (1983). *Legal rights and mental health care.* Boston: Lexington.

Hyman, M. D. (1970). Some links between source economic status and untreated illness. *Social Science and Medicine, 4,* 387–399.

Kasteler, J., Kane, R. L., Olsen, D. M., & Thetford, C. (1976). Issues underlying prevalence of "doctor'shopping" behavior. *Journal of Health and Social Behavior, 17,* 328–339.

Kindig, D. A., & Lastiri, S. (1986). Administrative medicine: A new medical specialty? *Health Affairs, 5,* 146–156.

Kirk, S., & Greenley, J. R. (1974). Denying or delivering services: The access problem. *Social Work, 19,* 439–447.

Koos, E. (1954). *The health of Regionville: What the people thought and did about it.* New York: Columbia University Press.

Levine, S., & White, P. E. (1961). Exchange as a conceptual framework for the study of interorganizational relationships. *Administrative Science Quarterly, 5,* 583–601.

Liebermann, M. A., Borman, L. D., Bond, G. R., Antze, P., & Levy, L. H. (1979). *Self-help groups for coping with crises: Origins, members, processes, and impact.* San Francisco: Jossey-Bass.

Lorber, J., & Satow, R. (1977). Creating a company of unequals: Sources of stratification in a ghetto community mental health center. *Sociology of Work and Occupations, 4,* 281–302.

Lorber, J., & Satow, R. (1978). Cultural congruity and the use of indigenous paraprofessionals in community mental health work. *Sociological Symposium, 23,* 17–26.

Mechanic, D. (1976). *The growth of bureaucratic medicine.* New York: Wiley.

Merton, R. K. (1968). *Social theory and social structure.* New York: Free Press.

Meyer, M. W. (1975). Organizational domains. *American Sociological Review, 40,* 599–615.

Mott, B. J. F. (1968). *Anatomy of a coordinating council.* Pittsburgh, PA: Pittsburgh Press.

Nagi, S. Z. (1974). Gate-keeping decisions in service organizations: When validity fails. *Human Organization, 31,* 47–58.

Noyes, R. W., Levy, M. I., Chase, C. L., & Vory, J. R. (1974). Expectation fulfillment as a measure of patient satisfaction. *American Journal of Obstetrics and Gynecology, 118,* 809–814.

Olsen, D. M., Kane, R. L., & Kasteler, J. (1976). Medical care as a commodity: An explanation of the shopping behavior of patients. *Journal of Community Health, 2,* 85–91.

Papper, S. (1970). The undesirable patient. *Journal of Chronic Diseases, 22,* 777–779.

Parkin, D. M. (1976). Survey of the success of communications between hospital staff and patients. *Public Health, 90,* 203–209.

Perrow, C. (1979). *Complex organizations.* Glenview, IL: Scott, Foresman.

Peyrot, M. (1982). Caseload management: Choosing suitable clients in a community health clinic agency. *Social Problems, 30,* 157–167.

Rein, M. (1980). Fact and function in human services organizations. *Sociology and Social Research, 65,* 78–93.

Robinson, D. (1971). *The process of becoming ill.* London: Routledge & Kegan Paul.

Rosengren, W. R. (1970). The careers of clients and organizations. In W. R. Rosengren & M. Lefton (Eds.), *Organizations and clients* (pp. 117–135). Columbus, OH: Merrill.

Ross, C., & Duff, R. (1982). Returning to the doctor: The effects of client characteristics, type of practice, and experiences with care. *Journal of Health and Social Behavior, 23,* 119–131.

Rothman, D. J. (1971). *The discovery of the asylum.* Boston: Little, Brown.

Rothman, D. J. (1980). *Conscience and convenience: The asylum and its alternatives in progressive America.* Boston: Little, Brown.

Rubington, E. (1965). Organizational strains and key roles. *Administrative Science Quarterly, 9,* 350–369.
Sapolsky, H. M. (1977). America's socialized medicine: The allocation of resources within the veteran's health care system. *Public Policy, 25,* 359–382.
Schulz, R., Greenley, J. R., & Peterson, W. (1984). Differences in direct costs between public specialty hospital and private community general hospital acute in-patient services. *Inquiry, 21,* 380–393.
Schwartz, B. (1974). Waiting, exchange, and power: The distribution of time in social systems. *American Journal of Sociology, 79,* 841–870.
Schwartz, B. (1975). *Queuing and waiting.* Chicago: University of Chicago Press.
Scott, R. A. (1969). *The making of blind men.* New York: Russell Sage Foundation.
Sills, D. L. (1957). *The volunteers.* Glencoe, IL: Free Press.
Stanton, E. (1970). *Clients come last.* Beverly Hills: Sage.
Tessler, R. C., Killian, L. M., & Gubman, G. D. (1987). Stages in family response to mental illness: An ideal type. *Psychosocial Rehabilitation Journal, 10,* 3–16.
Thompson, F. (1981). *Health policy and the bureaucracy.* Cambridge, MA: MIT Press.
Thompson, J. D. (1962). Organizations and output transactions. *American Journal of Sociology, 68,* 309–324.
Thompson, J. D. (1967). *Organizations in action.* New York: McGraw–Hill.
Ware, J. E., Snyder, M. K., & Wright, W. R. (1976). *Development and validation of scales to measure patient satisfaction with health care services.* Carbondale: Southern Illinois University School of Medicine.
Wasserman, H. (1971). The professional social worker in a bureaucracy. *Social Work, 16,* 89–95.
Weber, M. (1946). On bureaucracy. In H. H. Gerth & C. W. Mills (Eds.), *From Max Weber.* New York: Oxford University Press.
Wilensky, H., & Lebeaux, C. N. (1958). *Industrial society and social welfare.* New York: Free Press.
Wilkie, C. V., & Notkin, H. (1958). Community organization for health: A case study. In E. G. Jaco (Ed.), *Patients, physicians and illness* (pp. 148–159). Glencoe, IL: Free Press.

CHAPTER 13

The Design of Physical Environments and Health Behavior

Bruce A. Whitehead, Alice E. Fusillo, and Stephen Kaplan

INTRODUCTION

During the dramatic era of the conquest of infectious disease, the health sciences could with some justification consider environmental psychology a "frill." The traditional medical model emphasizing diagnosis and treatment of sickness in terms of acute, specifically biological causes (Mechanic, 1978) was unquestionably successful. The tendency of people to avoid doctors and medical facilities until they were acutely sick may have been understandable in such circumstances. While not conducive to preventive care, this tendency did serve to concentrate the efforts of an acute sick-care system upon those it would benefit most (Garfield, 1970). The benefits of this model of medical care were both quantitatively measurable (Dauer, Korns, & Schuman, 1968) and prominent in medicine's public image (Klein, 1972). These initial successes would probably have overshadowed any attempt to measure quantitatively and analyze the effects of the environment in which health care takes place.

If a way to solve problems is widely and successfully applied, it will tend to eliminate the type of problem it can solve. In this sense, the traditional medical model may to some extent become a victim of its own success. This model will continue to play an important role (Mortimer, 1978), of course, but its role will become less exclusive in the United States as problems less amenable to the medical disease model alone increasingly burden the health care system (Boden, 1976). Since the first Surgeon General's report on health promotion and disease prevention (U.S. Public Health Service, 1979), there has been a well-established consensus that the major health problems of the United States warrant greater emphasis on people who are not acutely sick. The National Commission on the Cost of Medical Care (1978) has recommended the involvement of health-related institutions in producing a population that better understands self-care and healthful life-styles. Efforts to provide incentives, or motivate people to adopt such preventive behaviors are

This chapter reflects the views of the authors only. It does not reflect the views of the U.S. Department of Health and Human Services.

BRUCE A. WHITEHEAD • College of Information Studies, Drexel University, Philadelphia, Pennsylvania 19104. ALICE E. FUSILLO • U.S. Department of Health and Human Services. STEPHEN KAPLAN • Department of Psychology, University of Michigan, Ann Arbor, Michigan 48109.

increasingly justified on the basis of economics alone. This is especially true for the economics of health maintenance organizations, which struggle to provide incentives for patients to adopt preventive care behaviors (Fuchs, 1974).

PARTICIPATORY HEALTH BEHAVIOR

Some recommendations for preventive care, such as early detection screening programs, depend upon getting nonsick patients to come to a health care facility. For other recommendations, the role of the facility would be to give people a sense of participation in and an understanding of their own health care that will motivate their behavior outside the facility. In either case, the people served will need to play a more active role in their own care. The knowledge and attitudes they acquire during visits to the facility will be crucial in developing this role. Creating a motivation for people to learn about and participate in their own health care is particularly difficult because of the amorphous nature of the threat. In successful public health programs of the past, the threat was often a highly visible infectious disease caused by a specific imageable "germ," and the public could see a direct cause-and-effect connection between the specific action recommended and the specific disease it would prevent. For many current health care problems, nearly the opposite is true. At the time in a person's life when diet, smoking, and exercise habits are being formed, degenerative diseases are an unfamiliar, probabilistic threat decades in the future. In this respect they are similar to certain natural hazards studied by Kates (1962). Kates's study suggested that the perception of such a probabilistic threat is much less tangible (and therefore less motivating) if it is not expected to occur within the usual time span of human planning activities. In particular, the possible effects of one's own activities upon such threats tend to be poorly perceived, allowing a somewhat fatalistic attitude to prevail. Any tendency for a similar attitude to develop toward long-term health risks would obviously be reinforced by a medical model in which one leaves the understanding and control of one's health entirely in the hands of the physician.

Under these circumstances, the psychological impact of the health care environment is no longer a peripheral issue. The staggering economic and human costs of acute curative care for degenerative diseases have necessitated a major effort toward health promotion and disease prevention. Specific recommendations along these lines are now supported by the health care community. But as we have seen, there are motivational prerequisites to the role that ordinary people must take in these recommended actions. The psychological impact of the health care environment, affecting people's understanding and sense of participation, must be considered. Unless these prerequisites are met, the effort toward health promotion and disease prevention will fail.

The preventive model thus requires research on the physical design of the health facility as it relates to participatory health behavior. Two major directions for this research appear particularly promising. The first concerns the relationship of human needs to the spatial arrangement of the physical environment. In this domain, hypotheses applicable to health facility design may be derived from basic research in cognitive and environmental psychology. These hypotheses may be tested by observation, simulation, and subsequent inclusion in the design of selected health care facilities on an experimental basis.

A second, complementary direction for research lies in the process by which health facilities are designed. This approach would develop research models for pretesting a facility design through the participation of prospective consumers. Although the use of functional and psychological analysis can greatly aid in effective environmental design, pretest and field evaluation provide complementary information vital to a good fit. Fortunately, there are a variety of promising new procedures that extend the possibilities beyond after-the-fact, better-luck-next-time data collection. Prospective evaluation techniques might be based on simulation or substitutes for experience of various kinds. Pertinent here are games, physical models, and sketches that take advantage of the human bias toward the visual approach, in addition to more traditional procedures such as questionnaires and interviews. A convergent analysis based upon these different research methods would allow information about human needs to be collected in a form useful for the design process.

HUMAN NEEDS AND THE PHYSICAL ENVIRONMENT

Let us now explore how the design of a health facility might either encourage or discourage people's sense of participation in and understanding of their own health care. In addressing this issue, we will consider three fundamental questions about the relation between human cognition and the environment:

1. How do people prefer to relate to their physical environment?
2. How do people develop an understanding of a particular environment, such as a health facility?
3. What physical characteristics of a hypothetical environment (such as a proposed health care facility) must be represented to allow prospective evaluation of that environment?

Kaplan and Kaplan (1982) presented a synthesis of environmental psychology which directly bears on these questions. To address the first question, we may begin with a few simple facts about the way in which people prefer to relate to their environment (S. Kaplan & Kaplan, 1982).

People care to make sense out of their world. They are reassured by the presence of the familiar. They want to be able to predict what might happen next. To choose knowledgeably among courses of action, and to predict the consequences of one's actions are among the universal human desires identified in Cantril's (1966) multinational survey. People care about being able to act effectively on their environment, to exert a reasonable degree of control over what goes on about them. Nursing home residents given responsibility for making their own decisions have been found to be more alert and more involved in social activities than a comparison group who were encouraged to assume that the staff would care for them (Rodin & Langer, 1977). The residents who were encouraged to make their own decisions subsequently showed greater health improvements and a lower death rate than the comparison group.

It is often the case, however, that the individuals in a medical setting sacrifice their grasp, their control, their understanding, in return for expert care (Korsh & Negrete, 1972). Of course, some acutely sick hospital patients may be in no shape to understand and guide their own affairs. Often they may be only too glad to relinquish control and responsibility under such circumstances. But the entire concept of a prevention-oriented, education-providing facility, not solely concerned with the critically ill, seems quite foreign to this pattern.

The central principle here is that humans are active, thinking, capable organisms who greatly prefer, under a wide range of circumstances, to be treated as active, thinking, capable organisms (Antonovsky, 1979). They are often resentful and incompetent when treated like incompetents. Being told exactly what to do and no more, being expected to respond in terms of narrow categories and no more, is in effect equivalent to being treated like an IBM card or a thing, no matter how well-meaning the source of this treatment (Beer, 1974). Lack of individuality and personal control is unfortunately a pervasive aspect of many hospital environments (Cohen, Evans, Stokols, & Krantz, 1986). This aspect of the hospital environment has been studied by means of presurgical interventions which provide preparatory information to the patient. While the results of these studies (reviewed by Cohen *et al.*, 1986) are mixed, it appears that information about what will be experienced, when combined with guidance on possible coping mechanisms, may have a beneficial effect on postoperative recovery. People greatly appreciate circumstances which expand their capacities, which offer them greater grasp, greater control in areas of interest or concern to them. Wolk and Telleen (1976) compared two residential settings which differed greatly in the amount of control exercised by residents over the activities in their lives. In one setting, the residents lived in an institution in which all basic needs were met through organized staff procedures; in the other setting, individuals lived in separate dwellings and took individual responsibility for most of their activities. Wolk and Telleen found that life satisfaction and developmental task accomplishment (both measured by questionnaires) were greater in the less constrained setting. Although the samples in this study were not random, the results corroborate those of Rodin and Langer (1977). Taken together, the studies above suggest that the educational component of preventive medicine has greater potential if offered in settings which encourage individuals to take responsibility for their own care. Further studies which directly test this hypothesis are a promising direction for future research.

This approach is not limited to preventive care but has great potential for all types of health care services. In the care of the dying, Kron (1978) described the importance of environmental psychology in the design of hospices. Some of these facilities have been designed to encourage participation of patients in their own care. In some cases, the design of the facility allows patients to create a homelike atmosphere and provides for family participation in the life of the patient. In Buckingham's (1982) study, both patients and primary care providers in a hospice reported less friction and greater satisfaction in their relationships with spouse, children, and other family members than did those who were not in a hospice.

One factor considered in the design of such facilities is the anxiety that people are likely to feel when entering the facility, and when entering a room where a dying person will be encountered. Appropriate placement of windows can allow people to see portions of the interior of a building before entering it, and to see the interior of a room before entering it. In this arrangement, the patient's privacy is protected by an anteroom which gives visitors a brief opportunity to become accustomed to the setting before entering (Kron, 1978).

Bazell (1971) provided another example of the power of treating people as thinking, discerning humans. East Harlem residents, hired to do apartment repairs and maintenance work, were also taught the public health implications of their work. The pride and quality of work that resulted provides an indication of how profound the effect of this realization can be. Although the East Harlem project was not a controlled study, the results are consistent with those of the other studies discussed above (Rodin & Langer, 1977; Cohen *et al.*, 1986; Wolk & Telleen, 1976) regarding the role of personal responsibility. The untested implication of these studies is that personal responsibility for behavior and personal understanding of the health consequences of one's behavior may both be significant factors in facilitating preventive health behaviors. Further study is needed to clarify the interaction of these two factors in influencing health behavior. The argument here is for treating humans as alert, flexible, information-processing, feedback-sensitive organisms who do almost anything better and more willingly—even taking care of themselves—when they know what they are doing.

This approach has many ramifications and is applicable at many different scales of design. Thus, for example, at the scale of the waiting room, the preference for the familiar, even including people like oneself and from one's own community, has important implications. A small waiting room that is not general-purpose but oriented to a particular, focused community might be a far more acceptable entry point for many people. Hypotheses such as this need to be tested in the evaluation of alternative designs. Although it might appear that the inefficiency of very small health care facilities rules out such a design, a radial grouping of small waiting rooms can be served by common central facilities. As another example, designing a staff conference room to be used for community meetings at night would encourage people to become familiar with the facility under nonthreatening circumstances. People would learn to find their way to and about the facility and have the opportunity to identify the facility with community participation and social support.

The desire to make sense out of one's environment, to be able to predict what might happen next, also has clear design consequences (S. Kaplan, 1973). It is not unusual for a hospital to have a series of routes marked only by colored lines along the corridors. The patient is apt to feel disoriented with such an arrangement, not to mention the likelihood of forgetting which of several colored lines was being followed. Such a procedure provides little information about the layout of the space and about the different areas one will come in contact with. It would not be difficult to make spaces clearly differentiable not only by the use of color schemes (Birren, 1979) but also by texture, style, and arrangement of furniture, and to use pictorial symbols to help guide the way. Cohen *et al.* (1986) reviewed evaluations of health facility designs in which the rearrangement of space serves purposes such as increasing privacy or facilitating social activities, but studies are needed which specifically evaluate orientation and way-finding in health facilities. Providing some information about where one is and where one is going does not seem inappropriate for a capable, spatially oriented organism.

There is also the vital problem of locating the facility in space within the community (Carp, 1975). Here again the concepts of familiarity and predictability might be used to locate the facility in a way which enhances its acceptability. If the health care facility is placed in a setting that is already part of a resident's "mental map," many aspects that might otherwise present problems will be partially avoided. The implication that preventive health behavior may be facilitated in this way is a promising topic for further research. For example, in a self-contained community built around a central point or room, the best location might be in that center or immediately adjacent to it. An ideal location within this central area would be near schools and recreation centers. In these cases it is usually easy to establish communication and interaction with health workers and teachers. Being close to a recreation area helps to remove the stigma or reduce the feeling of fear associated with a treatment center area. Being near shopping centers increases physical accessibility. With the specialization of communities as described by Coleman (1971), the proper embedding of health facilities within a community requires a different set of considerations for each type of community. But in any event, to enhance the accessibility and awareness of the existence of the facility, its identifiability is important.

While criteria based on environmental psychology can be applied to any facility used by humans, there are also more specific ways of evaluating a particular type of facility based on its functions and the needs of the people served. In housing facilities for the elderly, Moos and Lemke (1980) developed measures of the physical environment along nine empirically derived dimensions. Two of the dimensions (physical amenities and social-recreational aids) measure richness of the physical environment; three (prosthetic aids, orientational aids, and safety features) measure aids to daily activities; two (architectural choice and space availability) measure potential flexibility of the environment; and two measure staff facilities and community accessibility. Of these nine dimensions, Moos and Igra (1980) found physical amenities, social-recreational aids, architectural choice, and space availability to be significant predictors of the quality of the social environment.

In institutional settings, the influence of the physical environment on behavior may be conceptualized in terms of the congruence, or fit, between the particular needs of an individual and the particular characteristics of the specialized facility. Kahana (1974) investigated the congruence between characteristics of the individual and characteristics of the environment in nursing homes. This was done by developing separate measures of individual characteristics, based on interviews, and environmental characteristics, based on observations of the facility. Measures were developed for several dimensions, of which change versus sameness, privacy, dependency, order versus disorder, stimulation, affect, and motor control are representative components. Congruence between the individual and the environment in privacy, motor control, and stimulation were found to be significant predictors of the residents' morale in Kahana's study. Along similar lines, Carp (1978) measured the congruence between desired and actual levels of activity, each determined by structured interviews. Based on this congruence measure, Carp found that a physically improved residential setting for the elderly afforded increased levels of activity for an 8-year follow-up period. Although the activities measured were not specifically health behaviors, they were accompanied by a significant lowering of the residents' death rate, suggesting that opportunities for activity provided by the physical environment can promote behaviors which improve long-range health.

COMPREHENSION OF THE ENVIRONMENT

Let us next consider the physical environment of health care from the perspective of cognitive psychology. Based upon experience over a period of time, each person develops a mental image to represent objects, places, and activities. Representation of a location and how to get there can be referred to as a cognitive map. As S. Kaplan (1978) described more fully, the cognitive map is the information structure a person has about the environment. This structure is a set of mental images of recurring objects and events. Based upon one's experience, positive or negative feelings can become associated with these images in the cognitive map. As the cognitive map structure becomes more organized, less information is needed each time to find one's way, to make sense of objects or events, and to motivate appropriate behavior.

The psychological mechanisms for such representations of spatial information were reviewed in depth by Feldman (1985). Recent evidence on the underlying neural mechanisms is presented by Hein and Jeannerod (1983). Shepard (1984) discussed how the representation of spatial information is derived from interaction with the physical environment. From a broader perspective, Carver and Scheier (1981) integrated cognitive psychology into a synthesis of the literature on the regulation of human behavior.

Milgram, Greenwald, Kessler, McKenna, and Waters (1972) pointed out the various aspects of mental maps employed by different individuals to get from one point to another or to locate themselves in the environment. They discussed two main cognitive structures which lead to different strategies. First, an individual may proceed on the basis of a series of operations or cues. Here the use of signs would be important. Second, one may be guided by generalized images. This strategy allows for alternate routes to the same place and is particularly aided by distinctiveness and well-differentiated spaces.

Appleyard (1969) tested the seven attributes that Lynch (1960) stated affected a building's visibility. Inhabitants of four residential areas of a city in Venezuela were asked to tell what places in the city they remembered best, to draw a map showing the location of those places, and to recall places along a given road. Movement around a building; contours in terms of separate or isolated buildings; size in terms of bulk and height of buildings; considerable complexity or extreme simplicity in shape; and brightness of the buildings were significantly related to recall of the location of buildings. In contrast, verbal signs on buildings and the quality, i.e., condition, landscape, or use of expensive materials in buildings were not found to be significant for recall of location. Weisman (1981) similarly found that verbal signs alone cannot compensate for a cognitive map based upon poor environmental information. The implication here is that the design of a health facility can either help or hinder the efforts of personnel within it to give people feelings of responsibility and control over their own health. As a simple hypothesis, one might expect a preventive education program to have less influence on people who have gotten disoriented or confused on their way to the program. Such a hypothesis would not be difficult to test.

It is important to note that individuals observe the world and set up conceptual models from the viewpoint of their particular patterns of behavior (Lewis, 1961, 1965; Schorr, 1966; Strauss, 1970). Here, too, people behave and make predictions in terms of how they have perceived and coded past experiences. In designing health care facilities it would thus be necessary to be aware of characteristics of cognitive maps that derive from the life-styles of particular groups.

Although we have tried to provide some illustrations here of the ramifications of this approach—an approach that takes people's cognitive nature seriously—the greatest contribution will have to be made by those designers and researchers who approach the health care facility challenge alert to the implications of this approach.

CONSUMER PARTICIPATION IN THE DESIGN PROCESS

Skilled observation of existing facilities and the application of theory developed in the context of the larger field of human–environment relations can contribute substantially to the design of the effective health care facility. But to the designer of a particular health facility, the potential consumers of the intended services constitute another important source of information. How can information be gathered from these people in a way that can meaningfully influence the design process?

This question is a difficult one for two reasons. First, prospective consumers cannot react to a facility in the planning stages as easily as they can later when the facility is in actual operation. This difficulty might be phrased as a mismatch between the information obtainable prospectively and that obtainable retrospectively. The second difficulty is the familiar mismatch between the layman and the expert planner or designer. The information presented by the professional is typically too complex, too technical, or too detailed to be grasped by ordinary people. Conversely, the people to be served may not be able to translate their concerns into the explicit design criteria needed by the professional.

Both types of mismatch can become painfully obvious when public input is solicited through the usual channel of an open hearing on a proposed project. Typically, a presentation is made and people are given the opportunity to rise up and have their say. The people responding do not always understand the material presented to them, nor are they necessarily sufficiently articulate to make their own concerns understood. Evaluating an environment which only exists on paper would be difficult even if there were not also problems of different terminology, different modes of expression, different requirements for detail, and different axes to grind. The setting is often conducive to rhetoric, to the recitation of extraneous but popular clichés, to the reiteration of personal antipathies, and to polarization and confrontation. It is no wonder that design professionals are not universally enthusiastic about this particular innovation.

The open-ended community forum and the survey research instrument might profitably be viewed as opposite extremes of a continuum, defined by the degree to which the information-gathering process is structured by the expert. Such a view raises the possibility of developing a method more centrally placed on this continuum. Such a method might use the concepts developed in the last section to address both the mismatch between expert and layman and the mismatch between prospective and retrospective evaluation.

It is not difficult to think of criteria that an information-gathering method would ideally meet (R. Kaplan, Kaplan, & Deardorff, 1974; S. Kaplan, 1977). First, alternative environmental arrangements should be presented in a fashion which makes them graspable and which leads to reactions closely approximating those to be found in such an environment in reality. Presumably such a presentation would take advantage of the visual mode, because people comprehend the visual so effectively. Second, the setting should be structured to ensure that the potential consumers participate not merely in the discussion, but in the simulated environment as well. It is probably necessary to "put oneself into" the setting in order to obtain a realistic and empathic assessment of that possible environment. Third, reactions of participants should be called for that are appropriate to their future role in the facility. Participants must have a clear idea of what kind of help is expected of them if they are to make an effective contribution. It is also necessary to recognize that people typically handle certain types of judgements far more readily and confidently than others. And finally, it must be remembered that people are sensitive to the availability of genuine choices and resent being overly constrained. Questionnaires, as is well known, surprisingly often lead to hostility merely because the choices are so limited.

The most familiar form of substitute experience or environmental simulation is the game, and in recent years, games have been used with considerable effectiveness to simulate a wide range of environmental circumstances. On the other hand, the concept of a game tends to create images of a highly structured and rule-oriented arrangement. The immediacy of payoff that tends to characterize games may detract from their validity in studying preventive health behaviors with very long-term payoffs. Games can be structured to ensure involvement of the participants, but at the risk of creating a different level of involvement than would occur in an actual health facility. While games may be effective in certain environmental simulations, informal and flexible procedures which are more readily devised will often be more appropriate for evaluating health facility designs.

Games are often inadequate in the mode of presentation of the to-be-simulated environment. It would seem that much more could be done with various forms of visual presentations, including slides, graphics, and simple models (R. Kaplan, 1978). The possibility that participants could communicate a great deal through the manipulation of small figures through various alternative layouts also deserves careful study. In early phases of work in this area it seems entirely appropriate that a method or pair of methods used to evaluate alternative health care facility designs could be evaluated as models of participation at the same time.

The research questions involved in participatory design are not just issues of method, but are fundamentally issues of how the physical environment is represented in the mind. From this perspective, a visual model of a facility creates a representation in the prospective user's mind. To be effective, this representation must be similar to that produced by the actual facility when it is complete and operational. The research question is this: In what way must the two representations be similar to ensure that an evaluation of the model accurately predicts the evaluation of the facility itself? While this question has not been answered completely, there is certainly evidence (reviewed by S. Kaplan & Kaplan, 1982) that the representation of spatial relationships evoked by the model is crucial. This is not surprising in light of the fact that humans possess a rapid parallel-processing system specifically for perceiving and representing the spatial arrangement of the physical environment (Sagi & Julesz, 1985). It seems clear that spatial relationships are represented not in terms of a precise Euclidean metric (Moar & Bower, 1983), but rather in terms of more global and topological relationships (Chen, 1982; Brown, 1984) involving the behavioral possibilities afforded by the environment (Gibson, 1979).

Thus, it makes sense that a simple spatial model of a proposed physical environment can facilitate prospective evaluation by potential users. Such a model is likely to be effective if the viewer can sense the behavioral possibilities and constraints inherent in the proposed spatial arrangements. In light of what we have said about the way humans prefer to relate to their environment, it would not be surprising if such spatial arrangements affect how the facility is evaluated, and ultimately how it is used.

Simple spatial models have been used successfully in the evaluation of design alternatives by prospective users. R. Kaplan *et al.* (1974) compared simple models with highly detailed models in eliciting people's reactions to housing developments. Ratings of suitability for various functions (such as privacy, raising children, meeting people, and getting where one wanted to go) were not affected by the level of detail of the model presented. In R. Kaplan's (1980) study of design alternatives for an urban park, citizens had no difficulty providing preference ratings based on photographs of simple scale models. A follow-up study (R. Kaplan, 1980) showed high user satisfaction with the resulting park, and a surprising amount of interest in participating in the maintenance of the park. These same techniques could be applied to the design of a health facility without adding significantly to the cost of the facility. One might hypothesize that health behaviors not directly motivated by acute medical problems (such as participating in an early detection screening program, or participating in and following the advice of an education program) would be those most likely to be affected by people's attitude toward the physical environment in which the program is offered. A primary care facility might therefore be the most fruitful setting in which to study the effects of user participation in the design process.

It should be noted in passing that the same conceptions of humans as active processors of the environment that were raised in the previous sections also apply to the development of participatory design methods. Here too, people care to understand what is going on, and they care to know if their activity is having a genuine impact upon the environment. Thus, people have been known to become angry over graphics they cannot understand. Likewise, game rules that make no sense to the players or that unreasonably restrict their options are unlikely to be received with enthusiasm. The connection between the participants' input and ultimate design decisions should be made clear.

CONCLUSION

The central concern of this chapter has been to enlarge the concept of preventive health behavior to include people taking responsibility for and actively participating in their own health care. We have focused on the way in which the physical environment of the health facility can affect and be affected by such participatory behavior. To address these issues from the perspective of environmental and cognitive psychology, we have explored two directions for further research. The first is to investigate how the design of a health facility can influence people's sense of participation in and understanding of their own health care. The second is to investigate how characteristics of a design can be represented in the planning stage to allow prospective evaluation of the facility by the people it will serve.

The two major research directions we have explored ultimately converge. Environmental simulation or substitute experiences serve not only as a fascinating methodological challenge for data collection, but also as a way to enhance that very participation that theory leads us to believe humans are both capable of and concerned about. The conception of humans as cognitive, cognizant, competent organisms thus ramifies throughout theory, data collection, and application.

Efforts to provide effective health care while trying to hold down the costs cannot simply be mandated, unless the mandate addresses underlying causes. One such causative factor, the design of the health care environment, presents an opportunity to make significant improvements at little additional cost. Considering the magnitude of health care expenditures caused by inadequate participation of people in their own health care, and the potential influence of health facility design on such behaviors, a modest research program relating environmental psychology to health facility design would appear to be a wise investment.

REFERENCES

Antonovsky, A. (1979). *Health, stress, and coping.* San Francisco: Jossey–Bass.

Appleyard, D. (1969). Why buildings are known. *Environment and Behavior, 1,* 131–156.

Bazell, R. J. (1971). Urban health and environment: A new approach. *Science, 174,* 1005–1006. (Reprinted in S. Kaplan & R. Kaplan (Eds.), *Humanscape: Environments for people.* North Scituate, MA: Duxbury Press, 1978)

Beer, S. (1974). *Designing freedom.* New York: Wiley.

Birren, F. (1979). Human response to color and light. *Hospitals, 53,* 93–96.

Boden, L. I. (1976). The economic impact of environmental disease on health care delivery. *Journal of Occupational Medicine, 18,* 467–476.

Brown, C. M. (1984). Computer vision and natural constraints. *Science, 224,* 1299–1305.

Buckingham, R. W. (1982). Hospice care in the United States: The process begins. *Omega, 13,* 159–171.

Cantril, H. (1966). *The pattern of human concerns.* New Brunswick, NJ: Rutgers University Press. (Excerpts from Chapter 16 reprinted in S. Kaplan & R. Kaplan (Eds.), *Humanscape: Environments for people.* North Scituate, MA: Duxbury Press, 1978)

Carp, F. M. (1975). Life style and location within the city. *Gerontologist, 15,* 27–34.

Carp, F. M. (1977). Impact of improved living environment on health and life expectancy. *Gerontologist, 17,* 242–249.

Carp, F. M. (1978). Effects of the living environment on activity and use of time. *International Journal of Aging and Human Development, 9,* 75–91.

Carver, C. S., & Scheier, M. F. (1981). *Attention and self-regulation: A control-theory approach to human behavior.* Berlin: Springer-Verlag.

Chen, L. (1982). Topological structure in visual perception. *Science, 218,* 699–700.

Cohen, S., Evans, G. W., Stokols, D., & Krantz, D. S. (1986). *Behavior, health, and environmental stress.* New York: Plenum Press.

Coleman, J. S. (1971). Community disorganization and conflict. In R. K. Merton & R. Nisbet (Eds.), *Contemporary social problems.* New York: Harcourt, Brace, & Jovanovich.

Dauer, C. C., Korns, R. F., & Schuman, L. M. (1968). *Infectious diseases.* Cambridge, MA: Harvard University Press.

Feldman, J. A. (1985). Four frames suffice: A provisional model of vision and space. *The Behavioral and Brain Sciences, 8,* 265–289.

Fuchs, V. R. (1974). *Who shall live? Health, economics, and social choice.* New York: Basic Books.

Garfield, S. R. (1970). The delivery of medical care. *Scientific American, 222*(4), 15–23.

Gibson, J. J. (1979). *The ecological approach to visual perception.* Boston: Houghton Mifflin.

Hein, A., & Jeannerod, M. (1983). *Spatially oriented behavior.* Berlin: Springer-Verlag.

Kahana, E. (1974). Matching environments to needs of the aged: A conceptual scheme. In J. F. Gubrium (Ed.), *Late life: Communities and environmental policy* (pp. 201–214). Springfield, IL: Thomas.

Kaplan, R. (1978). Participation in environmental design: Some considerations and a case study. In S. Kaplan & R. Kaplan (Eds.), *Humanscape: Environments for people* (pp. 427–438). North Scituate, MA: Duxbury Press.

Kaplan, R. (1980). Citizen participation in the design and evaluation of a park. *Environment and Behavior, 12,* 494–507.
Kaplan, R., Kaplan, S., & Deardorff, H. L. (1974). The perception and evaluation of a simulated environment. *Man–Environment Systems, 4,* 191–192.
Kaplan, S. (1973). Cognitive maps, human needs, and the designed environment. In W. F. Preiser (Ed.), *Environmental design research.* Stroudsburg, PA: Dowden, Hutchinson, & Ross.
Kaplan, S. (1977). Participation in the design process: A cognitive approach. In D. Stokols (Ed.), *Perspectives on environment and behavior: Theory, research, and applications* (pp. 221–234). New York: Plenum Press.
Kaplan, S. (1978). On knowing the environment. In S. Kaplan & R. Kaplan (Eds.), *Humanscape: Environments for people* (pp. 54–58). North Scituate, MA: Duxbury Press.
Kaplan, S., & Kaplan, R. (1982). *Cognition and environment: Functioning in an uncertain world.* New York: Praeger.
Kates, R. W. (1962). *Hazard and choice perception in flood plain management* (Research Paper No. 78, Department of Geography). Chicago: University of Chicago Press.
Klein, A. E. (1972). *Trial by fury: The polio vaccine controversy.* New York: Scribner's.
Korsh, B. M., & Negrete, V. F. (1972). Doctor–patient communication. *Scientific American, 227*(2), 66–75.
Kron, J. (1978). Design a better place to die. In H. D. Schwartz & C. S. Kart (Eds.), *Dominant issues in medical sociology* (pp. 548–554). Reading, MA: Addison–Wesley.
Lewis, O. (1961). *The children of Sanchez.* New York: Vintage.
Lewis, O. (1965). *Five families.* New York: New American Library.
Lynch, K. (1960). *The image of the city.* Cambridge, MA: MIT Press.
Mechanic, D. (1978). *Medical sociology* (2nd ed.). New York: Macmillan Co.
Milgram, S., Greenwald, J., Kessler, S., McKenna, W., & Waters, J. (1972). A psychological map of New York City. *American Scientist, 60,* 194–200.
Moar, I., & Bower, G. H. (1983). Inconsistency in spatial knowledge. *Memory & Cognition, 11,* 107–113.
Moos, R. H., & Igra, A. (1980). Determinants of the social environments of sheltered care settings. *Journal of Health and Social Behavior, 21,* 88–98.
Moos, R. H., & Lemke, S. (1980). Assessing the physical and architectural features of sheltered care settings. *Journal of Gerontology, 35,* 571–583.
Mortimer, E. A. (1978). Immunization against infectious disease. *Science, 200,* 902–907.
National Commission on the Cost of Medical Care. (1978). *Vol. 1: Commission recommendations; Task force reports; Research agenda.* Monroe, WI: American Medical Association.
Rodin, J., & Langer, E. J. (1977). Long-term effects of a control-relevant intervention with the institutionalized aged. *Journal of Personality and Social Psychology, 35,* 897–902.
Sagi, D., & Julesz, B. (1985). "Where" and "what" in vision. *Science, 228,* 1217–1219.
Schorr, A. L. (1966). *Slums and insecurity* (U.S. Department of Welfare, Social Security Administration Research Report No. 1). Washington, DC: U.S. Government Printing Office.
Shepard, R. N. (1984). Ecological constraints on internal representation: Resonant kinematics of perceiving, imagining, thinking, and dreaming. *Psychological Review, 91,* 417–445.
Strauss, A. (1970). Life styles and urban space. In H. M. Proshansky, W. H. Ittleson, & L. G. Rivlin (Eds.), *Environmental psychology: Man and his physical setting* (pp. 303–312). New York: Holt, Rinehart, & Winston.
U.S. Public Health Service, Office of the Assistant Secretary for Health and Surgeon General. (1979). *Healthy people: The Surgeon General's report on health promotion and disease prevention* (DHEW (PHS) Publication No. 79-55071). Washington, DC: U.S. Government Printing Office.
Weisman, G. D. (1981). Way-finding and the built environment: An evaluation of architectural legibility. *Environment and Behavior, 13,* 189–204.
Wolk, S., & Telleen, S. (1976). Psychological and social correlates of life satisfaction as a function of residential constraint. *Journal of Gerontology, 31,* 89–98.

Cultural Determinants

The selection of materials on the cultural determinants of health behavior, as these are presented here, reflects the "pattern theory" of culture (e.g., Singer, 1968) which views culture as consisting of explicit or implicit patterns of and for behavior, acquired and transmitted by symbols, and constituting the distinctive achievements of human groups. Such patterns include: norms; standards for behavior; ideologies; justifications and rationalizations of selected ways of behaving; patterns of, for, and about behavior in a variety of areas; artifacts and traditional ideas.

Unfortunately, much research that has been labeled or indexed as cultural or sociocultural is simply demographic. There is, however, a rather small universe of research that deals with culture in terms more congruent with the broader, "pattern" definition. Moreover, culture permeates other levels of determinants of health behavior. Cultural values, norms, and expectations shape individual belief systems, life-styles, family interactions, role systems, social organization, and institutions.

To the degree that there are identifiably different pattern systems within a larger system, often associated with ethnic backgrounds, religions, and race, these can be thought of as distinctive subcultures. It is often through observations of subcultural differences that the impact of culture is itself appreciated. The term *cultural,* however, can be used to embrace subcultural effects.

Saunders (1954) was among the earliest researchers to show how cultural factors impinge on a variety of health-related behaviors. The importance of cultural influences on perspectives of health, illness, and disease have already been discussed in Chapter 1. Other cultural influences can be observed in beliefs that underlie utilization of services, and in responses to pain and to symptoms and signs of illness. The totality of a culture's beliefs and behaviors related to health, and its sanctioning and organization of healing practices are referred to as a "health culture." A health culture has meaning and integrity for its members.

HEALTH BELIEFS AND UTILIZATION

Concepts of cultural patterning were implicit in Suchman's research on social organization and use of health services (1965/1972), which was discussed in an earlier section.

Farge, for example (1978), was unable to replicate the significant linkages between all three of the Suchman medical orientation variables, but did observe a relationship between skepticism of medical care and dependency in illness. Moreover, the few observed linkages between social group and medical orientation variables related to ethnic exclusivity only, and were opposite in direction to Suchman's findings, e.g., high ethnic exclusivity was related to *greater* knowledge of health and disease. Farge reasoned for the development of a model of Chicano health care, based on Geertsen's model (Geertsen, Klauber, Rindflesh, Kane, & Gray, 1975), that would include the positive effects on medical orientation of maintaining Mexican cultural traditions in the home, and of self-determination.

Berkanovic and Reeder's (1974) review of the literature suggested that cultural factors may selectively determine the psychological cost of using certain services, misfitting expectations and priorities of professionals and consumers, and differences in vulnerability to the "ego assault" of interventions and treatments. These cultural differences were believed to be more important in utilization of health services than income.

Berkanovic and Telesky (1985) found that although Mexican-Americans, black Americans, and white Americans do not show differences in reporting of illnesses, days in bed or of restricted activity due to illness, or in frequency of seeking medical attention for illnesses, the factors that lead to seeking medical care differ among blacks than among whites and Mexicans. These observations suggest cultural and ethnic variability in the decision processes underlying utilization.

Cassel (1957) reported on the way in which cultural beliefs about foods may hinder acceptance of new, improved dietary patterns. For example, although milk had historically been an important part of the diet of the Zulu and other Bantu-speaking peoples of Africa, attempts to restore their milk consumption to healthy levels were impaired by their cultural beliefs about menstruating women coming in contact with milk herds, and about drinking milk only from the herd of a kinship group. Other cultural beliefs impeded the introduction of green vegetables and new grains.

Davis (1984) reported consistent anecdotal evidence that Newfoundland women exhibit a culturally patterned complaint of "nerves." For these women, nerves may mean any number of stresses or complaints. They can elicit concern from others, and—with proper etiquette—can be choreographed by the woman to manipulate her friends and family into assuring that she seek care. Davis additionally pointed out that physicians who are unaware of the meaning of "nerves" will not understand the woman's complaint and will not respond to it appropriately.

Hoppe and Heller's (1975) study of the Mexican-American cultural value of familism showed that it was not necessarily a barrier to use of scientific medical services, but rather served as a support for coping mechanisms. Moreover, familism was positively related to the timing of prenatal care, although not to use of curative services.

Welch, Comer, and Steinman (1973) systematically explored the effect of cultural beliefs about doctors and health care, social characteristics, and financial factors among Mexican-Americans. Their data suggested that assumptions about the impact of cultural factors on attitudes and use of health care should be questioned. Involvement with Mexican-American culture did not appear to explain as much as did social status and economic factors.

Jenny's observations about cultural conceptions of beauty (1975), which often lead people into painful and traumatic scarification processes, have implications about the acceptability and use of orthodontic services, above and beyond considerations of health and occlusion.

Too often, culture and race are used interchangeably in an inappropriate way. Scott's research (1974) carefully avoided the all-too-prevalent confusion of race, ethnicity, and culture. Her examination of five distinct black ethnic groups all living in close proximity—

Bahamian, Cuban, Haitian, Puerto Rican, and southern United States Blacks—revealed that they maintained culturally distinct beliefs about health, illness, and health care, and used a variety of available health systems, both traditional and "scientific." Kleinman and Lukoff's (1978) research demonstrated cultural differences in frequency and type of drug use in West Indian blacks, American blacks, and American whites, as well as different sources of influences on drug use.

Strauss's research (1976), while confounding economic and class factors with racial identity, nonetheless pointed out differences in perceptions between blacks and whites in the area of dental services. Blacks to a higher degree anticipate that a tooth will be extracted, and show more concern for the value of maintaining dental health.

Oller (1984) observed that within Judaism, anything that promotes health is advocated. Moreover, there is no endorsement of risk-taking behavior. Oller also noted that there is an overconcern with pain and symptoms, together with an accepted use of the physician as a way of dealing with stress.

Patrick, Sittampalam, Somerville, Carter, and Bergner (1985) demonstrated that although there was general agreement between British and American respondents in the values attached to aspects of health status, particularly where severe dysfunction was involved, there were some disagreements in areas where dysfunction was minimal.

Uyanga (1983) observed marked differences in conceptions of illness and health, as well as use of health services between rural and migrant-urban Nigerians. The rural residents were more likely than the migrant-urban residents, for example, to attribute illness to anger of the gods, or witchcraft, and use traditional healers who share personal relationships and symbol systems with them. However, among the migrants, when modern hospital treatment fails, traditional healers are sought.

Segall's chapter examines cultural differences in beliefs about the sick role, and the implications of these differences for other health behaviors such as lay consultation.

RESPONSES TO PAIN, SIGNS, AND SYMPTOMS

Zborowski's seminal analysis (1952) of ethnic differences in interpretation of, and response to, pain in Americans of Jewish, Italian, Irish, and "Yankee" backgrounds was a landmark study in generating research increasing understanding of cultural determinants of health behavior. Greenblum's study (1974) took a critical look at ethnic differences, reexamining Zborowski's conclusions about responses to pain as well as Suchman's conclusions (1965/1972) on the relationship between ethnicity, social status, and social integration and acculturation, and reported that ethnic differences in health behaviors diminish with increasing acculturation and upward social mobility.

Koopman, Eisenthal, and Stoeckle (1984) found that while older Italian-American women were more likely to report pain than older Anglo-American women, this ethnic difference was not observable among younger women or among men. The effects of acculturation are apparently mediated by age and gender.

Guttmacher and Elinson's observations (1971) of how diverse ethnic and religious groups differentially attribute illness to personal behaviors that depart from group patterns or subcultural norms, shed additional light on the effect of cultural factors in tolerating deviance through medicalizing it.

HEALTH CULTURE

Durie's (1985) elaboration of the Maori conception of health leads to an awareness that health pervades the totality of Maori culture. For the Maori, health involves spiritual, mental (psychic), somatic (physical), and family dimensions. The spiritual dimension includes not only religious beliefs, but beliefs about humans and their needs to be linked spiritually with their environment; the mental dimension embraces styles of thinking that go beyond Western linearity and analysis, and emphasizes holistic and synthetic thought; the somatic dimension extends beyond the traditional Western concern for the body to include concern for ritualized behaviors relating to a variety of bodily functions, particularly to the preparation and eating of food; the family dimension provides the Maori with much of their sense of identity and rootedness. Within the somatic dimension they have a highly polarized view of activities that involve food preparation and cleanliness, and maintain beliefs and behaviors that keep these two functions separated. Accordingly, a highly sanitized hospital setting with a hidden bedpan or urinal close to the eating tray will be perceived by them as *un*hygienic and hazardous. Moreover, by moving away from a strictly personal view, such as that found in Western societies, the Maori conception embraces and assigns high priority to community concerns such as pollution of streams, and to children's health.

Fabrega and Hunter's investigation (1977, 1978) of the Ladino population in a Mexican town is an interesting example of cultural patterns in relation to health and illness. Observations revealed a consistency—or a patterning—in beliefs about how personality and emotional factors contribute to both susceptibility and severity of certain diseases (1978). In other words, a "lay theory" of disease was maintained by members of this culture. Furthermore, there was consistency in the way this population perceived specific diseases to have effects on daily behavior (1977).

Kleinman and Sung (1979), in their analysis of the success of "indigenous healers," provided insight into how healing itself must be considered as a part of the entire social system, and must be seen not only as a way of controlling the sickness, but of providing meaning to the individual's experience of the sickness. Eisenberg and Kleinman (1981), paradoxically, warn against the reverse ethnocentrism involved in "the celebration of the wisdom of *the* folk healer as part of the myth of a Golden Age. . . . Healing ceremonies can be efficacious, but hardly substitute for anti-biotics or surgery . . ." (p. 10).

Young's decision-tree analysis (1981) of nonuse of physicians in a rural Mexican community, moved beyond the more typical study of demographic characteristics to relate this nonuse to a broader context of cultural beliefs related to the effectiveness of alternative, traditional healers. Young pointed out that the cultural tradition itself is less important than is the belief in the effectiveness of a particular curer—for a specific condition. Related to such findings are the observations of Martin, Martinez, Leon, Richardson, and Acosta (1985), who noted the distribution of reports of folk illnesses, e.g., "susto" (trauma, fright), and found that those physicians who reported receiving more of such reports were more sensitive in "psychosocial orientations" and were closer to Hispano-Mexican culture.

Hagey's (1984) narrative of the way in which urban Canadian Ojibway Indians view diabetes provided evidence that the illness is viewed as a metaphor in terms of a total cultural phenomenon: it represents concerns about stress, balance, and imbalance, and is "personified" in cultural legends about Windigo, a mythological gluttonous figure who represents the Ojibway conception of lack of morality, namely excess, or lack of balance or harmony.

Another way of viewing "health culture" is provided by Frankle and Heussenstamm's observations (1974) of youth culture and food zealotry, involving vegetarianism, natural and organically grown foods, and Zen macrobiotic diets.

Ostrowska's (1983) integration of data related to how patient characteristics, perceptions of availability of care, confidence in medical institutions, and availability of care alternatives were related to responses to illness, formed the basis for her delineation of contemporary Polish health culture. Among her findings were the association between lack of confidence in medical institutions and medical care, and delay in seeking such care and use of self-care.

Weidman's chapter synthesizes and amplifies the discussion of "health culture"; considers cultural differences in health and medical beliefs, and culture-bound syndromes; introduces the important concepts of "emic" and "etic" approaches, and "the transcultural perspective"; and discusses their implications for health professionals and health institutions.

CULTURAL PLURALISM

Durkin-Longley (1984) pointed out that medical pluralism, defined as the "coexistence in one society of divergent medical traditions" (p. 867), is more the norm than the exception in complex societies, and that there are regularities in the way the different medical practices are used. She noted two basic patterns of use: multiple therapeutic use, referring to use of more than one therapeutic system during a single illness, and illness-specific use, referring to use of specific therapies for the treatment of specific disorders. Her analysis of use of healers in Nepal revealed that although patients' reports of why they sought treatment substantiate illness-specific use, their actual behavior was consistent with multiple therapeutic use. Moreover, there was no consensus among respondents about which types of illnesses required which specific therapies. She did observe, however, that patients used multiple therapies to deal with different aspects of chronic conditions, i.e., one healer for medication, and another to build strength or to deal with stresses.

REFERENCES

Berkanovic, E., & Reeder, L. G. (1974). Can money buy the appropriate use of services? Some notes on the meaning of utilization data. *Journal of Health and Social Behavior, 15,* 93–99.

Berkanovic, E., & Telesky, C. (1985). Mexican-American, Black-American and White-American differences in reporting illnesses, disability and physician visits for illnesses. *Social Science and Medicine, 20,* 567–577.

Cassel, J. (1957). Social and cultural implications of food and food habits. *American Journal of Public Health, 47,* 732–740.

Davis, D. L. (1984). Medical misinformation: Communication between outport Newfoundland women and their physicians. *Social Science and Medicine, 18,* 273–278.

Durie, M. H. (1985). A Maori perspective of health. *Social Science and Medicine, 20,* 483–486.

Durkin-Longley, M. (1984). Multiple therapeutic use in urban Nepal. *Social Science and Medicine, 19,* 867–872.

Eisenberg, L., & Kleinman, A. (1981). Clinical social science: Is medical practice impeded by "too much science"? In L. Eisenberg & A. Kleinman (Eds.), *The relevance of social science for medicine*. Dordrecht: Reidel.

Fabrega, H., Jr., & Hunter, J. E. (1977). The effects of disease on behavior: Analysis of Ladino medical beliefs. *Ethos, 5,* 119–137.

Fabrega, H., Jr., & Hunter, J. E. (1978). Judgements about disease: A case study involving *Ladinos* of Chiapas. *Social Science and Medicine, 12,* 1–10.

Farge, E. J. (1978). Medical orientation among a Mexican-American population: An old and a new model reviewed. *Social Science and Medicine, 12,* 277–282.

Frankle, R. T., & Heussenstamm, F. K. (1974). Food zealotry and youth: New dilemmas for professionals. *American Journal of Public Health, 64,* 11–18.

Geertsen, R., Klauber, M. R., Rindflesh, M., Kane, R. L., & Gray, R. (1975). A re-examination of Suchman's views on social factors in health care utilization. *Journal of Health and Social Behavior, 16,* 226–237.

Greenblum, J. (1974). Medical and health orientations of American Jews: A case of diminishing distinctiveness. *Social Science and Medicine, 8,* 127–134.

Guttmacher, S., & Elinson, J. (1971). Ethno-religious variation in perceptions of illness: The use of illness as an explanation for deviant behavior. *Social Science and Medicine, 5,* 117–125.

Hagey, R. (1984). The phenomenon, the explanations and the responses: Metaphors surrounding diabetes in urban Canadian Indians. *Social Science and Medicine, 18,* 265–272.

Hoppe, S. K., & Heller, P. L. (1975). Alienation, familism and the utilization of health services by Mexican Americans. *Journal of Health and Social Behavior, 16,* 304–314.

Jenny, J. (1975). A social perspective on need and demand for orthodontic treatment. *International Dental Journal, 25,* 248–256.

Kleinman, A., & Sung, L. H. (1979). Why do indigenous practitioners successfully heal? *Social Science and Medicine, 13B,* 7–26.

Kleinman, P. H., & Lukoff, I. F. (1978). Ethnic differences in factors related to drug use. *Journal of Health and Social Behavior, 19,* 190–199.

Koopman, C., Eisenthal, S., & Stoeckle, J. D. (1984). Ethnicity in the reported pain, emotional distress and requests of medical outpatients. *Social Science and Medicine, 18,* 487–490.

Martin, H. W., Martinez, C., Leon, R. L., Richardson, C., & Acosta, V. R. (1985). Folk illnesses reported to physicians in the lower Rio Grande Valley. *Ethnology, 24,* 229–236.

Oller, D. T. (1984). Jewish genetic diseases and Jewish illness behavior: A review of selected sociocultural literature. *Jewish Social Studies, 46,* 177–187.

Ostrowska, A. (1983). Elements of the health culture of Polish society. *Social Science and Medicine, 17,* 631–636.

Patrick, D. L., Sittampalam, Y., Somerville, S. M., Carter, W. B., & Bergner, M. (1985). A cross-cultural comparison of health status values. *American Journal of Public Health, 75,* 1402–1407.

Saunders, L. (1954). *Cultural difference and medical care: The case of the Spanish-speaking people of the Southwest.* New York: Russell Sage Foundation.

Scott, C. S. (1974). Health and healing practices among five ethnic groups in Miami, Florida. *Public Health Reports, 89,* 524–532.

Singer, M. (1968). Culture: The concept of culture. In D. L. Sills (Ed.), *International encyclopedia of the social sciences* (Vol. 3). New York: Macmillan Co. and Free Press.

Strauss, R. P. (1976). Sociocultural influences upon preventive health behavior and attitudes towards dentistry. *American Journal of Public Health, 66,* 375–377.

Suchman, E. A. (1972). Social patterns of illness and medical care. In E. G. Jaco (Ed.), *Patients, physicians and illness: A sourcebook in behavioral science and health* (2nd ed.). New York: Free Press. (Reprinted from *Journal of Health and Human Behavior,* 1965, *6,* 2–16)

Uyanga, J. (1983). Rural–urban migration and sickness/health care behaviour: A study of eastern Nigeria. *Social Science and Medicine, 17,* 579–583.

Welch, S., Comer, J., & Steinman, M. (1973). Some social and attitudinal correlates of health care among Mexican Americans. *Journal of Health and Social Behavior, 14,* 205–213.

Young, J. C. (1981). Non-use of physicians: Methodological approaches, policy implications and the utility of decision models. *Social Science and Medicine, 15B,* 499–507.

Zborowski, M. (1952). Cultural components in responses to pain. *Journal of Social Issues, 8,* 16–30.

CHAPTER 14

Cultural Factors in Sick-Role Expectations

Alexander Segall

SOCIOCULTURAL DETERMINANTS OF HEALTH-RELATED BEHAVIOR

"Every human society faces the prospect of sickness and each one has developed its own general cultural adaptations for it, which constitute its solutions" (Simmons & Wolff, 1954, p. 74). Culture serves as a subtle, but systematic influence upon the way in which the members of any society perceive the world around them. The distinctive way of life which characterizes a particular group or subgroup of a society includes the health-related behavior of its members. For example, "cultures and subcultural groups vary in the extent to which they perceive a set of circumstances as constituting illness or health, abnormality or normalcy, as calling for action or disregarding" (King, 1962, p. 67).

The cultural context shapes prevailing beliefs regarding the cause of illness and appropriate forms of treatment. Whether a person is sensitive to feelings of discomfort, how symptoms are perceived and evaluated, and whether or not the individual decides to seek medical care are largely a matter of cultural prescription. Even the individual's view of the physician as a relevant helper depends in part upon cultural background. In other words, what should be done about a given condition once it has been defined as an illness is culturally prescribed. The type of treatment activity selected, the extent to which emotional expression is expected during sickness, and the emphasis placed upon individual versus collective decision-making are all part of the cultural tradition of the group. Thus, lay conceptions of health and illness and beliefs regarding the management of an illness experience are to a certain extent cultural phenomena.

The impact of culture upon health and illness behavior has been well summarized by Saunders (1954, p. 143). In his words, "an individual thus has cultural guides that enable him to know when he or others may be regarded as sick, something about the cause and nature of the sickness, what may be done to alleviate or remedy the condition, and the behavior expected of him and of others in the situation." It is evident that culture plays a broad part in shaping peoples' ideas about health and illness and their subsequent treatment activities. More precisely, however, what empirical evidence is there that culture determines definitions of health and responses to illness?

Investigations of the influence of cultural factors on health-related behavior have typi-

---

ALEXANDER SEGALL • Department of Sociology, University of Manitoba, Winnipeg, Manitoba, R3T 2N2, Canada.

cally focused upon subcultural units such as ethnic or religious groups. A variety of subcultural differences have been identified in selected aspects of health and illness. For example, it has been shown that particular cultural groups are characterized by distinctive patterns of disease (Graham & Reeder, 1979; Harwood, 1981). In other words, the incidence and prevalence of certain conditions such as cancer and heart disease vary among different ethnic groups. One possible interpretation offered is that group customs (e.g., dietary, hygienic, educational, religious) may predispose one to, or protect the individual from a given disease.

A number of other studies have focused upon cultural differences in the expression of symptoms associated with illness/disease (Croog, 1961; Zola, 1966). These studies indicate that the number of symptoms reported and the readiness of the individual to present pain as a symptom varies among different ethnic groups. Pain sensitivity and styles of pain expression have been subjected to detailed analysis (Zborowski, 1969). Zborowski contended that uniformities in behavioral responses to pain exist among the members of different ethnic groups and constitute an important part of the individual's cultural experience. Furthermore, he argued that there are ethnic differences in the meaning attached to pain and underlying attitudes toward pain. A number of experimental studies have also investigated the relationship between subcultural factors and pain (Sternbach & Tursky, 1965; Sternbach, 1968) and generally support Zborowski's field study.

Finally, the sociocultural determinants of willingness to consult a physician and to utilize health care facilities have received considerable research attention (Harwood, 1981; Mechanic, 1963; Plaja, Cohen, & Samora, 1968; Reeder & Berkanovic, 1973; Suchman, 1964). A variety of sociomedical differences have been reported among the ethnic groups studied including: (1) knowledge of disease and its prevention; (2) attitudes toward formal care (e.g., medical skepticism); and (3) responses to illness (e.g., physician contact and acceptance of dependency in illness). In summary, the evidence indicates that there are important sociocultural differences not only in medical orientation, but also in actual utilization patterns.

Sociomedical research has shown that within any given society, there may be found a number of distinct conceptions of sickness and sociocultural patterns of help-seeking behavior. It is reasonable, therefore, to anticipate the existence of a variety of subcultural beliefs regarding behavior appropriate for the sick role. Consequently, it is important to examine the extent to which the set of behavioral expectations embodied by the sick role concept is actually representative of different segments of the overall population.

SITUATING THE SICK ROLE IN A SOCIOCULTURAL CONTEXT

Parsons's sick role concept has been described as "the most important single theoretical contribution to medical sociology to date" (Cockerham, 1983, p. 1516). It has also been claimed (Johnson, 1975) that medical sociology, through this concept, has been able to make one of its few substantial contributions to general sociological theory. In addition, Parsons's (1951) formulation of the sick role has stimulated an extensive body of empirical research (see Levine & Kozloff, 1978, for a review). However, despite the obvious importance of Parsons's ideas and the impact which he has had on the development of medical sociology, the sick role concept has also prompted frequent critical commentary (Gallagher, 1976; Gerhardt, 1979; McCormack, 1981; Segall, 1976a).

Limitations of the Parsonian Sick Role Model

For example, Parsons's sick role has been accused of suffering from "socio-centricity" (Butler, 1970), because it failed to consider adequately the potential influence of sociocultural heterogeneity upon the behavioral pattern expected of the sick person. To illustrate the importance of this point, Butler argued unequivocally that the behavior expected of the sick person, as described by Parsons, cannot be taken as the role prescription for all types of illness in diverse sociocultural contexts. Indeed, Parsons's model was based, not upon systematic observation of human behavior, but upon an abstract set of hypothesized institutionalized expectations. In other words, in outlining the basic features of the sick role, Parsons presented his views on how a sick person should ideally behave. This ideal set of role expectations may not necessarily correspond to the ways in which people really behave when they experience illness. It has been claimed (Gordon, 1966) that uncritical acceptance of this ideal-type model has drawn investigators' attention away from exploring sociocultural variations in sick-role behavior. Consequently, the task still remains to determine the extent to which Parsons's conceptual model is empirically valid and whether sick-role expectations are affected by sociocultural factors.

In addition, Parsons's views have been widely criticized for presenting a relatively undifferentiated picture of the social structure of health care. For example, in describing the reciprocal relationship embodied in the sick role concept, Parsons focused essentially upon the physician and largely ignored the fact that different types of health care practitioners and lay persons may perform a therapeutic role. The Parsonian conceptual framework attributed a central position to the physician and professional health care and overlooked the fact that lay persons are active primary health care providers. Thus, an important flaw in Parsons's approach is that, on the one hand, it overestimates the therapeutic impact of the physician and medical institutions, while on the other hand, it underestimates the part played by the family and lay support systems in self-provided health care. Consequently, Parsons's sick role model has been characterized as "medico-centric" (Gallagher, 1976) and its apparent "professionalist bias" (Honig-Parnass, 1981) has diverted attention from a systematic exploration of lay participation in the illness process.

Redefining the Rights and Duties of the Sick Role

In Parsons's model the occupant of the sick role is, by definition, a potential patient. However, it is both theoretically and practically possible to enter and exit the sick role without seeking professional medical help and becoming a patient. In fact, the majority of family illness episodes are self-managed and are never brought to the attention of a health care professional. Therefore, it is important to distinguish conceptually between the sick role and the patient role. It is time "for a redimensionalization of the sick role concept" (Honig-Parnass, 1981, p. 622). In other words, there is a need to reformulate the behavioral pattern associated with the status of the sick person in contemporary society. There must be an improved specification of the range of behavior appropriate for the sick person, as well as the various conditions under which the sick role may be legitimately performed.

It is clear that the sick role (as conceived by Parsons) is not a unitary concept that applies equally well to all people who experience illness. In fact, it seems that empirically the ideal model of the sick role is not often fully realized. The dimensions of the sick role vary extensively and do not necessarily always occur together. For example, Twaddle (1969, p. 113) concluded his exploration of sick role variation by stating that "while Parsons may have successfully described the nature of the sick role, as defined by many Americans, when the elements he posited are treated discretely, the total configuration seemingly applies to only a minority." Similarly, Arluke, Kennedy, and Kessler (1979) found that the four sick-role expectations were completely uncorrelated to each other and concluded that Parsons's model is valid only if the normative components of the sick role are treated as discrete and unrelated dimensions. In their own words, these findings ''seem to throw the unidimensionality of Parsons' sick-role concept completely into doubt'' (p. 32).

In other words, it seems that respondents agree that each of the individual behavioral dimensions outlined by Parsons may apply to the sick person, but these four expectations together do not comprise a patterned role. As previously stated, Parsons's model is not a unitary construct, but in fact embodies aspects of both the sick role and the patient role. Close examination reveals that the four rights and duties described by Parsons are not reciprocal in nature. The rights of the sick person (i.e., exemption from responsibility for the condition and from usual well roles) translate into duties for lay others. For example, relatives and friends may help with child care or household duties when an individual is sick or co-workers may take on additional duties if the illness results in an absence from work. In contrast, the duties of the sick person (i.e., obligation to get well and to seek technically competent help) translate into rights for medical practitioners. The sick person is expected not only to seek the services of a physician, but also to cooperate in the process of trying to get well. According to the Parsonian model, this means becoming a patient and participating in the doctor–patient relationship by exposing oneself to the manipulations of health professionals, deferring to competent professional authority, and following the physician's orders.

A redefinition of the rights and duties associated with the social position of the sick person involves situating the sick role completely within the context of informal, lay caregivers (i.e., family and friends). A reformulated sick role concept would include a reciprocal set of expectations regarding the behavior of the person who is sick and the lay significant others with whom the person interacts. Physician contact and the utilization of professional health services would thus be interpreted as patient role behavior and not sick role behavior. The new sick role concept would consist of the following rights and duties: the right to be exempt from responsibility for the condition and from performing usual well roles, and the right to become dependent on lay others; along with the duty to view the condition as undesirable and to strive to overcome it, and the duty to engage in self-care and self-health management and to make use of lay others as health resources. This nonprofessional reconceptualization of the sick role should more accurately reflect the everyday illness experience of the individual and more fully recognize the pervasive nature of self-provided health care.

Redefining the rights and duties of the sick role in this manner should also facilitate a better understanding of the social context within which health and illness occur. In other words, sick role behavior can now be removed from the physician's office and the hospital and situated within the context of the family, informal social networks, and the broader sociocultural environment. Parsons acknowledged that the sick role is affected by the nature and severity of the individual's illness. However, it is important to recognize that sick-role behavioral expectations and performance are also affected by social, cultural, and personal factors. All of these factors interact with each other to shape the many contingencies which in turn influence the rights and duties of the sick role. For example, social factors (i.e., sex, age, marital status, employment status, education, income) along with cultural factors (religion, ethnicity) combine to give meaning to lay definitions of health and illness and ultimately to variations in the exemption of the sick individual from responsibility for the condition and from performing usual well roles. Similarly, these sociocultural factors structure general value orientations (e.g., instrumental activism, self-reliance), as well as attitudes toward health care alternatives (e.g., self versus professional care) which may affect the extent to which the sick person feels an obligation to try to get well, assumes personal responsibility for managing the illness experience, and utilizes available help sources.

EXPLORING SOCIOCULTURAL FACTORS AND SICK-ROLE BEHAVIORAL EXPECTATIONS

Very few studies have attempted to determine whether systematic sociocultural differences exist in sick-role behavioral expectations. Instead, the general tendency has been to operate on the assumption that the expected sick role behavior described by Parsons is the same for all members of society. As a result, a limited number of studies have focused upon group variations in the behavioral pattern associated with the status of the sick person, whereas most have concentrated upon willingness to adopt the sick role. Consequently, it still remains to be determined whether people view the sick role in terms of the behavioral dimensions identified in the conceptual model (either Parsons's original one or the reformulated version), and whether these views are affected by sociocultural factors.

A Review of Existing Research

Although quite limited and rather unclear, the existing research evidence offers little support for Parsons's sick role model. For example, Twaddle (1969) examined sick role variations and found that many of the respondents he interviewed did not perceive the rights and duties of the sick role in a manner consistent with Parsons's conceptualization. In fact, he concluded that when the sick role dimensions are combined, a number of different configurations emerge, of which Parsons's model is only one, although the behavioral expectations associated with these alternative sick roles are not yet clearly understood. While Twaddle did attempt to investigate religious, ethnic, and educational differences in expected and actual sick role behavior, the findings of this study are restricted by the nature of the sample used (i.e., a small sample of older, married men).

Despite the limitations of Twaddle's study, his findings are supported by Berkanovic's (1972) subsequent examination of the validity of the sick role concept. Berkanovic attempted to test the assumption that the features which Parsons identified at a structural level and presented as comprising an "ideal typical" sick role accurately reflect the nature of the content of lay expectations regarding the behavior of people who are sick. Again there are methodological problems with this study (i.e., the use of an availability sample, and inconsistencies in the data collection procedures). However, the findings presented indicate that the sick role, as conceived by Parsons, is not an adequate unit of analysis for the social psychological study of sick-role behavioral expectations. Berkanovic concluded by recommending that the assumption that this theoretical construct adequately describes the features of lay expectations regarding the sick person's behavior should be seriously questioned and subjected to further rigorous validation.

Segall (1976b) explored the sick-role expectations held by hospitalized female patients and found only one clear-cut area of agreement between the respondents' perception of how a person should behave when sick and the Parsonian model. The vast majority of the patients (84%) agreed that to be ill is "inherently undesirable," and that the occupant of the sick role should strive to achieve a state of "good health." In other words, the sick person has an obligation to try to get well. This is consistent with Twaddle's earlier finding that subjects responded without exception in a manner which was consistent with the expectation that illness should be defined as undesirable (although their responses to the other dimensions of the sick role were more variable). It is important to note that while few of the patients included in these studies disagreed completely with Parsons's conception of the sick role, their responses did not strongly support the behavioral dimensions of this role as originally outlined.

Segall's study (1976b) was designed to determine not only how closely actual perception of the rights and duties of the sick role corresponds to the Parsonian model, but also whether systematic sociocultural differences exist in the behavioral expectations associated with this role. To achieve the second objective, the views expressed about each of the four behavioral dimensions of the sick role were analyzed in terms of the respondents' ethnic/religious affiliation. Anglo-Saxon Protestant patients generally perceived the sick role more in terms of the Parsonian ideal type model than did Jewish patients although the differences between the two groups were not statistically significant. In one case (i.e., exemption from responsibility for the incapacity), the pattern was reversed. The Anglo-Saxon Protestant patients expressed the view that a person can do many things to maintain a state of good health. For these patients, the individual was viewed as capable of exercising a good deal of control over the condition, whereas the Jewish patients were more likely to exempt the sick person from responsibility for illness. Basically, however, the two groups of patients were found to share essentially the same expectations in regard to the sick role.

If ethnic/religious affiliation exerted a uniform influence on the members of each subcultural group, a high degree of homogeneity might have been expected in sick-role expectations. However, this was simply not the case. In fact, a good deal of intragroup variation was noted in a number of instances. Factors such as socioeconomic status and country of birth help to explain many of the differences found within ethnic groups. Overall, these findings suggest that the relative explanatory power of ethnic/religious group affiliation may not be as great as other sociocultural factors (such as total family income) in accounting for differences in sick-role behavioral expectations.

Arluke *et al.* (1979) extended this body of research in their more recent effort to uncover empirical differences in acceptance of the four sick-role expectations across various sociocultural groups. This study made use of the same research instruments used earlier by Segall (1976b) but increased the sample size from 70 to approximately 500. The sociocultural predictors examined include: sex, age, marital status, family size, education, income, employment status, and religion. In general, Arluke *et al.* found that respondents who are older, retired or unemployed, of low income, living alone, and Jewish tend to agree most with the expectation that people who are experiencing illness are not responsible for their condition. The religious difference is consistent with the data reported by Segall. Agreement with the expectation that the sick person has a right to be exempt from usual well role responsibilities is more characteristic of people who live with more than one other person than of those who live either with one other person or alone. This behavioral expectation did not vary in terms of any of the other sociocultural factors measured. Turning to the duties of the sick role, Arluke *et al.* found that respondents who are female, younger, more educated, and live alone tend to agree more than others with the expectation that the sick person should try to get well. Agreement with the expectation that the sick person has a duty to seek professional help is more characteristic of older rather than younger respondents. Again this expectation did not correlate with any of the other sociocultural factors. The finding that sick role duties do not vary by religion is consistent with Segall's (1976b) data. In summary, Arluke *et al.* found that sick-role scale scores correlated only weakly, although significantly, with selected sociocultural factors.

As a further test of the relationship between sociocultural factors and sick-role behavioral expectations, Arluke *et al.* entered all of the predictors simultaneously into a dummy variable regression analysis and found that only age, family size, and income were significantly related to at least one of the sick role components. However, they felt that this was sufficient evidence that acceptance of Parsons's model is not equal in all segments of society and concluded that "these findings argue against the existence of a completely universalistic pattern of agreement with the four sick-role expectations" (p. 33). At the same time, Arluke *et al.* contended that their findings support the Parsonian model of normative consensus regarding appropriate sickness behavior, even across sociocultural categories, as long as the expectations are considered discretely. In other words, it seems that the specific behaviors encompassed by the Parsonian model are individually perceived as relevant to the sick person, but do not cumulatively add up to a patterned set of role expectations.

Some Recent Empirical Evidence

It is important to note that the participants in the studies by Segall (1976b) and Arluke *et al.* (1979) were drawn from hospitalized patient populations. In Segall's study the patients were interviewed while still in the hospital, and in Arluke and colleagues' study recently discharged hospital patients completed a self-administered questionnaire. In both cases then, respondents had already demonstrated that they were willing to become dependent on medical practitioners and hospital staff for their health care. In other words, all of the respondents were actually playing (or had just finished playing) the role of hospital patient. In Parsons's terms, they had adopted the sick role and, therefore, might be expected to display greater acceptance of the Parsonian model than would be found in the general population. Thus, these studies are limited by the fact that: (1) the hospitalization experience of the individuals may have contributed to the development of similar sick-role expectations, and (2) the findings cannot be generalized to nonpatient populations.

In view of the medicalized nature of Parsons's definition of the behavior expected of a sick person, it could be argued that it is appropriate to explore role expectations by studying hospital patients. However, it must be recognized that in doing so, it is the patient role and not the sick role which is thus the object of investigation. The proper study of the sick role requires: a clear conceptual distinction between the sick role and the patient role, the reformulation of a nonprofessional, nonmedicalized set of behavioral dimensions for the sick role, and a large population-based sample to validate empirically the rights and duties of the sick role and to assess the extent to which lay expectations are affected by sociocultural factors.

The revised sick role concept described earlier in this chapter was incorporated in a recent community survey of lay health beliefs and self-care practices. Information on sick-role expectations was collected as part of the 1983 Winnipeg Area Study, which is an annual survey of the residents of Winnipeg, Canada. Winnipeg is a mid-western Canadian city situated in the southern portion of the province of Manitoba with a population of approximately 600,000. A random cross-sectional sample of 701 addresses was selected from all dwelling units listed in the 1982 property tax assessment file for the City of Winnipeg. Nursing homes and temporary residences were excluded from the sample. The household was the primary sampling unit and one adult per household was selected for a 1-hour interview. The eligibility criteria were that the dwelling was the individual's usual place of residence and the person was between 18 and 80 years of age. All of the interviews were conducted in the respondents' home during February and March 1983. A total of 524 respondents were interviewed for a response rate of 75%. The sample was compared to the adult population of Winnipeg (using 1981 *Census of Canada* statistics) and was found to be quite representative of the city on a number of characteristics such as age, sex, and household size (Segall & Currie, 1983).

What are the sociodemographic characteristics of the respondents who participated in this survey? Of the respondents 56% were female and 44% male. Close to half of those in the sample (47%) were between 25 and 44 years of age and the median age was 39 years. Single respondents made up 18% of the sample; 63% were married or living in a common-law relationship. The remaining 19% were either divorced, separated, or widowed. Forty-one percent of the respondents had attended or completed high school. Twenty-four percent had obtained, or been exposed to a university education; 18% had not gone beyond the junior high school level. The mean number of years of school completed by the respondents was 12. Half of the respondents were employed on a full-time basis at the time of the survey. The employment status of the others was: part-time (9%), unemployed (6%), retired (11%), in school (4%), or keeping house (18%). A fairly high proportion (84%) of the respondents provided information about their income and the median household income reported was in the $24,000 to $25,999 range. Responses to the question on religious preference revealed that: 30% of the respondents were Roman Catholic or Ukrainian Catholic, 16% were United Church members, 9% were Anglican, and 6% six percent were Lutheran. A number of other religions were cited by less than 5% of the respondents (e.g., Jewish, Mennonite). Fourteen percent stated that they have no religious preference. Respondents who considered their ethnic identity to be Canadian represented 36% of the sample. Others identified their ethnicity as English, Scottish, or British (9%), Ukrainian (7%), French or French-Canadian (6%), and German (4%). No other ethnic group was cited by more than 2% of the respondents. The majority of the participants in the survey (77%) were Canadian-born.

The rights and duties of the revised sick role investigated in this study include: the right to be exempt from responsibility for usual well roles and to depend on informal care-givers for assistance; and the duty to try to get well by seeking the help of nonprofessional lay significant others. In the modified sick role, the rights of the sick person continue (as Parsons suggested) to be partially dependent upon the person fulfilling the obligations. However, in this case the reciprocal behavioral expectations are restricted to the two participants directly involved in this role relationship. It is equally important to learn if the general public believes that the sick person is entitled to relinquish well roles and become dependent upon informal care-givers, and the frequency with which they actually consult significant lay others when they experience health problems.

To measure sick-role expectations, respondents were asked to indicate their level of agreement with a series of statements about the behavior expected of a sick person. These items were factor analyzed and a scale was developed which focused upon the right of the occupant of the sick role to: *role release* ("A person should try to keep up with his/her routine schedule even when not feeling well," "I find it very hard to give in and go to bed when I feel sick"); and *dependency* ("The trouble with being ill is that you have to depend on other people," "When I think I am getting sick, I find it difficult to talk to others about it"). In addition, willingness to adopt the sick role was measured by asking the respondents whether they speak to any of the following about their health problems: husband/wife, children, parents, brothers or sisters, friends, neighbors, co-workers.

To examine the potential influence of sociocultural factors upon sick-role expectations and performance, information was also collected about each respondent's sex, age, marital status (married, common-law, single, divorced, widowed, or separated), education (elementary or less, junior high school, some high school or graduated, postsecondary, some university or graduated), income (total annual family income), employment status (employed full-time, part-time, unemployed, retired, in school, or keeping house), religion (religious preference, strength of religious preference, and perceived importance of religion), and ethnicity (ethnic self-identity, perceived importance of ethnic identity, and ethnic generation).

What type of sick-role expectations were found in this community survey? Respondents were very divided in their views about the right of the sick person to be relieved of usual well-role responsibilities. Approximately 47% agreed with the items which focused upon keeping up one's routine schedule and/or going to bed when sick, and an equal proportion disagreed. The same response pattern was found for the item about depending upon other people when you are ill. Only the final indicator of the dependency which accompanies occupying the sick role revealed a clear pattern. Approximately two-thirds of the respondents (64%) indicated that they would have no difficulty in discussing their condition with others if they were not feeling well.

This was further reflected by the number of lay significant others actually consulted for assistance with health problems. Only 7% of the respondents stated that they spoke to no one at all. The rest of the participants in the survey consulted at least one other person and typically discussed their health problems with three members of their informal social network (i.e., the mean score was 2.6). The respondents were asked a series of follow-up questions such as: How often and why do you speak to these people? How much do these discussions generally influence the action you take to deal with your health problems? Space limitations do not permit a full presentation of the findings. Briefly, it is worth noting that the individual's spouse was the lay significant other most frequently utilized as a health resource (92%). In order of frequency, the respondents also consulted other family members: parents (47%), children (45%), siblings (40%). Among the nonfamily informal care-givers available, the respondents made the most use of friends (56%) and co-workers (44%), and seldom spoke to neighbors (17%) about health problems.

In summary, it seems that there is fairly widespread agreement that the sick person has the right to depend on lay others, at least for informal consultations. However, opinions were very divided about whether the person occupying the sick role has the right to expect that lay others will assume some of his/her usual responsibilities in the event of illness. Overall there appears to be a lack of normative consensus about sick-role behavioral expectations. Can this variation in responses be accounted for by sociocultural factors? To try to answer this question, a correlational analysis was performed using the sick role measures and the sociocultural factors selected for investigation in this study. Furthermore, all of the sociocultural factors were entered into a dummy variable regression analysis as a further test of their influence on sick-role expectations and performance.

Age, employment status, education, and income were all significantly ($p = .01$) related to sick-role expectations. In other words, those who believe that the sick person is entitled to role release and dependency tend to be younger respondents who are gainfully employed and enjoy a higher socioeconomic status. No statistically significant differences were found in terms of the other sociocultural factors measured (sex, marital status, religion, and ethnicity). The results of the regression analysis suggest that age is the single most important predictor of sick-role expectations. Furthermore, they indicate that those who are employed on a full-time basis and have higher levels of formal education and income differ in their views about the behavioral dimensions of the sick role from those individuals with lower socioeconomic status, even within the same ethnic/religious categories.

Marital status, employment status, income ($p = .01$), and age ($p = .03$) were significantly related to the number of nonprofessional lay significant others consulted for assistance with health problems. Younger, married respondents who are gainfully employed and receiving higher levels of income are the ones who most frequently speak to lay others about their health problems. Again, sex, religion, and ethnicity did not correlate with this sick role dimension. According to the regression analysis, marital status is the best predictor in this case. Obviously, being married ensures the availability of at least one other layperson to serve as a health resource (particularly for men). Although certain sociocultural factors seem to be important, a great deal of the variance in the behavioral expectations associated with the revised sick role concept remains unexplained and awaits further research.

FUTURE SICK ROLE RESEARCH

This discussion vividly illustrates the need for further specification of the behavioral expectations embodied by the sick role, as well as a need for a better operationalization of this concept and the development of improved measurement techniques. For example, willingness to adopt Parsons's sick (patient) role has traditionally been measured by physician contact (Battistella, 1970; Mechanic & Volkart, 1961; Petroni, 1969a,b; Phillips, 1965). In this research, respondents who indicated that they would seek medical help under a specified set of circumstances were considered to have a high willingness to adopt the sick role. Although the number of recent studies using the sick role concept has decreased, Parsons's influence and this operational definition are still evident. For example, Wolinsky and Wolinsky (1981) operationalized the process of legitimizing the sick role as the physician's issuance of a prescription for the patient. Clearly this indicates the individual's willingness to accept the patient role and not necessarily the sick role! It must be recognized that although the occupant of the patient role must be willing to utilize professional health care services, this is not a prerequisite for adopting the sick role. As stated previously, it is possible to enter and exit the sick role without consulting a physician.

The revised sick role outlined earlier in this chapter emphasizes the importance of learning whether or not sick persons are prepared to stop performing certain daily activities (depending on the nature and severity of the illness) and to rely upon informal care-givers for their well-being. Studies designed to measure willingness to adopt the sick role must strive to find out if the person is actually ready to give up usual well role responsibilities and at the same time become dependent upon lay health resources. There is some evidence that research on sick-role expectations is beginning to reflect this shift in emphasis and incorporate into the analysis factors such as the extent of dependency granted to the ill and the support provided by nonprofessional significant others (Honig-Parnass, 1983). Future attempts to explore willingness to adopt the sick role must develop more comprehensive measures of these behavioral expectations. Focusing on role release and dependency should facilitate renewed interest in the sick role concept and improved linkage between this theoretical construct and the growing body of research literature on self-care health behavior.

Gallagher pointed out some time ago that Parsons's sick role paradigm failed "to account for preventive health care, or health maintenance, as an element of normative lay conduct" (1976, p. 209). By redefining the expectations of this role and recognizing that the behavior of the sick person typically takes place within the context of the family and informal social networks, it may also be possible to build a bridge between the sick role concept and health behavior. The two are not mutually exclusive, and the revised sick role may be related not just to health restoration, but also to health protective behavior. Parsons's formulation assigned a position of central importance to the physician and the utilization of professional health care services and thus stimulated a large body of empirical research which focused upon the individual's willingness to adopt the sick role, and in rare cases studies of the individual's tendency to relinquish the status of the sick person and exit from the sick role (Brown & Rawlinson, 1975). The revised concept recognizes the vital part played by the layperson as a primary health care provider (and not just a consumer of professional services) and may stimulate research which focuses upon the individual's efforts to maintain health and avoid entering the sick role. If sick-role expectations are reconceptualized to include self-provided care and the use of lay significant others as health resources, then it may be possible to link behavior intended to keep one out of the sick role to health maintenance activities.

In this way, improved theoretical refinement within medical sociology may be achieved, along with a more integrated approach to studying the psychosocial process of becoming and being ill. Furthermore, it has been recognized for many years that health and illness behavior are influenced by social and cultural factors. Reformulating the behavioral expectations of the sick person may lead to the realization that sick role behavior is also embedded in a sociocultural context. Ultimately then, the sick role concept may contribute to a better understanding of the ways in which different groups of people think and behave when dealing with health and illness in their daily lives.

Despite the extensive body of research evidence currently available, many important questions remain unanswered. Perhaps the most urgent question concerns the distribution of behavioral expectations regarding the occupant of the sick role in different segments of the population. What importance is attached in various sociocultual contexts to the basic sick role components, and to what extent do normative definitions of the rights and duties of the sick person vary? What specific behavioral expectations are associated with membership in different social groups? Can the influence of social factors (such as education, occupation, and income) be isolated from cultural factors (such as ethnicity and religion) as determinants of sick-role behavioral expectations? These questions must be answered before it will be possible to demonstrate clearly that this conceptual model contributes to a greater understanding of the expectations and role performance of the sick person and reflects the nature of sociocultural variation in this type of health-related behavior.

REFERENCES

Arluke, A., Kennedy, L., & Kessler, R. C. (1979). Re-examining the sick-role concept: An empirical assessment. *Journal of Health and Social Behavior, 20,* 30–36.

Battistella, R. M. (1970). Status consistency: Health status and adoption of the sick role among late adulthood persons. *Medical Care, 8,* 333–342.

Berkanovic, E. (1972). Lay conceptions of the sick role. *Social Forces, 51,* 53–64.

Brown, J., & Rawlinson, M. (1975). Relinquishing the sick role following open-heart surgery. *Journal of Health and Social Behavior, 16,* 12–27.

Butler, J. R. (1970). Illness and the sick role: An evaluation in three communities. *The British Journal of Sociology, 21,* 241–261.

Cockerham, W. C. (1983). The state of medical sociology in the United States, Great Britain, West Germany and Austria: Applied vs. pure theory. *Social Science and Medicine, 20,* 1513–1527.

Croog, S. H. (1961). Ethnic origins and responses to health questionnaires. *Human Organization, 20,* 65–69.

Gallagher, E. B. (1976). Lines of reconstruction and extension in the Parsonian sociology of illness. *Social Science and Medicine, 10,* 207–218.

Gerhardt, U. (1979). The Parsonian paradigm and the identity of medical sociology. *Sociological Review, 27,* 229–251.

Gordon, G. (1966). *Role theory and illness: A sociological perspective.* New Haven, CT: College & University Press.

Graham, S., & Reeder, L. G. (1979). Social epidemiology of chronic disease. In H. E. Freeman, S. Levine, & L. G. Reeder (Eds.), *Handbook of medical sociology* (pp. 71–96). Englewood Cliffs, NJ: Prentice–Hall.

Harwood, A. (1981). *Ethnicity and medical care.* Cambridge, MA: Harvard University Press.

Honig-Parnass, T. (1981). Lay concepts of the sick-role: An examination of the professionalist bias in Parsons' model. *Social Science and Medicine, 15A,* 615–623.

Honig-Parnass, T. (1983). The relative impact of status and health variables upon sick-role expectations. *Medical Care, 21,* 208–224.

Johnson, M. L. (1975). Medical sociology and sociological theory. *Social Science and Medicine, 9,* 227–232.

King, S. H. (1962). *Perceptions of illness and medical practice.* New York: Russell Sage Foundation.

Levine, S., & Kozloff, M. A. (1978). The sick role: Assessment and overview. *Annual Review of Sociology, 4,* 317–343.

McCormack, T. (1981). The new criticism and the sick role. *Canadian Review of Sociology and Anthropology, 18,* 30–47.

Mechanic, D. (1963). Religion, religiosity, and illness behavior. *Human Organization, 22,* 202–208.

Mechanic, D., & Volkart, E. H. (1961). Stress, illness behavior and the sick role. *American Sociological Review, 26,* 51–58.

Parsons, T. (1951). *The social system.* New York: Free Press.

Petroni, F. A. (1969a). Social class, family size and the sick role. *Journal of Marriage and the Family, 31,* 728–735.

Petroni, F. A. (1969b). Significant others and illness behavior: A much neglected sick role contingency. *Sociological Quarterly, 10,* 32–41.

Phillips, D. L. (1965). Self-reliance and the inclination to adopt the sick role. *Social Forces, 43,* 555–563.

Plaja, A. O., Cohen, L. M., & Samora, J. (1968). Communication between physicians and patients in outpatient clinics: Social and cultural factors. *Milbank Memorial Fund Quarterly, 46,* 161–213.

Reeder, L. G., & Berkanovic, E. (1973). Sociological concomitants of health orientations: A partial replication of Suchman. *Journal of Health and Social Behavior, 14,* 134–143.

Saunders, L. (1954). *Cultural differences and medical care.* New York: Russell Sage Foundation.

Segall, A. (1976a). The sick role concept: Understanding illness behavior. *Journal of Health and Social Behavior, 17,* 163–170.

Segall, A. (1976b). Sociocultural variation in sick role behavioural expectations. *Social Science and Medicine, 10,* 47–51.

Segall, A., & Currie, R. F. (1983). *Selected findings from the 1983 Winnipeg Area Study* (Winnipeg Area Series Report No. 1). University of Manitoba: The Institute for Social and Economic Research.

Simmons, L. W., & Wolff, H. G. (1954). *Social science in medicine.* New York: Russell Sage Foundation.

Sternbach, R. A. (1968). *Pain: A psychophysiological analysis.* New York: Academic Press.

Sternbach, R. A., & Tursky, B. (1965). Ethnic differences among housewives in psychophysical and skin potential responses to electric shock. *Psychophysiology, 1,* 241–246.

Suchman, E. A. (1964). Sociomedical variations among ethnic groups. *American Journal of Sociology, 70,* 319–331.

Twaddle, A. C. (1969). Health decisions and sick role variations: An exploration. *Journal of Health and Social Behavior, 10,* 105–114.

Wolinsky, F. D., & Wolinsky, S. R. (1981). Expecting sick-role legitimation and getting it. *Journal of Health and Social Behavior, 22,* 229–242.

Zborowski, M. (1969). *People in pain.* San Francisco: Jossey–Bass.

Zola, I. K. (1966). Culture and symptoms: An analysis of patients' presenting complaints. *American Sociological Review, 31,* 615–630.

CHAPTER 15

A Transcultural Perspective on Health Behavior

Hazel H. Weidman

INTRODUCTION

An explicit transcultural perspective on health behavior has emerged since the mid-1970s. It rests upon an enduring and widely scattered research literature, primarily from the field of anthropology, the central, unifying concept of which is the concept of culture. Secondarily, it has come from the fields of sociology, psychology, social work, nursing, and medicine, the research protocols of which, increasingly, have incorporated culture as a significant variable. There is every indication that the findings of transculturally oriented research will have a profound impact upon the provision of orthodox health care and the training of biomedical health professionals in the future (e.g., Harwood, 1981; Helman, 1984; Kleinman, 1980; Lefley & Pedersen, 1986).

Both culture-specific and cross-cultural research strategies have encouraged a shift from a unicultural to a transcultural paradigm. The unicultural research paradigm derives its concepts, meanings, methods, and discriminant power from Western cultural traditions that gave rise to science as a method of knowledge construction (Wober, 1969, calls it "centricultural." We would call it "culturi-centric"). The dominant tradition within the community of scientific investigators has been to apply this approach as valid in all cultural contexts and to interpret findings in ways that are meaningful within the investigator's own cognitive framework. From a transcultural posture, however, this type of knowledge construction represents an "emic" system (a way of knowing from a cultural "insider" perspective) that is stretched in the direction of an "etic" system (a way of knowing from a cultural "outsider" perspective) through the methods of "science" (e.g., Harris, 1976). The fact that both culture-specific and cross-cultural research have brought us to the point of recognizing the crucial distinction between emic and etic perspectives is a major accomplishment of anthropological inquiry and anthropological method, the strength of which lies in the elicitation of emic or within-culture data.

DEFINITION OF "TRANSCULTURAL PERSPECTIVE"

As used herein, "transcultural" implies a perceptual stance and research posture that is detached or "alienated" but equidistant from two or more cultural units, however they

HAZEL H. WEIDMAN • Office of Transcultural Education and Research, Department of Psychiatry, University of Miami School of Medicine, Miami, Florida 33101.

may be defined (Weidman, 1986). The concept implies comparable respect for and commitment to understanding the complexities and meaning of health behavior in each social context under investigation. The comparison is overtly cross-cultural, with the characteristics of neither unit of the contrasted pair slighted by being allowed to remain "understood" or implicit.

A transcultural perspective is an observational stance which allows the simultaneous assessment of behavior in two or more cultural or subcultural systems, one of which, ideally, is always the investigator's own. When the focus is on groups, the "cultural" aspect of the term "transcultural" is self-evident. When the focus in on the individual, the transcultural posture becomes a "transperson" stance. Whether transcultural (culture as a group variable) or transpersonal (culture as an individual variable), it is a perspective that is not easily achieved. It requires a new definition of reality and, when translated into behavior, an expansion of the moral universe within which one functions (Weidman, 1976a,b, 1981, 1983).

When one is able, conceptually and perceptually, to juxtapose knowledge of cultural behavior manifested by members of another group with knowledge of cultural behavior manifested by oneself and members of one's own group, a genuine transcultural posture has been achieved. The intent of transculturally oriented research is to assess in a nonbiased, strictly comparable way, human behavior as it is shaped and guided by diverse assumptions, values, attitudes, and rules for achieving various goals, good health and a sense of well-being among them, however these may be defined.

One central task of such a research approach is to develop concepts which can be applied universally, without skewing the data by constraints imposed by uniculturally biased views and instruments. Since the time of Rivers (1926), theoretical trends in medical anthropology have advanced the concepts of "medicine" or "ethnomedicine" and "health culture" as the primary categories of comparison. Wellin (1977) traced aspects of the evolution of the former; Weidman and Egeland (1973) outlined some of the developments leading to the latter. Whichever central theoretical orientation is utilized, however, health behavior is understood as reflecting a social institution of central importance in all human societies.

THE HEALTH CULTURE CONCEPT

Since 1968 the author has utilized the concept of "health culture" in preference to that of "medicine" or "medical system" because of the confusion the latter terms tend to generate in the minds of those who automatically link "medicine" with medical orthodoxy, or the biomedical system of Western industrialized societies (Weidman & Egeland, 1973). In the author's view the health culture concept allows us to elicit reliable within-culture, meaning-centered, data from groups different from our own while, at the same time, ensuring that our own within-culture understandings of health behavior are made explicit in a comparable way. The following pages will be devoted to the health culture concept and others that contribute toward such a research goal.

While the terms "macro" and "micro" have been used in diverse ways (e.g., Baer, 1982; Baer, Singer, & Johnsen, 1986; Janzen, 1978a,b), for the purposes of this chapter, macro-level concepts are those that apply to health behavior understood in terms of group or system phenomena; micro-level concepts are those that apply to health behavior understood in terms of individual actions or interactions. Important macro-level concepts for this chapter include those of *culture* and *health culture*. Micro-level concepts, on the other hand, include *health behavior* as it pertains to specific dimensions of the health culture concept: (a) the cognitive dimension and (b) the social system dimension.

Macro-Level Concepts

The macro-level concept of *culture* may be defined as a society's repertoire of patterns for cognition, affect, and behavior (Harris, 1971, p. 624). As such it provides the framework within which individuals in various positions in the status hierarchy and/or positions of centrality or marginality in a social system learn specific ways of thinking, feeling, and behaving. In this respect culture is a group concept. However, once such patterns are learned by individuals (in somewhat idiosyncratic configurations but within the limits of culturally acceptable norms), culture may be conceived of as an internal guidance system influencing all aspects of cognition, affect, and behavior, including health-related awarenesses, emotions, understandings, and preferred strategies for ensuring a long, healthful, and productive life.

Health culture at the macro level may be defined as those patterns drawn from a society's entire repertoire which relate specifically to the maintenance of well-being and problems of sickness with which people cope in traditional ways within their own social networks and institutional structures (Weidman, 1978, p. 13).

Micro-Level Concepts

As every society includes persons with various degrees of specialization related to health and illness, we may define *health behavior* as "the procedures used by both lay persons and specialists [in the context of culture and health culture] to promote health, prevent sickness, and remedy sickness" (Polgar, 1963, p. 398). The bracketed addition to this definition emphasizes that transculturally oriented research on health behavior must always include an emic or within-culture perspective as a central focus or a complement to assessments based upon outside observer categories, interests, and methods.

"Culture" and "health culture" may be utilized in health behavior research as either group or individual variables. And "health behavior" as an individual variable becomes a group variable to the extent that such behavior is assessed within the context of diverse cultural and health cultural systems.

Because the health culture concept plays such an important unifying and integrating role in transculturally oriented research on health behavior, it will be of value to illustrate specific cognitive dimensions of health culture as they influence health behavior in clinical contexts and in the quest for cure of "sickness," however defined within specific social, cultural, economic, political, and ecological settings.

Analytic Dimensions of Health Culture

There are two aspects of the health culture concept that require elucidation. One relates to cognition and conceptual structure (the meaning-centered aspect of health culture); the other relates to social system functioning or networks of relationships that influence health behavior and states of health. Not only do social networks have an impact upon procedures to maintain health and prevent illness, they also, in various configurations of social roles with various degrees of specialization, become activated and directed toward remediation once an individual is defined as having become "ill" or as having a "disease" (e.g., Eisenberg, 1977; Kleinman, 1980; see also Sullivan, 1986, and Van Leeuwen, 1987, for discussions of the mind–body dualism in relation to distinctions between "illness" and "disease"). Both cognitive and social system components are involved in the learning and manifestation of all health behavior, but for purposes of analysis, it is helpful to keep them distinct.

SYMPTOMS AND CARE-SEEKING

The Cognitive Dimension

The cognitive aspect of health culture includes world view, values, and beliefs; guidelines for health action related to health maintenance as well as illness prevention and remediation. Such health culture cognitive processes are involved in every aspect of health behavior from preferred body image (Massara & Stunkard, 1979), to diet (Messer, 1984) and nutrition (Farb & Armelagos, 1980), to proper amounts of rest and exercise, to appropriate ways to express pain (Sargent, 1984; Zborowski, 1969), to specific home remedies (Evans, Kileff, & Shelby, 1982), to valued therapeutic techniques (e.g., Ito, 1985), to coping with chronic disease or disability (Alexander, 1982) and the management of death and bereavement (e.g., Palgi & Abramovitch, 1984). In this chapter, however, the significance of a transcultural perspective on health behavior will be illustrated by focusing upon the presentation of symptoms in clinical contexts, the organization of symptoms into conditions that have labels, perceptions of bodily functioning, natural/unnatural distinctions in etiological considerations, the "culture-bound" nature of specific syndromes, and symbols of power in the healing process.

The illustrations provided are drawn from transculturally oriented research in five ethnic groups in inner city Miami (Weidman, 1978). The low-income groups studied over a 5-year period were Bahamian, black American, Haitian, Cuban, and Puerto Rican. Although it would be extremely informative to contrast the five groups on each point to be discussed, space limitations preclude such treatment. In order to enhance the flow of discourse and ensure a sense of coherence, examples will be provided from the Black American group primarily.

Symptoms

There is a substantial research literature on the topic of symptomatology (e.g., Low, 1985; Zola, 1973). Among many other findings, one that is relevant here is that complaints are presented to health professionals in culturally patterned ways. Most certainly that was the case in our Miami research. Although we did not focus upon differential presentations of symptoms related to identically diagnosed conditions, we were struck by the great specificity of symptoms presented by the two Hispanic groups (which included subjects of both Negroid and Caucasoid physical type) in contrast to those presented by the three black groups. Members of both Hispanic groups were articulate and expansive in describing their complaints. Although Puerto Ricans offered a slightly larger number of symptoms than did the Cubans, both groups provided more symptoms in richer detail than did the three black groups (see Escobar, 1987, for confirmation of this type of health behavior for Hispanic psychiatric patients).

Perhaps the most globally presented complaint offered by black Americans was that of "hurting all over." Beyond that, however, it was common for black American participants in the study to describe their problems in very general terms. For example, "My side hurts," or "I have pain on the left side of the stomach," with "stomach" implying the abdominal cavity and "pain" being largely undifferentiated.

The great attention given by orthodox health professionals to the characteristics of pain as a discriminating factor in diagnosis (Fabrega & Tyma, 1976) was not matched by the black Americans in the Miami study. Their attention was focused upon other concerns, such as the wrong food they may have eaten, the impact of environmental conditions, or the effect of strained interpersonal relationships upon the body and, even more importantly, upon the behavior of blood—its movement, its volume, its purity, its sweetness, its viscosity, and the amount of heat it contained. Pain was a general indicator that something could be wrong, but aside from noting its presence there was no cultural emphasis upon describing precisely its quality, duration, periodicity, or intensity. Nor was there a cultural emphasis upon pain in relation to specific organs within the body; there were, for the most part, more "regional" concerns, more "directional" or movement-oriented concerns, or more global ones. This disparity between health practitioner and black American attention to specificity of symptoms, anatomical features, and the quality of pain suggests the type of influence that health cultural traditions have upon something so basic to health care as the presentation of symptoms in biomedical clinical contexts. The issues may be different, however, in the contexts of other health cultural traditions.

Conditions

In addition to a global presentation of complaints as a characteristic of the health behavior of low-income black American patients in Miami, symptoms were found to be clustered together in ways that are "atypical" by biomedical standards. One such example is the inclusion of "the smell of blood" or "the taste of blood in my mouth," along with "headaches" and "dizziness" as potential indicators of a black American condition that is labeled "high blood." Both the atypical symptom of the "smell of blood" and the label "high blood" may be dismissed by clinicians, but when blood pressure readings reveal systolic and diastolic blood pressure above nationally standardized norms, such patients are diagnosed as having a biomedical condition labeled "hypertension." It is considered to be a disease that is treatable but incurable and, therefore, chronic. The best that can be hoped for is "management" of the disease. The patient is placed on medication for life and given specific instructions regarding weight, diet, exercise, and so forth. Adherence to specific prescriptions and proscriptions is seen as contributing to "control" of the condition and leading to the prevention of complications such as stroke or cardiovascular disease.

Most health professionals who treat black American patients are aware of the popular label of "high blood" that such patients assign to this condition. The erroneous assumption is made that, even though different labels are given by black American patients to the biomedical condition of hypertension, they really mean the same thing. Not so. Snow (1974, 1983), working with black American groups in Arizona and Michigan, and Weidman (1978), working with black American populations in inner-city Miami, independently described the cognitive processes related to clusters of blood beliefs, including "high blood" on the one hand and "low blood" on the other. Such beliefs relate to perceptions of bodily functioning that are very different from those of health professionals in the orthodox, biomedical system (see Snow, 1974 for black American blood beliefs; also Weidman, 1978, pp. 451–576, for a fuller description of the blood paradigm, based upon data from black Americans, Bahamians, and Haitians in inner-city Miami).

Perceptions of Bodily Functioning

High blood is perceived to be blood that has moved from the lower part of the body toward or into the head. It is often considered, also, as being too hot and too thick. High blood is seen as an acute condition that can be corrected by remaining calm to keep the blood from being heated, stirred up, and rushing to the head; by reducing the amount of spices used in preparing foods, because they heat up the blood, and by eliminating some of the foods that are considered to be blood builders, because they generate "too much blood" and, with the spices, help to thicken it. "Too much blood" represents too great a volume of blood in the body; it presses toward the head. "Hot blood" is turbulent blood that moves toward the head. "Hot blood" also becomes "thickened"; so that the particular characteristics of "high blood" represent risk factors not only for stroke, but also for aberrant affect and even mental disorder.

In addition to changed behavior and alterations in diet, specific home remedies such as boiled aloe water (aloe is a succulent, bitter-tasting, cactus-like plant), and vinegar or Epsom salts in water, may be taken to "cool" and "thin" the blood and "bring it down." High blood is seen as just one of the temporary states that can develop in the dynamic blood system that is responsive to many life processes and circumstances. The blood may go up, but it can be brought down again by the proper health behavior. So many factors influence the state of the blood, however, that this is no simple task. Emotional states related to life events and tension in interpersonal relationships are believed to have a direct impact upon the blood. Impurities introduced via food, liquids, the environment, and personal contact with others all are believed to have an impact upon the state of the blood which, for good health, must be maintained in a clean, rich, full-bodied state that nourishes all of the parts of the body in a steady, health-sustaining fashion. Because medication for high blood pressure is perceived to "bring the blood down," there may be a reluctance to continue its use over long periods for fear it will cause "low blood."

What is perceived to be "low blood," for many low-income black American patients, is often diagnosed by biomedical practitioners to be "anemia" of various types. For orthodox health professionals, common forms of anemia represent reductions below normal of erythrocyte, hemoglobin, or hematocrit levels. Such conditions, generally, are considered to be correctable.

Although there are some correspondences between biomedical definitions of anemia and black American definitions of low blood, the latter is perceived to be a type of imbalance in the state of the blood that is just the opposite of high blood. Low blood is cool, weak, and thin. It is present in insufficient amounts to nourish all parts of the body equally; consequently, it renders one vulnerable to many other health-threatening assaults. Low blood is seen as causing some of the same kinds of symptoms as does high blood, i.e., weakness, dizziness, and even "passing out." Its remedy lies with proper blood-building strategies in the form of special food, teas, and tonics. Like "high blood," it is seen as a temporary state that can be corrected by "doing right" insofar as health behavior is concerned. And "doing right" may include both a greater range of activity and activity of a different order from that prescribed by biomedical practitioners, although there may, indeed, be meaningful overlap.

As we have seen, within the black American health cultural tradition, specific sets of symptoms are perceived to be worrisome. Many efforts may be initiated to alleviate them before they are brought to orthodox health professionals. Various tentative diagnoses may be held in mind as individuals present their symptoms in clinic settings. Regardless of the manner in which the symptoms are presented, they are transformed, through physical examination and laboratory findings, into signs of disease. In one instance, the diagnosis of hypertension is made; in the other the diagnosis of anemia. These are immediately "back translated" into "high blood" on the one hand and "low blood" on the other.

The within-culture meanings given to these states will have an impact upon the strategies adopted to correct them. There may or may not be full adherence to the regimen outlined by orthodox health professionals. Frequently, many compromises and adjustments are made by black American patients to accommodate the logical requirements of their own better known and understood health cultural tradition rather than to accept at face value all of the intricacies of the less well understood health cultural tradition of biomedicine. At times the latter is abandoned in favor of the former, and the quest for therapy is resumed with specialists in one or more of the other health care networks that are always available in pluralistic social settings. The important point to note is that in the case of high blood/hypertension and low blood/anemia, there are sufficient similarities that high blood and low blood are not considered to be "culture-bound syndromes."

From a transculturally oriented epistemology we might have to argue that both high blood and low blood on the one hand and hypertension and anemia of the other hand do, indeed, represent syndromes that are bound to the black American health cultural tradition in the first instance and to the orthodox biomedical health cultural tradition in the second instance.

Most clinicians and scientific investigators work comfortably within the epistemological framework of biomedicine, however. They tend to see "high blood" and "low blood" as popular misnomers for the disordered biological states of "hypertension" and "anemia." A great deal of effort goes into health education about these conditions, and, most certainly, biomedical terms and bits of biomedical knowledge are incorporated into the patients' cognitive system. This is evident, for example, when black American patients speak with authority about the loss of potassium that can occur with the use of "water pills" (diuretics) in the management of hypertension. The power of their own cognitive systems is revealed, however, when they go on to emphasize that salt is not the problem in dietary control of high blood; rather, it is spices that are so harmful. Furthermore, by remaining calm, they can control their "pressure." This allows them to discontinue medication which, if taken continuously, may lose its efficacy or contribute to other problems (Scott, 1981).

Culture-Bound Syndromes

There are other clusters of symptoms in black American communities constituting syndromes that might qualify as "culture-bound" disorders. The so-called "culture-bound syndromes" are those that are experienced by members of a particular group for which their health cultural traditions provide explanations and therapeutic measures, but which are not found universally or among all segments of every population (*Culture, Medicine, and Psychiatry,* 1987; *Social Science and Medicine,* 1985). "Falling out" is one such syndrome reported in our Miami research that has been described elsewhere (Weidman, 1979). It is a state of collapse into an altered state of consciousness, in which the individual is aware of events occurring at the moment but is powerless to speak or move. There may be convulsive movements. The eyes may be open but not "seeing." There is no bowel or bladder incontinence. "Fainting" or "syncope" are inaccurate labels, because there is no loss of consciousness.

The behavioral complex represents accepted and even expected behavior in specific social settings, such as at funerals, at the point of receiving shocking news, or when the mother of the bride is overcome during her daughter's wedding ceremony. It is behavior that is sought after during religious ceremonies or gospel concerts, because, in those settings, it signifies the presence of the Holy Spirit. But when the same behavior is unanticipated and occurs unpredictably under ordinary circumstances, then falling out begins to be defined as an unwelcome symptom that something is wrong. Too much heat from the sun may be seen as a contributing factor. Either high blood or low blood may be considered as possible causes of the episodes. Efforts may be taken to correct such imbalances, but if the seizure-like states continue, falling out begins to be considered a sickness, and the search for remediation begins.

When such patients enter the orthodox health care system, there is no acceptable way to treat them. Their symptoms cannot be translated into signs of disease in any of the divisions of the biomedical system. If the diagnosis of functional disorder is made, this suggests that nothing can be done, because psychotherapy offers little help for conditions so labeled. As the diagnostic process continues and the laboratory tests repeatedly show negative results, the patient's anxiety level generally mounts. In the view of many low-income black American patients, the fact that the doctors "don't know what is wrong" reinforces the possibility that the illness is an "unnatural" one, caused by spiritual activity of some sort, possibly sent via malign magic by some envious person or enemy, with the help of a specialist in rootwork, e.g., a root doctor; a root man or root woman.

At this point, the orthodox health care system becomes irrelevant. It has no techniques for dealing with illnesses perceived to be spiritually caused. Since traditional black American health culture does make the distinction between naturally and unnaturally caused illness and also assumes that every illness has a cure, the black American patient who considers the falling out episodes to be malignant will, in all likelihood, seek a religious cure through prayer and the power of God or through a root doctor who, with sufficient power, may be able to manipulate the spirit world to the benefit of the client by successfully reversing the malevolent process. We shall return to this point following a brief discussion of sources of power in healing.

Symbols of Power in Healing

Glick has argued that the idea of power—its source, its use, its distribution, and its control—offers a focal point around which descriptive materials related to "medical systems" might be organized for comparative purposes (Glick, 1977). Turner, on the other hand, has provided extensive materials on symbols in ritual healing (Turner, 1967). Our discussion of the cognitive aspects of the health culture concept might usefully contrast some of the symbols that reflect the source of power utilized within the biomedical health cultural tradition and some that reflect the source of power utilized by specialists within the black American health cultural tradition.

The symbols of power within the biomedical tradition are clearly evident in the associations linked to the physician's white coat (e.g., Helman, 1984, pp. 125–126). These include specialized training at an advanced level, a hard-won license to practice medicine, membership in an elite professional organization, control over knowledge that is largely inaccessible to those not entitled to wear the white coat, power to take a medical history, obtain privileged information, conduct invasive physical examinations, marshal the power of biotechnology in the diagnostic and therapeutic process, and make decisions that influence outcomes of life or death.

In addition to the white coat, there are other symbols of power, e.g., the stethoscope, the blood pressure cuff, and many other complex pieces of equipment. There are diplomas, certificates, and other framed testimonies to the degree of learning that has been achieved. There are the physical trappings of the office. The peer review process suggests the extent to which only a circumscribed body of knowledge may be drawn upon for the proper practice of medicine. Such knowledge is scientifically rational, oriented toward objective, numerical measurements, focused upon physiological and chemical processes of the body. It recognizes diseases as biological entities with their own natural histories, and, historically, it has separated the mind from the body (Fabrega & Silver, 1973; Helman, 1984; see also Sullivan, 1986, and Van Leeuwen, 1987, for recent discussions on this point). Biomedical practitioners function as intermediaries and power brokers on behalf of their clients, with biomedical knowledge as the medium through which the power is expressed.

In contrast, witness, through the eyes of one of the Miami research assistants, the symbols of power of one of the most sought-after black American healers in the United States (Weidman, 1978, pp. 717, 727–728). This minister in Georgia is described as owning "half of the town" in which he resides and functions as a minister in one of the larger churches. On one particular day, 28 Greyhound, Trailway, and other private buses were seen at his healing center "in the bush" along with "about three hundred cars" and "people everywhere." Upon arrival, several travelers said, "Thank God, we are on Holy ground."

This minister is said to be "powerful and wise, a born healer." He is considered to be a man of God who specializes in "all religious matters, no matter what they might be." He is said to be the seventh son of a seventh son, an ascribed status which confers special powers of healing, clairvoyance, and prophecy. He preaches and holds church services every day, seven days a week. In addition, he is led by the spirits—seven of them—with which he was born, as evidenced by the seven veils (cauls) over his face at birth. People respect him highly, because "you tell him nothing; he tells you everything."

Our research assistant sat quietly with other clients on benches against the walls of the waiting room of the small church where this healer saw his clients. There was a sign proclaiming "Silence," and on the walls were pictures of Jesus with a flock of sheep and Jesus with his disciples. But, upon entrance into this man's office, our research assistant "was afraid." She described a man sitting behind a desk in a big black chair. The carpet on the floor was black, as was the ceiling. The curtains were white against orange and pink walls, and, overhead, there was a white cross on the ceiling. There were seven skulls in the room, and on the desk a lighted lamp, ethereal in movement and effect, suggesting the presence of seven spirits inside. Accoutrements of the office included, in addition to a bible, a bathtub for medicinal baths, a hospital bed for patients to lie on while being massaged with healing oil, a safe, and a television set turned very low. Around the room candles were burning, and on the desk was an open money box along with papers and a box full of mail requests for prayers and other forms of therapeutic assistance from the healer.

Within the world view of many black Americans this setting symbolizes power—the power of God, the bible, the cross, and Jesus; the power of spirit protectors and spirit messengers, the power of sacred healing oils, the intrinsic power of medicinal plants used in cleansing and purifying baths, the power of the number "seven," related to the seven African powers, the special inheritance of power by the seventh son of a seventh son, and the gift of healing through seven "veils" and, therefore, seven spirits, not just the one veil that ordinarily symbolizes the power to heal. Here are the powers from God, the spirit world, and nature, manifested in the sacred "bush" and manipulated to the benefit of patients who understand their illnesses to be intricately interrelated with the social, natural, and supernatural realms that reflect their world view and cognition of reality. In addition, the colors, themselves, symbolize the transition from the blackness of evil, through reddish hues of healing power (symbolizing, in its full-bodied state, blood, strength, and life) to the whiteness of purity and God. And at the center sits the man who functions as intermediary and power broker on behalf of the client. The medium through which his power is expressed is that of the legitimate power of God on the one hand and the illegitimate power of the spirits on the other.

In the context of a world view in which the nature of man is seen to be unpredictable and potentially harmful, the environment as capable of penetrating body tissues and causing sickness, interpersonal relationships as capable of disrupting the normal state of the blood, and the self as more "acted upon" than "actor," then issues of power must be and are highly salient in the therapeutic traditions of black American health culture (see Snow, 1974, 1978, 1983; Weidman, 1978). As an example, in a case in which this author and research project staff were involved as "culture brokers," the power of biomedicine was having little therapeutic benefit. The patient's condition was deteriorating. He was helped to secure the services of black American traditional healers whose power was of a different order, and he recovered (Rubin & Jones, 1979). Given the convergences that are occurring in the social and medical sciences (Fabrega, 1977; Locke & Colligan, 1986; Rossi, 1986; Scheper-Hughes & Lock, 1987), this should come as no surprise.

It was noted above that health behavior always includes both cognitive and social system aspects of health cultural traditions. When we focus upon the cognitive dimension, world view, values, beliefs, symbols, and meanings are at the fore. They represent "figure"; social system aspects represent "ground." The distinction is apparent at this juncture. When we shift from cognitive considerations to those of status and role, the social system becomes figure, and the cognitive system becomes ground. We would have to argue, then, that from a transcultural perspective the black American healer whose symbols of office have been described is just as much a specialist in a social system comprised of health/illness-related roles as is any renowned biomedical practitioner. He does not meet the culture-specific requirements of "professionalism" as outlined by Freidson (1970); yet he is, most certainly, a professional within his own, historically anchored, black American health cultural tradition. He is in a socially sanctioned position of "therapist," and he is a repository of specialized health cultural knowledge.

It should be noted that this view contrasts with that of a host of researchers who have uncritically accepted a unicultural (culturi-centric) classification of specialists into three types: professional, folk, and lay, with only biomedical specialists being considered "professional" (see Helman, 1984, as an example). Although this may be acceptable within a particular health cultural tradition, where core/periphery or dominant/variant distinctions, legitimately, are made (e.g., Lock, 1986), it is unacceptable to apply such a classificatory scheme across the boundaries (permeable though they may be) of historically disparate health cultures.

The Social System Dimension

The social system aspect of the health culture concept refers to the organization of health care, or, the health care delivery system of a group. Such a system, from a within-culture view, is comprised of both laypersons and specialists, with varying types of health-related knowledge and reflecting varying levels of status and degrees of power. The system, itself, may be embedded in the general social organization of a group—without an immediately apparent structure as is the case for the Bushmen of the Kalahari Desert in Africa (e.g., Katz, 1982). Or, it may be highly organized and visible as a well-defined subsystem within a society, as is the case for both dominant (e.g., biomedicine) and variant (e.g., chiropractic) health cultural traditions in the United States and many other nations of the world. Depending upon the complexity of the society, and the vantage point from which one views the structure and functioning of health care systems, there may be one or many systems. In order to understand the operation of a health care system, however, one must become familiar with both informal networks and organized sets of health/illness-related roles and behaviors.

The cognitive and social system components in every type of health behavior are less easily separated into distinct analytic parameters in relation to health maintenance and illness prevention than in relation to help-seeking and remedial behaviors. One reason is that health maintenance is integral to individual adaptive behaviors within the context of family, community, culture, and health culture. Consequently, the characteristics of such behavior are embedded within the norms for acceptable functioning in specific social contexts. Cognitive and social system characteristics are immediately present and inextricably intertwined. However, from the point at which a symptom emerges as "a deviation from the culturally and historically variable standard of normality established by everyday experience" (Freidson, 1970, p. 285) and triggers a help-seeking response (Zola, 1973), health behavior becomes specifically focused upon the goal of a return to the prior state of wellness or, lacking that, to the maintenance of as optimal a level of functioning as possible.

At the "lay" end of the lay–specialist continuum is the therapy management group, i.e., ''the set of individuals who take charge of therapy management with or on behalf of the sufferer'' (Janzen, 1987, p. 68). The therapy management group may be a very limited set of individuals or a rather extensive one. At the ''specialist'' end of the continuum may be a whole range of persons with varying types and degrees of health-related knowledge. From a within-culture perspective, such persons may be claimed as ''one's own'' or as belonging to ''other'' health cultural traditions, depending upon circumstances which change through time. In the instances of ''high blood'' and ''low blood'' described above, orthodox health professionals may be seen as part of the black American health care delivery system. However, in the instance of ''falling out'' that comes to be understood as an ''unnatural'' sickness, orthodox health professionals may be seen as ''not knowing'' and ''not understanding'' and, therefore, not one of the types of specialists in their own, traditional, health care system.

A number of conceptual models have been developed to guide research on that process variously called ''help-seeking'' or ''health-seeking'' behavior. Most are rational, linear models that differentially assess the cognitive and social system characteristics of the process (e.g., Chrisman, 1977; McKinlay, 1981). Those of Kleinman (1980) and Janzen (1987), however, warrant consideration here.

Kleinman's (1980) model is strictly cognitively oriented. It argues that individual explanatory beliefs (influenced by family as well as popular explanatory beliefs) represent the keys to understanding help-seeking behavior. Because these beliefs or ''models'' are the ''notions about an episode of sickness and its treatment'' (Kleinman, 1980, p. 105), they offer explanations that guide individual and family choices among available therapies and therapists. The study of such patient and family explanatory models, Kleinman suggests, ''tells us how they make sense of given episodes of illness and how they choose and evaluate particular treatments'' (p. 105). In many respects, the concepts of ''explanatory models'' and ''semantic illness networks'' (Good, 1977) provide specific labels for aspects of cognition within what has been, herein, the cognitive component of health culture.

It is of interest to note that the Chrisman, McKinlay, and Kleinman models focus heavily upon individual health behavior, with group activity or social networks being both supportive and yet peripheral. Such conceptualizations are compatible, indeed, with the focus upon the individual in general American culture.

Janzen's model (1987), however, emerged from research in Africa, where the family has a far more important role in therapy management than is the norm for the United States. In this model the individual sufferer recedes into the background while the group moves to the fore—a model, incidentally, that is observed frequently for Cubans and other Hispanics in Miami, but also for many immigrant groups in multiethnic urban settings in the United States.

Janzen's model thus emphasizes the concept of the ''therapy management group'' which includes components of cognitive structuring, but which stresses social relationships and interactions. He emphasizes the need to examine the ''cumulative, microhistorical character of social relations and personal exchanges'' (p. 76) to understand how each decision and action shapes successive stages of knowledge, perception of events, diagnosis of the condition, and the social field around sufferer, family, and practitioners. He sees the concept of ''therapy management'' as holding promise for ''contextually sensitive analyses of the relationships among cultural assumptions and values, behavioral processes, and social and economic structures that influence the therapeutic process'' (p. 68). Janzen's ''therapy management process'' in relation to an individual sufferer is extremely compatible with the concept of health culture.

HEALTH MAINTENANCE BEHAVIOR

Each of these models is of value in assessing various aspects of *help-seeking* behavior. None incorporates very well either the cognitive or the social system aspects of *health maintenance* behavior. As such behavior represents the greatest percentage of all health behavior, we need a model that takes health maintenance and illness prevention into consideration as well as behavior directed toward remediation

THE HEALTH CARE SYSTEM

The utilization patterns observed within a particular group contribute to our knowledge of the more formal aspects of the health care system. A shift to another level of analysis allows identification of the range of specialists functioning within that social system and, therefore, its degree of complexity. By moving to yet another type of organizational analysis, we are in a position to ascertain the roles and role-related behaviors of specialists predominant in various segments of the health care system. These include therapeutic techniques employed, organizational modes and administrative structures, variations in the social context of curing, patient–healer interactions, forms of payment for services, referral networks to and among various healers, recruitment into the healer role, the training of candidates for such roles, credentialing, and relationships to the orthodox biomedical system and other health care systems that abound in pluralistic urban settings the world over (see Leslie, 1980, on issues of "medical" pluralism).

When theories of illness, disorder, and general misfortune are considered in relation to therapeutic techniques utilized by various specialists in the health care system, then cognition and meaning again move to the fore but at a different level of sophistication and complexity from that considered in relation to household remedies and health maintenance in the home, for example (see Fabrega & Silver, 1973, and Garro, 1986, on this point). Thus, the health culture concept comfortably unifies and integrates a multitude of theoretical orientations in health behavior research that remain segmented and distinct, without it. This discussion has been necessary, because a transcultural perspective on health behavior requires that individual behavior be understood within the context of culture and health culture from both a cognitive and a social systems point of view. Because of space limitations, our discussion of the social system component of black American health culture will move directly to a brief description of types of healers identified.

Types of Specialists and Roles

It is important to note, first, that the Miami research into the social system component of health culture in each of the five groups under study documented the presence of a range of specialists functioning in a variety of roles. Aside from orthodox health professionals available within each of the communities studied, the most highly specialized practitioners of the traditional systems of care were *espiritistas* in the Puerto Rican community, *santeras* and *santeros* in the Cuban community, *houngans* and *mambos* in the Haitian community, spiritualists and *root doctors* in the black American community, and spiritualists and *obeah* men and women in the Bahamian community. A brief description of the range of health/illness-related roles identified in the black American group is provided. Recruitment into such roles is based upon gifts of healing, although self-teaching, apprenticeships, and formal training may accompany the process of professionalization.

First are those "divinely gifted" persons who work within the family and neighborhood but have not yet adopted the specialist role of "herbalist" for a wider circle of clients.

The expertise of these ''Daddys'' and ''Mamas'' lies in their knowledge and use of medicinal plants in the preparation of more specialized remedies than are known to most members of the group.

Second are the faith healers, whose therapeutic techniques are linked closely to God, the Bible, and healing oils. The Holy Spirit is the only spirit acknowledged by these specialists. They are seen as being born with a gift of faith healing, and they transmit their healing powers from God directly to the patient by means of a ''laying-on'' of the hands. They may or may not be gifted, also, in the use of medicinal plants; although the former is very likely.

Third are the spiritualists, whose healing power also comes from God and the Bible plus a reliance on one or more personal, helping spirits representing the ''loving dead.'' These are ''far sighters'' whom Hall and Bourne (1973) called ''neighborhood prophets.'' ''Far sighters'' are ''wise'' women and men. They, also, were born with a special gift from God. Some are born with a veil; others are born with a veil in combination with other auspicious indicators of special status, such as birthdays including the magical numbers of 7 and 9. They are able to make predictions about events and foretell the future for individuals. As their power comes directly from the spirits, much of their diagnostic and therapeutic knowledge becomes manifest through dreams. Far sighters are considered to be ''wise,'' because they are in greater control of life circumstances than are ordinary persons. Through spirits, they can see further into the future than can others. Consequently, they are in a position to forestall the occurrence of some type of misfortune that is coming to someone. This ability allows them to create ''changed conditions'' with a better outcome for the client in the form of greater health and well-being.

Fourth are the root doctors, also born with the gift to heal. These are men and women of God who utilize spirits as messengers of evil as well as good. In addition to healing oils, bush medicines, baths and teas, incense and candles, and so forth, they use the most powerful parts of medicinal plants or ''bush,'' i.e., the roots. Furthermore, they work with the most dangerous of spirits, the angry dead, to control conditions on this earth, either to make them turn ''bad'' or to make them return to ''good.'' Despite working with both good and evil, there is no moral conflict on the part of such specialists about being the channels through which such power flows.

The individuals with healing powers greater than those of the average person may or may not move into fully professional roles and develop extensive practices. If they do, however, there is great freedom to incorporate additional healing techniques in an eclectic fashion. Such openness and flexibility introduces a great deal of variation in the trappings of office, titles, and therapeutic techniques employed. But power is inherent in the universe, and those with special gifts of healing are in a position to augment their power in whatever manner they choose. From an outside-observer perspective, this makes classification difficult. From a within-culture perspective, it reflects a coherence that illustrates the impact of culture as an integrated symbol and meaning system.

A great deal more might be said about the social system aspects of black American health culture, but the point that needs to be made here is that from a within-culture perspective, knowledge of such a system may be obtained by observing where members of a particular group go for therapeutic action by specialists and under what circumstances. By classifying the criteria that define such specialization, one begins to grasp not only the range of types of healers that may be identified, but also the source of power that legitimizes their status. Although space does not allow a discussion of processes of professionalization, it is evident that the criteria are very different from those supporting specialists in the orthodox biomedical health care system.

METHODOLOGICAL ISSUES

A transcultural research perspective on health behavior has far-reaching consequences for our research methodologies, the instruments we employ, and the questions we ask. Such a research posture prohibits an unquestioning acceptance of established unicultural research methodologies. It raises questions about the cross-cultural validity of the basic concepts utilized for comparison, and it argues, for example, that not only is distress expressed in culture-specific idioms for which direct translations may be impossible, but also that symptoms, emotions, and illnesses "are constituted as fundamentally different forms of social reality" (Kleinman & Good, 1985, p. 492).

This means that, no matter how much we modify our instruments to make them more culturally sensitive, we can never see, through them, into the symbol and meaning system of another cultural tradition. They do not allow us to ferret out the repertoire of patterns guiding the behavior of participants in such systems or to construct the world view they hold in expression of those patterns. The values supporting them are anchored in the larger cultural context that supports and gives high status to the community of investigators (Young, 1980).

Inasmuch as our sensitivities have increased regarding the social construction of knowledge generally, and scientific knowledge specifically (e.g., Wright & Treacher, 1982), it is no longer acceptable to (a) utilize the definitions, categories, and meanings from one cultural tradition, at a particular point in its history, (b) attempt to operationalize these into an "etic" language considered to be relatively culture-free and, then, (c) apply them anywhere. Nowhere has this been more cogently argued than in the recent transcultural psychiatric literature (Kleinman & Good, 1985).

Obeyesekere (1985), for example, indicated that a South Asian male suffering from a constellation of symptoms which includes drastic weight loss, sexual fantasies, night emissions, and urine discoloration would be diagnosed as having a disease called "semen loss." Operationally, this constellation of symptoms can be found in every society; therefore, one might conclude that "semen loss" is a universal disorder and that many Americans could be identified as suffering from this condition. Obeyesekere acknowledged that the problem with this formulation is that although such symptoms exist randomly in every group, they have not been fused, everywhere, into the same conception of disorder. He continued as follows:

> Yet if I were to employ the methodological norms implicit in the several Diagnostic and Statistical manuals and apply them from a South Asian perspective to the rest of the world (as Western psychiatrists do for depression), then it is incontrovertible that "semen loss" *is* a disease and is universally found in human populations. 1985, pp. 136–137).

Despite the difficulties involved, many efforts are under way to develop cross-culturally valid instruments to be used, etically, from a transcultural posture (e.g., Lonner & Berry, 1986; Triandis & Berry, 1980).

One example of creativity and ingenuity in research strategies comes from a large cross-cultural, multidisciplinary program project on ethnicity and health among low-income elderly that is being undertaken in Miami from an explicit transcultural research paradigm. It combines emic and etic data-gathering procedures. The project attempts, by means of an ongoing longitudinal inquiry, to integrate findings from research focused upon both cognitive and social system aspects of health culture on the one hand and the findings from research oriented toward sociological, psychological, nutritional, physiological, and immunological assessments of health behavior on the other. It is essential to constantly integrate the two types of data being collected so that interpretation of both emic and etic findings will be informed by the strengths of both research traditions.

NEW RESEARCH DIRECTIONS

A transcultural perspective on health behavior has been shown to be a productive research orientation (e.g., Harwood, 1981; Kleinman & Good, 1985). Such research will have an impact upon orthodox health professional behavior. The first impact will be experienced in the cognitive realm related to biomedical research—through recognition that culture influences health behavior at every level of functioning. Beyond that, however, the impact, as a consequence of changed cognition, will be experienced, also, in the social system component of biomedical health culture. Each of these points will be touched upon briefly.

Cognitive Directions

Kleinman (1980), speaking as a physician and anthropologist, argued that the cognitive aspects of health culture (explanatory models and semantic illness networks, in his terms) constitute the symbolic pathways that link culture and physiological functioning. The term "pathways" in biomedicine refers to the ways attitudes or emotions are processed by the body in creating physiological or biochemical changes (Cousins, 1986). Kleinman's remarks, therefore, fit well into the framework of the new field of biomedicine called "psychobiology" or "psychoneuroimmunology." This field has not yet moved to include culture as a crucial variable in the shaping of attitudes and emotions, but this will become an extremely important research area in the future.

Scheper-Hughes and Lock (1987), for example, reviewed some of the literature illustrating the ways in which emotions entail not only feelings, but also cognitive orientations, public morality, and cultural ideology. These authors considered the emotions, so constructed, to be the link missing from diverse theoretical orientations—the link that is capable of bridging mind and body, and also functioning as the "mediatrix" of the individual "mindful body," the social body, and the body politic.

Rossi (1986), on the other hand, saw no mysterious gap between mind and body. He argued convincingly that memory, learning, and behavior that are encoded in the limbic–hypothalamic system of the brain, function as the major information transducers forming the mind–body connection. He also presented evidence from several basic biomedical research traditions that this major pathway coordinates all of the "messenger molecules" of mind–body communication via the autonomic, endocrine, immune, and neuropeptide systems.

Locke and Colligan (1986) reviewed psychoneuroimmunology research findings that further demonstrate the influence of mental activity upon physical states and, therefore, upon health and illness. Clearly, the mind and body, conceptually, are being reunited as a "mindful body," to use Scheper-Hughes and Lock's apt phrase. Convergence among the biological, psychological, and social science disciplines suggests that the theoretical orientations are now in place to examine health behavior in all of its interlocking parameters from culture to immunology and from wellness to death. As that is the case, it may be anticipated that the linkages between cultural, social, psychological, and biological processes in relation to both the maintenance of health (or wellness) and remediation (or healing) will become central issues in health behavior research. Now that biomedical science has disproved one of its basic tenets and legacies from the past, i.e., that mind and body are separate, it will be possible to examine such issues within other healing traditions as well as that of biomedicine. The evidence comes from "hard science" that the body is a mindful one. General acceptance of this emergent scientific fact will open the way for serious inquiry, in cultural context, of wellness and processes of healing that are understood far less well than those of pathophysiology and biological repair. Such health behavior research, of necessity, will be organized as truly well-integrated multidisciplinary projects such as the one being undertaken in Miami, mentioned earlier in relation to methodological issues in transculturally oriented research.

Social System Dimensions

Cognitive changes in a health cultural tradition require, for internal consistency, a social structure that allows new conceptualizations to be expressed in behavior and institutional form. Meaning-centered research from a transcultural perspective points directly to negotiation and mediation as the keys to improved health care in multiethnic settings (e.g., Katon & Kleinman, 1981; Harwood, 1981; Weidman, 1975, 1976a,b, 1982). Acceptance of such research findings influences the manner in which biomedical practitioners define their professional roles and interact with patients in clinical contexts. The process of moving from cultural awareness to cultural knowledge reinforces the mediating attributes of the health professional role and encourages adoption of a transcultural perceptual posture.

The biomedical practitioner who functions from a transcultural posture becomes, in this author's theoretical model, a "culture broker" (Weidman, 1973, 1975, 1976b). The culture broker health professional is simultaneously: (a) "third party" observer of the professional's own interactions with patients, (b) mediator, at the conceptual level, of the social and cognitive gaps that may exist between the two, (c) interpersonal negotiator between the two, based upon cognitive assessments of similarities and differences, and (d) behavioral mediator as required by the extent of noncongruence between the health cultures (cognitive and social system) and explanatory models (Kleinman, 1980) of self as practitioner and that of the patient (Rubin & Jones, 1979; Weidman, 1979, 1983). Although the patient is always the final arbiter of clinical decisions, the clinician in a transcultural "culture broker" position, nevertheless, has many more options for negotiating strategies than a uniculturally oriented practitioner, because when reality is defined from a transcultural posture, the moral universe within which one functions is markedly expanded. What is considered unacceptable care, uniculturally, may become culturally appropriate care, transculturally.

There is evidence from the literature of the value of new culture broker roles in orthodox health care and, also, of the attributes of health professional roles in the direction of culture brokerage. Such value has been demonstrated in community mental health care and in cross-cultural training in Miami (Lefley, 1986; Lefley & Bestman, 1984; Weidman, 1982, 1983). Culture brokerage has been incorporated into nursing as a nursing intervention (Tripp-Reimer & Brink, 1986). Community health aides for the elderly are being defined as culture brokers (Moldy, 1981–82). Culture brokerage has been included as a specific change strategy in applied anthropology (Van Willigan, 1986). And there is beginning to be sufficient experience with the concept, the role, and role attributes in health care that issues of ambiguity and conflict are beginning to be addressed (Kaufert & Koolage, 1984).

This suggests that the *concept* of culture brokerage between clients and health professionals, the creation of a new health professional *role* of culture broker, or the incorporation of new culture brokerage *attributes* into ordinary clinical and community roles, together constitute both conceptual and social pathways that link the transcultural perspective as a perceptual and research posture to behavior in a social role based upon that same perspective. An extremely rich research area in the future, then, will be to examine changes in health behavior and in professional–patient interactions in the context of a system that is underdoing such a major paradigm shift.

We need to understand, also, the crucial interactions between the conceptual and social system sides of clinical phenomena for both patient and practitioner. This will be achieved through research focused upon biomedical health culture itself—the tradition upon which this section is focused. At issue is the accommodation of health professional roles and the structure of the health care system to a changing knowledge base that incorporates culture and social process as important influences upon health behavior. The extent of the accommodations that may be required for maximum therapeutic efficacy in a multicultural world are only now being explored (Lefley & Bestman, 1984; Lefley & Pedersen, 1986; Sussex & Weidman, 1975; Weidman, 1975, 1982, 1983).

All of the specific health behavioral research issues that, heretofore, have been examined primarily from a unicultural (culturi-centric) research posture now need to be reexamined from a transcultural research stance that incorporates the most sophisticated and refined emic and etic methodological approaches that can be devised.

REFERENCES

Alexander, L. (1982). Illness maintenance and the new American sick role. In N. Chrisman & T. Maretzki (Eds.), *Clinically applied anthropology* (pp. 351–367). Dordrecht: Reidel.

Baer, H. A. (1982). On the political economy of health. *Medical Anthropology Newsletter, 14*(1), 1–2, 13–17.

Baer, H. A., Singer, M., & Johnsen, J. H. (1986). Introduction: Toward a critical medical anthropology. *Socal Science and Medicine, 23*(2), 95–98.

Chrisman, N. J. (1977). The health seeking process: An approach to the natural history of illness. *Culture, Medicine and Psychiatry, 1,* 351–377.

Chrisman, N., & Maretzki, T. (Eds.). (1982). *Clinically applied anthropology*. Dordrecht: Reidel.

Cousins, N. (1986). Foreword (p. vii). In E. L. Rossi, *The psychobiology of mind–body healing*. New York: Norton.

Culture, Medicine and Psychiatry. (1987). Special Issue on Culture Bound Syndromes, *11*(1).

Eisenberg, L. (1977). Disease and illness: Distinctions between professional and popular ideas of sickness. *Culture, Medicine and Psychiatry, 1,* 9–23.

Escobar, J. I. (1987). Cross-cultural aspects of the somatization trait. *Hospital and Community Psychiatry, 38*(2), 174–180.

Evans, R. E., Kileff, C., & Shelby, K. (1982). *"That was all we ever know": Herbal medicine, a living force in the Appalachians* (Readings and Perspectives in Medicine, No. 4). Durham, NC: Duke University Medical Center.

Fabrega, H., Jr. (1977). Culture, behavior, and the nervous system. *Annual Review of Anthropology, 6,* 419–455.

Fabrega, H., Jr., & Silver, D. (1973). *Illness and shamanistic curing in Zinacantan*. Stanford: Stanford University Press.

Fabrega, H., & Tyma, S. (1976). Language and cultural influences in the description of pain. *British Journal of Medical Psychology, 49,* 349–371.

Farb, P., & Armelagos, G. J. (1980). *Consuming passions: The anthropology of eating*. Boston: Houghton Mifflin.

Freidson, E. (1970). *Profession of medicine: A study of the sociology of applied knowledge*. New York: Dodd, Mead.

Garro, L. (1986). Intracultural variation in folk medical knowledge: A comparison between curers and noncurers. *American Anthropologist, 88,* 351–370.

Glick, L. B. (1977). Medicine as an ethnographic category: "The Gimi of the New Guinea Highlands." In D. Landy (Ed.), *Culture, disease, and healing: Studies in medical anthropology* (pp. 58–70). New York: Macmillan Co.

Good, B. J. (1977). The heart of what's the matter: The semantics of illness in Iran. *Culture, Medicine, and Psychiatry, 1,* 25–58.

Hall, A. L., & Bourne, P. G. (1973). Indigenous therapists in a southern Black urban community. *Archives of General Psychiatry, 28,* 137–142.

Harris, M. (1971). *Culture, man, and nature*. New York: T. Y. Crowell.

Harris, M. (1976). History and significance of the emic/etic distinction. *Annual Review of Anthropology, 5,* 329–350.
Harwood, A. (Ed.). (1981). *Ethnicity and medical care.* Cambridge, MA: Harvard University Press.
Helman, C. G. (1984). *Culture, health and illness: An introduction for health professionals.* Littleton, MA: PSG Publishing.
Ito, K. L. (1985). Ho'oponopono, "To make right": Hawaiian conflict resolution and metaphor in the construction of a family therapy. *Culture, Medicine and Psychiatry, 9*(2), 201–217.
Janzen, J. M. (1978a). The comparative study of medical systems as changing social systems. *Social Science and Medicine, 12*(2B), 121–129.
Janzen, J. M. (1978b). *The quest for therapy in Lower Zaire.* Berkeley: University of California Press.
Janzen, J. M. (1987). Therapy management: Concept, reality, process. *Medical Anthropology Quarterly* (New Series), *1*(1), 68–84.
Katon, W., & Kleinman, A. (1981). Doctor–patient negotiation and other social science strategies in patient care. In L. Eisenberg & A. Kleinman (Eds.), *The relevance of social science for medicine* (pp. 253–279). Dordrecht: Reidel.
Katz, R. (1982). *Boiling energy: Community healing among the Kalahari Jung.* Cambridge, MA: Harvard University Press.
Kaufert, J. M., & Koolage, W. W. (1984). Role conflict among "culture brokers": The experience of native Canadian medical interpreters. *Social Science and Medicine, 18*(3), 283–286.
Kleinman, A. (1980). *Patients and healers in the context of culture: An exploration of the borderland between anthropology, medicine, and psychiatry.* Berkeley: University of California Press.
Kleinman, A., & Good, B. (1985). *Culture and depression.* Berkeley: University of California Press.
Lefley, H. P. (1986). The cross-cultural training institute for mental health professionals: Reeducating practitioners in cultural and community perspectives. In H. P. Lefley & P. B. Pedersen (Eds.), *Cross-cultural training for mental health professionals* (pp. 89–111). Springfield, IL: Thomas.
Lefley, H. P., & Bestman, E. W. (1984). Community mental health and minorities: A multiethnic approach. In S. Sue & T. Moore (Eds.), *The pluralistic society* (pp. 116–148). New York: Human Sciences Press.
Lefley, H. P., & Pedersen, P. B. (Eds.). (1986). *Cross-cultural training for mental health professionals.* Springfield, IL: Thomas.
Leslie, C. (Ed.). (1980). Special issue. Medical pluralism. *Social Science and Medicine, 14B*(4), 191–296.
Lock, M. (1986). The anthropological study of the American medical system: Center and periphery. *Social Science and Medicine, 22*(9), 931–932.
Locke, S., & Colligan, D. (1986). *The healer within.* New York: New American Library.
Lonner, W. J., & Berry, J. W. (Eds.). (1986). *Field methods in cross-cultural research.* Beverly Hills: Sage.
Low, S. M. (1985). Culturally interpreted symptoms or culture-bound syndromes: A cross-cultural review of nerves. *Social Science and Medicine, 21*(2), 187–196.
Massara, E. B., & Stunkard, A. J. (1979). A method of quantifying cultural ideals of beauty and the obese. *International Journal of Obesity, 3,* 149–152.
McKinlay, J. B. (1981). Social network influences on morbid episodes and the career of help seeking. In L. Eisenberg & A. M. Kleinman (Eds.), *The relevance of social science for medicine* (pp. 77–107). Dordrecht: Reidel.
Messer, E. (1984). Anthropological perspectives on diet. *Annual Review of Anthropology, 13,* 205–249.
Moldy, D. M. (1981–82). The community health aid [sic] as cultural broker. *Practicing Anthropology, 4*(1), 16–18.
Obeyesekere, G. (1985). Depression, Buddhism, and the work of culture in Sri Lanka. In A. Kleinman & B. Good (Eds.), *Culture and depression* (pp. 134–152). Berkeley: University of California Press.
Palgi, P., & Abramovitch, H. (1984). Death: A cross-cultural perspective. *Annual Review of Anthropology, 13,* 385–417.
Polgar, S. (1963). Health action in cross-cultural perspective. In H. Freeman, S. Levine, & L. G. Reeder (Eds.), *Handbook of medical sociology* (pp. 379–419). Englewood Cliffs, NJ: Prentice–Hall.
Rivers, W. H. R. (1926). *Psychology and ethnology.* New York: Harcourt Brace Jovanovich.

Rossi, E. L. (1986). *The psychobiology of mind–body healing*. New York: Norton.
Rubin, J. C., & Jones, J. (1979). Falling-out: A clinical study. *Social Science and Medicine, 13B*(2), 117–128.
Sargent, C. (1984). Between death and shame: Dimensions of pain in Bariba culture. *Social Science and Medicine, 19*(12), 1299–1304.
Scheper-Hughes, N., & Lock, M. M. (1987). The mindful body: A prolegomenon to future work in medical anthropology. *Medical Anthropology Quarterly, 1*(1), 6–41.
Scott, C. S. (1981). *Health cultural beliefs* [Videotape]. Miami: Department of Psychiatry, University of Miami School of Medicine.
Snow, L. F. (1974). Folk medical beliefs and their implications for care of patients: A review based on studies among Black Americans. *Annals of Internal Medicine, 81*, 82–96.
Snow, L. F. (1978). Sorcerers, saints, and charlatans: Black folk healers in urban America. *Culture, Medicine and Psychiatry, 2*, 60–106.
Snow, L. F. (1983). Traditional health beliefs and practices among lower class Black Americans. *The Western Journal of Medicine, 139*(6), 820–828.
Social Science and Medicine. (1985). Special section on New Approaches to Culture Bound Mental Disorders, *21*(2), 163–228.
Sullivan, M. (1986). In what sense is contemporary medicine dualistic? *Culture, Medicine and Psychiatry, 10*(4), 331–350.
Sussex, J. N., & Weidman, H. H. (1975). Toward responsiveness in mental health care. *Psychiatric Annals, 5*(8), 8–16.
Triandis, H. C., & Berry, J. W. (1980). *Handbook of cross-cultural psychology: Vol. 2. Methodology*. Boston: Allyn & Bacon.
Tripp-Reimer, T., & Brink, P. J. (1986). Culture brokerage. In G. M. Bulechek & J. C. McCloskey (Eds.), *Nursing interventions: Treatments for nursing diagnoses*. Philadelphia: Saunders.
Turner, V. W. (1967). *The forest of symbols*. Ithaca, NY: Cornell University Press.
Van Leeuwen, E. (1987). Comment on Mark Sullivan: "In what sense is contemporary medicine dualistic?" *Culture, Medicine and Psychiatry, 11*(2), 251–259.
Van Willigan, J. (1986). *Applied anthropology: An introduction*. Boston: Bergin & Garvey.
Weidman, H. H. (1973, March). *Implications of the culture-broker concept for the delivery of health care*. Paper presented at the annual meeting of the Southern Anthropological Society, Wrightsville Beach, NC.
Weidman, H. H. (1975). Concepts as strategies for change. *Psychiatric Annals, 5*(8), 17–19.
Weidman, H. H. (1976a). The constructive potential of alienation: A transcultural perspective. In R. S. Bryce-Laporte & C. Thomas (Eds.), *Contemporary perspectives on alienation* (pp. 335–337). New York: Praeger.
Weidman, H. H. (1976b). On getting from "here" to "there" [Guest Editorial]. *Medical Anthropology Newsletter, 8*(1), 2–7.
Weidman, H. H. (1978). *Miami health ecology project report, Vol. I: A statement on ethnicity and health*. Miami: University of Miami School of Medicine, Department of Psychiatry.
Weidman, H. H. (Ed.). (1979). The transcultural perspective in health and illness. Special issue. *Social Science and Medicine, 13B*(2), 85–167.
Weidman, H. H. (1981). Dominance and domination in health care: A transcultural perspective. In M. S. Staum & D. E. Larson (Eds.), *Doctors, patients, and society: Power and authority in medical care* (pp. 133–143). Waterloo, Ontario: Wilfrid Laurier University Press.
Weidman, H. H. (1982). Research strategies, structural alterations and clinically applied anthropology. In N. Chrisman & T. W. Maretzki (Eds.), *Clinically applied anthropology* (pp. 201–241). Dordrecht: Reidel.
Weidman, H. H. (1983). Research, service and training aspects of clinical anthropology: An institutional overview. In D. B. Shimkin & P. Golde (Eds.), *Clinical anthropology: A new approach to American health problems?* (pp. 119–153). Lanham, MD: University Press of America.
Weidman, H. H. (1986). Attaining the transcultural perspective in health care: Implications for clinical training. In H. Lefley & P. Pedersen (Eds.), *Cross-cultural training for mental health professionals*. Springfield, IL: Thomas.
Weidman, H. H., & Egeland, J. A. (1973). A behavioral science perspective in the comparative approach to the delivery of health care. *Social Science and Medicine, 7*(11), 854–860.

Wellin, E. (1977). Theoretical orientations in medical anthropology: Continuity and change over the past half-century. In D. Landy (Ed.), *Culture, disease and healing: Studies in medical anthropology* (pp. 47–58). New York: Macmillan Co.

Wober, M. (1969). Distinguishing centriculture from cross-cultural tests and research. *Perceptual and Motor Skills, 28,* 488.

Wright, P., & Treacher, A. (Eds.). (1982). *The problem of medical knowledge: Examining the social construction of medicine.* Edinburgh: Edinburgh University Press.

Young, A. (1980). The discourse on stress and the reproduction of conventional knowledge. *Social Science and Medicine, 14B,* 133–146.

Zborowski, M. (1969). *People in pain.* San Francisco: Jossey–Bass.

Zola, I. K. (1973). Pathways to the doctor: From person to patient. *Social Science and Medicine, 7,* 677–684.

PART III

HEALTH BEHAVIOR AND THE CARE DELIVERY SYSTEM

So far health behavior has been examined along a continuum of personal and social determinants, with individual health behaviors considered as outcomes or dependent variables. Part III deals with the encounter between the individual and the institutions of the health care system: physicians and other professional care-givers, clinics, and hospitals; and with how the interactive aspects of such encounters determine health behaviors. The material is organized into two categories: perceptions and interactions, and power, compliance, and control. Such a grouping is arbitrary, because the issues related to one topic overlap appreciably with the issues related to the others.

Perceptions and Interactions

PERCEPTIONS

Encounters between individuals and the health care system are mediated by perceptions. Perceptions include beliefs, expectations, evaluations, and other cognitive elements discussed earlier in this book, particularly in Chapters 1, 2, and 3. Patients and clients enter the encounter with their own personal—often idiosyncratic—perceptions of their conditions, of medical and other health professionals, and of the institutions in which care is sought or provided. Lederer's (1952) much-referred-to synthesis of the sick person's perspective identifies the constricted view of the world, the concreteness, the anxiety, the need for reassurance, the ego-centricity, and the ambivalence toward the physician, that characterize the experience of feeling sick. Professionals enter these encounters with *their* perceptions of patients in general, of particular patients, of the patient's condition, of themselves and other professionals, and of the institutions in which they conduct their work.

Anderson and Helm (1979) noted that the differential appraisals within the professional–layperson encounter are inevitable. The initial "realities" of the encounter are different for each. Patients initially perceive their conditions in an immediate, personal, subjective manner, and are often in a state of crisis. Physicians perceive the patient as typifying an instance of some condition. For the patient, the encounter is exceptional, evoking anxiety and concern for expenses; for the physician, the encounter is routine (p. 263). The encounter often culminates in what Anderson and Helm termed a "negotiated reality."

Research related to such perceptions can be grouped under four headings: client perceptions of professionals, professional perceptions of clients, incongruities in perceptions, and perceptions of satisfaction.

Client Perceptions of Professionals

Among the earliest reports of client perceptions of professionals is Freidson's seminal study (1961) of patients enrolled in New York City's Health Insurance Plan (HIP), and of patients of private practitioners (1961, Chapter 3). Freidson showed that patients were slightly more likely to perceive the private practitioners as taking greater personal interest in them, but that the HIP physicians were perceived as providing more competent care.

Adamson and Watts (1976) found that maternity patients perceived maternity nurse practitioners to be especially helpful in providing information and support, and to be more helpful than physicians in several ways, e.g., showing concern and reassurance, and providing information and explanations.

In a population of London dental patients, Liddell and May (1984) found that perceptions of the patients' regular dentists were more favorable, e.g., more competent, more likeable, more careful, less indifferent, less mercenary, and less unsympathetic, than perceptions of dentists in general. Moreover, these perceptions were related to age and gender, as well as to prior frightening dental experiences. Strauss (1976) observed that black patients have different perceptions of dentists and of dental treatment than do white patients, that they are more likely to expect to have an extraction, that they expect the dental treatment to be painful, and are less likely to express criticism of the professional. In a different vein, Rosen (1977) found that women who were experiencing unwanted conceptions, who had a regular physician, and who chose to terminate the pregnancy, did not perceive their primary care physicians as a source of advice in relation to their pregnancy.

Finally, in the context of examining "doctor-shopping" behavior, Kasteler, Kane, Olsen, and Thetford (1976) observed that patients have begun to perceive their physicians as "commodities," rather than as "gods."

Professional Perceptions of Clients

Professionals often demonstrate stereotyping in their perceptions of patients. McCranie, Horowitz, and Martin (1978) reported on the degree of gender-based stereotyping in medical diagnosis; misdiagnosis having a high potential for inappropriate and unsatisfactory encounters between female clients and male medical practitioners. The researchers' vignette-based study failed to show differential psychiatric diagnoses based on gender, but they acknowledged the problem of generalizing from such simulations to real encounters. On the other hand, Verbrugge (1984) was able to demonstrate that while men and women are equally likely to receive a psychiatric primary diagnosis, women are more likely to receive a secondary psychiatric diagnosis; that some differences exist in the kinds of services that are made available to men and to women, if not in the amounts of such services; that nonpsychiatrists are less equitable in their treatment of the genders than are psychiatrists; and that distressed women receive more care.

The issue of stereotyping also arises in Frazier, Jenny, Bagramian, Robinson, and Proshek's (1977) examination of the congruence between dentists' views of patients' beliefs and values, and the patients' actual beliefs and values. Data revealed that practitioners' inferences are influenced by patients' socioeconomic status. McKinlay (1975) reported that physicians, particularly older ones, underestimated patients' grasp of the meanings of a range of medical terms. Moreover, the physicians continued to use these terms, even though they believed (mistakenly) that patients would not understand them.

Gerbert (1984), using videotaped simulations demonstrating three combinations of patient likeability and competence, observed that aspects of these patient characteristics had an effect on case management. For example, recommendations for psychological referral were less likely to be made for likeable patients; and that likeable-competent patients were more often encouraged to maintain close contact with the physician's office.

Ghodse (1978, 1979) observed that emergency room physicians and nurses in London Accident and Emergency Departments varied in their perceptions of drug-overdose patients. Patients who overdosed accidentally on prescription medication were perceived more favorably than those who took an overdose in a suicide attempt, or those who were drug-dependent. Moreover, the recommendations for further treatment reflected these differential perceptions.

Similarly, Roth (1986) identified instances of moral evaluation of clients in emergency room settings, demonstrating that professional staff members were not morally neutral in how they perceive patients, and that there was consensus that some categories of patients, e.g., drunks, are less deserving of emergency room care, and that others, e.g., unusual cases, are more deserving.

Leiderman and Grisso (1985) identified the "Gomer" (*G*et *O*ut of *M*y *E*mergency *R*oom; *G*rand *O*ld *M*an of the *E*mergency *R*oom) phenomenon and showed that ambiguity of diagnosis and impairment of both adult social role functioning and mental status were more likely to lead to a patient being perceived and labeled as a Gomer, with ensuing problems of patient management and failure to respond to treatment. Gomers were no more likely to be seriously ill initially than comparable controls, but they remained longer in the hospital and experienced mental deterioration to a greater degree.

In a study of nurses in public and community health agencies, Keith and Castles (1975) examined how environmental and workplace characteristics relate to the professional's fears and rejections of patients, and to the emergence of stereotyping on the part of professionals.

Westbrook, Nordholm, and McGee (1984) demonstrated that Australian and Swedish nonphysician health professionals (physiotherapists, occupational therapists, nurses) showed differences in their perceptions of patients that reflected their cultural differences in beliefs about responsibility for health. Australians viewed patients more favorably, as more likely to need counseling, as more dependent, and as more poorly adjusted than did the Swedes. Australians, moreover, were more likely to speak with patients about feelings.

In their factor analysis of physicians' views of patients, Ford, Liske, Ort, and Denton (1967) demonstrated a consensus that effective practice depends on patients being cooperative with treatment, well-adjusted, responsive to treatment, expressive of appreciation, and believers in their physicians' skills.

Wills's literature review of how different helping professions view their clients (1978) demonstrated a general pessimism about clients, particularly in relation to treatability, manageability, and likeability.

The technology of measuring professional perceptions is slowly emerging. Ashworth, Williamson, and Montano (1984) developed and began the validation of a self-report instrument measuring physicians' perceptions about psychosocial aspects of care, including perceptions of the physician's role, perceptions about what patients want and do not want, and perceptions about physicians' reactions to patients as persons.

Incongruent Perceptions

As shared or overlapping perceptions are presumed to facilitate satisfactory and productive encounters, the degree to which patient and professional perceptions are incongruent may impede appropriate interactions and consequently may have a negative or unanticipated effect on health behavior and ultimately upon health status. Innes (1977) identified factors in the training of physicians that lead to failures of the physician to perceive the patient appropriately, i.e., to perceive the patient as a product of situational as well as dispositional factors, and to be sensitive to patient feelings and emotional states. Innes further observed that such failures lead to inadequate communication which in turn fails to satisfy patient needs and generates failure to comply with aspects of treatment.

On the basis of a latent structure analysis of the "normative conflict" between physicians and patients, Sawyer (1980) concluded that despite evidence that physicians know that incongruity exists between their own and their patients' perspectives and norms, physicians continue to ignore patients' perceptions and assume that a "normative consensus" exists.

Hill's (1978) observations of patients in rehabilitation programs demonstrated that their perceptions of themselves, and of physicians, were often determined by the policies of the rehabilitation unit in relation to authority, and patient participation in their own care. She reasoned that the policies and perceptions of the care unit may be incongruent with, and detrimental to, the entire rehabilitation process.

Kahn, Anderson, and Perkoff (1973) observed that laypersons' perceptions of the worsening of conditions and their subsequent use of emergency rooms for treatment were incongruent with the perceptions of physicians. Finally, Strull, Lo and Charles (1984) noted incongruence between physicians' and patients' perceptions of the decision-making process, and of their respective responsibilities in it. Physicians were observed to underestimate patients' desires for information, and, seemingly in contrast to other findings, to overestimate patients' desires to be active participants.

Perceptions of Satisfaction

Patients' perceptions of satisfaction—their positive evaluations or assessments of care—have been a major focus of health behavior research. Satisfaction is complexly determined. It involves trust, patient characteristics and needs, as well as their perceptions of physicians' technical and interpersonal skills together with their perceptions of whether or not they are responding appropriately to treatment.

Caterinicchio (1979) used path analysis to develop a model for predicting the degree of trust in patient–practitioner interactions based on continuity, frequency, and success of treatment, as well as for predicting the relationships between perceived trust, anxiety, tolerance of pain, and perceived health outcomes. The findings demonstrated that trust, once established, continues even in the face of subsequent negative experiences.

Kasteler *et al.* (1976) demonstrated that the degree to which patients have confidence or trust in their physician's competence; the degree to which they are impressed with the physician's personal characteristics; and the convenience of location and office hours, are all important determinants of "doctor shopping," the degree to which individuals will change physicians and systematically seek out new ones.

Ross (e.g., Ross & Duff, 1982; Ross, Mirowsky, & Duff, 1982) analyzed how patient satisfaction leads to patients returning to the physician, and related both of these to the interaction between the characteristics of the patient and of the practice setting, e.g., continuity of care, or small or large setting.

In addition, Mirowsky and Ross (1983) showed that the relationship between satisfaction and use of pediatric services resembles a self-regulatory system: although increased levels of satisfaction led to increased use of services, at some point, increased use eventually resulted in diminished satisfaction, which then led to a reduction in use.

Hall, Roter, and Rand (1981) developed ingenious techniques to filter-out the expressive qualities of speech from the verbal content. In a study of the qualities of oral communication between patients and physicians, they observed, paradoxically, that patients' contentment was positively related to physicians showing anger toward them; the anger being interpreted as reflecting a firm but fair attitude. Buller and Buller (1987) observed that patients' satisfaction with care was positively related to the degree of "affiliativeness" in their physicians' communications, and negatively related to the degree of "control" in such communications.

Locker and Dunt (1978) systematically reviewed problems in the conceptualization and measurement of satisfaction. Zyzanski, Hulka, and Cassel (1974) devised a psychometrically sound, and widely used scale to measure satisfaction with medical care in general, but it does not deal with care provided by individual physicians or health professionals.

INTERACTIONS

Complementing individual and health professional perceptions of one another are interactional characteristics such as role relations, and information sharing and communication.

Role Relations

Szasz and Hollender (1956/1975) described three basic models of physician–patient role relationships: activity–passivity, guidance–cooperation, and mutual participation. Each model specifies a different view of the hierarchy or symmetry in the relationship, and allows for the satisfaction of different physician needs. For example, in the activity–passivity model, physicians can presumably gratify their needs for mastery and express their feelings of superiority. Danziger's (1986) study of pregnant women showed the differential interactional outcomes depending on whether the model accepted by the physician was congruent or incongruent with that accepted by the patient.

In a study of physicians in a health maintenance organization, Barr and Steinberg (1985) identified two independent role dimensions: colleague dependency and client dependency; and observed that there was no unitary conception of the physician role, but rather that some saw themselves as bureaucrats, whereas others saw themselves as unhampered by nonmedical restraints. They did see themselves as moderately colleague-dependent, although few participated in organizational decision-making.

Drew, Stoeckle, and Billings (1983), analyzed gift-giving to physicians in relation to physician–patient roles and suggested that the gift-giving process contains elements of needs for reciprocity as well as elements of attempts to change the status and power imbalance of the relationship.

Shelp (1984) argued moreover that courage should be an important component of the physician's role, particularly in relation to the risks of medical uncertainty, in contexts where there is no cure. Such courage on the physician's part is presumed to elicit similar courage on the part of the patient facing pain and death. In relation to uncertainty, especially in the context of biomedical innovations leading to prenatal detection of inherited diseases, Sorenson (1974) showed that the traditional role relationship between physicians and patients was changing. The increased uncertainty was bringing about greater patient participation, and less authoritativeness on the part of the physician.

Todd and Still's (1984) observations of four general practitioners working with terminally ill patients suggested the appropriateness of physicians expanding their narrowly defined traditional role as *medical* practitioner to include the role of *counselor,* as their task was no longer one of treating or curing medically, but of helping the patient cope with the task of dying.

Information Sharing and Communication

Hauser (1981) provided an overview of empirical studies on interaction, particularly in relation to information exchange, and Stiles, Putnam, and Jacob (1982) analyzed frameworks for conducting interviews. Armstrong's (1984) analysis of changes in physician interviewing styles pointed out that the old "medical gaze" which went hand in hand with the physician's aggressive interrogation of an essentially passive, inchoate patient, followed by a physical examination, has evolved into a clinical perspective that allows greater amounts of input from the patient, and a greater appreciation of the patient's view.

Nonetheless, despite such changes, information sharing and communication between physician and patient remain problematic. Boreham and Gibson's (1978) exploration of information gathering and communication processes revealed that laypersons typically have been passive as information gatherers, despite changes in access to care, in the narrowing of the knowledge gap between professionals and clients, in the increasing chronicity—and thus increased needs for knowledge and information—of conditions that bring patients in for care, and the increasing degree to which poor communication is a source of patient dissatisfaction.

Moreover, Wartman, Morlock, Malitz, and Palm (1981) cautioned that physicians' prescriptions of medication may, in fact, become a substitute for meaningful communication with patients.

Hayes-Bautista's (1978) nontraditional conceptual paradigms for understanding the layperson–professional encounter is derived from a sociology of knowledge perspective. He pointed out that physicians and patients derive their knowledge and information from very different sources, and that the attributes of their knowledge are different. Such differences lead to difficulties in effective communication.

Helman (1985) analyzed four components of the communication process: the patient's view of the origin, significance, and effects of a condition; the physician's view of these; the physician's view of the patient's view; and the congruity of these three views. The physician is more likely to have a "disease" view, focusing on specific "objective" pathology, whereas the patient is more likely to have an "illness" view, reflecting "subjective" feelings and experiences. Moreover, Helman observed that although physicians and patients might be in marked agreement on diagnosis and other components of the encounter, physicians showed limited knowledge of patients' explanatory beliefs, but that their knowledge of patients' views was greater for patients who had completed college than for those who had not.

Heszen-Klemens and Lapinska (1984) observed how the way in which Polish physicians interacted with their patients had implications for patient behavior. The Bales Interaction Process Analysis technique showed, for example, that recall of instructions was greater when such instructions occurred more frequently in physicians' communications, when patients were allowed to act as partners in the encounter, when they asked more questions, and when the physician was friendlier. Recall worsened when the total amount of advice given by physicians (physician directiveness) increased.

Stewart's (1984) analysis of patient-centered behaviors showed that physicians asking patients for opinions and help resulted in increased patient satisfaction. Moreover, where physicians allowed patients to show negative feelings, satisfaction was greater.

Mathews's (1983) literature review identified a number of problem areas in the communication process, and emphasized the importance of shared knowledge, status, role, and ideology, and institutional restraints on sharing information.

Tuckett and Williams (1984) provided a literature review of attempts to measure explanation and information-giving, and emphasized the need to improve and develop procedures to do so, particularly in relation to the "meaning" of the information sought and provided. Buijs, Sluijs, and Verhaak (1984) developed a technique for assessing physicians' interview styles in relation to information-gathering in the two distinct phases of the consultation process: diagnosis and prescribing. Physicians vary along the dimension of use of patient-centeredness and doctor centeredness, depending on their use of patient's knowledge and experiences in relation to their own.

Roter's and Ben-Sira's chapters both integrate a number of issues relevant to perceptions and interactions. Roter discusses reciprocity between the task and socioemotional domains of the encounter, and the implications of this reciprocity for patient behavior. In complementary fashion, Ben-Sira elaborates on the relationship between patient affective needs, perceptions of physician affective behavior, and patient satisfaction, and discusses professional perceptions and behaviors that lessen the likelihood that the patient will be satisfied.

REFERENCES

Adamson, T. E., & Watts, P. A. (1976). Patients' perceptions of maternity nurse practitioners. *Public Health Reports, 66,* 585–586.

Anderson, W. T., & Helm, D. T. (1979). The physician–patient encounter: A process of reality negotiation. In E. G. Jaco (Ed.), *Patients, physicians and illness* (3rd ed.). New York: Free Press.

Armstrong, D. (1984). The patient's view. *Social Science and Medicine, 18,* 737–744.

Ashworth, C. D., Williamson, P., & Montano, D. (1984). A scale to measure physician beliefs about psychosocial aspects of patient care. *Social Science and Medicine, 19,* 1235–1238.

Barr, J. K., & Steinberg, M. K. (1985). A physician role typology: Colleague and client dependence in an HMO. *Social Science and Medicine, 20,* 253–261.

Boreham, P., & Gibson, D. (1978). The informative process in private medical consultations: A preliminary investigation. *Social Science and Medicine, 12,* 409–416.

Buijs, R., Sluijs, E. M., & Verhaak, P. F. M. (1984). Byrne and Long: A classification for rating the interview style of doctors. *Social Science and Medicine, 19,* 683–690.

Buller, M. K., & Buller, D. B. (1987). Physicians' communication style and patient satisfaction. *Journal of Health and Social Behavior, 28,* 375–388.

Caterinicchio, R. P. (1979). Testing plausible path models of interpersonal trust in patient–physician treatment relationships. *Social Science and Medicine, 13A,* 81–99.

Danziger, S. K. (1986). The uses of expertise in doctor–patient encounters during pregnancy. In P. Conrad & R. Kern (Eds.), *The sociology of health and illness: Critical perspectives* (2nd ed.). New York: St.

Drew, J., Stoeckle, J. D., & Billings, J. A. (1983). Tips, status and sacrifice: Gift giving in the doctor–patient relationship. *Social Science and Medicine, 17,* 399–404.

Ford, A. B., Liske, R. E., Ort, R. S., & Denton, J. C. (1967). *The doctor's perspective: Physicians view their patients and practice.* Cleveland: The Press of Case Western Reserve University.

Frazier, P. J., Jenny, J., Bagramian, R. A., Robinson, E., & Proshek, J. M. (1977). Provider expectations and consumer perceptions of the importance and value of dental care. *American Journal of Public Health, 67,* 37–43.

Freidson, E. (1961). *Patients' views of medical practice.* New York: Russell Sage Foundation.

Gerbert, B. (1984). Perceived likeability and competence of simulated patients: Influence on physicians' management plans. *Social Science and Medicine, 18,* 1053–1059.

Ghodse, A. H. (1978). The attitudes of casualty staff and ambulance personnel towards patients who take drug overdoses. *Social Science and Medicine, 12,* 341–346.

Ghodse, A. H. (1979). Recommendations by accident and emergency staff about drug-overdose patients. *Social Science and Medicine, 13A,* 169–173.

Hall, J. A., Roter, D. L., & Rand, C. S. (1981). Communication of affect between patient and physician. *Journal of Health and Social Behavior, 22,* 18–30.

Hauser, S. T. (1981). Physician–patient relationships. In E. G. Mishler, L. R. Amarasingham, S. T. Hauser, R. Liem, S. D. Osherson, & N. E. Waxler (Eds.), *Social contexts of health, illness, and patient care.* London: Cambridge University Press.

Hayes-Bautista, D. E. (1978). Chicano patients and medical practitioners: A sociology of knowledges paradigm of lay-professional interaction. *Social Science and Medicine, 12,* 83–90.

Helman, C. G. (1985). Communication in primary care: The role of patient and practitioner explanatory models. *Social Science and Medicine, 20,* 923–931.

Heszen-Klemens, I., & Lapinska, E. (1984). Doctor–patient interaction, patients' health behavior and effects of treatment. *Social Science and Medicine, 19,* 9–18.

Hill, C. E. (1978). Differential perceptions of the rehabilitation process: A comparison of client and personnel incongruity in two categories of chronic illness. *Social Science and Medicine, 12,* 57–63.

Innes, J. M. (1977). Does the professional know what the client wants? *Social Science and Medicine, 11,* 635–638.

Kahn, L., Anderson, M., & Perkoff, G. T. (1973). Patient's perceptions and uses of a pediatric emergency room. *Social Science and Medicine, 7,* 155–160.

Kasteler, J., Kane, R. L., Olsen, D. M., & Thetford, C. (1976). Issues underlying prevalence of "doctor-shopping" behavior. *Journal of Health and Social Behavior, 17,* 328–339.

Keith, P. M., & Castles, M. M. (1975). Fear and rejection of patients by health practitioners. *Social Science and Medicine, 9,* 501–505.

Lederer, H. D. (1952). How the sick view their world. *Journal of Social Issues, 8,* 4–15.

Leiderman, D. B., & Grisso, J.-A. (1985). The Gomer phenomenon. *Journal of Health and Social Behavior, 26,* 222–232.

Liddell, A., & May, B. (1984). Patients' perceptions of dentists' positive and negative attributes. *Social Science and Medicine, 19,* 839–842.

Locker, D., & Dunt, D. (1978). Theoretical and methodological issues in sociological studies of consumer satisfaction with medical care. *Social Science and Medicine, 12,* 283–292.

Mathews, J. J. (1983). The communication process in clinical settings. *Social Science and Medicine, 17,* 1371–1378.

McCranie, E. W., Horowitz, A. J., & Martin, R. M. (1978). Alleged sex-role stereotyping in the assessment of women's physical complaints: A study of general practitioners. *Social Science and Medicine, 12,* 111–116.

McKinlay, J. B. (1975). Who is really ignorant—physician or patient? *Journal of Health and Social Behavior, 16,* 3–11.

Mirowsky, J., & Ross, C. E. (1983). Patient satisfaction and visiting the doctor: A self-regulating system. *Social Science and Medicine, 17,* 1353–1361.

Rosen, R. H. (1977). The patient's view of the role of the primary care physician in abortion. *American Journal of Public Health, 67,* 863–865.

Ross, C. E., & Duff, R. S. (1982). Returning to the doctor: The effect of client characteristics, type of practice, and experience with care. *Journal of Health and Social Behavior, 23,* 119–131.

Ross, C. E., Mirowsky, J., & Duff, R. S. (1982). Physician status characteristics and client satisfaction in two types of practice. *Journal of Health and Social Behavior, 23,* 317–329.

Roth, J. A. (1986). Some contingencies of the moral evaluation and control of clientele: The case of the hospital emergency service. In P. Conrad & R. Kern (Eds.), *The sociology of health and illness: Critical perspectives* (2nd ed.). New York: St. Martin's Press.

Sawyer, D. (1980). Normative conflict and physician use: A latent structure approach. *Journal of Health and Social Behavior, 21,* 156–169.

Shelp, E. E. (1984). Courage: A neglected virtue in the patient–physician relationship. *Social Science and Medicine, 18,* 351–360.

Sorenson, J. R. (1974). Biomedical innovation, uncertainty, and doctor–patient interaction. *Journal of Health and Social Behavior, 15,* 366–374.

Stewart, M. A. (1984). What is a successful doctor–patient interview? A study of interactions and outcomes. *Social Science and Medicine, 19,* 167–175.

Stiles, W. B., Putnam, S. M., & Jacob, M. C. (1982). Verbal exchange structure of initial medical interviews. *Health Psychology, 1,* 315–336.

Strauss, R. P. (1976). Sociocultural influences upon preventive health behavior and attitudes toward dentistry. *American Journal of Public Health, 66,* 375–377.

Strull, W. M., Lo, B., & Charles, G. (1984). Do patients want to participate in medical decision making? *Journal of the American Medical Association, 252,* 2990–2994.

Szasz, T. S., & Hollender, M. H. (1975). A contribution to the philosophy of medicine: The basic models of the doctor–patient relationship. In T. Millon (Ed.), *Medical behavioral science.* Philadelphia: Saunders. (Reprinted from *Archives of Internal Medicine,* 1956, *97,* 585–592).

Todd, C. J., & Still, A. W. (1984). Communication between general practitioners and patients dying at home. *Social Science and Medicine, 18,* 667–672.

Tuckett, D., & Williams, A. (1984). Approaches to the measurement of explanation and information-giving in medical consultations: A review of empirical studies. *Social Science and Medicine, 18,* 571–580.

Verbrugge, L. M. (1984). How physicians treat mentally distressed men and women. *Social Science and Medicine, 18,* 1–9.

Wartman, S. A., Morlock, L. L., Malitz, F. E., & Palm, E. (1981). Do prescriptions adversely affect doctor–patient relationships? *American Journal of Public Health, 71,* 1358–1361.

Westbrook, M. T., Nordholm, L. A., & McGee, J. E. (1984). Cultural differences in reactions to patient behaviour: A comparison of Swedish and Australian health professionals. *Social Science and Medicine, 19,* 939–947.

Wills, T. A. (1978). Perceptions of clients by professional helpers. *Psychological Bulletin, 85,* 968–1000.

Zyzanski, S. J., Hulka, B. S., & Cassel, J. C. (1974). Scale for the measurement of "satisfaction" with medical care: Modifications in content, format and scoring. *Medical Care, 12,* 611–620.

CHAPTER 16

Reciprocity in the Medical Encounter

Debra L. Roter

HISTORICAL PERSPECTIVE

Respect for the therapeutic power of the physician–patient relationship was well noted in antiquity and has been recognized in modern times. However, it is only since the mid-1960s that the actual dynamics of the therapeutic dialogue have been observed in any systematic manner. The evolution of methodological and technological sophistication has made observation and analysis easier over the years, and indeed, the number of empirical studies of physician–patient communication doubled between 1982 and 1987 to over 60 (Roter, Hall, & Katz, 1987a).

Several reviews of this body of work have been undertaken (Wasserman & Inui, 1983; Inui & Carter, 1985; Pendleton, 1983; Tuckett & Williams, 1984) but a resulting synthesis has been lacking; this is a difficult body of work to review. The predominantly exploratory nature of this research, which is almost entirely of the kind in which everything tends to be correlated with everything else (Hall, Roter, & Katz, 1988), contributes to an overwhelming number of results with which to contend. The results appear so confusing that Inui and Carter (1985), in reviewing this literature, characterized the findings as producing a "Rorschach test" for readers in which overall interpretations are as apt to reveal something about the reader as about the results themselves.

Nevertheless, a brief review of the three most often applied systems will be presented in an attempt to highlight methods of investigation and patterns of results which have provided a consistent thread through the literature. Further, several general conclusions will be drawn from the broad literature, based on quantitative summary of research findings, to illustrate that the collective body of research has greater order and consistency than prior reviews would suggest. Moreover, this review will demonstrate not only that unifying themes in the literature exist, but that these themes support a theory of interpersonal exchange within the medical encounter based on the concept of reciprocity.

Interaction Process Methods

Concerned with group dynamics, Bales (1950) developed an analysis scheme for assessing patterns of interaction, communication, and the decision-making processes of small

DEBRA L. ROTER • Department of Behavioral Sciences and Health Education, Johns Hopkins University School of Hygiene and Public Health, Baltimore, Maryland 21205.

groups. Since its original conceptualization, Bales's scheme has been more widely applied and modified than any other single approach to increase understanding of the dynamics of the medical encounter. Bales's approach focuses on ways in which the process and structure of communication among persons in a group reflects how they differentially participate in problem-solving. The theoretical rationale of Bales's method conceives of problem-solving in two domains: the task area and the socioemotional area. Interaction is described in terms of 12 mutually exclusive categories; 6 are conceived as affectively neutral and ascribed to the task dimension (i.e., gives suggestion or asks for orientation) and 6 are equally divided into positive and negative affective categories and ascribed to the social–emotional dimension (i.e., agrees or disagrees; shows tension release or shows tension).

Analysis using Bales's method is based on literal transcripts of the verbal events of the encounter which are operationally defined as the smallest discriminable speech segment to which the rater can assign classification. A unit may be as short as a single word or as long as a lengthy sentence; compound sentences are usually divided at the conjunction and sentence clauses are scored as separate units when they convey a single item of thought or behavior.

Application of Bales's System to Medical Encounters

In the first study to apply Bales's system to medical interactions, Davis (1968, 1971) audiotaped the concluding segment of 154 physician–patient visits at their first encounter, and subsequently recorded the entire follow-up visit for 80 of these pairs. Based on Bales's analysis of the audiotape transcripts, Davis manipulated the basic 12 category scores to derive indexes of communication difficulty and used factor analysis to reveal underlying dimensions of communication. These variables were then correlated with compliance with taking medication.

First visits, probably because they were recorded only in part, were unrelated to compliance. However, for revisits, Davis found that patients' compliance with taking medication was greatest when patients and physicians engaged in joking and laughter and when patients sought and received physicians' suggestions. Noncompliance was more likely when patients and physicians expressed disagreement.

Furthermore, visits characterized by physicians seeking information from patients without giving them any feedback were more likely to promote noncompliant behavior than any of the other communication patterns identified. Davis termed this type of exchange "nonreciprocal informativeness" and concluded that the imbalance in information exchange during the medical encounter was probably viewed by patients as a physician failure to meet expectations regarding normal interactive exchange. This failure, Davis suggested, inspired a retaliation through patient failure to adhere to therapeutic recommendations.

In a second study using a slight modification of Bales's original approach, Freemon, Negrete, Davis, and Korsch (1971) analyzed transcripts of 285 audiotapes of pediatric, walk-in visits. Patterns of communication in which physicians were friendly and approving, informative, and not excessively questioning were positively associated with patient satisfaction and therapeutic compliance. Again, a finding consistent with Davis's nonreciprocal informativeness was found. Physicians who did not allow their question asking to dominate the visit, and who provided information to their patients, inspired the best results in terms of patient satisfaction and compliance with taking medication.

Roter's Interaction Analysis System

Roter (1977) substantially modified Bales's approach to study interaction dynamics in routine medical encounters in three primary ways. First, identification and classification of verbal events were coded directly from audiotapes, making transcription unnecessary. The unit of analysis remained quite similar to Bales's but coders "unitize" speech as they listen to the audiotape. Second, because coding was done directly from audiotapes rather than transcripts, assessment of the tonal qualities of interaction was possible. These tonal qualities transmit the emotional context of the visit, and coders are asked to rate both patient and physician on global affective dimensions such as anger, anxiety, dominance, friendliness, or interest. Finally, categories of interaction were more finely tailored to the substance of the medical encounter than Bales's categories, but generally reflected similar groupings. For instance, categories of information-giving, instructions and directions, and counseling were substituted for Bales's original categories of giving orientation, suggestion, and opinion.

This system was used in a study evaluating a health education intervention to increase patient question-asking during routine medical encounters (Roter, 1977). Question-asking is a problem-solving, task-focused behavior that is relatively rare for patients. The study found that question-asking was doubled in the experimental group but that this increase was achieved at some emotional cost. Increased question-asking was associated with reduced patient sympathy and greater patient anger and anxiety during the encounter. It was also associated with reduced provider sympathy and increased provider anger and matter-of-factness. Experimental patients were less satisfied with their physician at an exit interview, but over the subsequent 6 months demonstrated significantly better appointment-keeping than the control group. Despite some of the negative affect produced in both patients and physicians, the increased appointment-keeping observed over the subsequent 6 months for this group of patients suggests that the task-focused behavior engaged in within the visit (e.g., question-asking) generalized to task-focused behavior subsequent to the visit, in the form of appointment-keeping compliance. Further, it was noted that patient satisfaction with the medical encounter was independent of the patient's commitment to task-focused behavior.

Verbal Response Mode

An alternative approach to Bales's process analysis and its derivatives, based on reference to linguistic theories, was introduced by Stiles, Putnam, Wolf, and James (1979) as the verbal response mode (VRM). This system is one in which segments of language, defined grammatically to be equivalent to one psychological unit of experience, form a taxonomy which implies a particular interpersonal intent or microrelationship between communicator and recipient. The taxonomy is based on the assignment of language segments to eight mutually exclusive categories by the source of experience, frame of reference, and focus. The categories include disclosure, questioning, edification, acknowledgment, advisement, interpretation, confirmation, and reflection.

The taxonomic groupings were used in studies to identify communication patterns related to patient satisfaction (Putnam, Stiles, Jacob, & James, 1985; Stiles, Putnam, Wolf, & James, 1979). These studies found that patient satisfaction was associated with communication patterns characterized by information exchange. Satisfaction was enhanced when patients were allowed to relate fully their medical history in the early part of the visit, without being impeded by close-ended questions, and when their physicians closed the visit with information-giving.

Inui, Carter, Kukull, and Haigh (1982) undertook an important comparative study of process analysis schemes contrasting Bales's original process analysis scheme, Roter's modification, and Stiles's VRM. The three interaction analysis systems were applied to 101 new-patient visits to a general medical clinic for which multiple outcomes had been determined. Within systems, cross tabulations and multiple regressions were performed to relate events during the encounter to outcomes. Across systems, multiple regression R^2 and R^2 adjusted (R^2_a) for the number of independent variables entering the analysis were used to characterize strength of relationships. Roter's system showed stronger relationships of knowledge (41% R^2, 27% R^2_a) and compliance (44% R^2, 28% R^2_a) to outcomes than did Bales's or Stiles's systems. R^2 for patient satisfaction was identical for Bales's and Roter's (35%) and greater than R^2 for Stiles's (14%).

GENERAL CONCLUSIONS DRAWN FROM THE LITERATURE

Additional methods for analyzing interaction are evident in the literature; however, none of these are widely applied and they infrequently appear in more than one or two studies. Although the other systems are comprised of unique configurations of variables, there are some categories of communication common to many of the systems.

In an attempt to summarize the common research findings represented in this body of literature, we have applied to it methods of META analysis (Hall *et al,* 1988). META analysis is the application of quantitative procedures for combining and comparing research results across studies. Because of the quantitative nature of this type of summary, stronger conclusions may be drawn regarding the state of the literature than through traditional literature reviews (Rosenthal, 1984). These methods included three kinds of analytic activities: exhaustive literature searches; the identification and conceptual grouping of variables addressed in the literature; and statistical summary of research results.

The literature review included a diligent search of the published, English-language literature for all studies which involved nonpsychiatric, medical encounters, for which there was a neutral observation (nonparticipant observers, audiotape, or videotape) and some result relating aspects of communication to patient or provider variables. Every variable addressed in a study was extracted, resulting in the identification of over 200 unique variables.

In order to facilitate conceptualization of the research domain and to make statistical summary possible, it was necessary to transform the many unique variables into meaningful groupings. This was accomplished by independent judges sorting variable descriptions, comparing their conceptual groupings and their assignment of variables to these groupings, and negotiating a consensus on five mutually exclusive categories: information-giving; question-asking; socioemotional behavior which included social conversation, positive talk, negative talk, and body movements; competence which included both a technical and an interpersonal dimension; and partnership-building. The last of these categories applies only to physician communication. The primary patient outcome variables considered were satisfaction, compliance, and recall of medical information transmitted during the medical encounter.

Of all the patient outcome variables considered, satisfaction had the most consistent relation to provider behavior. Satisfaction was best predicted by the amount of information given by providers during the medical encounter. It was also related to more communication overall, and particularly social conversation, conversation which could be construed as partnership-building, more immediate and positive nonverbal behavior, and positive talk. Satisfaction was also related to technical and interpersonal competence. Of the variables considered, only physician question-asking showed no relation to satisfaction.

Patient compliance was associated with patterns of provider behavior during the medical encounter which included more information-giving, fewer questions overall (but more questions about compliance in particular), more positive talk, and less negative talk. Finally, patient recall was best predicted by information-giving, less question-asking, more positive talk, and more partnership-building.

TOWARD A THEORY OF RECIPROCITY IN THE MEDICAL ENCOUNTER

Since the mid-1970s, Dr. Judith Hall and I have developed a conceptual framework for viewing the therapeutic relationship based on task-focused and socioemotional dimensions of behavior. Although explorations of these behaviors are often undertaken as if they were separate and distinct components of behavior, we suggest that they are integrated and largely inseparable in practice.

Task-Focused Domain

Physicians' task behaviors are defined as technically based skills used in problem-solving which comprise the base of the "expertness" for which a physician is consulted. These are essentially those behaviors which define the role of the physician and are close to the role conceptualizations proposed by Parsons (1951) and others (Bloom, 1963; Ben-Sira, 1980).

Much less attention has been devoted to a conceptualization of patient behavior *within* the medical encounter. We suggest that patient behavior also has a task dimension which reflects problem-solving skills. For instance, patient task behaviors include accurate and full reporting of current and past symptoms and medically relevant experiences, attentiveness, comprehension, and recall, and active participation in the care process. Further, although not directly articulated within the medical encounter, behaviors such as compliance, and utilization of care or services, are influenced by the dynamics of the encounter and may also be considered as part of patients' task functions.

Socioemotional Domain

The socioemotional dimension of behavior is more difficult to operationalize than the task dimension. Although patient behavior has received almost no attention in this regard, the role of affect in physician behavior has been considered from several viewpoints. Conceptualization of the appropriate expression of physician affect has varied tremendously from Parsons's (1951) view of affective neutrality, in which affect is controlled or ignored, to models in which expression of affect and task are distinguished as different types of communication which are both present during an interaction, but largely independent of one another (Bloom, 1963).

Our conceptualization differs from these models, and is premised on the belief that all face-to-face behavior, even that which is ostensibly neutral, carries affective content. This is true for both physicians and patients. The affective character of the interaction may be seen on three levels: (1) intrinsic, (2) conveyed, and (3) interpreted. The *intrinsic* level includes verbal exchanges with explicit socioemotional content such as social conversation, agreements, criticisms, statements of concern, reassurance, legitimation, partnership, and empathy. The basis of identification for these exchanges is face validity, i.e., the obvious and literal content of a communication.

The *conveyed* level of affect reflects those qualities of voice tone which carry emotional content. Our assessment process for this type of affect is to filter out the verbal content from audiotapes by passing them through an electronic band filter. This process preserves voice qualities such as syncopation, rhythm, and speed but obscures the verbal content. It is like listening to a conversation through a closed door, where one can hear only sounds, but not meaningful content. Independent raters have been shown to agree substantially on ratings of voice quality measured in this manner (Hall, Roter, & Rand,

Domain	Physician	Patient
Socioemotional	Explicit communication of affective content Conveyed affect (warmth, anxiety, empathy, dominance) Interpreted affect Interpersonal attitudes	Explicit communication of affective content Conveyed affect (warmth, anxiety, empathy, dominance) Interpreted affect Interpersonal attitudes Satisfaction Feelings of competence, confidence
Task	Question-asking Information-giving Counseling Management Treatment Referral Competence scores (tests of performance) Concordance on problem identification and treatment	Full and accurate report of medical symptoms Full and accurate report of medical history Comprehension and recall Compliance Alleviation of symptoms Improved functional status Improved social and work-related role performance Utilization Decreased morbidity Decreased mortality Concordance on problem identification and treatment

FIGURE 1. Exploration of the medical encounter.

1981). This conveyance of affect occurs during verbal exchanges that are intrinsically affective, as well as during the performance of task behaviors, i.e., giving information, counseling, and question-asking.

Finally, the *interpreted,* or attributed level of affect reflects the total impression created in the receivers of a communication. Particular communications may gain affective significance by virtue of attribution or interpretation that they do not possess either intrinsically or by how they are conveyed. For example, physicians who give information may be perceived as interested irrespective of whether they have expressed or conveyed interest through any other messages they may communicate to patients; or a patient may be perceived as bored or disinterested because of silence or a downward gaze of the eyes.

In addition to expressed emotion, interpersonal attitudes and satisfaction with the therapeutic relationship are also reflections of the socioemotional domain.

Conceptual Framework

Data accumulating from several years of research (e.g., Hall *et al.,* 1981, 1987; Roter *et al.,* 1987b) suggest that during the medical encounter, task behaviors and socioemotional communication by patients are fostered by parallel task behaviors and socioemotional communication by physicians.

Figure 1 displays a conceptual framework reflective of this perspective. The purpose of the framework is heuristic; its two dimensions separate physician and patient behaviors, as well as the task and socioemotional domains. Examination of Figure 1 suggests many important and largely uninvestigated relationships both between and within the four cells formed by these two factors.

Patient-Analogue Study

The framework may be viewed as a comprehensive matrix for hypothesis generation. With this framework in mind, we have conducted a patient-analogue study predicting relationships in the parallel and cross domains (Hall *et al.,* 1987; Roter *et al.,* 1987b).

The sources of data for these studies were audiotapes and transcripts of two different standardized patient cases presented by trained patient simulators to 43 primary care physicians. The simulated patients were four men in their late 50s each of whom in reality had a medical history consistent with one of the two scripted cases. The cases were designed to reflect a patient with chronic bronchitis in the first instance, and emphysema in the second. Both cases were exacerbated by smoking and prior noncompliance. The simulators were trained to represent the particulars of the scripted case fully and otherwise to react as they would in a medical encounter. They were instructed to answer questions in an open manner but not to initiate discussion regarding aspects of their medical history. Training was conducted by a team including a pulmonary specialist and behavioral scientists.

Transcripts of these audiotapes were scored, based on criteria generated by pulmonary experts, to determine physician proficiency in history-taking, physical examination, patient education, accuracy of diagnosis, and appropriate drug prescription. A score related to the number of relevant medical facts the physician should have elicited from the patient was also determined from the transcript. Transcripts were also subjected to analysis to assess the process and explicit content of the communication using the Roter method of interaction analysis.

Because there were no actual patients participating in this study, an attempt was made to explore likely patient reactions to the physicians' behavior in the recorded visits. This was done by by recruiting three different subjects to listen to each of the 86 audiotapes (total $N = 258$). The subjects were instructed to imagine that they were the patient, and afterwards, asked to rate the physicians on a variety of affective dimensions, to rate their satisfaction, and to complete an extensive recall measure of the medical information communicated to them during that visit. These subjects were "role-playing patients" and the results can only be described as likely patient outcomes. For this reason, the study must be considered an analogue and its results interpreted with some caution.

Finally, electronically filtered excerpts of the audiotapes were played to another group of 37 independent judges to assess voice quality.

Within-Domain Results

In regard to the task domains, we hypothesized that physician task relevant behaviors would predict parallel patient task behaviors. Our findings were quite convincing from the perspective of the role-playing patients and the performance of the simulated patients. Correlations between role-playing patient recall of medical information communicated to them and physician technical proficiency, information-giving, and counseling ranged from .40 to .71, all significant at the .01 level or lower. Correlations between information-giving and counseling and simulated patient disclosure were .42 and .37, respectively, again significant at .01. These findings suggest that patient and physician task domains are substantially related.

Within the socioemotional domains, we were particularly interested in conveyed affect and satisfaction. Satisfaction was measured by a single global item and two independent scales derived from factor analysis. The first scale was comprised of six items reflecting the physician's task or technical performance. The second scale was five items designed to reflect the physician's humaneness or interpersonal skill in the medical encounter.

We found that the role-playing patient ratings of satisfaction were related to aspects of affect conveyed through the filtered tape excerpts of physician speech. Excerpts rated high on anger and boredom were negatively correlated with satisfaction. When global satisfaction was more specifically broken down in terms of the two scales, anger was negatively correlated with both satisfaction dimensions ($-.30$, $p < .05$ for task, and $-.27$, $p < .10$ for humaneness) but boredom was negatively related only to the task dimension ($-.30$, $p < .05$). This implies that a physician who sounds angry will jeopardize patient satisfaction with his technical performance, as well as his interpersonal skills. Boredom conveyed through the physician's voice is likely to jeopardize patient satisfaction with only technical performance and does not appear to affect judgements of interpersonal skill.

In examining explicit verbal communication, we defined a socioemotional cluster to include social conversation, statements of approval, laughter and joking, and statements of agreement. This cluster was significantly correlated with technical performance satisfaction, but in the negative direction ($-.44$, $p < .01$) and unrelated to satisfaction with interpersonal skills.

Because voice quality and the socioemotional verbal cluster were uncorrelated, these effects are independent and therefore not two expressions of the same relationship. These results mean that physicians who engage in socioemotional conversation and *sound* bored are most likely to inspire patient dissatisfaction. This is reflected particularly in dissatisfaction with technical performance of care, implying that patients interpret this combination as a lack of technical proficiency rather than a lack of interpersonal skill.

The significant relations observed between role-playing patient and provider socioemotional behaviors support the prediction that behaviors within the socioemotional domain would be related. However, not all of the observed relations were as expected. Patient satisfaction with the task dimension of physician conduct is particularly sensitive to socioemotional verbal messages. As the socioemotional messages are nonmedical, by definition, a patient's negative view of this type of communication may reflect a perception of the physician as offtask or distracted, particularly when the physician sounded bored.

Satisfaction with the physician's interpersonal skills, on the other hand, appears adversely affected only by a physician who sounds angry, regardless of socioemotional verbal messages.

Cross-Domain Results

Most notable in this study are the cross-domain findings. There were no relationships uncovered between physicians' socioemotional behaviors and the role-playing patients' recall of medical information. We did find, however, a consistent pattern of association between physicians' task behaviors and role-playing patients' expressions of satisfaction.

Physicians' verbal behaviors categorized as information-giving and counseling, and physicians' actual clinical proficiency, were significantly related to role-playing patients' satisfaction with technical performance (correlations were .49 to .69, $p < .001$) but unrelated to their satisfaction with the physicians' interpersonal skills. However, these behaviors were also related to measures of interpreted affect. These are impressions of interest, calm, and friendliness attributed to the physician by the role-playing subjects.

The clinically proficient physician created an impression of interest (.54, $p < .001$), calm (.48, $p < .001$), and friendliness (.28, $p < .1$). Physicians who communicated relatively more medical information and devoted more communication to counseling were also perceived as interested and less bored than others (.39, .46, $p < .01$; and .28, $p < .1$, respectively).

We conclude from this that the manner in which task behaviors were performed was anything but neutral in its effect on patients. Substantial variation in physician voice quality *conveys* affective messages to patients during the performance of such routine task behaviors as information-giving and counseling. Moreover, patients *interpret* or attribute affective meaning to these behaviors by interpreting information-giving and counseling as behaviors which reflect physician interest in them.

In sum, these cross-domain findings are perhaps counterintuitive. Patient satisfaction and affective impressions of the physician were more strongly predicted by ostensibly neutral, task-oriented communications than by explicitly socioemotional communication or by nonverbal voice quality. We maintain that words reflecting socioemotional communication are not nearly as effective in conveying a consistent message of interest and concern as is task-oriented communication. These findings, however, are consistent with a growing literature demonstrating the efficacy of information-giving for a variety of therapeutic effects, including shortened hospital stays, decreased use of analgesics, and reduced patient anxiety, among others (Mumford, Schlesinger, & Glass, 1982). We suggest that the mechanism by which information achieves its therapeutic effects is both through the explicit content, as well as through the interpreted message of interest and caring.

META-Analysis Results

Because these findings were based on simulated patients and role-playing subjects, questions may be raised regarding generalizability. We explored this question by applying the results of our META analysis to our two-dimensional framework.

We found the strongest relationships between parallel domains. The median absolute correlation between physician task-related behaviors (information-giving, questions, and technical competence) and patient task behaviors (compliance and recall) was .24; the correlation between physician socioemotional behaviors (positive, social, and negative talk, interpersonal competence, and partnership-building) and patient satisfaction was .26. For cross-domains, we found that the median correlation between physician task behaviors and patient satisfaction was .22, but between physician socioemotional behaviors and patient task behaviors, only .10.

We believe than an explanatory mechanism for these patterns of results may be provided through the broad concept of reciprocity. (The concept of reciprocity is regarded as critically important to the understanding of social relations, yet remains remarkably ambiguous with few theorists posing an operational definition. For a history of the concept and attendent difficulties in definition, see the extensive discussion in Gouldner (1960).) Simply put, behaviors are generated by reciprocal, or like behaviors. Physician task behaviors and patient task behaviors reciprocate one another as do physician and patient socioemotional behaviors. We suggest, however, that reciprocated exchange is not equally operative across domains. We believe that physician task behaviors carry socioemotional significance for patients in two ways: through conveyance by voice quality and through interpretation. A physician who is proficient or informative, for instance, *sounds* interested and is *perceived* as interested and caring regardless of whether he or she expresses interest through specific socioemotional behaviors.

Because of the generalization of positive affect from the task domain, socioemotional reciprocation by the patient, expressed in satisfaction, can be expected. However, physicians' socioemotional behaviors do not convey sufficient task or technical significance to lead to a reciprocal task-relevant patient response. The physician who is socioemotionally expressive may inspire patient friendliness or liking, but this is not sufficient for a patient task response. Friendliness is not enough to motivate patients to attend to information, modify life-style, or adhere to a therapeutic regimen.

FUTURE DIRECTIONS

There are a number of fundamental issues with which the field of physician–patient interaction must contend for progress to continue; the need for guiding theoretical models, current methodological limitations, the application of research methods and results to physician training and assessment, and the changing nature of the therapeutic relationship are among these important considerations.

First and primary among these issues is the lack of theoretical models to guide investigators. This deficit has contributed to the largely exploratory nature of this work, resulting in a rather indiscriminate proliferation of findings with little conceptual framing of their meaning. In this regard the application of meta-analytic methods can be helpful in uncovering common underlying dimensions to this body of research.

Methodological limitations are evident in all systems of interactional analysis. There has yet to be developed a practical approach to accounting for interaction sequence in our analysis. A basic assumption has been that summary profiles based on frequencies of verbal behaviors during the encounter adequately reflect the communication process. However, as pointed out by Inui and Carter (1985), this is analogous to describing *Hamlet* as a play in which the principal characters include ghosts, witches, lords, ladies, officers, soldiers, sailors, messengers, and attendants—one of whom is already dead, one of whom dies by drowning, one by poisoned drink, two by poisoned sword, and one by sword and by drink!

The design of research in the field has been quite narrow, and almost entirely cross-sectional. Of the 61 studies reviewed by Roter *et al.* (1987a), only 2 followed the same patient–physician dyad prospectively, and that was only through two visits. Forty percent of the studies did not even specify whether the patient and physician were previously acquainted. Better specification of the ongoing relationship can be accomplished through more conscientious reporting by investigators and through more creative research designs.

Investigators have some responsibility to make their research methods and findings accessible to the clinical audience. Seven studies in the reviewed body of literature mentioned earlier (Roter *et al.*, 1987a) reflect some form of physician intervention, usually medical student or resident training. More intervention studies are needed in which teaching methods are evaluated in light of actual changes in physicians' communication style, and further, validated against changes in patient outcomes. Those physicians responsible for teaching clinical interviewing courses could particularly benefit from this area of work by collaborating with researchers to develop analysis schemes pertinent to quality of care assessment.

Application of research to patient interventions is also an important and relatively underdeveloped focus. The 3 studies of the 61 reviewed (Roter *et al.*, 1987a) that addressed patient interventions all found favorable effects. This is clearly an area that needs further elaboration and has tremendous potential for health education trials.

Finally, one further issue is worthy of consideration; the basic characteristics of the provider–patient relationship may be undergoing substantial evolutionary change (Inui & Carter, 1985). There is considerable evidence that patients are becoming more consumerist in orientation, and particularly the new generation of patients are likely to directly challenge physician authority within the medical encounter (Haug & Lavin, 1981). There is also evidence that physicians may be accommodating their patients with a more egalitarian relationship and tolerance for patient participation in decision-making. The implications of these changes are tremendous and they must be given full and serious consideration in conceptualizing how the patient–physician relationship may be articulated in the medical encounter.

In sum, important strides have been made in the understanding of physician–patient relations but challenges remain. The most significant of these is to push forward our conceptual and methodological imagination to approach the field in new and meaningful ways.

REFERENCES

Bales, R. F. (1950). *Interaction process analysis*. Reading, MA: Addison–Wesley.

Ben-Sira, Z. (1980). Affective and instrumental components in the physician–patient relationship: An additional dimension of interaction theory. *Journal of Health and Social Behavior, 21,* 170–180.

Bloom, S. (1963). *The doctor and his patient: A sociological interpretation*. New York: Russell Sage Foundation.

Davis, M. (1968). Variations in patients' compliance with doctors' advice: An empirical analysis of patterns of communication. *American Journal of Public Health, 58,* 274–288.

Davis, M. (1971). Variation in patients' compliance with doctors' orders: Medical practice and doctor–patient interaction. *Psychiatry in Medicine, 2,* 31–54.

Freemon, B., Negrete, V., Davis, M., & Korsch, B. (1971). Gaps in doctor patient communication. *Pediatric Research, 5,* 298–311.

Gouldner, A. W. (1960). The norm of reciprocity: A preliminary statement. *American Sociological Review, 25,* 161–179.

Hall, J. A., Roter, D. C., & Rand, C. S. (1981). Communication of affect between patient and physician. *Journal of Health and Social Behavior, 22,* 18–30.

Hall, J. A., Roter, D. L., & Katz, N. R. (1987). Task versus socioemotional behaviors in physicians. *Medical Care, 25,* 399–412.

Hall, J. A., Roter, D. L., & Katz, N. R. (1988). Meta-analysis of correlates of provider behavior in medical encounters. *Medical Care, 26.*

Haug, M. R., & Lavin, B. (1981). Practitioner or patient—Who's in charge? *Journal of Health and Social Behavior, 22,* 212–229.

Inui, T. S., & Carter, W. B. (1985). Problems and prospects for health services research on provider–patient communication. *Medical Care, 23,* 521–538.

Inui, T. S., Carter, W. B., Kukull, W. A., & Haigh, V. H. (1982). Outcome-based doctor-patient interaction analysis: I. Comparison of techniques. *Medical Care, 20,* 535–549.

Mumford, E., Schlesinger, H., & Glass, G. (1982). The effects of psychological intervention on recovery from surgery and heart attacks: An analysis of the literature. *American Journal of Public Health, 72,* 141–151.

Parsons, T. (1951). *The social system*. Glencoe, IL: Free Press.

Pendleton, D. (1983). Doctor–patient communication: A review. In D. Pendleton & J. Hasler (Eds.), *Doctor–patient communication* (pp. 5–53). New York: Academic Press.

Putnam, S., Stiles, W., Jacob, M., & James, S. (1985). Patient exposition and physician explanation in initial medical interviews and outcomes of clinical visits. *Medical Care, 23,* 74–82.

Rosenthal, R. (1984). *Meta-analytic procedures for social research*. Beverly Hills: Sage.

Roter, D. L. (1977). Patient participation in the patient–provider interaction. *Health Education Monographs, 5,* 281–315.

Roter, D. L., Hall, J. A., & Katz, N. R. (1987a). *Doctor–patient communication: A descriptive summary of the literature*. Unpublished manuscript.

Roter, D. L., Hall, J. A., & Katz, N. R. (1987b). Relations of physicians' task and socioemotional behaviors to analogue patients' satisfaction, recall, and impressions. *Medical Care, 25,* 437–451.

Stiles, W., Putnam, S., Wolf, M., & James, S. (1979). Interaction exchange structure and patient satisfaction with medical interviews. *Medical Care, 17,* 667–674.

Tuckett, D., & Williams, A. (1984). Approaches to the measurement of explanation and information-giving in medical consultations: A review of empirical studies. *Social Science and Medicine, 18,* 571–580.

Wasserman, R. C., & Inui, T. S. (1983). Systematic analysis of clinician–patient interactions: A critique of recent approaches with suggestions for future research. *Medical Care, 21,* 279–285.

CHAPTER 17

Affective Behavior and Perceptions of Health Professionals

Zeev Ben-Sira

INTRODUCTION

The first part of this chapter will probe into the accumulating evidence regarding the significance of physicians' "affective" (humane, person-oriented) behavior for the patients' well-being. That has been explained by the patients' likelihood to assess the quality of the treatment on the basis of the doctors' affective behavior, due to their inability to judge both the meaning of their somatic disturbance and the doctors' competence. The first part of this chapter addresses the question as to whether this type of layperson's assessments both of the effectiveness of the technical (instrumental) medical activities and of the physician's competence are dependent on the physician's formal qualifications (i.e., certified "specialists" *vis-à-vis* "generalists") and on the seriousness (verified professionally) of the patient's health condition (i.e., chronic disease). The second part summarizes accumulating evidence regarding physicians' likelihood both to recognize the therapeutic importance of, and to engage in affective behavior as a component of the medical intervention.

STRESS–DISEASE RELATIONSHIP AND THE PATIENTS' PERCEPTIONS

Coping Insufficiency and Disease: Analytical Framework

Stress–Disease Relationship. Accumulating evidence suggests that psychosocial stress eventually fulfills a causal contributory function in the onset and severity of disease (Jensen, 1981; Lown, 1983; Norbeck & Peterson-Tilden, 1983; Sklar & Anisman, 1981). According to this evidence, disease has been conceptualized as an expression of "breakdown" in the wake of a prolonged failure to restore the emotional homeostasis which has been disturbed due to insufficient coping with the demands of life (Antonovsky, 1979; Ben-Sira, 1985b; Cohen, 1985).

In addition to the contributory role of stress in the onset and severity of the disease,

ZEEV BEN-SIRA • School of Social Work, The Hebrew University of Jerusalem, Mount Scopus, Jerusalem 91905, Israel.

disease by itself may produce an array of stressors. The patients' perception of the severity and prognosis of their somatic disturbance, their incompetence to judge the quality and efficacy of the technical medical activities, and medicine's frequent inability to give an immediate solution to the somatic problem are evidently the most salient, disease-generated stressors (Ben-Sira, 1976, 1980a, 1982a,b; Cousins, 1983). Acknowledgment of the doctors' competence and of the effectiveness of the medical treatment may fulfill a reassuring, hence tension-alleviating function and consequently promote recovery. Yet patients lack the proficiency for judging both the physicians' competence and the effectiveness of the technical medical activities.

The Intimidating Potential of Fragmentary Knowledge. Emerging consumerist activities which are aimed at enhancing the patients' autonomy (Betz & O'Connel, 1983; Haug, 1976; Haug & Lavin, 1981) seem hardly efficacious for improving the patients' capacity of judging the complex nature of diagnoses and decisions based on medical knowledge. Moreover, diffusion of information through health education and the media has familiarized large parts of the population with the limitations of medicine and alerted them to occasional deleterious mistakes of physicians (Clute, 1963; Fitts & Fitts, 1955; Mechanic, 1976, p. 272; Wallis, 1986). Thus, diffusion of knowledge may frequently intimidate patients, rather than enhance their reassurance. Publication of "do-it-yourself" health handbooks (e.g., Sehnert & Eisenberg, 1975; Vickery & Fries, 1976) aimed at facilitating and legitimizing both self-care and some control over physicians' decisions in case they do turn to them for help (Haug, 1976; Hayes-Bautista, 1976), seem hardly likely to give reassurance when medical help is needed. In fact, such lay knowledge may increase the salience of somatic disturbances. Thus, when laypersons ultimately reach the point when professional help is necessary, it will largely be perceived as the result of their own failure to solve the problem. They will then be emotionally disturbed by its suspected seriousness—the latter evidently being the decisive factor in medical help-seeking (Ben-Sira, 1980b, 1982b; Kasteler, Kane, Olson, & Thetford, 1976; Wan & Soifer, 1974). Under such circumstances, patients may hardly feel able to "control" their doctors' medical activities. Indeed, there is evidence that the more patients perceive their condition as serious, and concomitantly believe in their doctors' competence, the less they are likely to question their authority (Haug & Lavin, 1981, p. 223).

Upon entering a relationship with a doctor, patients have two goals: a manifest goal of solving a somatic problem, and a latent one of seeking relief for their anxiety (Cartwright, 1976, p. 25), the latter evidently being the dominant (though latent) goal in help-seeking (Ben-Sira, 1976, 1980b). Yet, as medical intervention *per se* is frequently unable to provide an immediate solution to the problem, medical intervention as such is unable to relieve the patient's anxiety. Moreover, anxiety may increase as a result of conjecture about the possibility of mistakes, and of the patients' incompetence in judging the quality and efficacy of the medical activities (Ben-Sira, 1976, 1980a, 1982a,b; Ross, Wheaton, & Duff, 1981).

The Tension-Alleviating Function of Affective Behavior

Lay Judgment versus Professional Recognition of Competence. How, then, can the patient's anxiety be alleviated? Accumulating evidence shows that when the practitioner's specific professional activities are accompanied by "affective" behavior toward the patient as a human being, it may fulfill an anxiety-alleviating function (Kosa & Robertson, 1969). Evidently, patients lacking the competence for judging the *content* of the physician's medical activities, base their judgment on the *mode* of their presentation—hence, the physicians' *affective* behavior toward them. Affective behavior serves as a basis by which patients tend to judge the quality and efficacy of the medical intervention and hence gain reassurance (Ben-Sira, 1976, 1980a, 1982a,b; Leigh & Reiser, 1980, p. 292). Affective behavior then may contribute to promoting recovery (Egberg, Battit, Welch, & Battlet, 1964; Hall, Roter, & Rand, 1981; Hellerstein & Ford, 1960; Ley & Spelman, 1967; Ross *et al.*, 1981).

Empirical evidence regarding the patients' likelihood of judging medical competence on the basis of the physicians' affective behavior in ambulatory settings has so far been derived predominantly from general practice (Ben-Sira, 1976; 1982a; Hornung & Massagli, 1979). The main justifications for concentrating on this level of medical practice were both its being the first level to which suffering persons turn in their distress (Ben-Sira, 1980b; Tessler, Mechanic, & Dimond, 1976), and its "general" nature, which has often been interpreted as representing a comprehensive approach toward the patient as a human being *vis-à-vis* the presumed fragmental approach of specialists. Conceivably, however, in an era of specialization, "general" practice may be interpreted as lacking the specific competence for treating effectively these problems which the laypersons were incompetent to overcome (Clute, 1963; Hadley & Crispen, 1978; Korman, Pate, & Chapman, 1980; McPhee, 1984). Under these circumstances, the search for "clues" on the basis of which laypersons may assess the physicians' competence seems plausible.

Contrary to the "general" practitioner, "specialist" by definition, implies having the competence, recognized by the professional community, for treating a specific domain of somatic disturbances. Does this evident recognition of competence eliminate the patient's use of the physician's affective behavior as a basis for assessing the physician's competence?

In several studies, the crucial test of the importance of the physician's affective behavior has been the patient's choice of an alternative treatment agent when dissatisfied with the initial treatment agent. Evidence based on general practitioners revealed that dissatisfied patients preferred "affectively" oriented (private fee for service) practitioners over an "instrumentally" proficient agent (i.e., hospital outpatient facilities) as an alternative (Ben-Sira, 1976, 1982a). To what extent does this pattern apply also in case of dissatisfaction with specialists' ambulatory treatment?

Severity of the Somatic Disturbance and Choice of Alternative. Since the patients' anxiety is largely a consequence of their subjective lay assessments of both the meaning and the seriousness of their somatic disturbances, one way that physicians' affective behavior alleviates this anxiety is by providing reassurance about the significance of the disturbance. Preference for "affective" agents then is motivated by the search for such reassurance. What then would be the preferred alternative when the condition has already been expertly diagnosed? For a person with a chronic disease, for example, the occurrence of new symptoms is likely to be related to that disease and interpreted as indicative of further health deterioration. Preference for an alternative with the highest expertise and the best equipment i.e., the hospital's outpatient service—would then seem logical. To what extent would practitioners' affective behavior still be a significant factor in the choice between alternatives?

THE STUDY

Scope

The scope of this study is the extent to which the importance of the physician's affective behavior toward the patient is dependent on the physician's formally certified qualifications and on the seriousness of the patient's professionally verified health condition.

METHOD

Sample and Field Work. A representative sample of the adult (age 20+) Israeli Jewish population (N = 1141) (for specification of the sample see the Appendix) was investigated using a closed-ended questionnaire presented to respondents by interviewers in the respondents' homes during January 1981. The items concerning this specific study were part of a broader project on utilization patterns, and on perceptions of the medical services in Israel, commissioned by the Israeli Ministry of Health and carried out by the author in the Israel Institute of Applied Social Research.

Measures: (1) Satisfaction with the Physician's Behavior. Measures identical to those in previous physician–patient interaction studies (Ben-Sira, 1976, 1980a, 1982a) were employed for obtaining the layperson's assessment (i.e., satisfaction) of the physician's affective and instrumental (medical treatment) behavior. Two sets of identical items were employed for measuring the respondent's satisfaction with the general practitioners and specialists upon recent visits, as specified in the following two paragraphs.

(2) Instrumental Component (Medical Treatment). Three items were used as measures of the extent to which the patients' interactions with the physician satisfied their expectations regarding why they turned to the physician, namely solution of their health problem. Hence, the questions focused on the "content" of the practitioner's activities: (a) *skills* in coping with the problem posed ("Did the doctor give you a feeling that he knows how to cope with problems such as yours? 1 = always . . . 7 = never); (b) suitability of *treatment* ("Did the doctor give the required treatment? 1 = always . . . 7 = never); (c) *reassurance* potency of the treatment given by the doctor (Did the doctor give you a feeling of reassurance? 1 = always . . . 7 = never).

(3) Affective Component of the Treatment. Affective behavior was defined as behavior directed by the physician toward the patient as a person rather than as a "case." Here the focus is on the *mode* of the physician's behavior. Hence, respondents were asked about the extent to which their physicians: (a) allocate sufficient *time* for allowing satisfactory presentation and discussion of the patients' problems (1 = definitely sufficient time . . . 4 = much too little); (b) show sufficient *interest* in the patient as a person (. . . show interest in your personal problems? 1 = definitely sufficient time . . . 4 = much too little); (c) demonstrate sufficient *devotion* to the management of the problems presented; (d) *listen attentively* (1 = definitely sufficient time . . . 4 = much too little).

(4) Level of Professional Competence. Respondents were presented with a card showing a ladder of nine numbered rungs: 1 = highest possible . . . 9 = lowest level of professional competence, and were asked to evaluate the professional competence of the physicians of the clinic or health organization with which they were affiliated, based on their own experience.

(5) Preferred Solution for Unsatisfactory Treatment. In Israel, almost the entire population has health insurance on a completely prepaid basis which prescribes the patient's affiliation with a specific clinic or physician. If a patient takes the initiative in turning to an alternative agency when dissatisfied with a treatment, this requires a payment in addition to the monthly fees to the health insurance plan. The common alternatives are (a) a private practitioner, (b) a hospital's outpatient clinic, or (c) a hospital's emergency ward. As indicated in earlier studies (Ben-Sira, 1976, 1982a), the hospital's facilities are characterized

by a high level both of professional competence and of technology (*instrumental* component of treatment) yet lack the personal atmosphere (*affective* component) of the private practitioner. In contrast, the private practitioner lacks the easy access both to high-ranking professional advice and to advanced technology (*instrumental*), yet may be motivated, frequently because of self-interest (attracting clientele) (Ben-Sira, 1985a, 1986b,c; Hall, 1964), to demonstrate *affective* behavior. As in earlier studies (Ben-Sira, 1976, 1982a), turning to a private practitioner was used as a measure of preference for the *affective* component if dissatisfied with treatment (*instrumental*). Turning to one of a hospital's outpatient facilities was used as a measure of preference for the *instrumental*. Respondents were asked: "In the last year [12 months], when you were dissatisfied with the treatment by your general practitioner/specialist or when you thought that you would not get the required treatment, did you turn, on your own initiative and by paying for it, to a private practitioner/hospital outpatient clinic/hospital emergency ward? Responses were coded as follows: *Yes:* 1 = 4+ times . . . 4 = once; *No* = did you ever—when? 5 = during the recent two years? 6 = a longer time ago? 7 = never.

(6) Chronic Disease. The respondents were asked whether they suffer from one or more of the following physician-diagnosed chronic diseases: (a) high blood pressure, (b) heart disease, and (c) diabetes. These diseases were chosen because of their imminent potential of imposing an enduring threat of further deterioration of the health conditions (i.e., "stress potential") and their requiring periodic, professionally competent checkups.

Results

Satisfaction and Assessment of Professional Competence. For both general practitioners and specialists the strength of the relationship between assessment of professional competence and satisfaction with the physicians' "affective" behavior is similar to that for satisfaction with the instrumental behavior (Table 1). However, the correlations between satisfaction with "affective" behavior and the assessment of competence are weaker for specialists than for general practitioners (average correlations for specialists are .50 and .49 compared to .70 and .65 for general practitioners). This evidently reflects the impact, discussed earlier, of the specialist's reputation which, by definition, recognizes the specialist as more competent. This thus reduces the importance of patient satisfaction in the assessment of the specialist's competence.

Preferred Alternative. Despite the lesser importance of satisfaction in the assessment of the specialists' competence, dissatisfaction with their *instrumental* (i.e., medical) performance is nonetheless more likely to lead to an *affective* rather than an *instrumental* solution (μ_2 with private practitioner = −.39, with hospital outpatient clinic −.26, with emergency unit −.12). Similarly, dissatisfaction with general practitioners' instrumental performance is equally likely to result in an affective solution (μ_2 = −.39) (see Table 2).

Health Status and Preferred Alternative. Utilization of alternative treatment agents by dissatisfied chronically sick persons follows a pattern similar to that of others in the population (Table 3). Both the chronically sick and the others are more likely to turn, in the case of dissatisfaction, to a private practitioner (18% and 21%, respectively) than to a hospital's outpatient clinic (6% of chronically sick; 12% of the others), or to an emergency unit (10% and 13%, respectively). In proportional terms, when seeking an alternative, the chronically sick are relatively more likely than the others to prefer private practitioners over hospital outpatient facilities. Particularly noteworthy is the decrease in preference

TABLE 1. Correlations (μ_2)[a] between Patients' Assessment of Professional Competence and Satisfaction with Physicians' Instrumental and Affective Behavior (General Practitioners and Specialists)

Satisfaction with the physicians' behavior		Correlation (μ_2)[a] with assessed professional competence of:	
Component	Item	General practitioner	Specialist
Instrumental	Skills	.67	.53
	Treatment	.70	.50
	Reassurance	.74	.48
	Average μ_2	.70	.50
Affective	Time	.68	.49
	Interest	.58	.39
	Devotion	.71	.60
	Listening	.62	.48
	Average μ_2	.65	.49

[a] As in the previous studies (Ben-Sira, 1976, 1980a, 1982a), use was made of the Weak Monotonicity Coefficient (μ_2) (Guttman & Levy, 1975; Rave, 1978). The peculiar property of this coefficient is that it does not assume a linear relationship. This property is particularly appropriate in the social sciences where frequently linear relationships cannot be assumed. The formula for μ_2 is as follows: Given n pairs of observations on numerical variables (x,y), (x_i,y_i) $(i = 1, 2, \ldots, n)$, then:

$$\mu_2 = \frac{\sum_{h=1}^{n}\sum_{i=1}^{n}(x_h - x_i)(y_h - y_i)}{\sum_{h=1}^{n}\sum_{i=1}^{n}|x_h - x_i||y_h - y_i|}$$

for hospital outpatient clinics with the deterioration of the health status (12% of the dissatisfied without a chronic condition, compared to 8% with one, and 3% with two or three preferred a hospital outpatient clinic). Inferentially, then, it appears that for chronically sick persons, the "affective" component of the medical intervention is of even greater significance than for others.

TABLE 2. Average Correlations (μ_2) between Turning to Alternative Treatment Agents and Satisfaction with Physicians' Affective and Instrumental Behavior

	Average correlation (μ_2) between turning to alternative and satisfaction with			
	General practitioners'		Specialists'	
Alternative treatment agent	Instrumental behavior	Affective behavior	Instrumental behavior	Affective behavior
Private practitioner	−.39	−.14	−.39	−.16
Hospital outpatient clinic	−.21	−.16	−.26	−.13
Hospital emergency unit	−.25	−.15	−.12	−.07

TABLE 3. Preference (in Percents) of Alternative Treatment Agent in Case of Dissatisfaction with Physician according to Health (Numbers in Parentheses indicate *N*)[a]

Alternative treatment agent	Percentage reporting utilization of alternatives (last year) because of dissatisfaction				
	One chronic condition	Two or three chronic conditions	Total chronic conditions	No chronic conditions	Total population
Private practitioner	18	18	18	21	21
	(146)	(54)	(200)	(838)	(1038)
Hospital outpatient clinic	8	3	6	12	11
	(146)	(55)	(201)	(834)	(1035)
Hospital emergency unit	13	8	10	13	12
	(146)	(55)	(201)	(832)	(1033)

[a] *N* refers to number of respondents who reported having any contact with a physician during the recent 12 months. Differences in *N* due to "missing data" (no response).

THE PHYSICIANS' AFFECTIVE BEHAVIOR: IMPORTANCE AND DEMONSTRATION

The Need for Affective Behavior

Affective Behavior: A Universal Need in Medical Treatment. These data contribute further to the understanding of the importance of the physician's affective behavior for the patient's assessment of the physician's competence. They expand the conclusions of earlier studies (Ben-Sira, 1976, 1980a,b, 1982a,b). The significance of the physician's affective behavior for the patient's well-being is independent both of the physician's institutionally acknowledged competence (specialist) and of the severity of the somatic disturbance (chronic disease). Of particular significance is the proportionally lesser likelihood of dissatisfied chronic patients to prefer evidently proficient agents (i.e., hospital facilities) as a desired alternative. Their preference of an affective solution (i.e., private practitioner) alludes to the plight of the chronically sick person.

Chronic Disease and Affective Behavior. The case of chronic disease is particularly illustrative of the significance of incorporating affective behavior as an inherent component of the medical interventions. In terms of the prevailing approaches to the stress and disease relationship (Antonovsky, 1979; Ben-Sira, 1985b; Cohen, 1985), stress (i.e., unresolved "stressors") presumably played a contributory role in the etiology of conditions. Moreover, chronic disease, particularly the diagnoses presented herein (i.e., high blood pressure, diabetes, and heart disease), may impose additional, presumably insurmountable demands upon the afflicted individuals. Demands may emerge from their perceptions of their permanent impairment and from the constant fear of a further deterioration of their condition with its potential of depriving them abruptly or gradually of their control of their entire life. The afflicted individuals and their primary lay network may feel helpless and incompetent both to interpret the patients' sensations and to affect their physical conditions substantially. It follows then that any effort at improving, or at least arresting, the deterioration of the sick person's emotional state may point to the need for competent professional help. Indeed, as expected, visits to the physician increase with the deterioration of health conditions from an average of 10 yearly visits for those without any of these three conditions, to 38 for those suffering from all three. Interpretation of data from a recent study (Ben-Sira, 1984) suggests that for chronically sick persons, "professional emotional support, particularly that of a physician, is the most sought for, yet the least attainable, for alleviating the individual's distress" (p. 732).

The Physicians' Attitude toward Affective Behavior

Distinction between the Affective and Instrumental Components. Patients' perception of physicians' reluctance to incorporate affective behavior in medical treatment evidently conforms with physicians' attitudes on this issue. Evidence suggests that the physicians are less likely both to attribute therapeutic significance to, and to demonstrate, affective behavior than instrumental behavior (Ben-Sira, 1986a, p. 99). Moreover, the physicians sharply distinguish between the affective and the instrumental components of their activities—frequently perceiving one as contradictory to the other. Even specialists in family medicine—a recognized medical specialization that advocates a "biopsychosocial" approach—do not differ in their attitudes and likelihood of demonstrating affective behavior from other primary care physicians. They, even more than the others, differentiate between both aspects of intervention (Ben-Sira, 1985a). Evidence thus contradicts the ideology of family medicine—a model which advocates relating to the patients' and their families' psychosocial problems as an inherent component of medical interventions (Engel, 1977; Henao, 1985; Mauksch, 1974; Miller, 1972; Pattison & Anderson, 1978; Ransom, 1985). This trend presumably reflects the dominance of the biomedical model in medical practice (Eisenberg & Kleinman, 1981, pp. 11–12). The biomedical orientation, together with the necessity of commanding a constantly accumulating body of medical knowledge (Lown, 1983), leads to increasingly narrow and in-depth biomedical specializations. Schlesinger (1985, pp. 138–140) argued that "major advances in medical techniques generated a tendency to treat diseased organs without paying attention to the person . . . suffering from the disease." The patients' emotional disturbance, if the physicians are attentive to it, is often regarded as an obvious accompaniment of the somatic disturbance, hence "naturally" will be resolved upon the solution of that disturbance (Balint, 1957; Balint, Hunt, Joyce, Marinker, & Woodcock, 1970; Leigh & Reiser, 1980, p. 25). Emotional support activities may thus be considered by physicians as a time-consuming luxury, coming at the expense of treating the "real" medical problem (Tuckett, 1976, pp. 193–194). A dilemma of allocation of time between "instrumental" (biomedical) and affective behavior may indeed confront a physician in hospital wards, in particular when dealing with urgent life- or limb-saving procedures (Tuckett, 1976, pp. 193–194). Yet such a dilemma seems hardly relevant for ambulatory care. Thus, the biomedical orientation per se can hardly be considered a sufficient explanation for the frequent reluctance of ambulatory care practitioners (general practitioners or specialists) to demonstrate affective behavior. What then may account for such a reluctance?

Affective Behavior: A Reward-Depriving Input. Ben-Sira (1986a), in a recent study, suggested viewing the practitioner's reluctance to demonstrate "affective" behavior to be a consequence of the exchange relationship that characterizes the physician–patient interaction (Ben-Sira, 1972; Betz & O'Connel, 1983). In fact, inherent in the nature of affective behavior are several characteristics that may make it seem unrewarding—and consequently make the interaction with the patient seen as "punishing" (Ben-Sira, 1986a, pp. 88–104).

Affective behavior is essentially aimed at bridging the intimidating status-gap between the physician and the patient. Leigh and Reiser (1980, pp. 292–293) maintained that "the friendly and nonjudgmental, but at the same time professional interest and concern that are manifested toward the patient by the physician . . . provide an interpersonal base for reassurance and for the relief of tension . . . when [the patient] can share with the doctor personal worries, problems, guilts, and anxieties . . . [similarly] it is important for the physician . . . to share . . . [the] rationale, strategy, and meaning [of the diagnostic procedures] with the patient . . ." regarding the etiology, diagnosis, and treatment (DiMatteo & Friedman, 1980, p. 132; Ross *et al.*, 1981).

Essentially, then, affective behavior toward patients comprises both tolerance for (or even interest in) the patients' idiosyncratic viewpoints and provision of lay intelligible explanations (Ben-Sira, 1976, 1980a, 1982a). Physicians, however, may perceive such behavior as a threat both to their *expert authority* (Haug, 1976; Haug & Lavin, 1981; Stimson & Webb, 1979) and to the *competence gap*—a gap which legitimizes the physicians' dominance (Weitzkin & Stoeckle, 1976). Conceivably then, affective behavior is likely to be valued by physicians as depriving them of the rewards inherent in their superior status (Ben-Sira, 1986a, pp. 108–121). Dismissing as bothersome and time-wasting both the patients' plea for explanations and their offering—in the doctors' eyes—irrelevant information, may illustrate the practitioners' effort to maintain the rewarding competence gap (Weitzkin & Stoeckle, 1976). Insisting on bringing up questions and suggestions contrary to the physician's request, carries the danger of being labeled as "demanding" or even "noncooperative" patients. Noncooperation is frequently viewed by doctors as a serious obstacle to applying their expertise for the patients' benefit (DiMatteo & Friedman, 1980, pp. 49–50; Leigh & Reiser, 1980, p. 17). Hampering physicians from applying their expertise justifies defining such a patient as "bad," ultimately legitimizing the withdrawal of help. Evidence alludes that the "bad patient" label indeed fulfills a status-securing function (Ben-Sira, 1986a, pp. 108–121).

Institutionalized Ambulatory Care, Reward Deprivation, and Affective Behavior. Obviously, "status" is only one basically "extrinsic" reward. Evidently, practicing medicine has the potential of eliciting an array of "intrinsic" gratifications inherent in the application and advance of professional knowledge. That, however, requires a practice that has the potential of eliciting such rewards. It necessitates a type of practice offering professional challenges in terms of a diversity of relatively severe diagnoses, where success is within the bounds of possibility and the follow-up of improvement is both feasible and attributable to the practitioner's intervention. Hospital care of acute, relatively severe cases exemplifies such a type of stimulating practice. On the other hand, however, recent evidence (Ben-Sira, 1986b) suggests that ambulatory care (both general practitioners and specialists) has much less capability for eliciting such intrinsic rewards. Evidently, the least rewarded are the salary employed general practitioners and specialists in ambulatory facilities—as suggested by data from an Israeli study (Ben-Sira, 1986b). Being deprived of both intrinsic and extrinsic (monetary remuneration) rewards from interaction with their patients, they evidently are more likely than the others to seek their rewards in the status gap. Inferentially, then, they are less likely than the others to demonstrate the reward-depriving, affective behavior (Ben-Sira, 1986a, pp. 105–107).

The data showing the greater likelihood of private fee-for-service practitioners demonstrating affective behavior (Ben-Sira, 1986a, p. 106) thus seem rather plausible. For the private practitioner, affective behavior may fulfill a crucial role in the competition for clients (p. 107) and frequently providing some protection from consumerist groups' pressure (Haug, 1976; Haug & Lavin, 1981). The currently flourishing commercial advertisements of competing medical facilities in the United States, highlighting both their affective ("warmth") and instrumental ("excellence") qualities, confirm this. These conclusions are congruent with the evidence that patients are more satisfied with the care given by private fee-for-service practitioners when dissatisfied with the treatment rendered by the physicians in the health agency to which they are affiliated.

The data suggest also that the physicians are implicitly aware of the reward value of their affective behavior. However, in view of the biomedical approach which questions the therapeutic significance of affective behavior (Ben-Sira, 1986a, p. 99), physicians' readiness to provide such "rewards" is contingent on the profits they may derive from them.

Chronic Disease and Affective Behavior. The preceding analysis furthers understanding of the problems in incorporating emotional support in the medical care of the chronically sick. A chronic, incurable condition can hardly elicit the "intrinsic" rewards that are inherent in the challenge of curing severe cases which have some potential of recovery. Moreover, the physicians' recognition of their inability to improve the patients' condition substantially (i.e., curing them) with the help of medicine's present technology, and hence their inability to respond to the patients' pleas for help, may constitute a sense of failure to live up to their role (Tuckett, 1976, pp. 196–197). That in turn may lead to defensive behavior by avoiding as much as possible confronting the patient—a behavior which is frequently justified by the necessity to allocate the scarce resources (the doctors' time) mainly to those who are likely to benefit the most from the doctors' interventions.

Thus, both the "profitless," and frequently "punishing" interaction with chronically sick persons, and the *a priori* rejection of the therapeutic significance of "affective" behavior make the physician's capacities to alleviate a chronically sick person's emotional disturbance rather dubious.

Compensation by Other Health Professionals. Could other health professionals possibly compensate for the doctors' reluctance to demonstrate affective behavior? Evidence suggests that the effectiveness of such compensation by health professionals, such as social workers, is rather dubious (Ben-Sira and Kacen, 1988). This should be understood in light of the assumption that such anxiety will not be alleviated simply because of the emotional support of the affective behavior per se. It is rather because the alleviation of anxiety is presumed to be a result of its providing the patient with "clues" for assessing the technical medical (instrumental) activities—hence fulfilling a reassuring function for the patient (Ben-Sira, 1982b).

In light of the apparently unavoidable medicalization of everyday life (Illich, 1976), the relevance of affective behavior as a "clue" is evidently acceptable only if it is elicited by an agent recognized as competent for dealing with health care—namely a physician.

CONCLUSIONS

Accumulating evidence highlights the significance of incorporating affective behavior as an inherent component in medical interventions. The importance of this behavior for the patient's well-being is independent of the level of treatment and the seriousness of the health disturbance. In fact, it appears that the less the chances for cure are, the greater the importance of the physician's affective behavior.

Contrary to patients' needs, however, there are evidently forces inherent in the medical profession counteracting physicians' motivations to incorporate such behavior. The biomedical orientation which both directs the focus on the somatic disturbance rather than on the person, and requires increasingly narrowing specializations, evidently brings about depreciation of the therapeutic significance of affective behavior. That, together with its reward-depriving nature, make demonstration of affective behavior as part of the medical intervention rather dubious.

It should be pointed out that these conclusions are to a great extent inferred from the existing body of knowledge, but require further empirical verification. To the extent that empirical evidence from comprehensive studies supports these conclusions, insights may be drawn about the factors which could potentially enhance the likelihood of incorporating affective behavior as an inherent component of medical treatment. At this stage, following the inferences from existing evidence it may be suggested that both the biomedical orientation and reward-oriented professional dominance play a crucial role in the decline of the likelihood of demonstrating affective behavior. The fact that private fee-for-service solo practitioners and the physicians employed by competing facilities are more likely than others to integrate affective behavior because of its remunerative potential, may give rise to questions about whether advances of medical knowledge promise needed *health* care (*vis-à-vis medical* care)—health comprising more than merely organic functioning. The issue seems particularly problematic for those who are in the greatest need of it—such as lower-class or chronically sick patients.

Thus, questions may be raised as to the extent to which medical intervention is gauged at meeting the needs of health as defined by the WHO—health comprising "a state of complete physical, mental and social wellbeing."

Further study is needed to pry into the factors that may further the likelihood of viewing health care as an integrated psychosocial and biomedical endeavor.

APPENDIX: SAMPLE CHARACTERISTICS

A representative sample comprising 1200 Jewish adults (aged 20+ years) was systematically drawn from the Israeli voting register, which is the relatively most reliable updated listing of the Israeli population. In total, 1141 persons were interviewed. The composition of the interviewed population is representative of the heterogeneous character of the Israeli Jewish adult population. Thirty-two percent were Israeli born (12% of North African or Asian origin, 16% European or American origin, and 4% at least second-generation Israelis) and 69% were born abroad (30% in a North African or Asian country, 37% in Europe or America, and 2% of other origin). Fifty-five percent of the latter immigrated after the establishment of the State of Israel (in 1948), 27% in the years 1948–1954, and only 9% after 1968. About a quarter (26%) had no more than elementary schooling, 25% had some high school, 23% had complete high school, and 27% had studied 13 years or more (13% completed university); 41% were male, 59% female.

Nineteen percent of the respondents had at least one of the three physician-diagnosed chronic conditions: 14% had one, 4% two, 1% all three of them. Twelve percent had high blood pressure (8% reported only this diagnosis, 1% in conjunction with diabetes, 2% with heart disease, and 1% with both); 6% had diabetes (3% only diabetes, 1% with high blood pressure, 1% with heart disease, 1% with both), 7% had heart disease (3% only heart disease, 1% with diabetes, 2% with blood pressure, 1% with both).

REFERENCES

Antonovsky, A. (1979). *Health, stress and coping*. San Francisco: Jossey–Bass.

Balint, M. (1957). *The doctor, his patient and the illness*. New York: International Universities Press.

Balint, M., Hunt, J., Joyce, D., Marinker, M., & Woodcock, J. (1970). *Treatment and diagnosis*. Philadelphia: Lippincott.

Ben-Sira, Z. (1972). *The doctor–patient relationship: Collectivism or exchange*. Unpublished Ph.D. dissertation. Jerusalem: The Hebrew University [in Hebrew].

Ben-Sira, Z. (1976). The function of the professional's affective behavior in client satisfaction: A revised approach to social interaction theory. *Journal of Health and Social Behavior, 17,* 3–11.

Ben-Sira, Z. (1980a). Affective and instrumental components in the physician–patient relationship: An additional dimension of interaction theory. *Journal of Health and Social Behavior, 21,* 170–180.

Ben-Sira, Z. (1980b). Involvement with a disease and primary care utilization. *Sociology of Health and Illness, 2,* 247–276.

Ben-Sira, Z. (1982a). Lay evaluation of medical treatment and competence: Development of model of the function of the physician's affective behavior. *Social Science and Medicine, 16,* 1013–1019.

Ben-Sira, Z. (1982b). Stress potential and esotericity of health problems: The significance of the physician's affective behavior. *Medical Care, 20,* 414–424.

Ben-Sira, Z. (1984). Chronic illness, stress and coping. *Social Science and Medicine, 18,* 725–736.

Ben-Sira, Z. (1985a). Primary medical care and coping with stress and disease: The inclination of primary care practitioners to demonstrate affective behavior. *Social Science and Medicine, 21,* 485–498.

Ben-Sira, Z. (1985b). Potency: A stress buffering link in the coping–stress–disease relationship. *Social Science and Medicine, 21,* 397–406.

Ben-Sira, Z. (1986a). *Stress, disease and primary medical care*. Aldershot, England: Gower.

Ben-Sira, Z. (1986b). The plight of primary medical care: The problematics of committedness to practice. *Social Science and Medicine, 22,* 699–712.

Ben-Sira, Z. (1986c). The stress resolving component in primary medical care. *Stress Medicine, 2,* 339–348.

Ben-Sira, Z., & Kacen, L. (1988). Stressbewältigung bei chronischer Krankheit: Gruppengespräche und Zuwendung des Arztes aus der Sicht der Sozialarbeit. In C. Mühlfeld, H. Oppl, H. Weber-Falkensammer & W. R. Wendt (Eds.), *Brennpunkte Sozialer Arbeit* (pp. 69–84). Frankfurt am Main: Diesterweg.

Betz, M., & O'Connel, L. (1983). Changing doctor–patient relationships and the rise in concern for accountability. *Social Problems, 31,* 84–95.

Cartwright, A. (1976). What goes on in the general practitioner's surgery? In M. Acheson & L. Aird (Eds.), *Seminars in community medicine* (Vol. I, pp. 23–48). London: Oxford University Press.

Clute, K. F. (1963). *The general practitioner*. Toronto: University of Toronto Press.

Cohen, F. (1985). Stress and bodily illness. In A. L. Monat & R. S. Lazarus (Eds.), *Stress and coping: An anthology* (pp. 40–54). New York: Columbia University Press.

Cousins, N. (1983). *The healing heart*. New York: Norton.

DiMatteo, M. R., & Friedman, H. S. (1980). *Social psychology and medicine*. Cambridge, MA: Oelgeschlager, Gunn & Hain.

Egberg, S., Battit, G. E., Welch, C. E., & Battlet, M. K. (1964). Reduction of postoperative pain by encouragement and instruction of patients. *New England Journal of Medicine, 270,* 825–827.

Eisenberg, L., & Kleinman, A. (1981). Clinical social science. In L. Eisenberg & A. Kleinman (Eds.), *The relevance of social science for medicine* (pp. 7–20). Dordrecht: Reidel.

Engel, G. L. (1977). The need for a new medical model: A challenge for bio-medicine. *Science, 196,* 129–136.

Fitts, W. T., & Fitts, B. (1955). Ethical standards of the medical profession. *Annals of the American Academy of Political and Social Science, 297,* 25.

Guttman, L., & Levy, S. (1975). Structure and dynamics of worries. *Sociometry, 38,* 448–473.

Hadley, C. G., & Crispen, J. E. (1978). Unprofessional physicians—Some correlative data. *Western Journal of Medicine, 128,* 85–88.

Hall, J. A., Roter, D. L., & Rand, C. S. (1981). Communication of affect between patient and physician. *Journal of Health and Social Behavior, 22,* 18–30.

Hall, O. (1964). The informal organization of medical practice. *Canadian Journal of Economics and Political Science, 12,* 30–44.

Haug, M. R. (1976). The erosion of professional authority: A cross-cultural inquiry in the case of the physician. *Milbank Memorial Fund Quarterly, 54,* 83–105.

Haug, M. R., & Lavin, B. (1981). Practitioner or patient—Who's in charge? *Journal of Health and Social Behavior, 22,* 212–229.

Hayes-Bautista, D. E. (1976). Modifying the treatment: Patient compliance, patient control and medical care. *Social Science and Medicine, 10,* 233–238.

Hellerstein, H. H., & Ford, A. B. (1960). Comprehensive care of the coronary patient: Optimal (intensive) care recovery and reconditioning: An opportunity for the physician. *Circulation, 22,* 1166.

Henao, S. (1985). A system's approach to family medicine. In S. Henao (Ed.), *Principles of family medicine* (pp. 24–40). New York: Brunner/Mazel.

Hornung, C. A., & Massagli, M. (1979). Primary care physicians' affective orientation toward patients. *Journal of Health and Social Behavior, 20,* 61–76.

Illich, I. (1976). *Medical nemesis.* New York: Pantheon.

Jensen, M. M. (1981). Emotional stress and susceptibility to infectious diseases. In K. Bammer & H. Newberry (Eds.), *Stress and cancer* (pp. 59–70). Toronto: Hogrefe.

Kasteler, J., Kane, R. L., Olson, D. M., & Thetford, C. (1976). Issues underlying prevalence of doctor-shopping behavior. *Journal of Health and Social Behavior, 17,* 328–339.

Korman, M., Pate, M. L., & Chapman, T. S. (1980). Selection of primary care as medical career: Demographic and psychological correlates. *Southern Medical Journal, 73,* 924–927.

Kosa, J., & Robertson, L. S. (1969). The social aspects of health and illness. In J. Kosa, A. Antonovsky, & I. K. Zola (Eds.), *Poverty and health: A sociological analysis* (pp. 35–68). Cambridge, MA: Harvard University Press.

Leigh, H., & Reiser, F. (1980). *The patient.* New York: Plenum Press.

Ley, P., & Spelman, M. S. (1967). *Communicating with the patient.* London: Staples.

Lown, B. (1983). Introduction. In N. Cousins, *The healing heart* (pp. 11–28). New York: Norton.

Mauksch, M. O. (1974). A social science basis for conceptualizing family health. *Social Science and Medicine, 8,* 487–493.

McPhee, J. M. (1984, July). Heirs of general practice. *The New Yorker,* pp. 40–85.

Mechanic, D. (1976). *The growth of bureaucratized medicine.* New York: Wiley.

Miller, A. E. (1972). The expanding definition of disease and health in community medicine. *Social Science and Medicine, 6,* 573–581.

Norbeck, J. S., & Peterson-Tilden, V. (1983). Life-stress, social support, and emotional disequilibrium in complications of pregnancy: A prospective multivariate study. *Journal of Health and Social Behavior, 24,* 30–46.

Pattison, E. M., & Anderson, R. C. (1978). Family health care. *Public Health Reviews, 7,* 83–134.

Ransom, D. C. (1985). The evolution from an individual to a family approach. In S. Henao & N. P. Grose (Eds.), *Principles of family systems in family medicine* (pp. 5–23). New York: Brunner/Mazel.

Rave, A. (1978). Finding periodic patterns in time series with monotonic trend: A new technique. In S. Shye (Ed.), *Theory construction and data analysis in the behavioral sciences* (pp. 371–390). San Francisco: Jussey–Bass.

Ross, C., Wheaton, B., & Duff, R. S. (1981). Client satisfaction and the organization of medical practice. *Journal of Health and Social Behavior, 22,* 243–255.

Schlesinger, E. G. (1985). *Health care and social work practice.* St. Louis: Times Mirror/Mosby.

Sehnert, K. W., & Eisenberg, H. (1975). *How to be your own doctor.* New York: Grosset & Dunlap.

Sklar, S., & Anisman, H. (1981). Contributions of stress and coping to cancer development and growth. In K. Bammer & H. Newberry (Eds.), *Stress and cancer* (pp. 98–136). Toronto: Hogrefe.

Stimson, G., & Webb, B. (1975). *Going to see the doctor.* London: Routledge & Kegan Paul.

Tessler, R., Mechanic, D., & Dimond, M. (1976). The effect of psychological distress on physician utilization. *Journal of Health and Social Behavior, 17,* 353–369.

Tuckett, D. (1976). Doctors and patients. In B. Tuckett (Ed.), *Medical sociology* (pp. 190–224). London: Tavistock.

Vickery, D. M., & Fries, J. F. (1976). *Take care of yourself.* Reading, MA: Addison–Wesley.

Wallis, C. (1986, May 26). Weeding out the incompetent. *Time,* pp. 57–58.

Wan, T. T., & Soifer, S. V. (1974). Determinants of physician utilization: A causal analysis. *Journal of Health and Social Behavior, 15,* 100–108.

Weitzkin, H., & Stoeckle, J. D. (1976). Information control and the micropolitics of health care. *Social Science and Medicine, 10,* 263–276.

Power, Compliance, and Control

A power–authority differential is characteristic of most encounters between laypersons and professionals. Professionals have greater power and authority by virtue of their training, knowledge, and skill. In exchange for their services to community and society, professionals are accorded a preferred and special status, which reinforces and augments this power and authority. Often, the power of the health professional is invoked to influence the behavior of individual patients, particularly in relation to compliance with a specified regimen. Issues related to power can thus be considered in terms of the general power and authority of the professional, and in terms of patient compliance.

PROFESSIONAL POWER AND AUTHORITY

The professional power and authority of the physician can be observed in a number of ways. Stimson and Webb (1975), for example, demonstrated how physicians can control aspects of the encounter with patients by establishing clinic hours and appointment systems and thus limiting their availability. Patients, on their part, seek to counter this power by seeking additional information from other physicians they may be seeing, or from pharmacists who fill their prescriptions.

The relationship between power and information exchange and communication was examined by Shapiro and colleagues' (1983) case history study of Australian obstetrical cases. Women seldom received the information they sought or needed; those in public clinics apparently needing more and receiving disproportionately less than those in private care. Shapiro *et al.* interpreted their findings to indicate that physicians maintain their power by selectively managing discussions to avoid providing information. Examples of the power of physicians to stigmatize and label (or, conversely, to destigmatize), for example, are provided by Volinn's (1983) analysis of professional reactions to alcoholism and leprosy.

Gerson (1976) viewed illness and the physician–patient encounter in terms of a political process, involving conflict between the patient's needs and the physician's control over work, as well as allocation of scarce resources. Ermann's (1976) analysis of the shift from decision making by independent health care professionals who were presumed to be controlled by their clients, toward decisions made by physicians who are employees of hospitals and other large health care organizations, raised questions about what types of social institutions can provide appropriate countervailing power to serve as social controls in the health care area.

Haug's chapter elaborates on the changing power and authority of medicine and its implications for health behavior.

COMPLIANCE, ADHERENCE, CONTROL

Whether, and to what degree, persons perform medically recommended or prescribed activities, and how they relate to, and respond to medical regimens, are important factors in maintaining and improving health status, and critical areas of health behavior research. Yet, reports (e.g., Stimson, 1974) indicate that persons demonstrate great variability in the degree to which they exhibit such acceptance of medical regimens and prescribed activities. There is no neutral word to refer to this. The terminology—"compliance," "obedience," "adherence"—repeatedly emphasizes an implicit hierarchical authority structure, an implicit acceptance of the power and right of the professional to make demands, and an imperative for "submission" by the patient.

Although the literature on "compliance" deals with a variety of health behaviors, including weight control and smoking reduction, it is primarily concerned with proper acceptance of medication—particularly in the area of hypertension and diabetes—and with patients' keeping of appointments. Moreover, as Stimson (1974) pointed out, much of the literature reflects attempts to discover the nature of the patient "flaws" that account for the failure to comply. As a rule, compliance research does not deal with physicians' failure to keep appointments, i.e., patients having to wait an hour or more beyond a scheduled appointment time; or with physicians' failures to communicate clearly (e.g., McKinlay, 1975). It is implicit that compliance is normative and "good," and that noncompliance is deviant and "bad," and that pressures must be exerted to induce normative, good, compliant behavior.

Research on compliance can, for convenience, be considered in terms of whether it focuses on the individual, on system factors, or whether it addresses reconceptualization of compliance itself.

The individual. Much research dealing with the individual is derived from the health belief model. Becker, Drachman, and Kirscht (1974), for example, demonstrated the applicability of a modified health belief model as a predictor of how well mothers will engage in recommended behaviors relating to their child's health, such as giving medications and/or keeping appointments. Although their study introduced some health care system factors such as whether the same physician treated the child previously, the major focus is nonetheless on the mother's beliefs, such as whether she perceives that her child is resusceptible to the present illness, whether that illness is serious, and whether the prescribed medicine will be of benefit. Hartman and Becker (1978) found that perceived benefits and perceived barriers were the most important health-belief model variables in the prediction of compliance with hemodialysis.

On the other hand, Fincham and Wertheimer (1985) found the health belief model of limited value in predicting whether prescribed medications would be picked up from the pharmacist. And Kegeles and Lund (1984) explored health belief model variables as a way of increasing understanding of children's acceptance of a mouth-rinse program, but found that environmental reward contingency patterns were better predictors.

Among other approaches to compliance, Borkman (1976) identified how professional staff perceptions of patients' intelligence and grasp of instructions are related to compliance with hemodialysis regimens.

Dishman's (1982) study of compliance with an exercise regimen dealt with a large number of individual cognitive, motivational, and physiological characteristics, together with consideration of the exercise setting, and the interaction between the person and the setting. Although self-motivation seemed to show some promise as a predictor of compliance, most of the variables had little or no predictive value.

Focusing on individual characteristics seems to promise limited effectiveness in increasing compliance.

System factors. Moving beyond the individual, Lorber's (1975) study of the degree to which the behaviors of hospitalized surgical patients comply with—or disrupt—hospital routines demonstrated how such disruptions lead to differential responses by physicians and nurses, invoking labeling in terms of conformity or deviance. Her analyses showed how the task organization of the hospital setting, together with professionals' differential expectations for behavior and responses to pain for different categories of patients, enter into the labeling process.

Davis (1976) examined how the profession of dentistry functions as a social regulatory institution, and reasoned that compliance with dental regimens must be understood in terms of the degree of congruity that exists between the components of the provider system and the culture of the patient.

The relative importance of structural aspects of the health care system in determining levels of appointment-keeping was demonstrated by Hertz and Stamps' (1977) analysis of clients of a Model Cities Health Center. Hulka, Cassel, Kupper, and Burdette's (1976) systematic examination of how inadequate physician communications can influence acceptance of medication by patients with diabetes mellitus and congestive heart failure, further demonstrated the importance of the interaction between the system and the patient.

Interventions at the system level have been examined by Reid (1979), who showed that instructional materials were moderately successful on a short-term basis in maintaining adherence to an exercise program by firefighters; by Tagliacozzo, Luskin, Lashof, and Ima (1974), who showed that instructional interventions by nurses could improve compliance by increasing the patients' understanding of their condition; by Belisle, Roskies, and Levesque (1987), who reported very modest success for a "relapse-prevention" program to improve adherence to an exercise regimen; and by Roberts, Wurtele, and Leeper (1983), who raised questions about the value of specific forms of reminders in increasing the return rate of patients for TB screening.

Toward a reconceptualization of "compliance." Lipton and Hershaft's (1985) analysis of how dubious findings have been incorporated into medical practice on a large scale, raised the question of the value to the patient of compliance with medical regimens, and with it, the value of the medical perspective. For many patients, nonacceptance of a regimen is an appropriate and healthy behavior!

Conrad (1985) reasoned that an important issue in nonacceptance of medication is the meaning that the medication and the illness have for the patient. Within the context of epilepsy, Conrad demonstrated that taking medication may be associated with the stigma of the condition, and that not taking medication may represent attempts at self-regulation.

Hayes-Bautista's (1976) study of Chicano females led him to conclude that compliance or noncompliance is an outcome of negotiations between the patient and the physician and that noncompliance—sometimes considered in terms of decreasing or increasing the amount of medication taken—may reflect the patient's dissatisfaction with the treatment, as well as ways whereby the patient can control the treatment process.

Kotarba and Seidel (1984) demonstrated how some "pain management" clinics perceive the chronic pain patient to be in need of social control, and how the seminars presented on the management of such patients seem to equate compliance with social control. Patients are discredited, their presentations are distorted, their stories are listened to cynically. From Kotarba and Seidel's analysis, one can see that the issues are social and behavioral rather than medical; that compliance—or behaving properly—is a way of medicalizing a behavioral issue.

Stimson (1974) analyzed the legitimacy and "rationality" of the "view from the other side," the patient's views on medication, and showed how these may often vary from the perspectives of the physician. Moreover, from the patient's perspective, not taking medication can be seen to be rational and appropriate. Furthermore, Stimson and Webb (1975, p. 11) pointed out that the patient's decision whether or not to accept medication is a result of reappraisal of the recommendation in light of additional consultation with others, and attempts to make sense out of what the patient knows about the condition and the medication.

Waissman (1985) provided insights into what might be termed the ultimate act of noncompliance: a "strike" in which patients of a French hemodialysis clinic refused to accept their treatment. In this context, they were showing—at great risk—their disapproval of some clinic management policies, and were using noncompliance as a political tool, as a way of demonstrating their own social power.

Barofsky (1978) identified several alternate models of therapeutic relationships that could be substituted for the traditional model in which a powerful figure or institution requires compliant or conforming behavior. In such alternatives, coerciveness is increasingly replaced by self-management, and the relationship between the physician and the patient is that of a therapeutic alliance with the objective of increased self-care.

Regardless of whether the behaviors are referred to as compliance, adherence, or acceptance; or whether they are viewed in terms of physician, social, or patient control; the research and conceptualizing about how persons respond to medical or health regimens clearly indicates that a simple medical perspective is insufficient, and that the problem will not be resolved by technology or simple interventions. The problem clearly does not inhere in patient or client inadequacy; the problem is multifaceted, and emerges from interactions with the system. On the one hand, nonacceptance or nonadherence may not be a problem at all, but an appropriate means of adaptive behavior from the patient's perspective. On the other hand, where patients wish to accept or adhere, professionals must consider the importance of their own behavior, their communication, their role performance, and other system dimensions in order to increase the likelihood that such acceptance or adherence occurs.

Cole, Berger, and Garrity's chapter continues the movement away from a strictly medical conception of compliance, toward a broader view that encompasses engaging in safety behavior in occupation settings, and demonstrates the commonalities between occupational and medical considerations of compliance. The chapter is an innovative way of bringing together two areas of behavioral research that have too long been kept separate.

REFERENCES

Barofsky, I. (1978). Compliance, adherence and the therapeutic alliance: Steps in the development of self-care. *Social Science and Medicine, 12,* 369–376.

Becker, M. H., Drachman, R. H., & Kirscht, J. P. (1974). A new approach to explaining sick-role behavior in low-income populations. *American Journal of Public Health, 64,* 205–216.

Belisle, M., Roskies, E., & Levesque, J.-M. (1987). Improving adherence to physical activity. *Health Psychology, 6,* 159–172.

Borkman, T. S. (1976). Hemodialysis compliance: The relationship of staff estimates of patients' intelligence and understanding to compliance. *Social Science and Medicine, 10,* 385–392.

Conrad, P. (1985). The meaning of medications: Another look at compliance. *Social Science and Medicine, 20,* 29–37.

Davis, P. (1976). Compliance structures and the delivery of health care: The case of dentistry. *Social Science and Medicine, 10,* 329–337.
Dishman, R. K. (1982). Compliance/adherence in health-related exercise. *Health Psychology, 1,* 237–267.
Ermann, M. D. (1976). The social control of organizations in the health care area. *Milbank Memorial Fund Quarterly, 4,* 167–183.
Fincham, J. E., & Wertheimer, A. I. (1985). Using the health belief model to predict initial drug therapy defaulting. *Social Science and Medicine, 20,* 101–105.
Gerson, E. M. (1976). The social character of illness: Deviance or politics. *Social Science and Medicine, 10,* 219–224.
Hartman, P. E., & Becker, M. H. (1978). Non-compliance with prescribed regimen among chronic hemodialysis patients: A method of prediction and educational diagnosis. *Dialysis & Transplantation, 7,* 978–985.
Hayes-Bautista, D. E. (1976). Modifying the treatment: Patient compliance, patient control and medical care. *Social Science and Medicine, 10,* 233–238.
Hertz, P., & Stamps, P. L. (1977). Appointment-keeping behavior reevaluated. *American Journal of Public Health, 67,* 1033–1036.
Hulka, B. S., Cassel, J. C., Kupper, L. L., & Burdette, J. A. (1976). Communication, compliance, and concordance between physicians and patients with prescribed medications. *American Journal of Public Health, 66,* 847–853.
Kegeles, S. S., & Lund, A. K. (1984). Adolescents' acceptance of caries-preventive procedures. In J. D. Matarazzo, S. M. Weiss, J. A. Herd, N. E. Miller, & S. M. Weiss (Eds.), *Behavioral health: A handbook of health enhancement and disease prevention.* New York: Wiley.
Kotarba, J. A., & Seidel, J. V. (1984). Managing the problem pain patient: Compliance or social control. *Social Science and Medicine, 19,* 1393–1400.
Lipton, J. P., & Hershaft, A. M. (1985). On the widespread acceptance of dubious medical findings. *Journal of Health and Social Behavior, 26,* 336–351.
Lorber, J. (1975). Good patients and problem patients: Conformity and deviance in a general hospital. *Journal of Health and Social Behavior, 16,* 213–225.
McKinlay, J. B. (1975). Who is really ignorant—Physician or patient? *Journal of Health and Social Behavior, 16,* 3–11.
Reid, E. A. L. (1979). Exercise prescription: A clinical trial. *American Journal of Public Health, 69,* 591–595.
Roberts, M. C., Wurtele, S. K., & Leeper, J. D. (1983). Experiments to increase return in a medical screening drive: Two futile attempts to apply theory to practice. *Social Science and Medicine, 17,* 741–746.
Shapiro, M. C., Najman, J. M., Chang, A., Keeping, J. D., Morrison, J., & Western, J. S. (1983). Information control and the exercise of power in the obstetrical encounter. *Social Science and Medicine, 17,* 139–146.
Stimson, G. V. (1974). Obeying doctor's orders: A view from the other side. *Social Science and Medicine, 8,* 97–104.
Stimson, G., & Webb, B. (1975). *Going to see the doctor: The consultation process in general practice.* London: Routledge & Kegan Paul.
Tagliacozzo, D. M., Luskin, D. B., Lashof, J. C., & Ima, K. (1974). Nurse intervention and patient behavior: An experimental study. *American Journal of Public Health, 64,* 596–603.
Volinn, I. J. (1983). Health professionals as stigmatizers and destigmatizers of diseases: Alcoholism and leprosy as examples. *Social Science and Medicine, 17,* 385–393.
Waissman, R. (1985). A protest movement in a private clinic: An analysis of a patients' strike. *Social Science and Medicine, 20,* 129–132.

CHAPTER 18

Power, Authority, and Health Behavior

Marie R. Haug

INTRODUCTION

As we approach the end of the 20th century, few would argue that the relationship between physicians and patients in Western industrialized countries is the same as it was a generation ago. Witness the popularity of Dr. Seuss's *You're Only Old Once* (1986). As of this writing 34 weeks on the *New York Times* best seller list, it mercilessly and humorously pillories the impersonal assembly-line treatment of an elderly patient, by physicians who are uncaring, test-happy, and overspecialized.

The popular media remind the public that physicians can make dreadful mistakes and can be sued successfully for seven-figure damages, that some physicians are impaired by alcohol, drug abuse or old age, and that they can charge exorbitant or unwarranted fees; in short, that physicians are all too human. The patient who believed and trusted every word of the doctor and considered it a duty to comply with "doctor's orders" is gradually becoming obsolete, as people achieve more years of education and grow more medically sophisticated. Identifying and understanding these relatively recent developments calls for a review of the roots of physician power, and the sources of the challenges to that power.

THEORIES OF PROFESSIONAL POWER

Power is the ability to compel behavior in another, regardless of the other's own desires. It may take the form of raw force, which is rarely if ever a factor in professional–client relationships. In that context, the compelling force is authority, the right to rule that is accepted by others as valid and legitimate. Weber (1961) proposed three sources of such legitimated power: traditional, charismatic, and legal rational. Each is relevant to the role of the physician.

Traditional authority flows from past history and custom. In Britain, the practice of medicine was long identified with the aristocratic elite; only gentlemen with university degrees from Oxford or Cambridge were admitted to the Royal College of Physicians when it was founded in 1518 (Elliott, 1972; Haug, 1975). In the United States, after the Flexner report in 1910 shut off poor boys' pathway to medicine by exposing the inadequacy of the

MARIE R. HAUG • Center on Aging and Health, Case Western Reserve University, Cleveland, Ohio 44106.

proprietary schools, it was the sons from wealthy prestigious families with the wherewithal to be trained abroad, who came to dominate medicine (Kunitz, 1974). A history of upper-class position clothed physicians with the authority of status.

Charismatic authority was based on the extraordinary mystical quality of the priest and medicine man in earlier times. More recently, the image of the kindly, dedicated family physician carried the same mystique. Even today, some of that aura still clings to many practitioners (Coe, 1970), for example the famous heart surgeons who appear on television to explain their latest life-saving exploits. More generally applicable to all physicians is legal-rational authority. Licensure laws and regulations of various kinds prohibit the practice of medicine by anyone not properly credentialed. The power of the state backs the authority of physicians by giving them the sole legal right to act as doctors.

One source of power and authority that Weber did not capture is monopolized knowledge. Larson (1977) considered professional knowledge to be a form of property, a resource used to maintain power and eliminate competition by limiting access to training and thus to credentials. Parsons (1951) identified unshared knowledge as justifying the right of physicians to exercise control over their patients. His concept of the "sick role" long dominated sociological thinking on physician–patient relationships. In this model of the interaction, sick persons are excused from normal duties, provided they try to get well by seeking out a physician, and complying with the regimen prescribed.

Because of the "competence gap" between patients and doctors (Parsons, 1975), the knowledgeable practitioners must have full authority over the ignorant patients in order that the latter can be cured and resume their presickness roles and obligations. This model is congruent with the functionalist perspective, which holds that social life is made possible by shared values and interrelated functions that hold the system in equilibrium.

Although the sick role concept has been criticized as not applicable to chronic conditions, which characterize a major part of contemporary illness (e.g., Levine & Kozloff, 1978), its applicability even to acute conditions is currently being called in question, from two distinct but related directions. On the one hand, those who espouse a conflict model of society, criticize the sick role as assuming equivalence of purpose and values between physicians and patients. The potential for conflict inheres in any medical interaction (Freidson, 1970). Patients' perspectives and expectations often differ from those of the practitioner, on cultural or class grounds, and this mediates their acceptance of treatment recommendations and compliance with regimen (Mechanic, 1982). In the conflict situation, physicians use the tactic of information control to maintain their power, while patients attempt to limit that power by information-seeking, a process referred to as the "micropolitics" of the therapeutic encounter (Waitzkin & Stoeckle, 1976).

A consumerist perspective on the part of the patient also challenges the sick role model. "It focuses on purchasers' (patient's) rights and seller's (physician's) obligations, rather than on physician's rights (to direct) and patient obligations (to follow directions) . . ." (Haug & Lavin, 1981, p. 213). Just as consumers negotiate the terms of purchase of any commodity, patients can negotiate the terms under which they will buy the physician's advice, including both diagnosis and treatment plans. The negotiating model of physician–patient interactions defines how the conflict between the parties can be amicably resolved. For it to work, however, the patient needs to secure health information, make rational choices, and be ready to play an active role in determining the terms of care (Pratt, 1978).

Although the sick role and the negotiating model are the two major sociological images of authority in the physician–patient relationship, there is a third approach to physician power that has confused the issue. This approach emphasizes the work autonomy of the professional rather than his or her authority in interaction with clients or patients. Although the two concepts intertwine in practice, they are conceptually distinct as ideal types.

> While authority concerns power over others, autonomy is the power not to be compelled by others. Physicians have enjoyed both types: the right to give patients "doctor's orders" that will be accepted, and the right not to have anyone else, whether bureaucratic boss or fellow physician, interfere with their work (Haug & Lavin, 1983, p. 10).

Freidson, in his book *Professional Powers* (1986), reiterated the position taken in his earlier seminal works on the dominance of the physician in the medical arena (1970). His chief interest then was on the power of the physician over other occupations in the medical division of labor, involving both the authority to give orders, to nurses, paraprofessionals, and others, and the autonomy to be free from receiving orders from administrators or even from peers. Currently, Freidson (1986) focuses on the position of the physician in relation to administrative and supervisory personnel who often now control access to the tools and services needed to carry out medical work, more clearly a case of autonomy. On both flanks physician power is being eroded. Witness the increasingly successful battle of nurse-midwives to practice their trade without physician oversight and the growing "corporatization" of medical care under the rule of conglomerates that hedge physician autonomy (Salmon, 1984) even to the point that some predict physicians will become "proletarianized" (McKinlay & Arches, 1985).

At the same time, the negotiating model implicitly empowers patients to act as equals in any interaction with a health provider. By challenging physician authority, patients are asserting their right to be autonomous actors in a medical encounter. Perhaps as physicians' autonomy is being assailed by co-workers and administrators, their authority is being undermined by autonomy demands of their patients.

Empirical data to test the comparative validity of the two models—the sick role and the negotiating—are hard to come by, chiefly because of the lack of research on the shared power model. Some limited material on the attitudes and reported experiences of the public are available, however. It is useful in showing that characteristics of patients have an effect on the balance of power between the giver and the receiver of care. Still fewer data are available on physician characteristics that might tip that balance. Many studies seem to assume that physicians are undifferentiated monoliths, when in fact their differences in age, gender, specialty or beliefs can have a marked effect on the nature of the physician–patient relationship.

FACTORS IN PATIENT POWER

The age cohort of the patient is a critical variable in determining events in a medical encounter. The old-old cohort, those currently 85 and over, were born before technological and scientific developments produced dramatic changes in medical care. Buffeted by two major depressions, many could afford to use a physician's services only in desperate emergencies, when such help was seen as a lifesaver. Also older persons are more likely to have little education and to have been trained to accept the authority of person's higher on society's status ladder. Compare these attributes to persons now in their 20s and early 30s, who have heard about both medical miracles and medical mistakes, who are likely to have had at least a high school or perhaps some college education, and who appear to have little respect for authority.

Two studies, one a statewide and one a national sample of the public (Haug & Lavin, 1983), which assessed attitudes of challenge to physician authority as well as reported challenging behaviors, do indeed show differences by age. Those 18 to 34 were three to four times as likely as those aged 65 and over to claim willingness to question a physician's advice. Over half of the younger asserted that they had actually done so in the past, as against only a quarter to a third of those 80 and over. The age of the patient could well influence whether he or she acts out the sick role, or attempts to take a more egalitarian negotiating approach to the doctor (Haug, 1979). Although these earlier studies did not directly determine whether respondents had actually attempted to negotiate an acceptable diagnosis or treatment with their attending physician, by claiming they were willing to, or had actually challenged medical authority, they were showing that they did not accept the sick role model, with its requirement of unquestioning acceptance of the physician's advice.

Older patients may also be at a disadvantage in the power game because of the stereotypical attitudes of their practitioners. One study has shown that old people are less able than younger ones to get the doctor to listen to their problems, and attend to their concerns. Overriding the wishes of the patient in this way is evaluated as a subtle form of ageism, and "reflects a liability in power dynamics" (Greene, Adelman, Charon, & Hoffman, 1986, p. 121).

Gender and race characteristics could also be expected to affect the nature of the encounter. Because blacks, given the paucity of practitioners of their own race, are usually constrained to deal with white physicians, they may be more reserved, and less forthcoming in interacting with them (Santos, Hubbard, & McIntosh, 1983). Women make more physician visits than men (Verbrugge, 1985), and familiarity might foster a less submissive role despite the conventional wisdom that women are generally unaggressive. Indeed, female gender was related to challenging attitudes and behaviors in the state sample (Haug & Lavin, 1979), whereas race was unrelated in both surveys (Haug & Lavin, 1983).

Bridging the competence gap would empower the patient. Accordingly, those with higher education and better health knowledge should have the confidence to question what the physician suggests. And indeed, in the same two samples, this expectation was borne out, with respect to both attitudes and reported behavior. Those with more education and knowledge of health matters were consistently more challenging of physician authority. One facet of this knowledge concerns patient access to their own medical records. In applauding the passage of a New York State law mandating that patients be given such records, the sponsor of the legislation explicitly noted the relationship between knowledge and power. He commented that the law "says patients have a much larger role in making decisions about their treatment, that patients are equal to doctors and no longer subservient to their decisions" (Sullivan, 1986).

The role of the media in educating the public on health matters should not be underestimated. With the growing interest in health, TV specials on new discoveries, both technological and biomedical, are not uncommon and are available to members of all classes. "Doctor-books" and how-to-do-it manuals have proliferated in recent years, but are perhaps more appealing to the middle class than to other groups.

Szasz and Hollender (1956) were among the first to point out that the nature of the patient relationship could vary depending on the health condition of the patient, with an adult to adult, egalitarian interaction most common when the patient was not in dire physical straits. In this respect, a curious reversal in effect between attitudes and behaviors was found in the two samples. Persons who considered their health was excellent, or did not have a disabling chronic condition, were more apt to be willing to challenge a physician's authority, but those who assessed their health as poor or had a chronic condition that interfered with normal activity were *more* likely to have translated attitude into action, claiming to have openly disagreed with their caregiver in the past (Haug & Lavin, 1983). It is as if those who were not well believed they had not been satisfactorily treated, perhaps because they had not been "cured," and had at some point confronted the physician with this presumed failure.

This speculation is reinforced by the fact that in the state sample, where a question was asked about prior experiences with medicine, those who claimed they had been the victims of medical error were more likely to report challenging behavior (Haug & Lavin, 1979). Similarly, those who admitted that they often did not comply with medical regimen were also the most likely to be challengers (Haug & Lavin, 1983). Clearly, those dissatisfied with the treatment plans or outcomes of care were inclined to refuse to accept the physician's authority.

FACTORS IN PHYSICIAN POWER

Physician characteristics can either enhance or erode their power in relationships with patients. Unfortunately, the tendency to treat all physicians as undifferentiated actors has resulted in very little empirical data, forcing much of the following to be speculative. For example, we do not know what the effect of age is on physician power *vis-à-vis* patients. Older doctors may carry an aura of the wisdom of years, which enhances their authority, or may be considered out-of-date, which diminishes it. Newly minted doctors can be evaluated as greenhorns, or as being up on the latest medical breakthroughs, with opposite effects on their authority. There is some limited evidence on age effects on physician attitudes concerning the challenging patient. In a small state sample of 88 practicing physicians, those under 35 years of age were most apt to agree with a patient's right to challenge their authority, and to be willing to accommodate to such challenge (Haug & Lavin, 1983).

A few clues exist on the effects of provider gender. A recent analysis of actual interactions of patients with male and female physicians revealed that male physicians tend to interrupt their patients while they are talking more than they are interrupted by the patients. With women the opposite is true. Patients interrupt female physicians more than the latter interrupt them (West, 1984). Assuming that the act of interruption is an expression of dominance, these findings suggest the lesser power and authority of women. Such a conclusion also resonates with the stereotype of women as less aggressive and assertive than men, two behaviors that can express power. Supporting evidence comes from a study of practicing physicians (Heins, 1979), which found that women tended to take a more power-sharing, egalitarian approach than their male colleagues, a finding reaffirmed by Weisman and Teitelbaum (1985).

No one, to this writer's knowledge, has studied the effect of practitioner's race on power relations with patients. Given that black physicians are in the minority in the United States, cross-race interactions are most likely to involve white physicians and black patients. Such a mix would superimpose racial dominance on professional authority and exacerbate the power imbalance.

Another factor in the equation is what might be called the physician's practice style. Those who are willing and able to take the time to explore fully with the patient the various options for care and treatment, along with their rationale and possible effectiveness, at the same time respecting the patient's values and concerns, are acting in ways that diminish their power. As Waitzkin and Stoeckle (1976) pointed out, mystification and withholding of information are the major techniques used to maintain the professional's authority. Demystification tends to equalize the participants' power.

Medicine is not an exact science. There is a great deal of uncertainty, as to both correct diagnosis and effective treatment (Fox, 1957). Physicians whose style is to share this uncertainty openly with their patients may generate trust, but simultaneously are revealing that their claim to authority is not absolute. Indeed, it has been suggested that failure to be open is a sign of lack of confidence, or even incompetence. As one experienced British physician once commented, "Many doctors are authoritarian because . . . they are afraid to be found out as wrong . . . not as good as they should be" (Haug, 1976b, p. 30). Uncertainty becomes most obvious in treating chronic conditions like renal failure, or incurable diseases, like AIDS today. Physicians do not have a cure and cannot easily claim authority in such cases.

The time-orientation of the provider is another element of practice style. Fee-for-service doctors must fit many patients into a limited number of hours, in part for economic reasons. Those who handle an assembly line of patients in different cubicles, give short shrift to persons who ask a lot of questions and who want to be part of decision-making concerning their care, because they interfere with the flow. Patients have little time to exercise power in these circumstances. Indeed, in the previously reported state sample, practitioners who saw 50 or more patients a day were less likely to accommodate to patient challenge than those who saw fewer than 30 (Haug & Lavin, 1983).

Practice style is also linked to specialty. Family practice, because it is designed to take into account the sick person's social characteristics and the family situation, requires more input from the patient and thus should offer more opportunity for egalitarian interaction than is true of other specialties. This did not emerge in the state study where pediatricians and internists were more accommodating. Surgery probably offers the most clear-cut case of an authority-based practice style. The process of securing informed consent may be marked by persuasion rather than real information giving, and is often pro forma (Miller, 1986). The major interaction between physician and patient occurs when the latter is unconscious. In the course of a surgical procedure the physician makes decisions to excise or not to excise without consultation with the patient. In that context the physician's power is absolute.

CONTEXTS OF CARE

Organizational setting also makes a difference. In a competitive fee-for-service system it is conceivable that a practitioner would bow to patients' wishes in order to keep their business. If the predictions of a coming doctor glut prove true, such behavior could become common. On the other hand, "demanding," not at all submissive, patients have been identified in prepaid group plans, such as health maintenance organizations, because they feel free to invoke organizational rules to get their way (Freidson, 1973). Yet in the state study, the HMO-based physicians were more apt to accept patient challenge, although this could be because they tended to be younger (Haug & Lavin, 1983). Furthermore, the power relationship may shift depending on the locale of care. Patients seen in a hospital are less able to challenge their physician's demands than are patients in a physician's office (Goss, 1981). And physicians may be at a relative disadvantage in dealing with those patients seen in their own homes, their own familiar turf (Zola, 1986).

Even the societal context may affect the power balance. Although there appears to be little variation in physician–patient relations between Western industrialized countries (Haug, 1973, 1976a), in China the pattern has been markedly divergent. During the Mao period, the power of professionals was denigrated, and the experiential knowledge of the common folk valued over the academic knowledge of the physician (Gibson, 1970). Those findings, however, are impressionistic, or based on small samples. Cross-cultural and cross-national differences in physician–patient power relations remain largely unstudied.

THE NEW CONSUMERISM

Outlines of the new role of the patient as active consumer instead of the passive recipient of care began to sharpen in the late 1960s in the United States. It was a time of revolt against traditional authority, among students, antiwar activists, and feminists (Haug

& Sussman, 1969). Reeder (1972) was among the first specifically to identify patients as consumers in a changing physician–patient relationship. The general ferment of the times was fed with respect to the medical arena by the dawning discovery that physicians could make dreadful mistakes. One of the most dramatic of these errors was the use of the sedative thalidomide for pregnant women, with the result that their babies were born with flipperlike appendages instead of arms or legs. These and other mistakes in treatment sparked a surge of widely publicized malpractice suits, some of which produced large damage awards. Physicians, who public polls had shown were widely trusted figures, began to lose some of their respect among a sizable minority of the populace (Betz & O'Connell, 1983).

Concerns about the efficacy of medicine and the competence of physicians began to surface. In the statewide sample previously referred to, over a third of the public was skeptical of medicine's effectiveness and nearly two thirds had some doubt about physicians' efficacy as well. Indeed, over half were not sure that physicians in the main were competent or had real concern for their patients (Haug & Lavin, 1983). With such widespread doubts about practitioners' advice, it is small wonder that estimated rates of noncompliance run high: perhaps 60% of patients do not follow their doctor's advice, and 50% do not take prescribed medications as they have been instructed (Becker, 1985). Indeed, in a few cases, failure to follow a doctor's "orders" may be a conscious assertion of autonomy and independence (Marshall, 1981), and thus a challenge to the practitioner's authority. Generally, noncompliance is more likely to result from physician withholding of information or restricted responsiveness (Hauser, 1981), as well as high costs or unexpected side effects of a prescribed regimen.

How do physicians respond to these developments? In the first place, many recognize that patient attitudes toward them are changing. In the state study, 58% of the practicing physicians surveyed believed that patients were more challenging than in the past (Haug & Lavin, 1983). A similar perception was expressed as well by practitioners in Great Britain and the USSR (Haug, 1976a). Leaders in academic medicine have drawn the same conclusion: "the traditional conceptions of professional authority are being challenged by a more educated and more egalitarian society" wrote a Yale professor a decade ago (Pellegrino, 1977). Stoeckle at Harvard Medical School is among those who argue that these changes in patients' expectations require a more negotiating approach to arriving at a diagnosis and treatment plan (e.g., Lazare, Eisenthal, Frank, & Stoeckle, 1978; Lifton, 1979; Katon & Kleinman, 1980; Becker, 1985). In fact, it has been found that a physician's authoritarian stance may diminish the likelihood of patient compliance (Svarstad, 1986).

The extent to which rejection of physician authority and assertion of patient autonomy has become a popular theme is evidenced by media advice about the advisability of questioning doctors and seeking second opinions. Industry has now seen the advantage, in cost terms, of patients no longer meekly acceding to whatever a physician proposes to do. A business coalition recently placed an advertisement in a midwestern newspaper; headlined "take charge of your health care", it declared that "you can and should question your doctors about procedures, tests and courses of treatment . . ." (Health Action Council, 1986).

A recent study of medical students and their teachers, supported in part by NIMH Grant 5R01 AG04733, has shown that some academic physicians share these views about patient autonomy and are apparently passing on some of their opinions to their students (Lavin, Haug, Belgrave, & Breslau, 1987). Between the time they first entered medical school and 6 years later, when they had completed their first year of residency, 41% of the 124 students studied had changed their views and accorded less authority to physicians and more autonomy to patients than earlier. The greatest change occurred among those who originally had given little weight to patient rights (57%), or had believed that physicians should have authority in dealing with patients (64%). Factors that contributed to these changes included plans to enter specialties such as family medicine, humanitarian reasons for choosing a medical career, and a tendency to reject authority in general.

Although the direct effect of medical school faculty on individual students' shifts in attitudes could not be assessed, there is evidence that faculty support of patient autonomy was transmitted to the students. For example, on measures of belief in patient rights and criticism of physician authority, the mean scores of a sample of 121 faculty members were significantly more egalitarian than those of the students as they entered their medical training. By the end of their residency year, the students' mean scores had come closer to the faculty values, and indeed were no longer significantly different from the attitudes of their mentors. At least in the academic setting studied, the faculty was adapting to changes in the physician–patient relationship, and apparently transmitting these perspectives to the student body. How these attitudes will be maintained in the "real world" of practice is uncertain, however, and the potential topic of a follow-up study.

FUTURE OF POWER RELATIONS

What then is the future of physician power and patient autonomy? Will the sick role, authority-based model go into decline, and the negotiating model dominate? Although it is always dangerous to extrapolate current trends into the future, some tentative predictions are in order. Consumerism on the part of patients is not apt to decline, but whether it will be more dominant is problematic. There are likely to continue to be people more comfortable with a dependent patient role (Haug & Lavin, 1981). Increasing levels of public education will not catch up with constantly expanding medical knowledge. Yet many common acute illnesses are self-limiting, or easily treated with self-care. People are more and more learning to handle their chronic conditions, monitoring their health states on a day-to-day basis. Some physician books provide decision trees (a series of questions and possible answers about symptoms) to help a person decide if a problem is serious or not (Kunz, 1982).

The popularity of all forms of self-health care, from attention to diet and exercise to self-treatment for symptoms without resort to professional attention, is likely to continue. There is no evidence that lay medicine produces more ill effects than the iatrogenic problems resulting from faulty procedures and misdiagnoses of medical professionals (Light, 1983). Self-care has existed for many centuries and in many parts of the world. Its impact on the future power balance in the physician–patient relationship will probably be minimal. If anything, any effects are apt to be in the opposite direction. Unhappy experiences in dealing with a physician may well encourage self-care rather than submitting to an unpleasant interaction (Haug, 1986).

Two major societal developments will undoubtedly have an impact on physician–patient relationships in this country, as a result of their effect on the physician's own power and autonomy. The first of these is the bureaucratization of medicine, as it comes to be more and more a corporate enterprise, with a profit-making ethos (Starr, 1982; Salmon, 1984). As physician authority is being challenged by demands for patient autonomy, their own autonomy is being hedged by bureaucratic rules. At the moment this manifests itself most dramatically in care for the elderly in hospitals. Medicare payments are based on DRGs (diagnosis related groups), which determine reimbursible lengths of stay. The extension of such regulations to ambulatory care is already on the horizon. In large group practices, where profit-making is also a consideration, the control may take the form of allotting only so much time to any patient visit, regardless of the complaint.

The intrusion of economic constraints on clinical practice is not new, but the changes now taking place are more far-reaching and more intrusive than in the past (Luft, 1986). But no one has as yet considered their implications for physician–patient relationships. One can only speculate that limiting the physician's autonomy will of necessity reduce the range of available options in dealing with patient concerns; even if the physician wishes to follow the negotiating model, he or she will have fewer areas in which choices can freely be made. The potential is for an encounter in which conflicts are resolved by physician fiat, or by patient rejection.

The second of these societal developments is the technological revolution in medicine. It is hardly necessary to document the extent and force of these changes, which allow studies of the living brain in full color through positron emission tomography (PET) scans, permit heart transplants with cadaver or artificial hearts, provide kidney dialysis, and offer birth control through a pill. Computers have been programmed to take medical or psychiatric histories. Data have been stored, and updated as new discoveries are reported, to allow the split-second calculation of the most likely diagnosis and preferred treatment, given an input of a constellation of symptoms. Theoretically, a person who knows how to access the computer could be his or her own doctor (Haug, 1977), with attendant loss of physician power (Antley & Antley, 1973). Moreover, the physician's performance can be evaluated by computer, perhaps revealing the fallibility of medical decisions.

The impact of these developments on physician–patient relationships has been explicitly considered in two analyses. Reiser (1978) rejected the notion that turning over technical tasks to a computer will free physicians to give more attention to patients' social and psychological concerns. He believes the practitioner will become more technologically oriented by his or her attachment to "the machine at the bedside," and be even less open to nonbiological issues. Bursztajn, Hamm, and Gutheil (1984) are concerned that the two models of medical decision-making, which they call paternalism versus consumer preference and patient autonomy, can degenerate into the misuse of technology. "The use of technological aids (and technological mystification) to bolster the physician's authority is a commonly noted phenomenon. But . . . greater patient involvement in decisions may also be expressed as a clamor for technological placebos" (p. 180). This cautionary note is sounded in spite of the fact that these authors favor involving the patient in the process of decision-making, as providing a context of mutual support in openly sharing the inevitable uncertainty of medical diagnosis and treatment potential. If mutual trust can be established through joint decision-making, technology will be less likely to be used "as an escape from uncertainty" (p. 190).

What then is the forecast? Undoubtedly, physician autonomy will decline, and perhaps prestige as well (Freidson, 1985), whereas patient autonomy will show some staying power. What is unlikely is that the age of paternalism will return in full flower. Physician–patient relationships will not revert to the old form for everyone. The most likely outcome has been stated in an earlier paper: the "two competing models [will] apply differentially depending on the characteristics of the actors, their orientation to power and dependence, and the circumstances under which they meet" (Haug & Lavin, 1981).

UNANSWERED QUESTIONS

A rich agenda of research questions has been suggested by the present state of knowledge on power in physician–patient relationships. In the first place, we need to know whether a more egalitarian negotiating pattern of interactions actually occurs during therapeutic encounters. We need to know also what the barriers are and what facilitates mutual decision-making between physicians and patients, including the characteristics of both parties. Although there are some data on patient characteristics that foster autonomy in dealing with physicians, they concern attitudes and reported behaviors, rather than actual interactions. About physician characteristics the data are even more limited, and again do not involve their effect in real-life medical encounters. Studies of communication and language patterns during physician visits do not differentiate by type of practitioner. Clearly what is needed are studies that compare characteristics of actors and settings in the two types of interaction model, the sick role and the negotiating model.

The effects of cultural and societal contexts are also unknown. Do people with symptoms in Brazil, China, Morocco, Finland play out the sick role or do they succeed in relating to their care-givers in a give-and-take way? Nobody really knows.

Nor are we aware of the health outcomes of the two types of interaction. Whether a particular mode affects compliance is not the issue, as that word implies following a physician's prescriptions, and indeed compliance may not be relevant to health outcome. One of the most difficult measurement problems is finding an appropriate indicator for the outcome of care. Preventing mortality is a poor one for most illnesses, few of which are life-threatening. Termination of morbidity may be a better measure, but it often occurs regardless of treatment, although it could be delayed by inappropriate care. Patient and/or practitioner satisfaction with the interaction may be interesting to know, but whether it is a valid measure of health outcome is quite another matter.

The overarching research question restates the forecast as proposed by Haug and Lavin (1981) as a subject for inquiry: *Do* the competing models apply differentially, depending on the characteristics of the actors, their orientations to power and dependence, and the circumstances under which they meet? And one must add another: What difference does it make for patient health outcomes?

REFERENCES

Antley, R. M., & Antley, M. A. (1973). Automation: Its impact on the delivery of health care. *Computers and Automations, 22,* 13.

Becker, M. H. (1985). Patient adherence to prescribed therapies. *Medical Care, 23,* 539–555.

Betz, M., & O'Connell, L. (1983). Changing doctor–patient relationships and the rise in concern for accountability. *Social Problems, 31,* 84–95.

Bursztajn, H. J., Hamm, R. M., & Gutheil, T. J. (1984). The technological target: Involving the patients in clinical choices. In S. J. Reiser & M. Anbar (Eds.), *The machine at the bedside* (pp. 177–191). London: Cambridge University Press.

Coe, R. M. (1970). *The sociology of medicine.* New York: McGraw–Hill.

Elliott, P. (1972). *The sociology of professions.* London: Macmillan & Co.

Fox, R. (1957). Training for uncertainty. In R. K. Merton, G. Reader, & P. L. Kendall (Eds.), *The student physician* (pp. 207–241). Cambridge, MA: Harvard University Press.

Freidson, E. (1970). *Professional dominance.* New York: Atherton Press.

Freidson, E. (1973). Prepaid group practice and the new demanding patient. *Milbank Memorial Fund Quarterly, 51,* 473–488.

Freidson, E. (1985). The reorganization of the medical profession. *Medical Care Review, 42,* 11–35.

Freidson, E. (1986). *Professional powers.* Chicago: University of Chicago Press.

Gibson, G. (1970). *Chinese medical practice and the thoughts of Chairman Mao.* Paper presented at the Medical Sociology Section of the American Sociological Association, Washington, DC.

Goss, M. E. W. (1981). Situational effects in medical care of the elderly: Office, hospital and nursing home. In M. R. Haug (Ed.), *Elderly patients and their doctors* (pp. 147–156). New York: Springer.

Greene, M. G., Adelman, R., Charon, R., & Hoffman, S. (1986). Ageism in the medical encounter: An exploratory study of the doctor–elderly patient relationship. *Language and Communication, 6,* 113–124.

Haug, M. R. (1973). Deprofessionalization: An alternative hypothesis for the future. *The Sociological Review Monograph, 20,* 195–211.

Haug, M. R. (1975). The deprofessionalization of everyone. *Sociological Focus, 8,* 197–213.
Haug, M. R. (1976a). The erosion of professional authority: A cross-cultural inquiry in the case of the physician. *Milbank Memorial Fund Quarterly, 54,* 83–106.
Haug, M. R. (1976b). Issues in general practitioner authority in the national health service. *The Sociological Review Monograph, 22,* 23–42.
Haug, M. R. (1977). Computer technology and the obsolescence of the concept of profession. In M. R. Haug & J. Dofney (Eds.), *Work and technology.* (pp. 215–228). Beverly Hills: Sage.
Haug, M. R. (1979). Doctor patient relationships and the older patient. *Journal of Gerontology, 34,* 852–860.
Haug, M. R. (1986). Doctor–patient relationships and their impact on self care of the elderly. In B. Holstein, K. Dean, T. Hickey, & L. Coppard (Eds.), *Self care and health behavior in old age.* Copenhagen: Croom Helm.
Haug, M. R., & Lavin, B. (1979). Public challenge of physician authority. *Medical Care, 17,* 844–858.
Haug, M. R., & Lavin, B. (1981). Practitioner or patient—Who's in charge? *Journal of Health and Social Behavior, 22,* 212–229.
Haug, M. R., & Lavin, B. (1983). *Consumerism in medicine: Challenging physician authority.* Beverly Hills: Sage.
Haug, M. R., & Sussman, M. B. (1969). Professional autonomy and the revolt of the client. *Social Problems, 17,* 153–161.
Hauser, S. T. (1981). Physician–patient relationships. In E. G. Mishler, L. R. Amarasingham, S. T. Hauser, R. Liem, S. D. Osherson, & N. E. Waxler (Eds.), *Social contexts of health, illness and patient care* (pp. 104–140). London: Cambridge University Press.
Health Action Council. (1986, October 27). Take charge of your health care. *Cleveland Plain Dealer,* p. All.
Heins, M. (1979). Career and life patterns of women and men physicians. In E. C. Shapiro & L. M. Lowenstein (Eds.), *Becoming a physician* (pp. 217–235). Cambridge, MA: Ballinger.
Katon, W., & Kleinman, A. (1980). Doctor–patient negotiation and other social science strategies in patient care. In L. Eisenberg & A. Kleinman (Eds.), *The relevance of social science for medicine* (pp. 253–279). Dordrecht: Reidel.
Kunitz, S. T. (1974). Professionalism and social control in the progressive era: The case of the Flexner report. *Social Problems, 22,* 16–27.
Kunz, J. R. M. (Editor-in-chief). (1982). *The American Medical Association family medical guide.* New York: Random House.
Larson, M. S. (1977). *The rise of professionalism.* Berkeley: University of California Press.
Lavin, B., Haug, M. R., Belgrave, L. L., & Breslau, B. (1987). Change in student physicians' views on authority relationships with patients. *Journal of Health and Social Behavior, 28,* 256–272.
Lazare, A., Eisenthal, S., Frank, A., & Stoeckle, J. D. (1978). Studies on a negotiated approach to patienthood. In E. B. Gallagher (Ed.), *The doctor–patient relationship in the changing health scene* (pp. 119–139). Washington, DC: U.S. Government Printing Office.
Levine, S., & Kozloff, M. A. (1978). The sick role: Assessment and overview. In R. H. Turner, J. Coleman, & R. C. Fox (Eds.), *Annual review of sociology No. 4* (pp. 317–343). Palo Alto, CA: Annual Reviews.
Lifton, R. J. (1979). Advocacy and corruption in the healing professions. In W. Rogers & D. Barnard (Eds.), *Nourishing the humanistic in medicine* (pp. 53–72). Pittsburgh, PA: University of Pittsburgh Press.
Light, D. W. (1983). Lay medicine and the medical profession: An international perspective. In P. Herder-Dorneich & A. Schuller (Eds.), *Spontanität oder ordnung: Laienmedizin gegen professionelle systeme* (pp. 95–110). Stuttgart: Verlag W. Lohlhammer.
Luft, H. S. (1986). Economic incentives and constraints in clinical practice. In L. H. Aiken & D. Mechanic (Eds.), *Applications of social science to clinical medicine and health policy* (pp. 500–518). New Brunswick, NJ: Rutgers University Press.
Marshall, V. W. (1981). Physician characteristics and relationships with older patients. In M. R. Haug (Ed.), *Elderly patients and their doctors* (pp. 94–118). New York: Springer.
McKinlay, J. B., & Arches, J. (1985). Towards the proletarianization of physicians. *International Journal of Health Services, 15,* 161–195.

Mechanic, D. (1982). The epidemiology of illness behavior and its relationship to physical and psychological distress. In D. Mechanic (Ed.), *Symptoms, illness behavior and help seeking* (pp. 1–24). New Brunswick, NJ: Rutgers University Press.
Miller, B. L. (1986, October 24). *Autonomy and decision-making: The institution and the patient.* Paper presented at the Aging and Health Symposium on decision-making in long term care, Cleveland, Ohio.
Parsons, T. (1951). *The social system.* New York: Free Press.
Parsons, T. (1975). The sick role and the role of the physician reconsidered. *Milbank Memorial Fund Quarterly, 53,* 257–278.
Pellegrino, E. D. (1977). Medicine and human values. *Yale Alumni Magazine and Journal, 41,* 10–11.
Pratt, L. V. (1978). Reshaping the consumer's posture in health care. In E. B. Gallagher (Ed.), *The doctor–patient relationship in the changing health scene* (pp. 197–214). Washington, DC: U.S. Government Printing Office.
Reeder, L. G. (1972). The patient-client as consumer: Some observations on the changing professional–client relationship. *Journal of Health and Social Behavior, 13,* 402–416.
Reiser, S. J. (1978). *Medicine and the reign of technology.* London: Cambridge University Press.
Salmon, W. (1984). Organizing medical care for profit. In J. B. McKinlay (Ed.), *Issues in the political economy of health care.* New York: Tavistock.
Santos, J. F., Hubbard, R. W., & McIntosh, J. L. (1983). Mental health and the minority elderly. In L. D. Breslau & M. R. Haug (Eds.), *Depression and aging: Causes, care and consequences* (pp. 51–70). New York: Springer.
Seuss, Dr. (1986). *You're only old once.* New York: Random House.
Starr, P. (1982). *The social transformation of American medicine.* New York: Basic Books.
Sullivan, R. (1986, September 14). New York patients to have access to their medical records, *New York Times,* p. 30.
Svarstad, B. L. (1986). Patient–practitioner relationships and compliance with prescribed medical regimens. In L. Aiken & D. Mechanic (Eds.), *Applications of social science to clinical medicine and health policy* (pp. 438–459). New Brunswick, NJ: Rutgers University Press.
Szasz, T., & Hollender, M. H. (1956). A contribution to the philosophy of medicine: The basic models of the doctor–patient relationship. *AMA Archives of Internal Medicine, 97,* 585–592.
Verbrugge, L. M. (1985). Gender and health: An update on hypotheses and evidence. *Journal of Health and Social Behavior, 26*(3), 156–182.
Waitzkin, H., & Stoeckle, J. D. (1976). Information control and the micro-politics of health care: Summary of an ongoing research project. *Social Science and Medicine, 10,* 263–276.
Weber, M. (1961). Legitimate order and types of authority. In T. Parsons, E. Shils, & D. Naegele (Eds.), *Theories of society* (Vol. I, pp. 229–235). New York: Free Press.
Weisman, C. S., & Teitelbaum, M. A. (1985). Physician gender and the physician–patient relationship: Recent evidence and relevant questions. *Social Science and Medicine, 20,* 1119–1127.
West, C. (1984). *Routine complications: Troubles with talk between doctors and patients.* Bloomington: Indiana University Press.
Zola, I. K. (1986). Reasons for non-compliance and failure of the elderly to seek care. In R. W. Moskowitz & M. R. Haug (Eds.), *Arthritis and the elderly* (pp. 72–84). New York: Springer.

CHAPTER 19

Analogues between Medical and Industrial Safety Research on Compliance Behavior

Henry P. Cole, Philip K. Berger, and Thomas F. Garrity

Medical care compliance refers to the extent to which a person's behavior coincides with medical or health advice. The advice is usually in the form of a prescription for the regular use of a medication or a regimen to change a life-style pattern, such as modification of diet, increasing exercise, flossing teeth, and similar activities designed to maintain or restore health.

In the industrial health and safety setting, compliance may be defined as the extent to which a worker's behavior coincides with performance standards that describe proper and safe execution of a task. For example, a safe and proper procedure for changing a light bulb in a factory ceiling receptacle may involve using a sturdy stepladder of the appropriate height and construction, and in a specified manner. A worker may or may not comply with the prescribed procedure. If a worker stands on the tines of a forklift and is raised up to the receptacle by another person to change the bulb, neither person would be complying with the prescribed safety practice for changing light bulbs.

In both the medical and the industrial health and safety settings, the degree of compliance depends not only upon the individual but also upon the social and organizational context, the nature and complexity of the prescribed activity, the level of the person's understanding of the risks involved, existing technology to reduce those risks, the availability of this technology to the individual, the influence of peers and authority figures, as well as the motives and choices of the individuals involved (Leventhal & Hirschman, 1982).

PURPOSE

In the fields of medicine, health, and primary prevention, there is a large body of research on techniques to change individual behaviors and life-styles. The research was stimulated by Public Health Service grants and other funds which became available after

HENRY P. COLE • Department of Educational and Counseling Psychology, University of Kentucky, Lexington, Kentucky 40506-0205. PHILIP K. BERGER • Martin School of Public Administration, University of Kentucky, Lexington, Kentucky 40506-0058. THOMAS F. GARRITY • Department of Behavioral Science, University of Kentucky, Lexington, Kentucky 40506-0086.

the Health Manpower Act of 1968 and the Comprehensive Health Manpower and Training Act of 1971 (Cole, 1978; Cooper, 1976). Much of this research focuses on modifying patterns of individual behavior and personal choice to increase adherence to health and/or safety practices in daily living (e.g., wearing seat belts, reducing smoking, taking medication for hypertension control, and modifying life-style patterns of exercise and diet).

Likewise, in the area of industrial safety and health, accidents, injuries, and occupational illnesses also have observable behavioral factors associated with them. Research has shown that accident and injury rates can be reduced by increasing worker adherence to safe and healthy work practices. A focus on altering worker behavior to achieve increased compliance with safe work practices, coupled with the more traditional approaches of engineering a safer workplace environment and enforcing health and safety rules, appears to be an effective way to lower injury and illness rates (Benfari, Eaker, & Stoll, 1981; Matarazzo, 1982; Watson, 1986).

A review of the literature in both fields clearly indicates that the extensive research about boosting patient compliance to medical care and health practice regimens is not generally known to researchers who study ways to boost compliance with healthy and safe work practices in industry. Likewise, most researchers in the medical and health compliance field are unfamiliar with the literature dealing with compliance with healthy and safe work practices in industrial production settings. Our goal was to examine research from both areas to (1) determine if there were common sets of principles and/or themes in those two research literatures on compliance and (2) to see whether the literatures could inform each other in terms of future research and practice agenda. The focus was upon well-conceptualized empirical studies in each field that demonstrated significant improvement in compliance with health and/or safety regimens. It is our hope that future intervention studies in both fields may profit from this synthesis.

METHOD

A multidisciplinary research team was formed. The team included health, educational, rehabilitation, and counseling psychologists, as well as medical sociologists, industrial health and safety experts, and engineers. The research team located and reviewed research about how medical and health personnel attempt to increase compliance with recommended regimens. The team also searched for applications of similar strategies used to increase worker compliance with safe work practices in underground coal mining, other mining, and other heavy industries. Computer searches of the world's research literature in both medical compliance and industrial safety and health were carried out in 17 major databases. Experts in these fields were also contacted and asked to identify exemplary studies that described effective health and safety intervention programs. These activities resulted in a 31-page bibliography concerned with increasing compliance to safety and health practices (Cole *et al.*, 1985).

Members of the research team met in a biweekly seminar over a period of 1 year. Key findings from well-designed studies in both the medical compliance and the industrial safety and health fields were reviewed, discussed, and compared. Eventually five areas of parallel findings concerning compliance behavior in both fields were identified. These areas are (1) typical rates of persons' compliance with health and/or safety practices, (2) the effects of acute versus chronic health and/or safety threats on compliance behavior, (3) phases over which compliance behaviors emerge and become institutionalized, (4) factors and conditions correlated with compliance rates, and (5) principles and procedures shown to be effective in boosting persons' typical compliance rates.

FINDINGS: PARALLELS IN COMPLIANCE BOOSTING RESEARCH

For medicine, behavioral intervention programs designed to enhance health have fallen into four general approaches (Benfari *et al.,* 1981). These include:

1. Interventions designed to modify individual physiological responses, such as relaxation training to reduce stress
2. Modification in the behavior of the health provider (e.g., dentist, nurse, physical therapist, physician, nutritionist) to make patient teaching more understandable and useful
3. Increasing the frequency of patient adherence to prescribed medical regimen (diet, exercise, medication)
4. Modification of clusters of individual's behaviors or life-style to reduce risk of illness or injury

The research in these areas may be relevant to thinking about individual workers' well-being at the workplace. For example, intervention programs that seek to lessen back and other skeletal muscular system injuries to laborers through individual physiological assessment and physical conditioning programs are examples of a physiological intervention. Programs that seek to improve the effectiveness of training staff, foremen, and management to communicate safety and health information, values, and policy to workers fall into the second category. Programs that seek to increase frequency of specific worker behaviors such as wearing safety glasses, or always looking before backing equipment fall into the third category. Safety education programs designed to promote increased worker perception of occupational hazards, ongoing corrective and preventive action to reduce risks, and the cooperative, vigilant, and consistent following of prescribed safe work practices fall under the fourth approach.

In the following sections a number of parallels between industrial and safety programs that increased workers' adherence to safe work practices and interventions that increased patients' compliance with medical or health regimens are described. Readers interested in a more detailed treatment should refer to the final project report (Cole *et al.,* 1985).

Frequency of Compliance

Research results in medical compliance often show approximately a third of the trained population complying routinely, a third occasionally complying, and the remaining third frequently not complying (Benfari *et al.,* 1981). There appear to be no comparable data on worker compliance with safe work practices. Nonetheless, similar patterns may exist among individual worker behavior. The prevailing viewpoint among experts in industrial safety is that many workplace accidents and illnesses occur because individuals do not routinely comply with prescribed safe work practices (Committee on Underground Coal Mine Safety, 1982, 1983; Watson, 1986). If, in fact, worker noncompliance is a major factor in accidents and occupational illness and the overall rates of noncompliance are similar to those reported in the medical literature, the need for improved preventive efforts could not be more starkly demonstrated.

Acute versus Chronic Health and Safety Threats

In the medical literature, research efforts to boost compliance can be divided into programs for acute conditions, chronic conditions, and primary prevention. Findings on patient adherence to medical regimens for treatment of acute health conditions do not generalize to regimens for chronic health conditions in which the immediate threats to life and health are not as pressing and there is less discomfort (Taylor, Lichtman, & Wood, 1984). Adherence in the workplace appears to more closely parallel the medical compliance situation for primary prevention and treatment of chronic health problems.

Industrial health and safety programs stress the routine practice of work procedures designed to prevent or lessen injuries and illness among workers. Yet the failure to follow a specific safe practice on a given occasion is only infrequently followed by a serious accident. In the case of inappropriate behaviors which have occupational health consequences, the disease may not become manifest for many years after the exposures occurred. An example is the cumulative and nonreversible respiratory disease that develops from failure to wear respirators in dusty environments. As a safety example, consider a worker in a mine or factory who may occasionally choose to cross a moving conveyor belt by crawling under or climbing over the belt, rather than complying with the safer practice of traveling to the nearest belt crossover point. For any given instance of improperly crossing a moving conveyor belt, the worker is not likely to become entangled, to fall, or to be injured. Similarly, the medical patient with hypertension or diabetes may not always comply with the medication and dietary regimens and not suffer immediate consequences from lack of adherence to the regimens. In both the industrial and the chronic illness cases, frequent noncompliance is statistically dangerous, but individual regimen violations typically have no immediate negative consequences. Furthermore, in both situations noncompliance may be immediately rewarding in terms of saving time and money and reducing physical discomfort.

Four Phases of Compliance

Learning to follow health or safety regimens routinely is a complex process that is acquired over a period of time. Research in both medical compliance and industrial safety suggests that it may be useful to conceptualize health and safety training as occuring over four phases (Brownell, Marlatt, Lichtenstein, & Wilson, 1986; Garrity, 1983). In the first phase (preparation), the individual must become aware of the risks to personal well-being and the value of the compliance procedure. In the second stage (activation), the patient or worker must become capable and willing to follow routinely practices that reduce health hazards. In the third stage (tailoring), some aspects of the health regimen, safety procedures, the job task, or the work station may have to be adjusted to make it easier for the person to comply routinely with the desired practice. In the last stage (sustenance), the patient or worker, as well as peers and supervisors, must internalize high standards (goals) for routinely monitoring and complying with the prescribed health or work practices. The conceptualization of four phases of compliance may be most useful as a way to think about what needs to be taught and what tasks need to be accomplished at each stage in the adoption of a health or safety regimen from initiation through habituation.

Correlates of Compliance

In both the medical and industrial safety literatures there are many descriptive studies that seek to determine what variables are correlated with individuals' compliance with health and safety practices. In both fields there are far fewer well-controlled long-term intervention studies that evaluate the effectiveness of various compliance-boosting strategies.

Descriptive studies in both fields point to some common setting characteristics associated with individuals' high rates of compliance. These studies reveal that important correlates of compliance tend to be: the level of support (organizational, technical, social,

TABLE 1. Characteristics of Safe Mines and Factories

Strong management commitment to safety
- Safety matters regularly included on meeting agenda
- Safety of workers viewed as management responsibility
- All levels of management committed to and involved in safety

Positive and proactive organizational climate
- Supportive and open relationship by management toward workers
- Frequent, easy, two-way communication among workers and managers

Management efficiency in planning and operations
- Good housekeeping and materials handling/storage
- Shared knowledge and well-coordinated activities among departments, workers, supervisors, and managers
- Good record-keeping in production, job performance, safety, and widespread sharing of this information
- Frequent use of data in planning and decision making

Decentralized wide involvement of persons in safety matters
- First-line supervisors and workers involved in daily inspections, hazard detection/corrections
- Top managers encourage widespread preventive/corrective safety activity and are themselves frequently involved
- Little reliance upon a central safety officer/staff to be mainly responsible for maintaining a safe work environment

Behavioral specificity in safety and job procedures
- Rules for proper task performance are clearly and operationally specified
- Regular and redundant communication of safety and proper job performance procedures by several means including:
    - Informal meetings/dialogue at the work section
    - Formal safety meetings
    - Posters including safety rules, procedures, reminders, and so forth
    - Formal investigation of accidents or near accidents
    - Consistent and fair enforcement of safety procedures

Stable work force
- Good worker morale and attendance
- Little employee turnover
- Experienced and older workforce

Strong financial solvency of the company
- Company/division is earning profits
- Good backlog of orders for products ensures future

and peer) available to assist the individual in complying; the ease or difficulty in complying (cost, required effort, intrusiveness of the health and/or safety practice, the complexity and side effects of the procedures); the technical competence and interpersonal skill of the health or safety trainer; the opportunity and willingness of the individual trainee to be involved in setting personal goals for compliance; and the trainee being frequently informed about the degree of success in achieving the goals. In neither field has compliance been found to be related to worker personality, character, or intelligence (Cole *et al.*, 1985).

Table 1 summarizes the major characteristics that distinguish mines and factories with good safety practices and records from those with poor records. These characteristics were abstracted from 12 major descriptive studies of pairs of safe and unsafe workplaces (Althouse & Hurrell, 1977; Cleveland, Cohen, Smith, & Cohen, 1979; Cohen, 1977; Committee on Underground Coal Mine Safety, 1982, 1983; Davis & Stahl, 1964; Demichiei, Langton, Bullock, & Wiles, 1982; Naval Ammunition Depot, Research and Development

Department, 1971; Pfeifer, Grether, & Grether, 1976; Sanders, Patterson, & Peay, 1976; Simonds & Shafai-Sahrai, 1977; Smith, Cohen, Cohen, & Cleveland, 1978). The studies were exceptionally thorough; they involved detailed reviews of company safety procedures, accident records, safety training and procedures, interviews with management, supervisors, and workers, and walk-through inspections at each site.

Although the results of correlational studies offer many ideas for developing safer work environments, there tend to be problems in implementing interventions based on these characteristics. Medical compliance interventions based on findings of correlational studies have often been disappointing and have not improved frequency of patient compliance with medical or health regimens (Haynes, Taylor, & Sackett, 1979). In addition, a number of the correlates of compliance in both the health care and industrial safety areas are not directly manipulable. For example, Cleveland *et al.* (1979) in their study of safety record-holding factories in the United States, found that financially strong companies, and factories located in a small rural community with a relatively homogeneous and stable work force, generally had good safety records. Such variables are not subject to manipulation by workers, industries, or researchers. Likewise in medical compliance research the degree of compliance is often dependent upon the economic, family, and community circumstances of individuals which are not manipulable by health providers. For example, poor people who live in remote areas of Appalachian eastern Kentucky often have difficulty complying with medical treatment regimens when needed care facilities and services are not locally available.

Principles and Procedures for Boosting Compliance

Principles that improved compliance with health and safety practices were abstracted from key empirical studies in both fields. Particularly helpful were nine well-designed studies that introduced safety programs into mines or factories and achieved major increases in workers' routine compliance with safe work practices (Cohen & Jensen, 1984; Komaki, Barwick, & Scott, 1978; Komaki, Heinzmann, & Lawson, 1980; Komaki, Collins, & Penn, 1982; Larson *et al.*, 1980; Reber & Wallin, 1984; Rhoton, 1980; Sulzer-Azaroff & de Santamaria, 1980; Uslan, Adelman, & Keller, 1978). Subsequently, the accident and injury rates dropped dramatically at most of these work sites. These and other behavioral intervention studies in other industrial settings, as well as research on successful interventions in medical compliance situations (Feuerstein, Labbe, & Kuczmierczyk, 1986; Haynes *et al.*, 1979; Leventhal, Zimmerman, & Gutmann, 1984), were carefully reviewed. General principles for boosting compliance in both settings were abstracted from this body of research literature. These principles are summarized in Table 2.

A set of common procedures used to implement effective behavioral safety programs is shown in Table 3. Although these procedures are more specific to increasing compliance with safe work practices, they share much in common with behavioral interventions that are effective in boosting patients' compliance with medical regimens (Benfari *et al.*, 1981; Garrity, 1981; Garrity, 1983; Garrity & Garrity, 1985; Haynes *et al.*, 1979).

The principles in Table 2 and the steps in Table 3 are well illustrated in a number of studies (Cohen & Jensen, 1984; Komaki *et al.*, 1978, 1980, 1982; Reber & Wallin, 1984). These studies took place in a large commercial bakery, a vehicle maintenance shop, a poultry processing plant, a farm machinery manufacturing plant, and in warehouses where heavy lift trucks were used. In all cases the safe work practices targeted for improvement were based upon analysis of past injuries. For example, in the vehicle maintenance shop, mechanics were frequently injured by falling when climbing on equipment by using jacks and jack stands instead of ladders. In the bakery one source of injuries resulted from workers climbing over or crawling under moving conveyor belts rather than using desig-

TABLE 2. Principles for Boosting Compliance

1. Foster the informed consent and the active participation of the client (worker or patient) in targeting specific behaviors as goals for increased compliance.
2. Elicit the help of the client's social group (family, friends, and co-workers) to help achieve increased levels of compliance with the prescribed procedure (regimen).
3. Target those behaviors that are linked to illness and injury; the ones in which compliance with a prescribed procedure will have the most impact on reducing risk.
4. Define each targeted behavior and procedure for compliance in specific and directly observable terms.
5. Focus the educational and training activities, and the monitoring of the client's performance, directly upon the specific targeted behaviors, not on the long-term therapeutic goals. (In a diet regimen, have patients monitor daily caloric intake or food eaten, not pounds lost. In a factory, monitor the number of times electrical circuits are locked out when working on electrical equipment, not the number of electrical accidents or electrocutions.)
6. Provide frequent cues to the client to help him or her remember to comply with the prescribed procedure. Good record-keeping, frequent feedback, and social support from peers and supervisors are good sources of cues.

nated crossing points. Other problem areas included slips and falls on walkways with clutter and oil spills, injuries from cleaning equipment that had not been shut down, and eye injuries from grinding and cutting metal without wearing safety glasses.

In these successful safety intervention programs, specific unsafe work practices were identified for each work section. These problem areas were then discussed with workers and supervisors from that section. Specific procedures for routinely carrying out each safe

TABLE 3. Steps in Developing Effective Behavioral Safety Programs

Phase 1—Preparation (antecedent activities)
- Target specific tasks that are:
  - Linked to past injuries
  - Behaviorally defined

Phase II—Instruction (educational activities)
- Hold a 30- to 40-minute meeting with workers and supervisors by sections where:
  - Baseline data are presented
  - Advantages of working safely are discussed
  - Each specific safety procedure is demonstrated
  - Compliance with safety practices is reinforced by supervisors by verbal praise, recognition, and so forth
  - Workers and supervisors are encouraged to publicly affirm high rates of compliance (90% or greater)
  - Procedures for the next phase are presented

Phase III—Implementation (behavioral feedback and institutionalization of activities)
- Continue observing, recording, and charting worker performance on targeted tasks three to four times weekly
- Display graphs of percent correct performance in the work section after each observation
- Continue holding monthly or biweekly safety meetings by sections where:
  - Graphs are discussed
  - Tailoring safe work procedures and/or the work station to overcome barriers to routine compliance is planned
  - New or potential hazards are identified

work practice were discussed and agreed to (e.g., using ladders for climbing, crossing conveyors only at designated points, wearing safety goggles for metal working). Workers in each section then saw a demonstration of the safe and unsafe procedures for each targeted task. Workers were asked to set and affirm high goals for working safely, e.g., at least 90% of the time. A simple performance checklist was developed for each of the targeted behaviors. An observer made an unannounced, randomly scheduled, walk-through inspection, typically about three times a week. Using the checklist, the observer openly recorded compliance or noncompliance with each targeted behavior for the workers on that section. Immediately following these random observation periods, the percentage of compliance with all targeted safe work practices was summed across all workers and tasks, calculated, and plotted on a graph. In the next phase, those data collected from regular observations of workers' performance on the targeted tasks for a period of a few weeks were displayed and discussed by supervisors and workers from each work section. Both groups were frequently surprised to learn that targeted safe work practices, such as looking when backing powered equipment, were followed only about 70% of the time. (A parallel finding exists in the medical compliance literature. Physicians typically overestimate the extent to which their patients comply with prescribed regimens (Inui, Yourtee, & Williamson, 1976).) The third phase continued the thrice weekly random observations of worker performance on the targeted tasks, but also provided immediate feedback of the compliance rate to the workers. The graphs and completed checklists were posted in the work section immediately following the observation periods. In addition to these procedures, Cohen and Jensen (1984) asked workers and supervisors to reaffirm their intention publicly to comply with the safe work practices and to model these for others in their daily activity. In all the studies, workers and supervisors showed much interest in the graphs, and the rate of compliance with the targeted safe work practices rapidly climbed to near 100% once the checklist and graph results were posted immediately following observation periods. In some cases the number of accidental injuries that resulted in lost time dropped by as much as 80%.

LIMITATIONS OF BEHAVIORAL STRATEGIES

Behavioral interventions to increase compliance with safe work practices are not substitutes for ergonomic or organizational interventions, nor for the enforcement of safety regulations. Rather, they are best used in conjunction with these more basic approaches as Teleky (1948) noted long ago. This point can be illustrated by the following example.

In a large study of Swedish woodsmen involved in tree-felling, it was determined that increased training in safe work practices would not likely lower the high injury rate for these workers. The tree-fellers already knew the safe practices for felling trees. They failed to work safely because of problematic production and organizational factors in the management of the industry, and because they lacked equipment such as that needed for safely dropping a felled tree that has become lodged in a second standing tree (Ostberg, 1980). In situations like this it would be foolish and irresponsible to propose a behavioral safety program as a solution to the problem. Rather, ergonomic, organizational, and legal approaches are required. However, once the workers' capability to fell trees safely is enhanced by these other means, behavioral strategies are useful in maintaining high levels of worker compliance with safe work practices.

Other interventions for improving health and safety in job performance in mines and other workplaces that depend more upon the training of managers in the economics of loss control (Peters & Schaffer, 1986), or upon supervisory training and improvement of management and labor relations (Blumberg, 1980; Fiedler, Bell, Chemers, & Patrick, 1984;

Trist, Susman, & Brown, 1977; Uslan *et al.*, 1978) have sometimes achieved increases in compliance with safe work practices as large as those observed in the behavioral studies that have been reviewed here. However, these other types of interventions tend to be oriented toward managers and not workers, to be complex, expensive, and require longer to implement than the more targeted behavioral approaches described earlier.

POTENTIAL FOR SHARING PERSPECTIVES

The first part of this chapter described many of the commonalities between the medical and industrial safety compliance literatures. These parallels are not unexpected given the similarities in social and behavioral science training received by researchers in both fields. This section takes a selective look at potentially fruitful research efforts which are underdeveloped in one or both of the medical and industrial safety literatures.

Fishbein and Ajzen's behavioral intention model has been widely used to predict medical compliance and preventive health behaviors but has not been applied to industrial safety and healthy work practices. Leventhal's focus on mental representations of diseases and symptoms and their relation to compliance with medical regimens has no parallel in the industrial safety/health literature. Finally, Locke's goal setting theory has seen little or no application in either of the two compliance literatures. Each of these perspectives will be examined briefly.

Behavioral Intentions

Compensatory models are used extensively to predict health-related behaviors. These models assume that the individual evaluates a range of attributes (e.g., costs, benefits, consequences) before deciding to engage in some activity. A perceived weakness on one attribute (e.g., high cost) can be compensated for by strength in other attributes (e.g., improved health). Expectancy value models are one class of compensatory models of judgment. In expectancy value models, judgments are based upon one's beliefs that engaging in a behavior (like working safely or dieting) will or will not lead to the attributes ascribed to that behavior, together with one's evaluation of the goodness or badness of that belief.

In the medical compliance literature, several value-expectancy theories have been applied to behaviors concerning adherence to medical regimens and engaging in preventive health behaviors. The most prevalent of those theories is the health belief model which is discussed elsewhere in this volume. In the past decade, Fishbein and Ajzen (1975), Triandis (1980, 1982), and Rogers (1983) proposed alternative value-expectancy theories which have received a good deal of empirical support as predictors of health-related behaviors (e.g., Jaccard, 1975; Montano, 1986; Oliver & Berger, 1979). These models have not been applied to the prediction of workers' compliance with safe or healthy work practices. The work environment, especially with the enactment of OSHA's hazard communication directive, is one in which rational choice models may be appropriate characterizations of decision behavior (Janis, 1984). For brevity, we will explore how Fishbein and Ajzen's behavioral intention model might be applied to compliance with safe work practices in an underground coal mine.

A basic safe work practice in underground coal mining is to travel *only* under supported mine roof. The roof is supported by mechanically installing long steel roof bolts that bind the rock layers together to prevent a roof fall. According to the Fishbein and Ajzen model, attitudes toward engaging or not engaging in a safe work practice are based on the person's evaluation of the act's consequences and the belief that acting will lead to these consequences. To illustrate, the consequences of walking through an area of unsupported roof in an underground coal mine might include:

1. A large fall of rock that could injure or kill the miner
2. No fall of rock or some minor flaking that would not cause injury
3. Increased production of coal because of time saved by traveling directly to the desired point rather than taking a safer but much longer route
4. Less expenditure of physical effort, especially when one is carrying a heavy load
5. Being cited for an unsafe act by a company or federal inspector, should the act be witnessed
6. Demonstration to others of lack of fear

A large roof fall may be evaluated as very dangerous but believed to be unlikely. The time and effort saved by taking a shortcut through an unbolted passage may be evaluated as desirable because increased production may result from time saved and the foreman may believe that the time saved is likely to yield production increases.

A subjective social norms component also influences the miner's intentions to comply. That is, the miner's beliefs about what significant others (co-workers, supervisors, family members, inspectors) expect in this situation and how those opinions are valued, influence the individual's intention to comply or not comply with the safety practice. Finally, the model includes one's sense of personal obligation, what one ought to do, as an influence on intentions and subsequent behaviors.

Fishbein and Ajzen posited three classes of conditions that influence the degree to which intentions to comply actually result in compliance. The first condition concerns the degree to which a general intention such as "work safely" is translated into a specific prescribed safety practice such as "never walk under an unsupported mine roof." General intentions often have little influence on compliance with specific healthy and safe work practices unless the linkage is made specific.

Second, Fishbein and Ajzen noted that behavioral intentions are not stable. They can change depending upon the time interval between the person's expression of the intention or goal (to work safely) and the opportunity to exhibit actions that uphold that goal. In addition, the worker's intentions to work safely are influenced by physical and organizational conditions in the workplace. If adequate roof bolting equipment and materials are not available, and good roof control plans are not specified and followed, the miner's intention may be compromised. Attempts to engage in a specific safe work practice, like never going under an unsupported mine roof, depend largely on the behavior of other persons and the adequacy of tools, materials, management procedures, and organization of the workplace. Peters (1983), Unger and Connelly (1983), the Committee on Underground Coal Mine Safety (1983), and others have noted the crucial role of appropriate organization, tools, and management procedures as prerequisites to workers' compliance with healthy and safe work practices.

The third condition noted in the Fishbein and Ajzen model concerns the individual's knowledge and skill levels. It is not sufficient to intend to comply with a safe work practice. One must also know how to do so. For example, much knowledge and skill are required to clean up a roof fall and restore mining operations without exposing oneself to unsupported roof and a second roof fall.

Finally, the model's implications for changing workplace behavior to increase frequency of safe work practices are straightforward. One can change components of behavioral intentions for the conditions that intervene between the worker's intention and the carrying out of the intended behavior. To modify behavioral intentions one should focus upon attitudes toward the specific safe acts of interest and the subjective norm, and/

or the personal norm that influence the worker's decisions to comply or not comply with specific safe work practices. The physical and organizational aspects of the workplace must support the worker's intentions to comply with safe work practices. From this latter perspective the usual means to boost compliance with such work practices is the reduction of hazards through engineering, educational interventions aimed at workers, management, and policymakers, as well as strong and consistent enforcement of health and safety laws. These latter topics are outside the scope of this chapter.

Representations of Illness/Health States

Leventhal's theory of self-regulated behavior includes a component called a schema or a mental representation of illness/health states and of health hazards in general. Illustrative research in this area includes papers by Leventhal and Nerenz (1985), Leventhal, Meyer, and Nerenz (1980), Leventhal, Safer, and Panagis (1983) and Meyer, Leventhal, and Guttman (1985). These schemata are persons' commonsense models of the health hazard and seem to be based on recollections of their personal experience with the hazard (Leventhal *et al.*, 1983). As schemata change, compliance strategies must likewise be modified.

We have been able to identify only a single study which could be construed as an attempt to develop an analogous cognitive map of accidents within a specific job. Roberts, Golder, and Chick (1980) modeled the cognitive space (i.e., schemata) of airplane pilot errors. Five of the six dimensions they identified through cluster analysis were:

1. Errors of decision
2. Errors of judgment
3. Errors of awareness
4. Errors of technique or skill
5. Normal and emergency procedures

The sixth dimension was unique to pilots' preflight procedures.

Roberts *et al.* employed multidimensional scaling on these clusters in terms of cognitive attributes of these errors. The six attributes included: (1) errors which could ruin your career, (2) errors which would embarrass you, (3) errors which would "rattle" you, (4) serious errors, (5) responsibility for the error, and (6) a positive affect from making an error. Pilots had a difficult time agreeing on which errors were "fun," i.e., produced a positive affect; otherwise there were high rates of agreement on the remaining cognitive attributes.

Leventhal and Nerenz (1985) laid out in great detail the research strategies necessary to capture such commonsense mental representations and Roberts *et al.* (1980) suggested a starting point in terms of analytic strategies and possible dimensions. The industrial safety and health field would do well to explore such a conceptual approach to enhance its understanding of why workers persist in engaging in what health and safety professionals agree are "obviously unsafe" work practices.

Goal Theory

A third perspective appears to hold the promise for conceptualizing both medical and industrial compliance, but has seen little application in either field. This is the concept of goal setting as developed by Locke (1968). Perceptions of successful or unsuccessful behavior are dependent, in large part, upon the goals and the criteria used to evaluate goal achievement. Here, we briefly review the following aspects of the goal setting process:

(1) goal difficulty, (2) goal specificity, (3) goal timeliness, (4) goal acceptance, and (5) the goal setting process. This discussion relies on review articles by Carver and Scheier (1982), Leventhal and Nerenz (1985), Locke (1980), Locke, Shaw, Saari, and Latham (1981), and Austin and Bobko (1985). It should be noted that the vast majority of studies on goal theory involve short time perspectives and very simple tasks. Little research has been done which mirrors the long-term and complex behaviors associated with compliance to many medical and industrial health and safety regimens. The theory is, nonetheless, a provocative one for both fields.

The conclusion of this research is succinctly stated by Leventhal and Nerenz (1985):

> Unreasonable goals—excessively abstract or demanding, unclear, and temporally inappropriate—doom the individual to conclude that his efforts cannot produce desired outcomes (p. 21).

The term *goal* refers to a desired level of outcome. That outcome could be defined in terms of a state of being (e.g., healthy, asymptomatic, not exposed to a hazard) or in terms of a level of task or behavior proficiency (e.g., proportion of times wearing a respirator, proportion of prescribed medications consumed).

The evidence from many studies is unequivocal that *difficult* goals lead to better performance than easy or medium goals (Austin & Bobko, 1985; Chidester & Grigsby, 1984; Locke *et al.,* 1981), provided the individual is involved in setting the goals and has the means to achieve them. Moreover, the more *specific* the goals, the better is the performance. That is, statements of intentions to accomplish a specific measurable outcome result in better performance than intentions simply to "do one's best." There is also some evidence to suggest that people who have complex, challenging, and specific goals become more proactive in developing strategies to accomplish those goals.

Goals, by themselves, are not sufficient to improve performance to its maximum. In order for behavior to change drastically, feedback or knowledge of results must accompany the goal setting and goal acceptance process (Locke *et al.,* 1981).

Locke *et al.* (1981) define goal acceptance as an agreement "to commit oneself to a goal assigned or suggested by another person." They conclude that:

1. The higher the expectations of success, the higher the acceptance of the goal
2. The higher the perceived value of the goal, the greater its acceptance

As Carver and Scheier (1982) noted, expectancy assessments are important in self-regulated behavior theory. Bandura (1982) also noted that communication strategies that get people to believe they possess the capabilities to achieve their goals can contribute to successful performance. In addition to expectations of success and the value attached to the goal, Locke *et al.* (1981) report that *personal goals are the best predictors of performance*. Hence, when a particular goal is one in which there is personal investment, goal-oriented performance is strongest.

Finally, there is the important issue of the goal setting process. Conventional wisdom and a variety of empirical studies emphasize the value of participative management strategies. Locke *et al.* (1981) and Austin and Bobko (1985) concluded that participation *per se* does not affect performance. Rather, participation may influence one or more of the following mechanisms:

1. Create positive attitudes which may serve to reduce conflict in the goal setting activity
2. Produce higher goals which in turn influence behavior
3. Reflect greater supportiveness by management or health care provider which results in enhanced goal acceptance which in turn leads to improved performance

4. Enhance performance because it results in a broader discussion of strategies that can be used to attain the goals

In terms of medical compliance, these generalizations suggest (1) that the patient–provider process be a collaborative effort in setting targets for compliance, and (2) that in some cases, groups of patients working collaboratively with a health care provider may produce better compliance outcomes than that obtained with one-to-one patient–provider interactions.

Finally, Austin and Bobko (1985) discussed some of the nuances of goal theory and identified gaps in the empirical literature. One particularly relevant issue which they raised is the potential dysfunctional consequences of substantially improving one's compliance performance but yet not attaining one's goal. Little is known about the consequences of simultaneously succeeding and failing at a task. In complex health regimens, compliance is likely to be incremental and thus be characterized by simultaneous success and failure.

The few well-designed studies which have incorporated components of goal setting theory, along with behavioral methods like those outlined in Table 3, show the merits of this union (Cohen & Jensen, 1984; Reber & Wallin, 1984). Cohen and Jensen increased the compliance rates of 98 forklift truck operators in two warehouses on 14 specific tasks, the improper performance of which had caused frequent accidents and injuries. The procedures used were nearly identical to those used in the Komaki *et al.* (1978, 1980, 1982) studies, with some important distinctions. Explicit treatment stages were added that included goal setting and affirmation, and informal peer modeling. These were combined with the operational specification of the targeted safe work practices and frequent performance feedback to the operators about their degree of skill and compliance with each safe work practice. Three months after the formal program and regular observations stopped, truck operators continued high rates of compliance. In the Komaki *et al.* and other earlier studies, compliance rates usually fell to preintervention levels once regular observation and feedback stopped. Cohen and Jensen (1984) suggested that goal setting, regular performance feedback, and modeling of safe work practices by workers and their supervisors can be explicitly developed as program intervention methods and serve to institutionalize high compliance rates in the absence of experimenters or special programs and personnel.

Cohen and Jensen attributed the endurance of safe work practices, after an intervention, to the habitual practice of procedures, and redefinition of group norms for workers and supervisors that dictate and model compliance with the proper work practices. This interpretation is consistent with the previously discussed models of compliance developed by Fishbein and Ajzen (1975) as well as Triandis (1982).

Although there is recognition in both the medical and work fields of the importance of goals and feedback, there is little in the way of empirical research on adopting or extending goal theory to the problem of enhancing compliance with behaviors which promote personal well-being.

CONCLUSION: POSSIBILITIES FOR FURTHER CONNECTIONS

In our review of the literature, we found a few well-conceptualized interventions to increase compliance with healthful and safe work practices in industrial settings. Counterparts to these few well-designed behavioral experiments in the medical field were scarce, perhaps because they are more difficult to implement. We also observed that the magnitude of the effect of the treatments for these few studies are larger than for similar studies in the medical field. Perhaps those who conceptualize and carry out health and medical regimens can be informed by those few industrial safety interventions that conceptualize changing specific behaviors through a broader social and organizational framework.

There are also parallels in the ethical issues involved in research and policy matters in both fields. Examination of commentary on ethical issues in compliance reveals that most of the ethical problems (and methods for dealing with these) in the medical and health compliance research area can also inform the ethics of industrial health and safety intervention programs (Jonsen, 1979; Levine, 1980). For example, to what extent is it ethical to pressure, punish, or mislead in order to improve compliance? How does one balance the values of freedom of choice versus avoidance of harm, or the worker's right to know versus being free from undue anxieties about health and safety conditions? In the current climate of more stringent hazard communication standards for workers and the movement for the public's right-to-know about workplace and environmental hazards, those concerned with these matters may find useful analogues in the more extensive medical ethics literature dealing with compliance issues.

Another area for crossover of concepts is in research methods. Sackett (1979) suggested that what has been learned in medical and health compliance research methods can be informed by (and help inform) similar compliance studies concerned with changing of life-styles and behavior patterns of persons in work settings. Indeed, until very recently attempts to use behavioral strategies in the workplace to increase compliance with safe work practices are noticeably absent in the industrial safety literature.

What we have learned about the similarities between compliance in the medical field and industrial safety and health can be succinctly summarized. Properly designed behavioral strategies are successful to the extent they call the clients' attention to specific ways in which they can think about and act to routinely comply with safe practices and to achieve goals they desire. Setting and achievement of specific goals, assistance in overcoming barriers, knowledge of one's progress in striving toward changes in life-style or work patterns can be helpful in both maintaining the person's performance and changing the person's thinking and feeling about the situation, helping the individual and the group to seek and achieve more self-direction of behavior and an increased sense of agency and responsibility. This is why these types of intervention strategies have come to be called "cognitive-behavioral" (Bandura, 1982; Turk, Meichenbaum, & Genest, 1983). This perspective and its methods apply to increasing compliance with medical, dietary, and exercise regimens as well as improving the degree of compliance with healthy and safe work practices in the home or factory. Staying on one's diet to control weight and blood pressure is not unlike following the work practice of wearing protective equipment like hard hats, safety goggles, and hearing protectors, and consistently following other detailed or time-consuming routines. In both cases, compliance occurs by individuals within intimate social groups and a larger physical, sociopolitical, and legal environment. In both spheres, compliance is undoubtedly aided by approaches that recognize this complexity and that seek to enhance the individual's sense of agency and capacity for self-direction and responsibility.

Acknowledgments

Dr. Cole currently heads, and Drs. Berger and Garrity are principals in IMMR/BRASH, the Behavioral Research Aspects of Safety and Health working group that operates under the auspices of the University of Kentucky Institute of Mining and Minerals Research. The research reported in this chapter was partially supported by U.S. Bureau of Mines contract PO333468 September 1983 to February 1985. The authors gratefully acknowledge the many ideas and suggestions contributed throughout the project by R. Michael Digman and William J. Wiehagen, the Bureau of Mines Technical Project officers, and the assistance of C. Dwight Auvenshine, Anthony B. Szwilski, Maria Hernandez,

David K. Blythe, and Warren E. Lacefield in the completion of the research activity upon which this chapter is based. The views presented herein are those of the authors and not necessarily those of the Interior Department's Bureau of Mines.

REFERENCES

Althouse, R., & Hurrell, J. J., Jr. (1977). *An analysis of job stress in coal mining*. Cincinnati: National Institute for Occupational Safety and Health.

Austin, J. T., & Bobko, P. (1985). Goal setting theory: Unexplored areas and future research needs. *Journal of Occupational Psychology, 58,* 289–308.

Bandura, A. (1982). Self-efficacy mechanism in human agency. *American Psychologist, 37,* 122–147.

Benfari, R. C., Eaker, E., & Stoll, J. G. (1981). Behavioral interventions and compliance to treatment regimens. *Annual Review of Public Health, 2,* 431–471.

Blumberg, M. (1980). Job switching in autonomous work groups: An exploratory study in a Pennsylvania coal mine. *Academy of Management Journal, 23,* 287–306.

Brownell, K. D., Marlatt, G. A., Lichtenstein, E., & Wilson, G. T. (1986). Understanding and preventing relapse. *American Psychologist, 41,* 765–782.

Carver, C. S., & Scheier, M. F. (1982). Control theory: A useful conceptual framework for personality-socio-clinical, and health psychology. *Psychological Bulletin, 92,* 111–135.

Chidester, T. R., & Grigsby, W. C. (1984). A meta-analysis of the goal setting-performance literature. In J. A. Pearce, II, & R. B. Robinson, Jr. (Eds.), *Academy of Management proceedings* (pp. 202–206). Boston: Academy of Management.

Cleveland, R., Cohen, H. H., Smith, M. J., & Cohen, A. (1979). *Safety program practices in record-holding plants* (NIOSH Publication No. 79-136). Morgantown, WV: National Institute for Occupational Safety and Health.

Cohen, A. (1977). Factors in successful occupational safety programs. *Journal of Safety Research, 9,* 168–176.

Cohen, H. H., & Jensen, R. C. (1984). Measuring the effectiveness of an industrial lift truck safety program. *Journal of Safety Research, 15,* 125–135.

Cole, H. P. (1978, March 28). *Roles and contributions of educational and counseling psychology to the health care professions*. Paper presented at the annual meeting of the American Educational Research Association, Toronto, Canada. (ERIC Document Reproduction Service No. ED 153 042).

Cole, H. P., Berger, P. K., Garrity, T. F., Auvenshine, C. D., Szwilski, A. B., Hernandez, M., Blythe, D. K., & Lacefield, W. E. (1985). *Generalization of medical and health compliance research to coal mine safety* (Final Report, Contract No. P0333468). Pittsburgh, PA: Bureau of Mines.

Committee on Underground Coal Mine Safety. (1982). *Toward safer underground coal mines*. Washington, DC: National Academy Press.

Committee on Underground Coal Mine Safety. Commission on Engineering and Technical Systems. (1983). *Fatalities in small underground coal mines* (OFR 124-83). Pittsburgh, PA: Bureau of Mines.

Cooper, T. (1976). Editorial. *Commitment, 1,* 2.

Davis, R. T., & Stahl, R. W. (1964). *Safety organization and activities of award-winning companies in the coal-mining industry* (Information Circular No. 8224). Pittsburgh, PA: Bureau of Mines.

Demichiei, J. M., Langton, J. F., Bullock, K. A., & Wiles, T. C. (1982). *Factors associated with disabling injuries in underground coal mines*. Arlington, VA: Mine Safety and Health Administration.

Feuerstein, M., Labbe, E. E., & Kuczmierczyk, A. R. (1986). *Health psychology: Psychobiological perspective*. New York: Plenum Press.

Fiedler, F. E., Bell, C. H., Jr., Chemers, M. H., & Patrick, D. (1984). Increasing mine productivity and safety through management training and organization development: A comparative study. *Basic and Applied Social Psychology, 5,* 1–18.

Fishbein, M., & Ajzen, I. (1975). *Belief, attitude, intention and behavior*. Reading, MA: Addison–Wesley.

Garrity, T. F. (1981). Medical compliance and the clinician–patient relationship: A review. *Social Science and Medicine, 15E,* 215–222.

Garrity, T. F. (1983). Enhancing dental compliance: Suggestions for patient education at various stages of compliance. In R. Moretti & W. A. Ayer (Eds.), *The President's conference on the dentist–patient relationship and the management of fear, anxiety, and pain* (pp. 27–33). Chicago: American Dental Association.

Garrity, T. F., & Garrity, A. R. (1985). The nature and efficacy of intervention studies in the National High Blood Pressure Education Research Program. *Journal of Hypertension, 3* (Suppl. 1), 91–95.

Haynes, R. B., Taylor, D. W., & Sackett, D. L. (1979). *Compliance in health care*. Baltimore: The Johns Hopkins University Press.

Inui, T. S., Yourtee, E. L., & Williamson, J. W. (1976). Improved outcomes in hypertension after physician tutorials: A controlled trial. *Annals of Internal Medicine, 84,* 646–651.

Jaccard, J. (1975). A theoretical analysis of selected factors important to health education strategies. *Health Education Monographs, 3,* 152–167.

Janis, I. L. (1984). The patient as decision maker. In W. D. Gentry (Ed.), *Handbook of behavioral medicine* (pp. 326–368). New York: Guilford Press.

Jonsen, A. R. (1979). Ethical issues in compliance. In R. B. Haynes, D. W. Taylor, & D. L. Sackett (Eds.), *Compliance in health care* (pp. 113–120). Baltimore: The Johns Hopkins University Press.

Komaki, J., Barwick, K. D., & Scott, L. R. (1978). A behavioral approach to occupational safety: Pinpointing and reinforcing safe performance in a food manufacturing plant. *Journal of Applied Psychology, 63,* 434–445.

Komaki, J. L., Collins, R. L., & Penn, P. (1982). The role of performance antecedents and consequences in work motivation. *Journal of Applied Psychology, 67,* 334–340.

Komaki, J., Heinzmann, A. T., & Lawson, L. (1980). Effect of training and feedback: Component analysis of a behavioral safety program. *Journal of Applied Psychology, 65,* 261–270.

Larson, L. D., Schnelle, J. F., Kirchner, R., Jr., Carr, A. F., Domash, M., & Risley, T. R. (1980). Reduction of police vehicle accidents through mechanically aided supervision. *Journal of Applied Behavior Analysis, 13,* 571–581.

Leventhal, H., & Hirschman, R. S. (1982). Social psychology and prevention. In G. S. Saunders & J. Suls (Eds.), *Social psychology of health and illness* (pp. 183–226). Hillsdale, NJ: Erlbaum.

Leventhal, H., Meyer, D., & Nerenz, D. (1980). The common sense representation of illness danger. In S. Rachman (Ed.), *Medical psychology* (Vol. 2, pp. 7–30). New York: Pergamon Press.

Leventhal, H., & Nerenz, D. R. (1985). The assessment of illness cognition. In P. Karoly (Ed.), *Measurement strategies in health psychology* (pp. 517–554). New York: Wiley.

Leventhal, H., Safer, M. A., & Panagis, D. M. (1983). The impact of communications on the self-regulation of health beliefs, decisions, and behavior. *Health Education Quarterly, 10,* 3–29.

Leventhal, H., Zimmerman, R., & Gutmann, M. (1984). Compliance: A self-regulation perspective. In W. D. Gentry (Ed.), *Handbook of behavioral medicine* (pp. 369–436). New York: Guilford Press.

Levine, R. J. (1980). Ethical considerations in the development and application of compliance strategies for the treatment of hypertension. In R. B. Haynes, M. E. Mattson, & T. O. Engebretson, Jr. (Eds.), *Patient compliance to prescribed acute hypertension medication regimens: A report to the National Heart Lung and Blood Institute* (NIH Publication No. 81-2102). Bethesda, MD: National Institutes of Health.

Locke, E. A. (1968). Toward a theory of task motivation and incentives. *Organizational Behavior and Human Performance, 3,* 157–189.

Locke, E. A. (1980). Latham versus Komaki: A tale of two paradigms. *Journal of Applied Psychology, 65,* 16–23.

Locke, E. A., Shaw, K. N., Saari, L. M., & Latham, G. P. (1981). Goal setting and task performance: 1969–1980. *Psychological Bulletin, 90,* 125–152.

Matarazzo, J. D. (1982). Behavioral health's challenge to academic, scientific, and professional psychology. *American Psychologist, 37,* 1–14.

Meyer, D., Leventhal, H., & Gutmann, M. (1985). Common sense models of illness: The example of hypertension. *Health Psychology, 4,* 115–135.

Montano, D. E. (1986). Predicting and understanding influenza vaccination behavior. *Medical Care, 24,* 438–453.

Naval Ammunition Depot, Research and Development Department. (1971). *Survey of human factors in underground bituminous coal mining* (RDTR No. 184). Craine, IN: Department of the Navy, Ordinance System Command.

Oliver, R. L., & Berger, P. K. (1979). A path analysis of preventive health care decision models. *Journal of Consumer Research, 6,* 113–122.

Ostberg, O. (1980). Risk perception and work behavior in forestry: Implications for accident prevention policy. *Accident Analysis and Prevention, 12,* 189–200.

Peters, R. H. (1983). Activities and objects most commonly associated with underground coal miners' back injuries. In J. M. Peay (Ed.), *Back injuries: Proceedings of the Bureau of Mines Technology Transfer Symposia* (IC 8948). Pittsburgh, PA and Reno, NV: Bureau of Mines.

Peters, R. H., & Schaffer, L. (1986). *Field test of a model health and safety program for the mining industry* (IC 8948). Washington, DC: Bureau of Mines.

Pfeifer, C. M., Jr., Grether, S., & Grether, C. B. (1976). *Psychological, behavioral, and organizational factors affecting coal miner safety and health* (Contract No. HSM 99-72-151). Columbia, MD: National Institute for Occupational Safety and Health, Westinghouse Behavioral Service Center.

Reber, R. A., & Wallin, J. A. (1984). The effects of training, goal setting, and knowledge of results on safe behavior: A component analysis. *Academy of Management Journal, 27,* 544–560.

Rhoton, W. W. (1980). A procedure to improve compliance with coal mine safety regulations. *Journal of Organizational Behavior Management, 2,* 243–249.

Roberts, J. M., Golder, T. V., & Chick, G. E. (1980). Judgment, oversight, and skill: A cultural analysis of P-3 pilot error. *Human Organization, 39,* 5–21.

Rogers, R. W. (1983). Cognitive and physiological processes in fear appeals and attitude change: A revised theory of protection motivation. In J. T. Cacioppo & R. E. Petty (Eds.), *Social psychophysiology* (pp. 153–176). New York: Guilford Press.

Sackett, D. L. (1979). Methods for compliance research. In R. B. Haynes, D. W. Taylor, & D. L. Sackett (Eds.), *Compliance in health care* (pp. 323–333). Baltimore: The Johns Hopkins University Press.

Sanders, M. S., Patterson, T. V., & Peay, J. M. (1976). *The effect of organizational climate and policy on coal mine safety* (Contract No. HO242039). Crane, IN: Naval Weapons Support Center, Applied Sciences Department.

Simonds, R. H., & Shafai-Sahrai, Y. (1977). Factors apparently affecting injury frequency in eleven matched pairs of companies. *Journal of Safety Research, 9,* 120–127.

Smith, M. J., Cohen, H. H., Cohen, A., & Cleveland, R. J. (1978). Characteristics of successful safety programs. *Journal of Safety Research, 10,* 5–15.

Sulzer-Azaroff, B., & de Santamaria, M. C. (1980). Industrial safety hazard reduction through performance feedback. *Journal of Applied Behavior Analysis, 13,* 287–295.

Taylor, S. E., Lichtman, R. R., & Wood, J. V. (1984). Compliance with chemotherapy among breast cancer patients. *Health Psychology, 3,* 553–562.

Teleky, L. (1948). *History of factory and mine hygiene*. New York: Columbia University Press.

Triandis, H. (1980). Values, attitudes, and interpersonal behavior. In D. Levine (Ed.), *Nebraska symposium on motivation* (Vol. 17, pp. 195–259). Lincoln: University of Nebraska Press.

Triandis, H. (1982). A model of choice in marketing. In L. McAlister (Ed.), *Choice models for buyer behavior* (pp. 147–162). Greenwich, CT: JAI Press.

Trist, E. L., Susman, G. I., & Brown, G. R. (1977). An experiment in autonomous working in an American underground coal mine. *Human Relations, 30,* 201–236.

Turk, D. C., Meichenbaum, D., & Genest, M. (1983). *Pain and behavioral medicine.* New York: Guilford Press.

Unger, R. L., & Connelly, D. J. (1983). Materials handling methods and problems in underground coal mines. In J. M. Peay (Ed.), *Back injuries: Proceedings of the Bureau of Mines Technology Transfer Symposia* (IC 8948). Pittsburgh, PA and Reno, NV: Bureau of Mines.

Uslan, S. S., Adelman, H. M., & Keller, R. S. (1978). *Testing the effects of applied behavioral analysis and applied behavioral management techniques on the safe behaviors of salt mine personnel* (Final Report, Contract No. J0166137). Pittsburgh, PA: Bureau of Mines.

Watson, C. E. (1986). Does behavior based safety management work? *Professional Safety, 31*(9), 20–25.

PART IV

HEALTH BEHAVIOR: ITS RELEVANCE AND FUTURE

Ways in which knowledge generated by health behavior research is relevant for the training of health professionals, for health promotion and health education programs, and for clinical settings have already been addressed explicitly in several of the preceding chapters. The chapters by Ben-Sira and Roter, for example, point to the need for physicians to be more aware of, and sensitive to the affective dimensions of their interactions with patients, as these can have an important effect on the technical dimensions of therapy. Furthermore, much health behavior research had roots in applied settings. The health belief model, for example, originated in attempts to understand, and thereby increase public response to appeals to participate in preventive screening programs (e.g., Rosenstock, 1974), and as the chapter by Kirscht indicates, continues to be heavily involved in predicting, understanding, and improving responses to a variety of health promotion appeals. Similarly, as Lau's chapter reveals, research on health locus of control is often conducted in the context of health promotion programs; and the chapter by Sallis and Nader refers to educational programs intended to promote health behavior.

Moreover, clinical applications can integrate knowledge about physician (or professional)–patient (client) relationships, and about health education strategies, with the complexity of issues related to compliance with, acceptance of, or adherence to medical regimens. Cole, Berger, and Garrity identify some of these compliance applications in their chapter; others are discussed in the material introducing the section on "Power, Compliance, and Control." Clinical applications themselves often involve educational efforts, but for these discussions, clinical applications refer essentially to those that involve therapeutic interventions or regimens for a medically defined condition.

Because health behavior does not yet have an established identity, its knowledge is often broadly referred to as behavioral or social science knowledge. Health behavior knowledge is a special subset of behavioral or social science knowledge. Understandably, literature addressing the linkages between health behavior and professional training, health promotion and health education, and clinical applications, often uses these terms interchangeably. Yet, regardless of how it is referred to, and despite an increasingly impressive accumulation of empirical data, the application and integration of knowledge generated by health behavior research is far less than might be hoped for or expected.

TRAINING OF HEALTH PROFESSIONALS

The need for increasing the social and behavioral science content in the training of health professionals, particularly in medicine and dentistry, has long been documented. Discussions of such needs have involved both general and specific content.

General Content

Millon (1975) listed several indictments of the narrow scientism of the typical medical curriculum, based on its failure to include a broad spectrum of social and behavioral science knowledge. Grinker (1975) argued for a "systems theory" approach to medical thinking, and attacked the historical "atomistic" perspective of medicine and medical training which results in patients being thought of as specific disorders or organs. He urged that patients' emotions and thoughts, frustrations, disappointments, and hopelessness be considered along with their somatic complaint or symptom. Knowles, as far back as 1968 (1968/1975), stated that "medicine is a social as well as a physical and biological science, and that it needs the humanities and social sciences and the effects of their study as never before in . . . history" (p. 7). Such content, he urged, should be part of the premedical program, and the medical curriculum as well. Knowles identified historical barriers that have prevented this from happening, but encouraged medical education to incorporate this content nonetheless.

In their cogent overview of medical practice, Eisenberg and Kleinman (1981) noted a historical concern about physicians who demonstrate an overly narrow disease focus, rather than a broader, more person-oriented one. However, they argued that this divergence in perspectives reflected community and societal factors more so than flaws in medical education. They noted, though, that contemporary medical education's emphasis on increased specialization and increased technology has exacerbated this divergence, and expressed concern that medical interventions may be less effective because of it. They advocated increased social and behavioral science content in medical training as a way of countering this narrowness, and thus assuring that medicine can deliver its technological skills with increasing effectiveness.

Dentistry. Kegeles and Cohen (1971) concluded that social science research has had a "humanizing force for the profession" of dentistry, and anticipated that incremental research findings will ultimately have an impact upon dental curricula. They noted, however, that social science research findings have not had an appreciable impact upon dental education, nor have social scientists teaching within dental schools, although the number of social scientists employed in dental contexts has increased. In the years since Kegeles and Cohen's report, little has changed appreciably in the degree to which health behavior knowledge has been incorporated in the training of dental professionals.

Specific Content

More specific to health behavior, Mechanic and Newton (1965/1975) urged, for example, that physicians need to understand dimensions of illness behavior, the significance to the patient of the presenting symptoms, the dynamics of the process of eliciting relevant information from patients, and the social and institutional context in which medicine is practiced, and that medical education should incorporate such content.

Petersdorf and Feinstein (1981) documented the inclusion of medical sociology content in medical curricula, defining medical sociology to include a broad range of health behavior topics, including: personal, family, societal, institutional, and community effects on health and illness; and the interpersonal aspects of medical practice. Although this content was included in somewhat systematic ways in a number of curricula, it was absent from a far larger portion. Petersdorf and Feinstein further noted that the enthusiastic supporters of medical sociology content "were not nearly as eloquent in expounding their positive views, as the detractors were in relieving themselves of their negative biases" (p. 40).

Segall (1984), addressing the importance of educating physicians for clinical prevention, identified physician–patient interactions, including communication and decision processes; support of family and friends; and patient motivation as areas where physicians require increased knowledge and sensitivity, and which should be targets of medical school curricula.

Additional health behavior domains relevant to physicians, dentists, and nurses, and thus appropriate targets for their training, are how they perceive patients (e.g., Tannenbaum, Weschler, & Massarik, 1961/1975); communication with patients (e.g., Elder, 1963/1975), including the relationship between social factors and communication (e.g., Schatzman & Strauss, 1975); and different models of professional–patient interaction (e.g., Szasz & Hollender, 1956/1975).

The chapter by Baumgart and Costello describes the gap between what is hoped for, in relation to incorporating health behavior knowledge in medical and nursing training, and the degree to which it actually exists, along with an analysis of some of the factors that serve as barriers to increasing their presence.

Health Promotion and Health Education

Understandably, many important health promotion and health education campaigns are based on research establishing the health risk of certain behaviors such as smoking and cholesterol intake. This health-risk perspective, however important in understanding the behavioral concomitants of disease, is not, as Chapter 1 points out, the perspective on health behavior taken in this book. Moreover, arguments have been made (e.g., Fielding, 1977) that overidentification with risk factors and disease are inappropriate, ineffective approaches to health promotion campaigns.

Health behavior, as this book approaches it, as a body of basic knowledge, clearly has relevance for such programs. Simonds (1984) acknowledged health education's increasing emphasis on the determinants of human behavior, and on health behavior research. Green (1984) similarly noted that effective models for health education require greater knowledge of the determinants of health behavior, including individual cognitive factors such as interests, attitudes, perceptions, beliefs, values, and motives; and skills at estimating risks or vulnerabilities, and recognizing symptoms; as well as social determinants such as peer influences.

Health behavior knowledge thus has implications both for the broad conceptions of what health education and health promotion programs should be like, as well as for specific aspects of the content and targets of such programs.

Broad Conceptions

Fielding (1977) pointed out problems resulting from health promotion becoming coopted as the preventive part of specific medical regimens, e.g., exercise or smoking-reduction programs being perceived as part of the regimen for heart disease, rather than as general health-promoting behaviors. Health promotion has thus acquired a disease-specific orientation and connotation. Fielding urged that health promotion programs begin to emphasize the nondisease factors that determine health behavior—e.g., patterns of reinforcement that increase the likelihood of such behaviors occurring; tax structures and insurance policy premiums that reward health-promoting behavior—which can be potent factors in moving health promotion away from risk-reduction, disease-specific models. Knowledge generated by health behavior research can identify the nondisease factors that generate and support preventive behaviors. Moreover, Fielding argued for the greater involvement of community groups in the planning of health promotion programs. Knowledge generated by health behavior research can determine how, and in what ways, social networks and other social and community factors support or impede preventive, health-promoting behaviors.

Knowledge generated by health behavior research was the basis for England's reasoning (1978) that it was necessary to cast off myths about the ease of establishing successful prevention programs in underdeveloped countries. Other myths, as well as untested assumptions, about health education and health promotion programs, were identified by Johnson (1981) on the basis of knowledge generated by health behavior research. Noting the *real* data on the age of onset of smoking, Johnson could use this knowledge base to urge that antismoking programs begin at an appropriate age, an age that is not *so* early that the program effects would boomerang. Johnson also used health behavior research data to argue against erroneous assumptions about the long-term effects of health as a value compared with the effects of social approval.

Love and Kalnins (1984) used knowledge generated by health behavior research to support "structuralist" approaches to health promotion programs, rather than the more traditional approaches which attempt to change individuals. In nutrition education, for example, structuralist programs would focus on the community, on the food industry, and on television advertising as ways of changing dietary patterns. Similarly, congruent with knowledge generated by health behavior research, Milio (1976) argued that health education becomes more effective if it is group focused, and if the group then serves as a social network to support norms that endorse health-generating behaviors. She further emphasized that health education be viewed as a way of developing options rather than as strategies for restricting choice.

Finally, Graham (1973), using health behavior research data, identified cultural barriers to acceptance of innovations in relation to engaging in new, preventive behaviors, and urged that campaigns designed to change behaviors, or to elicit innovative behaviors, be considered in relation to the cultural meanings of the new behavior.

Specific Content and Targets

Eardley and colleagues' (1985) study of attendance at British cervical screenings showed that those women most in need of the services were least likely to take the initiative in making the appointments, and might be most threatened by the screening procedure and its potential findings. Their data showed that such programs would be more successful if the providers took initiative both in identifying participants and in the appointment-setting process; and that information about the screening be more directed at the needs and fears of the target population.

Frazier (1978), basing her arguments on health behavior research data demonstrating the great difficulty of changing motives, and of overcoming the social and cultural barriers to care, urged health education programs to move away from traditional attempts to change individual motives through typical dental health education programs for school-age children. Instead, she favored changing community policies through the skillful use of group and community planning processes.

Based on health behavior research data, Jenny (1976) urged that dental health promotion campaigns become more ecologically focused, and deal with the family as a whole, and with the community, rather than attempt to change individual diet and other behaviors that place dental health at risk. Community values encourage families to use refined carbohydrates. School health materials are ineffective in this context. Furthermore, Jenny identified barriers to care that reduce the effectiveness of health education programs, and urged that services and facilities be brought closer to the population to be served.

In relation to health screening campaigns, Kirscht, Haefner, and Eveland (1975) stressed the importance of coordinating types of appeals with characteristics of a target population. Stahl, Lawrie, Neill, and Kelley (1977) similarly endorsed adapting specific techniques to the characteristics of their target areas in a community hypertension screening program. Health behavior research has an important contribution to make in generating knowledge of such target population characteristics.

McAlister, Puska, Salonen, Tuomilehto, and Koskela (1982) based their comprehensive approach to health promotion in the North Karelia Project, on knowledge generated by health behavior research. Knowledge about the difficulty of changing individual preventive behaviors, including use of preventive services, together with data on the existing beliefs in their target population, led them to develop a program aimed at changing larger system variables. Their internationally recognized project in Finland mobilized a variety of community resources in a successful attempt at changing risk factors for cardiovascular disease. Wherever possible, families were involved by including them in cooking demonstrations, or by encouraging spousal support in adherence to regimens. Environmental changes included implementation of restaurant policies on smoking and successful encouragement of the development of a sausage with lower fat content. Significant reductions in risk estimates based on smoking, serum cholesterol, and blood pressure were obtained over a 5-year period.

West, Graham, Swanson, and Wilkinson (1977) urged the need for follow-up health behavior data on smoking cessation. Nearly a decade later, Shumaker and Grunberg (1986) provided a systematic account of the factors involved in smoking relapse. Although the systemic effects of nicotine themselves require greater understanding, they operate in conjunction with a variety of behavioral cues (e.g., Pomerlau, 1986) and improving the success of interventions will require greater understanding of personal motivation, social support, and family determinants of health behavior (e.g., Brownell *et al.,* 1986).

Despite the demonstrated value of health behavior knowledge and perspectives, very few health promotion and health education programs systematically incorporate such knowledge in their planning or implementation.

Kolbe's chapter identifies a number of health behavior objectives for health promotion and health education, particularly at the national level in the United States. He systematically notes areas in which health behavior knowledge and conceptual models might be used to enhance health promotion programs. Of critical importance in the chapter are the methodological and conceptual improvements that are suggested for those behaviors that will be used to evaluate these programs. One can infer from the chapter that basic health behavior knowledge has both a large and an unrealized potential for enhancing such programs. It has a major role, but one yet to be played.

CLINICAL APPLICATIONS

Health behavior knowledge about physician and patient interactions, about how they communicate, and about their changing role patterns, has obvious relevance to clinical settings, as does knowledge about the issues involved in patients' adherence to, or compliance with medical regimens. Clinical issues related to self-management and to chronicity are two areas where knowledge derived from health behavior research has particular relevance.

Self-Management

Concern for self-management has been particularly notable in relation to youngsters who have asthma and diabetes.

Childhood Asthma. A number of educational programs were designed to improve and increase self-management and thus improve the social functioning of large numbers of youngsters, as part of a national effort (National Institute of Allergy and Infectious Diseases & Asthma and Allergy Foundation of America, 1981). The results of such programs were equivocal at best. Most of them focused on technology: on the visuals, books, and behavioral methodologies. Scant attention was paid to the broad spectrum of potential personal, family, social, and cultural determinants of self-management behaviors, to the apparent stability of health-related beliefs in young populations, to the meaning of the condition to the child, or to the child's actual motives (in contrast to those that are presumed to exist) that could be engaged in enhancing the self-management process (Gochman, 1981).

Analyses of these programs revealed the need for health behavior research perspectives in this area. Gochman (1981) identified specific ways in which health behavior knowledge might have improved the effectiveness of the programs; and Bruhn (1983), in a scholarly and integrative way, showed how health behavior theory might have been used as a framework for such programs and thereby enhance their effectiveness.

Juvenile Diabetes. The value of health behavior knowledge has had a greater systematic impact on studies of self-management of juvenile diabetes. Research using health locus of control measures (e.g., Moffatt & Pless, 1983), and social networks (e.g., Marrero *et al.,* 1982) have shown the value of both of these factors in improving the management of the condition.

Chronicity and Future Applications

Complementing the self-management of childhood conditions, there are an increasingly large number of adults facing chronic conditions, for whom issues of self-management are interwoven with issues of patient role and sick role, and with issues of relationships with professionals. This population provides an especially critical challenge for future applications for health behavior research. Gallagher's chapter demonstrates ways in which the management problems posed by chronic renal disease—where many of these issues come together—offer a promising arena for future investigations of the applications of health behavior knowledge and theory.

Although the practical value of health behavior research was not a primary concern of this volume, the increasing knowledge that it has generated, and the increasing refinement of its models and conceptualizations, raise questions about why it has not become more integrally a part of professional training, health promotion and health education programs, and clinical interventions. These questions pose a challenge for future health behavior researchers.

THE FUTURE OF HEALTH BEHAVIOR RESEARCH

The final chapter provides an integrative summary of some of the predominant themes identified in the individual chapters, some of the issues that health behavior research must face in relation to its future identity, and some areas where it might productively conduct future research.

REFERENCES

Brownell, K. D., Glynn, T. J., Glasgow, R., Lando, H., Rand, C., Gottlieb, A., & Pinney, J. M. (1986). Task Force 5: Interventions to prevent relapse. In S. A. Shumaker & N. E. Grunberg (Eds.), *Proceedings of the National Working Conference on Smoking Relapse. Health Psychology, 5*(Suppl.), 53–68.

Bruhn, J. G. (1983). Application of theory in childhood asthma self-help programs. *Journal of Allergy and Clinical Immunization, 72,* 561–577.

Eardley, A., Elkind, A. K., Spencer, B., Hobbs, P., Pendleton, L. L., & Haran, D. (1985). Attendance for cervical screening—Whose problem? *Social Science and Medicine, 20,* 955–962.

Eisenberg, L., & Kleinman, A. (Eds.). (1981). *The relevance of social science for medicine.* Dordrecht: Reidel.

Elder, R. G. (1975). What is the patient saying? In T. Millon (Ed.), *Medical behavioral science.* Philadelphia: Saunders. (Reprinted from *Nursing Forum,* 1963, *2,* 25–37).

England, R. (1978). More myths in international health planning. *American Journal of Public Health, 68,* 153–159.

Fielding, J. E. (1977). Health promotion—Some notions in search of a constituency. *American Journal of Public Health, 67,* 1082–1085.

Frazier, P. J. (1978). A new look at dental health education in community programs. *Dental Hygiene, 52,* 176–186.

Gochman, D. S. (1981). On labels, systems, and motives: Some perspectives on children's health behavior. In *Self-management educational programs for childhood asthma, 2,* Conference Manuscripts. Sponsored by Center for Interdisciplinary Research in Immunologic Diseases, University of California at Los Angeles; National Institute of Allergy and Infectious Diseases; Asthma and Allergy Foundation of America.

Graham, S. (1973). Studies of behavior change to enhance public health. *American Journal of Public Health, 63,* 327–334.

Green, L. W. (1984). Health education models. In J. D. Matarazzo, S. M. Weiss, J. A. Herd, N. E. Miller, & S. M. Weiss (Eds.), *Behavioral health: A handbook of health enhancement and disease prevention.* New York: Wiley.

Grinker, R. R., Sr. (1975). Biomedical education as a system. In T. Millon (Ed.), *Medical behavioral science.* Philadelphia: Saunders.

Jenny, J. (1976). Promoting dental health—An ecological approach. *The Dental Assistant, 45,* 14–20, 48–49.

Johnson, C. A. (1981). Untested and erroneous assumptions underlying antismoking programs. In *Promoting adolescent health: A dialog on research and practice.* New York: Academic Press.

Kegeles, S. S., & Cohen, L. K. (1971). Role of social sciences in dentistry. In N. D. Richards & L. K. Cohen (Eds.), *Social sciences and dentistry: A critical bibliography.* The Hague: A. Sijthoff.

Kirscht, J. P., Haefner, D. P., & Eveland, J. D. (1975). Public response to various written appeals to participants in health screening. *Public Health Reports, 90,* 539–543.

Knowles, J. H. (1975). Medical education and the rationalization of health services. In T. Millon (Ed.), *Medical behavioral science.* Philadelphia: Saunders. (Reprinted from J. H. Knowles (Ed.), *Views of medical education and medical care,* 1968, Cambridge, MA: Harvard University Press)

Love, R., & Kalnins, I. (1984). Individualist and structuralist perspectives on nutrition education for Canadian children. *Social Science and Medicine, 18,* 199–204.

Marrero, D. G., Myers, G. L., Golden, M. P., West, D., Kershnar, A., & Lau, N. (1982). Adjustment to misfortune: The use of a social support group for adolescent diabetics. *Pediatric Adolescent Endocrinology, 10,* 213–218.

McAlister, A., Puska, P., Salonen, J. T., Tuomilehto, J., & Koskela, K. (1982). Theory and action for health promotion: Illustrations from the North Karelia Project. *American Journal of Public Health, 72,* 43–50.

Mechanic, D., & Newton, M. (1975). Social considerations in medical education: Points of convergence between medicine and behavioral science. In T. Millon (Ed.), *Medical behavioral science*. Philadelphia: Saunders. (Reprinted from *Journal of Chronic Diseases*, 1965, *18*, 291–301)

Milio, N. (1976). A framework for prevention: Changing health-damaging to health-generating life patterns. *American Journal of Public Health, 66*, 435–439.

Millon, T. (1975). Behavioral perspectives in medicine. In T. Millon (Ed.), *Medical behavioral science*. Philadelphia: Saunders.

Moffatt, M. E. K., & Pless, I. B. (1983). Locus of control in juvenile diabetic campers: Changes during camp, and relationship to camp staff assessments. *Journal of Pediatrics, 103*, 146–150.

National Institute of Allergy and Infectious Diseases. (1981). *Self-management educational programs for childhood asthma, 2,* Conference Manuscripts. Sponsored by Center for Interdisciplinary Research in Immunologic Diseases, University of California at Los Angeles; National Institute of Allergy and Infectious Diseases; Asthma and Allergy Foundation of America.

Petersdorf, R. G., & Feinstein, A. R. (1981). An informal appraisal of the current status of 'medical sociology.' In L. Eisenberg & A. Kleinman (Eds.), *The relevance of social science for medicine*. Dordrecht: Reidel.

Pomerlau, O. F. (1986). Neuroregulators and the reinforcement of smoking. In S. A. Shumaker & N. E. Grunberg (Eds.), *Proceedings of the National Working Conference on Smoking Relapse. Health Psychology, 5*(Suppl.), 85–86.

Rosenstock, I. M. (1974). Historical origins of the health belief model. In M. H. Becker (Ed.), The health belief model and personal health behavior [Special issue]. *Health Education Monographs, 2*, 328–335.

Schatzman, L., & Strauss, A. (1975). Social class and modes of communication. In T. Millon (Ed.), *Medical behavioral science*. Philadelphia: Saunders.

Segall, A. (1984). Physician education in clinical prevention. In J. D. Matarazzo, S. M. Weiss, J. A. Herd, N. E. Miller, & S. M. Weiss (Eds.), *Behavioral health: A handbook of health enhancement and disease prevention*. New York: Wiley.

Shumaker, S. A., & Grunberg, N. E. (Eds.). (1986). *Proceedings of the National Working Conference on Smoking Relapse*. Supplement to *Health Psychology, 5,* entire issue.

Simonds, S. K. (1984). Health education. In J. D. Matarazzo, S. M. Weiss, J. A. Herd, N. E. Miller, & S. M. Weiss (Eds.), *Behavioral health: A handbook of health enhancement and disease prevention*. New York: Wiley.

Stahl, S. M., Lawrie, T., Neill, P., & Kelley, C. (1977). Motivational interventions in community hypertension screening. *American Journal of Public Health, 67*, 345–352.

Szasz, T. S., & Hollender, M. H. (1975). A contribution to the philosophy of medicine: The basic models of the doctor–patient relationship. In T. Millon (Ed.), *Medical behavioral science*. Philadelphia: Saunders. (Reprinted from *Archives of Internal Medicine*, 1956, *97*, 585–592)

Tannenbaum, R., Weschler, I. R., & Massarik, F. (1975). The process of understanding people. In T. Millon (Ed.), *Medical behavioral science*. Philadelphia: Saunders. (Reprinted from R. Tannenbaum *et al., Leadership and organization: A behavioral science approach, 1961,* New York: McGraw–Hill)

West, D. W., Graham, S., Swanson, M., & Wilkinson, G. (1977). Five year follow-up of a smoking withdrawal clinic population. *American Journal of Public Health, 67*, 536–544.

CHAPTER 20

Health Behavior Research and the Training of Health Professionals

Alice J. Baumgart and Edith A. Costello

By many measures, health behavior remains a neglected subject in the training of health professionals in North America even though it has been a prominent concern in social policy and popular culture for well over a decade. Yet the picture may not be as gloomy as seasoned critics have painted it. What they have tended to overlook is how new socioeconomic and political conditions have affected the landscape of health services and higher education during the 1980s. As is usual in such circumstances, thinking beyond old categories and perspectives has been required. There are many signs that the resulting shift in consciousness is beginning to lead to significant changes in the form and content of health sciences education including heightened interest among educators and practitioners in incorporating knowledge germane to an understanding of health behavior (Council of Ontario Universities, 1982; Mustard, 1987; Squires, 1987).

The purpose of this chapter is to examine these developments in the context of basic and continuing education for nurses and physicians. These two occupational groups not only account for over half of all health care providers in Canada and the United States, but they tend to be regarded by consumers as the most accessible and appropriate sources of help for a wide variety of health matters. As such, their education and training is where some of the most conspicuous problems and possibilities lie for disseminating the results of health behavior research.

To provide a backdrop and point of reference, the chapter begins with a brief profile of the medical and nursing workforce and the many dimensions of their education and training. This is followed by an examination of the progress being made in incorporating health behavior perspectives into medical and nursing curricula and ongoing development activities. The chapter concludes with a consideration of the socioeconomic trends and health needs which are contributing to the structural transformation of health care and health sciences education and so stimulating a greater interest in health behavior.

Because the authors are Canadian, both American and Canadian educational developments are discussed. These developments have many parallels, for the two countries share common cultural roots and their systems of medical and nursing education have a long history of people and ideas flowing back and forth across the border. Where substantial

ALICE J. BAUMGART and EDITH A. COSTELLO • School of Nursing, Queen's University, Kingston, Ontario K7L 3N6, Canada.

differences exist is in the economic climate of health care. Whereas the United States continues to rely heavily on private funding of health services, medical and hospital services for Canada's 25.5 million people are financed by a comprehensive government-administered health insurance scheme.

THE MEDICAL AND NURSING WORK FORCE

The 1960s ushered in a sustained period of expansion and diversification in medical and nursing education in North America. One of the most visible results was a more than doubling in the number of active physicians and nurses. By 1985, there were over 500,000 active physicians in the United States with close to 17,000 graduating medical students being added to this supply each year. In Canada, the physician work force numbered nearly 50,000 and the yearly output of medical schools, about 1700. About two-thirds of these practitioners earned their livelihood through office-based practice, with 22% functioning as family physicians in the United States and 50% in Canada. About 1.5% of the physician work force in the United States and 6% in Canada were engaged in medical teaching on a full-time basis in 1986.

In the mid-1980s the registered nurse work force outnumbered that of medicine's by about three to one, with 1.5 million active nurses in the United States and 180,000 in Canada. About two-thirds worked in acute care hospitals. Another 9% worked in nursing homes and about 10% in preventive services and community settings such as occupational and school health services and visiting nurse agencies.

Nurses are a more heterogeneous group educationally than physicians, with their initial preparation being from 2 to 4 years in duration and taking place in any one of three settings: hospital diploma schools, community college programs, and baccalaureate degree programs in colleges and universities. Until the 1970s, over 80% of all nurses received their training in hospital schools. Fewer than 5% were graduates of degree-granting institutions. By 1985, many hospital schools had been closed and the remaining ones accounted for only 15% of new graduates; four-year colleges and universities were producing about 37% of the 75,000 new nursing graduates in the United States and 20% of such graduates in Canada. The full-time faculty members in these three types of nursing education programs comprised about 1.5% of the total nursing work force in both countries.

The Educational Task

As these statistics suggest, educational activities in relation to the medical and nursing work force are of impressive dimensions. In addition to preparatory education and training, a wide variety of specialty qualifications have been pursued. Since the 1960s, there has also been an explosive growth of continuing education offerings to help practitioners keep abreast of new methods and knowledge. Beyond this, there is a whole array of in-service programming by hospitals and other health care agencies to meet institutional training needs.

It is on this scale, and against entrenched professional interests, that the research findings on health behavior produced in the last 20 years have had to enter medical and nursing education. How has health behavior as a special field of learning fared under these circumstances? We look first at medical education.

HEALTH BEHAVIOR AND MEDICAL EDUCATION

Clearly, the subject of health behavior did not enter medical education *de nouveau* in 1974 when the Lalonde Report, *A new perspective on the health of Canadians,* sparked an international shift in thinking about how to approach health problems. However, its origins are difficult to trace and beg for more systematic study. In a historical sense, the claim could be made that its roots go back to teachings associated with the Greek goddess Hygeia, the guardian of health, who symbolized the belief that good health was the result of leading a balanced life. In a formal scientific sense, the incorporation of the concept into medical teaching is probably a product of the last 20 years, and most probably followed the publication of the widely cited definition of health behavior by Kasl and Cobb in 1966, which used the term to denote primary preventive behaviors.

The manner in which health behavior has been addressed in medical education in Canada and the United States is also difficult to trace and begs for systematic study. A tentative outline may be placed together, however, by drawing on a variety of published materials and personal sources.

A useful starting point is recent literature examining the social construction of medicine and the history of behavioral science teaching; in particular, writings on attitudes toward the role of behavior in disease (e.g., see Bloom, 1986; Wright & Treacher, 1982). Although these accounts do not specifically address health behavior as an area of basic research, they provide an instructive lesson on medical education's long-standing indifference to knowledge about health, disease, and the healing relationship emanating from the behavioral and social sciences.

This indifference is reflected, for example, in the neglect of prevention and related subjects in formal medical curricula and the continuing separation of public health schools from the mainstream of health sciences education (Barker & Jonas, 1981; Freymann, 1975, 1981). As Freymann (1975) pointed out, although almost half of U.S. medical schools have departments of preventive medicine (with the first established at Harvard in 1910), these departments "played bit parts on the state of medical education" until the 1960s.

Flexner's enshrining of disease and the biological sciences in medical education has frequently been blamed for this state of affairs. Cassell (1986) took the analysis a step further. He contended that in subsequent decades, the phenomenal success of medical science and its attendant technology helped to consolidate an unreal connection between medicine and a conception of science founded on early 20th century orthodoxy. In Cassell's words, "science was the physician" and teaching people to be doctors was viewed as being synonymous with teaching them the so-called scientific basis of medicine. As a result, the behavioral aspects of medical care were not only actively demoted from importance but considered unworthy of scientific investigation. This may be seen in the stigmatizing of behavioral science in medical writings and teaching as "soft science" and "anecdotal," or as sloppy, unscientific medicine.

The Behavioral Movement in Medical Education

The full eclipse of the behavioral and social sciences was forestalled by the emergence in the 1950s of what has been called the behavioral movement in medical education (Badgley & Bloom, 1973), a movement marked by three distinct but associated trends. The first saw the expansion of psychiatry in medical education and with it, the forging of new teaching and research alliances between psychiatry and the fields of clinical psychology and medical sociology (Blackwell & Torem, 1982; Matarazzo, 1980). The intellectual importance of these efforts lay, in part, in their providing a safe haven for teaching of behavioral content in medical curricula. Of greater significance, the ties established with the behavioral and social sciences created an opportunity to introduce a different heritage of thought and values about behavior into medical education.

A second, parallel trend saw departments of preventive medicine expand to take on central roles in comprehensive care programs. These educational experiments, launched by medical programs at Western Reserve University, Cornell University, and the University of Colorado (Light, 1983) helped to redress the growing imbalance between hospital-based specialization and general ambulatory care. These experimental programs had as a key strategic objective the injecting of a strong preventive orientation into clinical medicine (Barker & Jonas, 1981). As in the case of psychiatry, behavioral and social scientists were called upon to assist with teaching undergraduate and graduate medical students, and to strengthen the generally weak research skills of physician faculty members employed by the growing number of independent departments of preventive medicine (Van Etten & Rutten, 1986).

By the end of the 1950s, departments of preventive medicine began focusing their attention on epidemiology, and to a lesser extent, community medicine and the provision of community health services. This tendency was reinforced by the Great Society debates of the 1960s as reform-minded faculty members became involved in experiments to improve access to, and the organization of health care for disadvantaged populations.

A third, more deeply rooted trend of the behavioral movement in medical education was the development, in the late 1950s and 1960s, of separate courses in behavioral science. To support such teaching, a number of medical schools established independent departments of behavioral science with faculty drawn from disciplines such as medical sociology, psychology, psychiatry, and anthropology (Badgley & Bloom, 1973; Blackwell & Torem, 1982). According to Bloom (1986), most of these departments were based on the model of the basic sciences and their faculty members were expected to take their place in teaching the basic science of human behavior in the preclinical years. These directions were strengthened by a number of factors that included the leadership and financial support received from private foundations such as the Russell Sage and Milbank foundations and the Commonwealth Fund; the sponsorship of powerful advocates in academic medicine; and the curriculum innovations piloted by new medical schools such as that at McMaster University (Bloom, 1986). As well, public disillusionment with physicians and the authority they wielded had become sharper. This converged with the more generous supply of resources in a period of economic prosperity to give behavioral science departments the room to maneuver advantageously. Their teaching and research functions received additional support from the rapid expansion of the study of health and health care services and the growing range of disciplines directing attention to health problems (Mechanic, 1983).

Predictably, the cost consciousness that followed the 1973 world oil crisis and economic recession provided a more critical climate for behavioral science teaching. There was less money, and correspondingly less tolerance for the perceived weaknesses of the pedagogical model which had been put in place in medical education during the previous decade. In almost every medical school, behavioral science teaching had also been forced into much more vigorous competition for curriculum time with an ever-burgeoning number of clinical specialty and subspecialty departments. This competition had been made tougher by the accumulation of other new demands on medical education including the increasing concern with changing demographics, ethical issues in medical practice, and the intensification of medicine observed in the proliferation of hospital intensive care units.

The effects of these pressures, although widely discussed by those involved, have not received much attention in print. Reference to the *1986–87 Curriculum Directory* of the American Association of Medical Colleges suggests that required and elective course work under rubrics such as social and behavioral sciences, medical humanities, or behavioral medicine is included in over 80% of Canadian and American medical curricula (AAMC, 1985). Over 90% of these schools also include instruction in community medicine or health care and epidemiology. Taken together, the hours of instruction on these subjects comprise less than 5% of total teaching time in any one of these programs. No program listed offered either required or elective courses labeled health behavior.

A common and rather pessimistic view of these shifts in circumstance and attitude is that they have provided the conditions for a return to the supremacy of the biomedical model. Clearly, this interpretation must be treated with respect. The historical trends just outlined tend to support it. The growing interest in the role of heredity and biochemical factors in disease and behavior, also lend credibility to this interpretation as does the grip of technology, reflected in the elevation of artificial heart recipients to the status of folk heros.

New Perspectives

But is there a brighter side to the incorporation of behavioral concepts and methods into medical training? Has the upsurge of policy interest in health behavior found its way into medical teaching? If one tallies up the reported changes, do they add up to minor or trifling tinkering, or a fundamental shift in direction? As already noted, these are difficult questions to answer. The changes in medical training since the mid-1970s have not been studied in a comprehensive fashion. Nor has much study been undertaken in relation to the diffusion of new ideas and technologies to physicians and the academic medical community (Feeny, Guyatt, & Tugwell, 1986; Greer, 1977). What scant evidence exists comes mainly from three sources: recent reports and studies of medical education and training; the sparse literature on the attitudes of medical students and practicing physicians toward the concepts of health promotion and disease prevention; and the much more speculative literature on the trajectory of social and economic change.

Behavioral issues have been a distinct current in most contemporary proposals for reform of medical education including that reflected in the World Health Organization's "Health for All" initiative (Bryant, 1984) and in the Association of American Medical Colleges' influential 1984 report on general professional education for the physician, popularly known as the GPEP Report (AAMC, 1984, 1986). The unfinished debate concerns how much emphasis should be given to them and where they should be incorporated. A popular stance sees a resurfacing of the idea of clinical prevention, i.e., the weaving of health promotion and disease prevention into the practice and teaching of all clinical departments. As White (1987) argued, "modern medical education cannot afford to rely exclusively on one department."

So much for the principle. What one does not yet see clearly is tangible evidence of the pragmatics. Teachers well versed in the research on health behavior are in short supply. Resources to support and help knit together an integrated approach across an entire medical curriculum are difficult to find.

There is also the lingering opposition of powerful teaching departments. An enlightening picture in this regard is provided by the questionnaire survey on the current status of medical sociology conducted by Petersdorf and Feinstein (1981). They reported attitudes ranging from expressions of outright hostility and apathy from the chairpersons of departments of medicine, to growing enthusiasm from departments of pediatrics and family medicine. This gradient of enthusiasm was evident in the low proportion of departments reporting formal instruction on behavioral topics in medicine (12%) as compared with family medicine (34%) and pediatrics (26%).

A somewhat more encouraging picture emerges from recently published surveys of the attitudes and activities of medical students and practising physicians. For example, a study of 154 physicians who had completed an internal medicine residency at 15 major teaching hospitals in 1982 showed a majority interested in knowing more about behavioral issues and health promotion topics (Linn, Brook, Clark, Fink, & Kosecoff, 1986).

Similarly, in a study of beginning and third-year medical students' attitudes toward prevention, Scott and Neighbor (1985) found that both groups were in agreement as to the importance of incorporating a wide range of preventive services into medical care and felt confident about the ability of physicians to provide those pertaining to health counseling, cancer detection education, and blood pressure control. Much less confidence was expressed about the ability of current medical education and medical practice to address adequately behaviors such as smoking cessation, weight reduction, and exercise. A small study of physicians completing a family medicine residency in Alabama produced similar findings, with 87% of them feeling comfortable with patient education and only 14% having confidence with more directive behavioral interventions such as stress management (Kirkland & Skelton, 1985). Greater physician receptivity to incorporating concepts of disease prevention into their practices may also account for the finding from a telephone survey of residents of the city of Edmonton, conducted in 1985, that 77% of respondents had had their blood pressure checked in the previous year (Kurji & Macdonald, 1986). Equally impressive in this survey was the high proportion of females (78%) who had been shown how to perform breast self-examination. Another indicator of the greater health behavior presence in medical education in the last few years is the increased emphasis it receives in licensing and certifying examinations and in the accreditation requirements for medical schools and hospitals (Bloom, 1986; Butzin, 1985). It is also interesting to note the appearance of textbooks with titles such as *Preventive Cardiology* (Fraser, 1986).

These findings underscore that although attitudes are changing, the knowledge of physicians about effective health promotion and disease prevention strategies still varies widely. What is impossible to untangle is the extent to which these changes are being driven by reforms in medical education or by shifts in societal perspectives about the health implications of behaviors such as smoking.

For practicing physicians, continuing medical education (CME) programs are logical sources for the knowledge and skills they require. The extent to which these needs are being addressed is difficult to judge. A tally of CME courses listed in the *Journal of the American Medical Association* from 1977 to 1979 showed an increase in prevention-oriented topics over this brief period but an infinitesimal number of such offerings (1.02% in 1979) (Weinberg & Andrus, 1982).

Reading the medical literature is also regarded as a valid means for meeting continuing education needs, and surveys of physician reading habits show that a majority subscribe to professional journals and spend time reading them (Stinson & Mueller, 1980). The medical literature is also considered an important learning resource in undergraduate and graduate medical training. To give an indication of the opportunities available to medical students and practising professionals to increase their knowledge of health behavior from this body of literature, the authors completed a MEDLINE search for health behavior-related articles in selected high-circulation journals in Canada and the United States for the period 1975–1985. As indicated in Table 1, the MEDLINE data base was searched for titles under eight subject headings deemed most pertinent to health behavior. The total number of articles catalogued in MEDLINE under each heading for the 11-year period are listed in the next-to-last column. This data base was then cross referenced with the seven popular medical and nursing journals to determine how many health behavior-related articles were in each. The results suggest just how difficult it would be for physicians who relied mainly on one or two journals in their personal libraries to find pertinent material on health behavior. In this 11-year period, patient compliance topics appeared 31 times in the *Canadian Medical Association Journal,* 58 times in *Journal of the American Medical Association,* 7 times in the *Journal of Medical Education,* and 44 times in the *New England Journal of Medicine*. Thus, if one subscribed to all four journals, one might expect to see one article on compliance in only one of them on a monthly basis.

TABLE 1. Total Number of Health Behavior-Related Articles from Selected Medical and Nursing Journals in MEDLINE according to Eight Health Behavior Subjects 1975–1985

	Total number of articles in selected journals 1975–1985								
	Medicine				Nursing				
Subject	*Canadian Medical Association Journal*	*Journal of the American Medical Association*	*Journal of Medical Education*	*New England Journal of Medicine*	*American Journal of Nursing*	*Canadian Nurse*	*Nursing Outlook*	Eleven-year total of listings for subject	Percent of total listings for this subject from these journals
Attitude to health	20	64	19	39	22	15	5	6312	2.9%
Behavioral medicine[a]	0	0	2	0	0	0	1	135[b]	2.2%
Health promotion[b]	14	14	3	11	1	16	4	1495[b]	4.2%
Life-style	31	40	14	25	42	25	2	5497	3.3%
Patient education	16	34	13	16	130	52	9	5888	4.6%
Patient compliance	31	58	7	44	21	6	4	4938	3.5%
Sick role	3	0	1	5	6	0	0	1442	1.0%
Social environment	5	6	9	10	8	6	4	5877	0.8%

[a] Term not used in MEDLINE before 1978.
[b] Term not used in MEDLINE before 1980.

A more promising avenue is suggested by the research on compliance with antihypertensive therapy, namely, the use of well-designed tutorials or training sessions for practising physicians. For example, Inui, Yourtee, and Williamson (1976) were able to demonstrate an impressive effect on patients' knowledge and compliance by providing physicians with a 1- to 2-hour tutorial in compliance-enhancing strategies.

HEALTH BEHAVIOR AND NURSING EDUCATION

We turn next to nursing. Nursing education enjoys two advantages over medical education in regard to incorporating health behavior research into its training programs. The first is the long association of nurses with the public health movement and their employment in sizeable numbers in health care agencies oriented toward health promotion and disease prevention. The second advantage is an intellectual one. Views of nursing's mission and theory base, from the time of Florence Nightingale, have assigned a much more central role to health behavior concepts than has generally been true in medical education.

The debate on how best to prepare nurses for changing health patterns is a perennial one. At the beginning of the century, many in-hospital training programs provided valuable firsthand experience on the process of comforting the sick, but prevention was beyond their scope. The American Society of Superintendents of Training Schools for Nurses established in 1912 the National League of Nursing Education to examine and advise on nursing education (Piemonte, 1976). This organization has done much to promote awareness that nurses prepared in a university setting have the benefits of taking a range of biological, physical, and social science courses. Disciplined study about human behavior, and health and society is presumed to provide the necessary foundation for preventive nursing practice.

Nursing has been primarily a female profession; thus, during the first half of this century there was slow headway in establishing university baccalaureate programs. This paralleled the extent to which all women have been somewhat nervously integrated into institutes of higher education. Slowly, academic administrators were persuaded that community health nurses, nurse teachers, and nurse administrators could benefit from knowledge being generated at schools of public health, business administration, policy planning, teaching/learning, and many related sciences.

The leading professional nursing associations in Canada and the United States now recognize that all nurses should be prepared in an accredited university program in order to function competently as collaborators with clients for behavior change. Professional nursing associations believe that curricula at the basic baccalaureate level should provide in-depth preparation to enable nurses to problem solve and make valid judgments about nursing practice (Torres, 1974).

Curricular Responses to the Surge of Interest in Health Behavior

Many nurses have gone beyond basic baccalaureate preparation in their quest to examine the discipline's *raison d'être*. Other sciences have been examined to determine their contribution to the process of nursing amid changing societal demands. As a result of the United States Surgeon General's report, *Healthy People* (1979), models have been proposed to guide curricula and practice. Assisting clients with self-care is a dominant theme in those nursing models designed to reduce mortality and morbidity (Neuman, 1982; Orem, 1980; Parse, 1981). However, operationalizing health behavior is proving a difficult task; hence, measuring the ultimate value of these models remains elusive (Pender, 1984).

Baccalaureate nursing programs, more so than diploma education, have included additional content regarding patient education and preventive measures (Camooso *et al.*, 1980). This has been in part a response to the need to prepare public health nurses to be effective teachers of mothers and children. Another pressure on the practice of nursing has been the need to focus on life skills training and fostering social supports for the deinstitutionalization of psychiatric patients, which began in the 1960s. Nursing education is beginning to respond, too, to the rapidly increasing number of very old people, meaning that chronic illness occupies a growing portion of peoples' life spans in the developed world (Fries, 1980). However, it was not until the 1970s that most nursing education took place outside of hospital settings. It is in college and university departments of political studies, anthropology, sociology, and psychology where students have the opportunity to interpret health-related behavior research. In these departments, for example, nursing students can critique the findings of studies relating social supports to pregnancy outcome (Nuckolls, Cassel, & Kaplan, 1972), or examine studies relating the family and health (Croog, Lipson, & Levine, 1972), or link mental and physical health among the elderly with the existence of social support networks (Lowenthal & Berkman, 1967; Schwartz, Henley, & Zeita, 1964). Although it cannot be assumed that this content is learned by all undergraduate nursing students, a recent survey of 18 baccalaureate programs indicated that these courses, among others, were required: general psychology (15 programs); sociology (11); developmental psychology (8); growth and development (3); anthropology (3); social psychology (2); and abnormal psychology (2) (Sohn, 1986).

In 1974, a committee of nursing and medical experts was convened by the World Health Organization to recommend ways in which nursing could impact on the health problems prevailing in developing and developed countries (WHO, 1984). It was recommended that there be a shift from traditional foci to nursing services that were responsive to community needs and that encompassed primary health care coverage for all. Then, in 1978, WHO identified primary health care as the key to obtaining health for all by the year 2000. In 1983, nine years after the first WHO expert committee had disbanded, a new expert nursing committee was charged with recommending practical and viable strategies and approaches for the reorientation of nursing education. The latter committee felt that nursing education should take place in a university, an institute of higher education, or other relevant educational establishment and that content should come from multidisciplinary sources in order to prepare nurses as agents of change.

Collaboration among the 1.5% of nurses who are educators, health care agency administrators, trustees of postsecondary education, and legislators has to follow in order to attain the recommended objective that all nursing education take place in universities or the equivalent. In Canada and the United States, nurses are still embroiled in debate about how to credit previous learning and experience to enable nurses to upgrade to baccalaureate status. Thus, educators are constrained from moving into serious planning to ensure that minimum nurse preparation includes behavioral science education at the baccalaureate level and that primary care be a curricular focus (Murphy, 1986; Richardson, 1986).

In spite of lack of consensus, health behavior content is becoming reality. A recent survey of 131 accredited four-year baccalaureate nursing degree programs in the United States examined the extent to which content on health promotion and prevention was included (Simson & Wilson, 1984). Among the 89% of schools responding, all offered courses on prevention. The prevention course content in order of those most frequently present were: wellness promotion; primary, secondary, and tertiary clinical prevention; health services delivery; epidemiology; biostatistics; social and behavioral sciences; and environmental and occupational health. Further survey questions led to the conclusion that these disease prevention and health promotion courses need to be more interdisciplinary and interdepartmental in nature and they should also focus on present and future health care needs of the elderly. Another survey of nursing education administrators concluded that in order to prepare practitioners for the health care system circa 1992, there must be increased integration of health promotion concepts into the system, growth in competitive incentive programs for clients, and an increased number of counselors to assist with those incentive programs (Snyder Hill, 1984).

Nursing is a practice discipline concerned with client well-being. The intent of most institutes of higher learning is teaching and research. What then do nursing faculty do to maintain competence and gain expertise in health behavior approaches to health maintenance and life-style modifications? Organizational realities in most instances separate educational institutes from practice settings. Thus, nursing faculty are frequently blamed for creating an education–practice gap. Since the 1960s a number of designs have been proposed and implemented to address this gap and to help faculty demonstrate what they teach in a wider context (Fagin, 1985; Jacobs, 1976).

It is probably safe to say that most university schools of nursing now have faculty who hold joint appointments with health care service agencies. These faculty can often spearhead research and teaching activities to enhance client health behaviors. Shortridge (1985) described a program where nursing students attend class on the same campus where they practice primary health care with their faculty in a practice setting. Nakagawa Kogan (1985) described another nurse practice center administered by faculty where, since 1979, numerous funded projects and theses have materialized from helping clients with self-management who suffered from such stress-related disorders as hypertension, insomnia, headache, anxiety, and muscle tension. Indeed, the many projects reported at the 1985 American Academy of Nursing's symposium on nursing faculty practice suggest that health behavior concepts are well on their way toward integration into nursing curricula, and faculty success with being change agents will depend on careful manipulation of structured variables (Barnard & Smith, 1985). This may also be a reflection that nursing programs need money to survive, hence the impetus for faculty to establish practice models.

Health Behavior Concepts and Practicing Nurses

Beyond these innovative curricula for nursing students, questions arise about how practicing nurses can incorporate health behavior concepts. The literature does not reveal estimates of numbers of obsolete or incompetent nurses in practice, but the issue sparked concern in the 1970s, so the states and provinces began the debate about whether there should be mandatory continuing education for relicensing. By 1986, many state licensing bodies required that nurses demonstrate evidence of having a minimum number of continuing education units (CEUs) prior to relicensure. This has meant a proliferation of planned and organized learning experiences and made nurses more aware of their special needs (Kuramoto, 1985). Three regional committees representing the American Association of Nursing are now charged with accrediting continuing education offerings.

Most studies on the subject of continuing education in nursing have examined characteristics of nurse learners, their learning needs, and teaching methods. Findings have not been generalizable to the CEU's impact on practice and on patient care (Cooper, 1983). It is acknowledged that there is a definite need to examine ways in which new findings from the behavioral sciences can be incorporated into the lifelong learning requirement of nurses.

One survey which included nurse practitioners in Alabama asked how they kept abreast of advances in their field (Stinson & Mueller, 1980). In addition to medical and nursing literature, these nurses spent 1 to 5 hours per week in discussion with colleagues, 5 to 10 hours per year at local professional meetings, 15 to 25 hours per year at state and national meetings, and 10 to 15 hours at CEU courses. The nature and content of the CEU courses in this survey were not disclosed. These practitioners further indicated that they spent an average of 5.5 hours per month reading relevant journals and another 1.6 hours per month using texts. At this juncture, it is important to note the amount of health behavior-related articles in three popular nursing journals in the period from 1975 to 1985 (Table 1). If one looks for articles with health behavior-related subject headings over an 11-year period in the *American Journal of Nursing, Canadian Nurse,* and *Nursing Outlook,* fewer than three articles per month deal with health behavior. It is speculative, therefore, which if any of these articles would be included in nurse practitioners' 5.5 hours a month of journal reading.

That health behavior concepts and communication skills are incorporated into the curricula of nurse practitioner education programs may account for some of these programs' positive effects. One study noted a drop in suicide rate of a prison staffed by nurse practitioners (Hastings *et al.,* 1980); another study demonstrated higher relief of symptoms of acute, minor illnesses of patients managed by nurse practitioners versus physicians (Komaroff, Sawayer, Flatley, & Browne, 1976); and others have demonstrated that nurse practitioners had higher rates of success than physicians in helping patients lose weight, comply with recommendations, and keep appointments (Watkins & Wagner, 1982). A problem with much of the reported nurse practitioner research is its lack of a base in theory. Molde and Diers (1985) speculated that practitioners in primary care have had less success with the "guidance-cooperation" model of communication dominant in medical practice than with the "mutual participation" model advocated in psychiatry and the social sciences. Some of the answers to how, why, with whom, and when might be better addressed by comparing the effectiveness of specific health behavior techniques with outcomes. Nurse practitioner studies have not yet indicated what style of practice enhances acceptance, satisfaction, and compliance.

Consumers are confronted daily with many choices that influence their health and welfare. For example, although in 1983 in America cigarettes continued to be the most widely advertized consumer product, similar marketing strategies taken up by the nonsmokers' rights movement have reduced the adult per capita consumption of cigarettes significantly from its peaks in the 1960s and 1970s (Warner, 1985). Heart disease projects in the United States and Finland have demonstrated clearly that consumer health behavior can be improved (Finnegan, 1985; Puska, McAlister, Pekkola, & Koskela, 1981). Acknowledgment of a consumerist ethic in the 1970s necessitated clearer articulation by nurses of standards of care. The American Hospital Association (1972) devised a Patient's Bill of Rights which recognizes that the institution and workers therein have clear responsibilities to their clients. Written into the standards of nurse practice acts in the 1980s are the nurses' teaching responsibilities and the patients' rights to all information necessary to give informed consent.

The effects on patient outcome of educational interventions have been the subject of increasing study since the 1970s. Much of this study has been generated by nurses in master's and doctoral programs. Starting with methodologically sound studies on structured presurgical intervention by nurses, researchers were able to demonstrate reduction in postoperative complications (Lindeman & Van Aernam, 1971; Lindeman, 1972). The nurse researchers began demonstrating that patients were eager to learn specific techniques such as deep breathing, range of motion exercises, and relaxation techniques preoperatively if they felt it would enhance their recovery. The shift to prospective pricing, or diagnostic-related groups (DRGs), for reimbursements for medical care in 1983 in the United States has forced a further critical examination of instructional resources for clients. Social scientists have fortuitously afforded the means through the process of meta-analysis which allows many studies to be combined and then examined to determine whether the difference between treatment and control groups favors particular interventions (Glass, McGaw, & Smith, 1981).

Three meta-analyses of the effects of education programs on client well-being demonstrate that health professionals, and in particular nurses, are having a significant positive effect by having clients actively participate in self-care activities preoperatively, and then transfering this learning to the period after the diagnostic or surgical event (Devine & Cook, 1983; Mumford, Schlesinger, & Glass, 1982; Smith & Naftel, 1984). Some of these benefits include: reduction in pre- and postsurgical self-reports of anxiety and pain; reduction in requirement of postoperative narcotics and hypnotics; and other external indicators of client recovery and reduction of complications. Of particular note, in these times of monetary constraint, are the reductions in days of hospitalization for patients receiving programmed intervention (Devine & Cook, 1983). When outcomes of nurse providers of instructional intervention were compared to those of others (such as dental students, psychologists, physicians, and anesthesiologists), the nurses had a significantly greater positive effect (Smith & Naftel, 1984). Common instructional resources used by these nurse researchers to prepare patients for stressful and invasive procedures included informative, psychotherapeutic, modeling, cognitive-behavioral, and hypnotic techniques (Anderson & Masur, 1983).

Health behavior is now being assisted by "behavioral high technology." A search of the database MEDLINE from the computerized system MEDLARS (Medical Literature Analysis and Retrieval System) revealed 336 citations from January 1977 through September 1982 on audiovisual aids, programmed instruction, and computer-assisted instruction (CAI) in patient education (Sparks, 1984). CAI in nursing education and patient education is a subject requiring much greater research into its effectiveness. In a comprehensive review of CAI in nursing education, Chang (1986) found there was little control over extraneous variables such as learning style, student aptitude, teacher bias, and reliability and validity of outcome measures, and concluded that CAI's contribution to nursing has been modest but the most consistent finding was a reduction in learning time. That the computer will play a greater part in the training of nurses, and in turn help with their health promotion function, goes without question. A continuing challenge is to help nurses become skilled in using computers.

The Future for Nursing

The roles and responsibilities of nurses have expanded considerably in the past 20 years and the profession continues to redefine essential elements for practice in the context of the tremendous growth in human knowledge and resulting amount of information to be learned (American Association of Colleges of Nursing, 1986). The domain of nursing is improving the health and functioning of people, and nurse theorists are helping to define what is nursing knowledge (Visintainer, 1986). Nurses borrow heavily, too, from other theorists who help to explain human behavior in the process of assessing, setting goals, and implementing patient care.

It has been noted that the effects of prospective pricing on health care in the United States, and continuing financial retrenchment in Canada, mean that hospitals are becoming critical care units, and that critical care is also becoming an ever-increasing part of care at home where clients have respirators and other complex forms of therapy (Shaver, 1986). However, professional nurses meet their clients in all phases of wellness, and as primary health providers they must help with health promotion and patient teaching wherever the encounter. One prediction is that by 1990, hospitals will be allocating 20 to 40 in-service hours, per month, per nurse in order to help them keep up with technology (McCormick,

1983). Improved CAI and increased access to computers in nursing programs will be of continuing importance.

Nurses will function in many sites: schools, work places, health centers, public health and home health agencies. Here there will be an increased demand to apply knowledge in reducing risk factors and maintaining health through contracting and counseling techniques for young and old. The rapidly increasing cohort of elderly in the population is creating greater pressure to understand their special learning and self-maintenance needs. Institutional practices such as specialized critical care units will mean varied educational roles for nurses in their interactions with patients and families. Two recent surveys in Canada and the United States demonstrate that health care institutes see themselves involved with health promotion activities not just for inpatients and outpatients, but also for their own employees, those of corporations, businesses, and other community groups (Ross *et al.,* 1985; Thompson, Davidson, & Le Touze, 1986).

In summary, this overview of nursing's attempt to integrate health behavior concepts over the years points to the need for continued definition of nursing relative to primary care and specialty practice. Trends and issues in health care indicate that nurse researchers and educators need to continue to try to operationalize health behavior; implement and evaluate innovative nurse practice-teaching models; examine the effects of CEUs on patient outcomes; research the effects of CAI in nursing and patient education; and contribute more health behavior content to leading journals. Rigorous, controlled, and well-thought-out research into nursing education and practice is indispensable.

FUTURE DIRECTIONS: THE TRAINING OF HEALTH PROFESSIONALS

The changes in medical and nursing education in Canada and the United States offer some signs that health behavior is being given a higher priority. Only the first few steps in a complex adoption and diffusion process have been taken, of course. These have moved the concept past the stages of reformist rhetoric and consciousness raising, but have stopped short of fashioning a workable pattern for building up the necessary skills and support structures. In part, this is attributable to the fact that there is still much to be accomplished in translating research findings about health behavior into a major practical technology. There is also the long list of barriers pulled out repeatedly by the critics of the existing health care system. A point less frequently highlighted is the unsettled question of whether or not health behavior strategies should be solidly integrated into the existing health care system. One group would seek to raise the prevailing level of knowledge and skills of existing health care workers (Frederiksen, Solomon, & Brehony, 1984). Another, building on the entrepreneurial and privatizing trends in health care, would press for alternate services in the open marketplace (Gaylen, 1985; Kiser, 1982; Stahl, 1984). A third, the opponents of greater medicalization, see the answers in the self-care and the self-help movement (Caporael-Katz, 1983; Angus & Manga, 1986). A middle ground is proposed by those who recognize that the skills called for are still in short supply. They propose a timely contribution to the change process through harnessing the unique capability of microcomputer technology, interactive telemedia, and other instructional media (Bell, 1986) to provide instructional and consultant services regarding health behavior change to practicing health professionals.

This degree of ferment provides a volatile and often confusing environment for both practitioners and educators. While the dangers of a return to an earlier indifference and hostility to health behavior concepts and methods are certainly there, the prospects for restoring the balance between health and disease in our health care systems seem to be supported by a series of shifts in public consciousness. The critique of health care and existing knowledge systems provided by feminist scholars is another force supportive of this change. The momentum of social forces attributable to demographic shifts and changing morbidity patterns is a third. Different structures are also developing to incorporate health behavior.

If change is viewed in these terms, it becomes possible to be guardedly optimistic that health behavior will receive due emphasis in future health sciences education in Canada and America.

REFERENCES

American Association of Colleges of Nursing. (1986). *Essentials of college and university education for professional nursing: Report to the membership*. Washington, DC: Author.

American Hospital Association. (1972). *A patient's bill of rights*. Chicago: Author.

Anderson, K. O., & Masur, F. T. (1983). Psychological preparation for invasive medical and dental procedures. *Journal of Behavioral Medicine, 6,* 1–40.

Angus, D. E., & Manga, P. (1986). National health strategies: Time for a new "new perspective." *Canadian Journal of Public Health, 77,* 81–85.

Association of American Medical Colleges. (1984). *Physicians for the twenty-first century: Report of the panel on the general professional education of the physician and college preparation for medicine*. Washington, DC.

Association of American Medical Colleges. (1985). *1986–87 curriculum directory* (15th ed.). Washington, DC.

Association of American Medical Colleges. (1986). Commentary on the report of the panel on the general professional education of the physician and college preparation for medicine. *Journal of Medical Education, 61,* 345–352.

Badgley, R. F., & Bloom, S. W. (1973). Behavioral sciences and medical education: The case of sociology. *Social Science and Medicine, 7,* 927–941.

Barker, W. H., & Jonas, S. (1981). The teaching of preventive medicine in American medical schools, 1940–1980. *Preventive Medicine, 10,* 674–685.

Barnard, K. E., & Smith, G. R. (Eds.). (1985). *Faculty practice in action*. Kansas City: American Academy of Nursing.

Bell, J. A. (1986). The role of microcomputers in patient education. *Computers in Nursing, 4*(6), 255–258.

Blackwell, G., & Torem, M. (1982). Behavioral science teaching in U.S. medical schools: A 1980 national survey. *American Journal of Psychiatry, 139*(10), 1304–1307.

Bloom, S. W. (1986). Institutional trends in medical sociology. *Journal of Health and Social Behavior, 27,* 265–276.

Bryant, J. H. (1984). Health services, health manpower, and universities in relation to health for all: An historical and future perspective [Commentaries]. *American Journal of Public Health, 74*(7), 714–719.

Butzin, D. W. (1985). Behavioral pediatrics in the examinations of the American Board of Pediatrics. *Developmental and Behavioral Pediatrics, 6*(4), 229–231.

Camooso, C., Green, M., Hoffman, F., Leuner, J., Mattis, C., Ptaszynski, E., Reiley, P., Silver, S., Winfrey, M., & Winland, J. (1980). Preventive health practices of generic baccalaureate nursing students. *Nursing Research, 29,* 256–257.

Caporael-Katz, B. (1983). Health, self-care and power: Shifting the balance. *Topics in Clinical Nursing, 5*(3), 31–41.

Cassell, E. (1986). The changing concept of the ideal physician. *Daedalus* (Cambridge, MA), *115,* 185–208.

Chang, B. L. (1986). Computer aided instruction in nursing education. In H. H. Werley, J. J. Fitzpatrick, & R. L. Taunton (Eds.), *Annual review of nursing research* (Vol. 4). New York: Springer.

Cooper, S. S. (1983). *The practice of continuing education in nursing*. Rockville, MD: Aspen.

Council of Ontario Universities. (1982). *Proceedings of the Conference on Health in the '80s and '90s and Its Impact on Health Sciences Education*. Toronto: Author.

Croog, S. H., Lipson, A., & Levine, S. (1972, February). Help patterns in severe illness: The roles of kin network, non family resources and institutions. *Journal of Marriage and the Family, 1972,* 32–41.

Devine, E. C., & Cook, T. D. (1983). A meta-analytic analysis of effects of psychoeducational interventions on length of postsurgical hospital stay. *Nursing Research, 32,* 267–274.

Fagin, C. M. (1985). Institutionalizing practice: Historical and future perspectives. In K. E. Barnard & G. R. Smith (Eds.), *Faculty practice in action*. Kansas City: American Academy of Nursing.

Feeny, D., Guyatt, G., & Tugwell, P. (Eds.). (1986). *Health care technology: Effectiveness, efficiency, and public policy*. Montreal: The Institute for Research on Public Policy.

Finnegan, J. R. (1985, November). *Community-wide health promotion: The Minnesota heart health program*. Paper presented at the fourth annual health promotion workshop of the Ontario Public Health Association and Ontario Ministry of Health, Toronto.

Fraser, G. E. (1986). *Preventive cardiology*. London: Oxford University Press.

Frederiksen, L. W., Solomon, L. J., & Brehony, K. A. (Eds.). (1984). *Marketing health behavior: Principles, techniques, and applications*. New York: Plenum Press.

Freymann, J. G. (1975). Medicine's great schism: Prevention vs. cure: An historical interpretation. *Medical Care, 13*(7), 525–536.

Freymann, J. G. (1981). The origins of disease orientation in American medical education. *Preventive Medicine, 10,* 663–673.

Fries, J. F. (1980). Aging, natural death, and the compression of morbidity. *New England Journal of Medicine, 303,* 130–135.

Gaylen, S. (1985). The coming of the corporation and the marketing of psychiatry. *Hospital and Community Psychiatry, 36*(2), 154–159.

Glass, G. V., McGaw, B., & Smith, M. L. (1981). *Meta-analysis in social research*. Beverly Hills: Sage.

Greer, A. L. (1977). Advances in the study of diffusion of innovation in health care organizations. *Milbank Memorial Fund Quarterly, 55,* 505–532.

Hastings, G. E., Vick, L., Lee, G., Sasmor, L., Natiello, T. A., & Sanders, J. H. (1980). Nurse practitioners in a jailhouse clinic. *Medical Care, 18,* 731–744.

Inui, T., Yourtee, E., & Williamson, J. (1976). Improved outcomes in hypertension after physician tutorials. *Annals of Internal Medicine, 84,* 646–651.

Jacobs, R. M. (Ed.). (1976). *A flexible design for health professions education*. New York: Wiley.

Kasl, S. V., & Cobb, S. (1966). Health behavior, illness behavior and sick role behavior. *Archives of Environmental Health, 12,* 246–266, 531–541.

Kirkland, K. B., & Skelton, J. B. (1985, June). Behavioral medicine education in the family medicine residency: A critical review. *Alabama Medicine, 1985,* 31–39.

Kiser, W. S. (1982). Buying and selling health care: A battle for the medical marketplace. *American College of Surgeons Bulletin, 70*(7), 2–8.

Komaroff, A. L., Sawayer, K., Flatley, M., & Browne, C. (1976). Nurse practitioner management of common respiratory and geritourinary infections, using protocols. *Nursing Research, 25,* 84–89.

Kuramoto, A. M. (1985). Research on continuing education in nursing. In H. H. Werley & J. J. Fitzpatrick (Eds.), *Annual review of nursing research* (Vol. 3). New York: Springer.

Kurji, K., & Macdonald, P. (1986). Health practices of Edmontonians. *Canadian Journal of Public Health, 77,* 320.

Lalonde, M. (1974). *A new perspective on the health of Canadians*. Ottawa, Canada: Ministry of National Health and Welfare.

Light, D. W. (1983). Medical and nursing education: Surface behavior and deep structure. *Handbook of health, health care, and the health professions* (pp. 455–478). New York: Free Press.

Lindeman, C. (1972). Nursing intervention with the presurgical patient: Effectiveness and efficiency of group and individual preoperative teaching—phase two. *Nursing Research, 21,* 196–209.

Lindeman, C., & Van Aernam, B. (1971). Nursing intervention with the presurgical patient: The effects of structured and unstructured preoperative teaching. *Nursing Research, 20,* 319–322.

Linn, L. S., Brook, R. H., Clark, V. A., Fink, A., & Kosecoff, J. (1986). Evaluation of ambulatory

care training by graduates of internal medicine residencies. *Journal of Medical Education, 61,* 293–302.
Lowenthal, M. F., & Berkman, P. L. (1967). *Aging and mental disorder in San Francisco: A social psychiatric study.* San Francisco: Jossey–Bass.
Matarazzo, J. D. (1980). Behavioral health and behavioral medicine: Frontiers for a new health psychology. *American Psychologist, 35*(9), 807–817.
McCormick, K. A. (1983). Preparing nurses for the technological future. *Nursing and Health Care, 4,* 379–382.
Mechanic, D. (Ed.). (1983). *Handbook of health, health care, and health professions.* New York: Free Press.
Molde, S., & Diers, D. (1985). Nurse practitioner research: Selected literature review and research agenda. *Nursing Research, 34,* 362–367.
Mumford, E., Schlesinger, H. J., & Glass, G. V. (1982). The effects of psychological intervention on recovery from surgery and heart attacks: An analysis of the literature. *American Journal of Public Health, 72,* 141–151.
Murphy, N. (1986). Collaboration between nurse educators in the use of nursing education resources for the year 2000. *Entry to practice newsletter* (Vol. 2, No. 5). Ottawa: Canadian Nurses Association.
Mustard, J. F. (1987). Achieving health for all: Implications for Canadian health and social policies. *Canadian Medical Association Journal, 136,* 471–473.
Nakagawa Kogan, H. (1985). Nurse practice centers: Ingredients of success. In K. E. Barnard & G. R. Smith (Eds.), *Faculty practice in action.* Kansas City: American Academy of Nursing.
Neuman, B. (1982). *The Neuman systems model: Application to nursing education and practice.* New York: Appleton–Century–Crofts.
Nuckolls, K., Cassel, J., & Kaplan, B. (1972). Psychosocial assets, life crisis, and the prognosis of pregnancy. *American Journal of Epidemiology, 95,* 431–441.
Orem, D. (1980). *Nursing: Concepts of practice* (2nd ed.). New York: McGraw–Hill.
Parse, R. R. (1981). *Man–living–health: A theory for nursing.* New York: Wiley.
Pender, N. J. (1984). Health promotion and illness prevention. In H. H. Werley & J. J. Fitzpatrick (Eds.), *Annual review of nursing research* (Vol. 2). Berlin: Springer.
Petersdorf, R. G., & Feinstein, A. R. (1981). An informal appraisal of the current status of medical sociology. In L. Eisenberg & A. Kleinman (Eds.), *The relevance of social science for medicine* (pp. 27–45). Dordrecht: Reidel.
Piemonte, R. V. (1976). A history of the National League of Nursing Education 1912–1932: Great awakening in nursing education. *Dissertation Abstracts International, 78,* 701B–702B. (University Microfilms No. 76-17, 291)
Puska, P., McAlister, A., Pekkola, J., & Koskela, K. (1981). Television in health promotion: Evaluation of a national program in Finland. *International Journal of Health Education, 25,* 238–250.
Richardson, S. (1986). Articulation and baccalaureate entry to practice: The Canadian context. *Nursing Papers, 18*(13), 47–58.
Ross, C. K., Sherman, S. L., Berg, L., Radbill, L., Lee, E., Giloth, B., Jones, L., & Longe, M. (1985). Health promotion programs flourishing: Survey. *Hospitals, 59*(16), 128–135.
Schwartz, D., Henley, D., & Zeita, I. (1964). *The elderly ambulatory patient.* New York: Macmillan Co.
Scott, C. S., & Neighbor, W. E. (1985). Preventive care attitudes of medical students. *Social Science and Medicine, 21*(3), 299–305.
Shaver, J. (1986). High touch nursing in a high tech world. *Canadian Nurse, 82,* 16–19.
Shortridge, L. M. (1985). Faculty practice in action: A nurse practice center. In K. E. Barnard & G. R. Smith (Eds.), *Faculty practice in action.* Kansas City: American Academy of Nursing.
Simson, S., & Wilson, L. B. (1984). Education in prevention, health promotion and aging in medical and nursing schools. *Gerontology and Geriatrics Education, 5*(1), 43–52.
Smith, M. C., & Naftel, D. C. (1984). Meta-analysis: A perspective for research synthesis. *Image: The Journal of Nursing Scholarship, 16,* 9–13.
Snyder Hill, B. A. (1984). A delphi application health care, practice, education and education administration; circa 1992. *Image: The Journal of Nursing Scholarship, 16,* 6–8.

Sohn, K. S. (1986). General education in nursing: Current practices and faculty attitudes. *Nursing Papers, 18*(4), 41–56.

Sparks, S. M. (1984). The National Library of Medicine's bibliographic databases: Tools for nursing research. *Image: The Journal of Nursing Scholarship, 16,* 24–27.

Squires, B. P. (1987). Medical education to achieve health for all. *Canadian Medical Association Journal, 136,* 474–475.

Stahl, D. A. (1984). Developing and marketing ambulatory care programs. *Nursing Management, 15*(5), 20–24.

Stinson, E. R., & Mueller, D. A. (1980). Survey of health professionals' information habits and needs. *Journal of the American Medical Association, 243,* 140–143.

Thompson, C., Davidson, S., & Le Touze, D. (1986, September). National survey reveals how hospitals are promoting health. *Dimensions, 1986,* 17–20.

Torres, G. (1974). *Faculty—curriculum development part IV: Unifying the curriculum—The integrated approach.* New York: National League for Nursing.

U.S. Department of Health, Education and Welfare. (1979). *Healthy people: The surgeon general's report on health promotion and disease prevention.* Washington, DC: U.S. Government Printing Office.

Van Etten, G., & Rutten, F. (1986). The social sciences in health policy and practice. *Social Science and Medicine, 22*(11), 1187–1194.

Visintainer, M. A. (1986). The nature of knowledge and theory in nursing. *Image: The Journal of Nursing Scholarship, 18,* 32–38.

Warner, K. E. (1985). Cigarette advertising and media coverage of smoking and health. *New England Journal of Medicine, 312*(6), 384–388.

Watkins, L., & Wagner, E. (1982). Nurse practitioner and physicians adherence to standing orders: Criteria for consultation or referral. *American Journal of Public Health, 72,* 55–57.

Weinberg, A., & Andrus, P. L. (1982). Continuing medical education: Does it address prevention? *Journal of Community Health, 7*(3), 211–214.

White, F. M. (1987). Prevention of diseases and promotion of health: An overview of medical education in Canada. *Forum, The Association of Medical Colleges, 20*(2), 1–3, 6.

World Health Organization Expert Committee. (1984). *Education and training of nurse teachers and managers with special regard to primary health care* (Technical Report Series No. 708). Geneva: World Health Organization.

Wright, P., & Treacher, A. (Eds.). (1982). *The problem of medical knowledge: Examining the social construction of medicine.* Edinburgh: Edinburgh University Press.

CHAPTER 21

The Application of Health Behavior Research

Health Education and Health Promotion

Lloyd J. Kolbe

HUMAN BEHAVIOR AND PUBLIC HEALTH

The great majority of the controllable risk factors associated with chronic diseases and traumatic injuries are behavioral in nature (National Center for Health Statistics, 1981; U.S. Department of Health, Education and Welfare, 1979). As a consequence, these risk factors, and the death and illness they cause, can be reduced by health promotion and health education interventions that apply the findings of behavioral research both to inform people about means to decrease behavioral risks, and to foster social and environmental changes that facilitate these behavioral changes. Health promotion and health education are based on knowledge generated by behavioral epidemiology as well as by basic health behavior research.

BEHAVIORAL EPIDEMIOLOGY

Much of what we know about the effects of behaviors on health has been determined through epidemiologic methods. Epidemiology has been defined as the study of the distribution and determinants of diseases and injuries in human populations (Mausner & Kramer, 1985). Behavioral epidemiology can be defined as the study of the distribution and determinants of *behaviors that influence* diseases and injuries in human populations.

Mason and Powell (1985) suggested that behavioral epidemiology may have two distinguishable, if not sequential, processes. As depicted in Figure 1, one process uses epidemiologic methods to assess the relationship between a given *behavior* and a given *disease* (R1). The other process uses epidemiologic methods to assess relationships between a given *behavior* and *determinants of that behavior* (R2). For both processes, means to measure the comparative incidence and prevalence of the *behavior* among populations are essential.

LLOYD J. KOLBE • Office of School Health and Special Projects, Division of Health Education, Center for Health Promotion and Education, U.S. Centers for Disease Control, Atlanta, Georgia 30333.

Behavioral determinants $\xleftrightarrow[R2]{}$ Behavior $\xleftrightarrow[R1]{}$ Health/disease

FIGURE 1. Two relationships of interest in behavioral epidemiology.

Relationships between behaviors and diseases (R1) are complex. Some behaviors may maintain health (e.g., consuming adequate dietary fiber); others may threaten it (e.g., consuming an excessive amount of saturated fat). Some behaviors may have a great influence on the incidence of a given disease (e.g., cigarette smoking and lung cancer); other behaviors may have a comparatively small influence (e.g., saccharin consumption and bladder cancer). Evidence associating some behaviors with certain diseases may be substantial (e.g., cholesterol consumption and atherosclerosis), whereas evidence associating other behaviors with certain diseases may be more tenuous (sodium consumption and high blood pressure). Some behaviors may influence diseases that are severe (e.g., adhering to an antimalarial chemoprophylactic regimen); other behaviors may influence diseases that are comparatively benign (e.g., drying the feet to prevent fungal infection).

Some behaviors are more prevalent in a population (e.g., marijuana use); others are more rare (e.g., heroin use). Some behaviors must be performed frequently (e.g., wearing a seat belt); others need be performed infrequently (e.g., getting vaccinated for measles). Some behaviors have a relatively short incubation period, and thus more immediately may

TABLE 1. A Typology of Health Behavior

Wellness behavior—any activity undertaken by an individual who believes himself to be healthy for the purpose of attaining an even greater level of health

Preventive health behavior—any activity undertaken by an individual who believes himself to be healthy, for the purpose of preventing illness or detecting it in an asymptomatic state (Kasl & Cobb, 1966a)

At-risk behavior—any activity undertaken by an individual who believes himself to be healthy but at greater risk than normal of developing a specific health condition, for the purpose of preventing that condition or detecting it in an asymptomatic state (Baric, 1969)

Illness behavior—any activity undertaken by an individual who perceives himself to be ill, to define the state of his health and to discover a suitable remedy (Kasl & Cobb, 1966a)

Self-care behavior—any activity undertaken by an individual who considers himself to be ill, for the purpose of getting well. It includes minimal reliance on appropriate therapists, involves few dependent behaviors, and leads to little neglect of one's usual duties

Sick-role behavior—any activity undertaken by an individual who considers himself to be ill, for the purpose of getting well. It includes receiving treatment from appropriate therapists, generally involves a whole range of dependent behaviors, and leads to some degree of neglect of one's usual duties (Kasl & Cobb, 1966b)

Reproductive behavior—any activity undertaken by an individual to influence the occurrence or normal continuation of pregnancy

Parenting health behavior—any wellness, preventive, at-risk, illness, self-care, or sick-role behavior performed by an individual for the purposes of ensuring, maintaining, or improving the health of a conceptus or child for whom the individual has responsibility

Health-related social action—any activity undertaken by an individual singularly or in concert with others (i.e., collectively) through organizational, legal, or economic means, to influence the provision of medical services, the effects of the environment, the effects of various products, or the effects of social regulations that influence the health of populations

influence prominent health conditions of a given age-cohort (e.g., unprotected sexual intercourse that leads to gonorrhea or unintended pregnancy). Other behaviors have a longer incubation period; consequently, the conditions they influence may not have clinical manifestations for 10, 20, or 30 years (e.g., cirrhosis from excessive alcohol consumption). Some behaviors may contribute to only one disease (e.g., skin cancers from excessive sunbathing); other behaviors may contribute to multiple diseases simultaneously (e.g., lung cancer, cardiovascular disease, and emphysema from smoking). Some diseases may result from the synergistic effects of multiple behaviors (e.g., esophageal cancer from smoking and excessive alcohol consumption). The results of epidemiologic, biophysical, and clinical research often are combined to test hypotheses about the extent to which various behaviors influence health.

HEALTH BEHAVIOR RESEARCH

Typology and Methods

Additional knowledge about behaviors that influence health is derived from basic health behavior research. Concepts from health behavior research provide the basis for the typology reflected in the nine categories of behaviors defined in Table 1 (Kolbe, 1984a,b). The first six categories include behaviors that influence the health of the individual performing the behavior. The last three categories include behaviors that influence the health of individuals other than the one performing the behavior. Programs and policies

TABLE 2. Methods to Measure Health Behavior

Category and method	Examples
Behavioral reports	
1. Self-report	24-hour dietary recall Health risk appraisal questionnaire
2. Report of others	Parental report of child oral hygiene habits Physician report of patient appointment-making and appointment-keeping behaviors
Physical measures of behavior	
3. Physiological markers	Thiocyanate measures of smoking behaviors Serum cholesterol measures of cholesterol consumption
4. Related health status	Frequency of diabetic or asthmatic emergencies to measure adherence to therapeutic regimen Weight gain or loss to measure adherence to dietary and exercise regimen
Observational measures of behavior	
5. Indirect observation	Analysis of supermarket or cafeteria inventories to measure customer selections Analysis of per capita consumption of tobacco, alcohol, butter, eggs, etc.
6. Direct observation	Observation of seat belt use Observation of aerobic activities among schoolchildren during recess or physical education classes

TABLE 3. Theoretical Stages of Smoking Behaviors

Smoking prevention			
Gordon (1986)	Never smokers	Triers	Current smokers
Leventhal & Cleary (1980)	Preparation	Initiation, becoming a smoker	Maintenance of smoking
	Primary prevention	*Secondary prevention*	*Tertiary prevention*
Smoking cessation			
Rosen & Shipley (1983)	Maintenance	Initial control	Initial decision
Bass (1982)	Maintenance	Behavior change	Motivation

that address the last three categories enable individuals and populations to make informed decisions about, for example, using alcohol or tobacco during pregnancy, proscribing the use of saccharin in foods, legislating the use of seat belts, regulating vehicle emissions and industrial wastes, improving access to medical services for the poor or elderly, and so forth.

Six separate methods can be used to measure health behaviors. These fall into three categories: behavioral reports, physical measures, and observational measures. Table 2 delineates these six methods and offers examples of each.

Conceptual Stages of Health Behaviors

Data from health behavior research indicate that the establishment and disestablishment of a health behavior pattern probably occurs in progressive stages. Just as disease prevention activities are designed specifically to target the primary, secondary, or tertiary stage of disease progression, interventions designed to reduce health risk behaviors can benefit by targeting specific stages in the progression of a behavior pattern. For example, as shown in Table 3, *smoking prevention* interventions might be more effective if formulated specifically to address either those who have never smoked, or those who may be just beginning to smoke (Gordon, 1986; Leventhal & Cleary, 1980).

In reverse progression, *smoking cessation* interventions might be most effective if formulated specifically to address either those who are smoking, those who have just begun to stop, or those who have stopped for some time (e.g., Rosen & Shipley, 1983). Thus, *primary prevention of risk behaviors* comprises interventions designed to preclude the *initiation* of a behavior pattern that adversely affects health. *Secondary prevention of risk behaviors* comprises interventions designed to preclude the *establishment* of a behavior pattern that adversely affects health, among those who have initiated the pattern, or among those identified as particularly prone to initiate the pattern. *Tertiary prevention of risk behaviors* comprises activities designed to enable those who have established a behavior pattern that adversely affects health to *disestablish* the pattern, and to maintain its disestablishment.

HEALTH PROMOTION AND HEALTH EDUCATION STRATEGIES

Given the evolution of our understandings about factors that influence health behaviors, the complexity of those factors, the right of populations to determine their own behaviors, and the various frameworks within which ideologies about health-related behaviors have developed, it is not surprising that (just as there are numerous definitions of health) there are numerous definitions of health promotion.

Three Definitions

Although most of these definitions address similar processes and outcomes, the first of the three definitions of health promotion that follow is representative of those that depict it to be primarily a process of medicine and public health.

In 1975, the U.S. National Conference on Preventive Medicine (The John E. Fogarty International Center for Advanced Study in the Health Sciences & The American College of Preventive Medicine, 1976) conceived health promotion to include:

> . . . in balanced proportion, all the means or strategies . . . of promotion: research, education for the health professions, public health, environmental protection, occupational health, consumer health education, health care (diagnosis and treatment of illness and disability), and health economics (organization and financing). (p. 87)

This first definition emphasizes medical treatment, and suggests that health promotion includes all traditional medical and public health activities. Knowledge of health behavior generated by research on how and why persons use health services, how they respond to regimens, and how they interpret signs and symptoms, particularly as these behaviors are related to, or determined by personal, family, or social factors, is critical to this conception of health promotion.

In contrast, in 1984 the European Working Group on Concepts and Principles of Health Promotion reasoned that

> basic resources for health are income, shelter and food. Improvement in health requires a secure foundation in these basics, but also: information and lifeskills; a supportive environment, providing opportunities for making choices among goods, services and facilities; and conditions in the economic, physical, social, and cultural environments (the "total" environment) which enhance health. . . .
>
> Health promotion is the process of enabling people to increase control over, and to improve, their health. (p. 2)

This second definition of health promotion emphasizes social reform. This definition was expanded in 1986 by the Ottawa Charter for Health Promotion which suggests that health promotion involves building healthy public policy, creating supportive environments, strengthening community participation, developing personal skills, and reorienting health services beyond providing clinical and curative care. This conception of health promotion provides the foundation for *Achieving Health for All: A Framework for Health Promotion* in Canada (Epp, 1986), which states:

> In summary, health promotion implies a commitment to dealing with the challenges of reducing inequities, extending the scope of prevention, and helping people to cope with their circumstances. It means fostering public participation, strengthening community health services and coordinating healthy public policy. Moreover, it means creating environments conducive to health, in which people are better able to take care of themselves, and to offer each other support in solving and managing collective health problems. (p. 12)

Knowledge of how community, institutional, and social policy factors determine health-related activities can be of great value to such health promotion activities.

Focusing more on health-related behaviors, Green (1979a) defined health promotion as

> . . . any combination of health education and related organizational, political, and economic interventions designed to facilitate behavioral adaptations that will improve or protect health. (p. 52)

This third definition emphasizes health behaviors, and is most consistent with Federal health promotion and disease prevention efforts in the United States (US DHEW, 1978) that differentiate among *preventive health services* (usually provided by medical personnel, including immunization, chemoprophylaxis, contraception, disease screening, and so forth); *health protection* (usually provided by regulations, including standards for air and water quality, occupational safety and health, building codes, and so forth); and *health promotion* strategies (that usually enable populations to improve health-related behaviors such as smoking, misuse of alcohol and drugs, dietary habits, exercise, seat belt use, and adherence to therapeutic regimens). Knowledge about how personal, family, social, and institutional factors serve as barriers to, or enhance, such behavioral adaptations or changes is critical to the development of effective health promotion programs.

Regardless of how health promotion is defined, *health education* is considered to be a critical *component* of it. In addition to empowering individuals to understand and modify behaviors that influence their health, health education drives the availability and quality of preventive health services, health protection, and health promotion programs alike to the extent that such programs are dependent on support from an informed public, organizational administrators, and institutional policymakers. Health education has been defined by the World Health Organization as any combination of planned activities leading to a situation where people want to be healthy; know how to attain health; do what they can individually and collectively; and seek help when needed (World Health Organization, 1981a,b). Health education also has been defined as any combination of learning opportunities designed to facilitate voluntary adaptations of behavior conducive to health (Green, 1979b).

Health promotion and health education programs can be implemented largely through five vehicles: schools, work sites, community agencies, medical care facilities, and media. The distinction between health promotion and health education may be illustrated by the school health promotion components and outcomes depicted in Figure 2 (Kolbe, 1986). The total school health promotion program can be seen to include eight interactive components that can influence not only the health behaviors and health status of school students, faculty, and staff, but also their cognitive performance (Kolbe, 1985; Kolbe *et al.*, 1986) and productivity (e.g., Blair *et al.*, 1986). The capacity for schools to improve the health behaviors of students thus is not determined by school health education programs alone. For example (as described in a succeeding section), school food service programs and school physical education programs may be more effective than school health education programs in modifying student and faculty dietary and exercise behaviors, respectively (Parcel *et al.*, 1987).

INCREASING THE EFFECTIVENESS OF HEALTH PROMOTION

The effectiveness of health promotion interventions might be increased in five ways: (1) by *improving the theory* on which interventions are based; (2) by *focusing interventions on priority behaviors* that most influence the health of populations; (3) by *focusing on high-risk populations;* (4) by focusing on *policies that influence health behaviors;* and (5) by *combining interventions* to attain complementary or synergistic effects. Each of these means increasingly is becoming the focus of research, and briefly is described in succeeding sections.

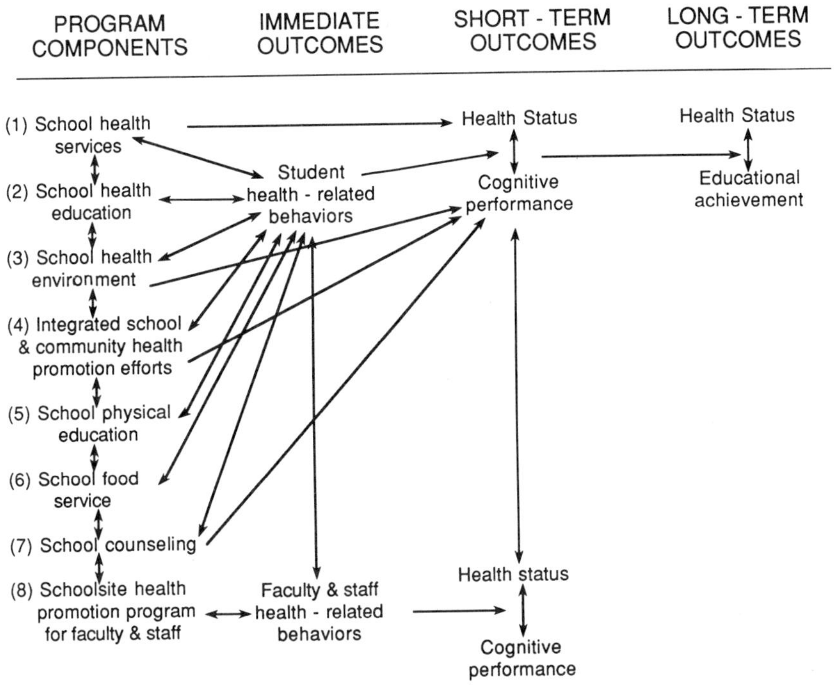

FIGURE 2. School health program components and outcomes.

Improving Theory

The effectiveness of a health promotion intervention might be increased by improving the theory on which the intervention is based: i.e., by more accurately describing and modeling the interacting determinants of a given health behavior, and by more accurately describing means by which those determinants can be influenced to modify the behavior. Theories and models that have been used to design and evaluate health education interventions have been described in detail in other chapters of this book (e.g., the health belief model, locus of control, attribution theory, social learning theory).

Especially as more theories and models are developed and refined, it may prove increasingly useful to synthesize one or more components from several theories to establish the most parsimonious model of a given health behavior within a given population (e.g., Kar, 1984). Indeed, there may be no one theory or model that can be universally applied to explain, or to develop interventions that might modify: (a) a great variety of health-related behaviors; (b) that are performed by populations that have very different socio-psychological characteristics (e.g., age, socioeconomic status); (c) that are performed in different contexts or situations; (d) that might be influenced by different types of interventions (e.g., social regulations, economic incentives, education); (e) implemented by various organizational vehicles (e.g., medical care facilities, schools, media, work sites). Instead, specific health-related behaviors more effectively might be explained and modified by integrating components from the range of existing models in order to generate the most parsimonious eclectic model of a specific behavior, performed by a targeted population, in identified contexts or situations, with specific types of interventions and organizational vehicles available.

Thus, for example, the PRECEDE model (Green, Kreuter, Deeds, & Partridge, 1980) might provide an organizing framework for developing a model of factors that influence safety belt use among adolescents. In general, PRECEDE suggests that three types of variables should be addressed to influence health behaviors. *Predisposing variables* include relevant knowledge, beliefs, attitudes, values, and skills that might be influenced by *direct communication* with the target population. *Reinforcing variables* include relevant attitudes and behaviors of significant others (including parents, peers, teachers, celebrities, and so on) as they are perceived to be important by the target population. Hence, *indirect communication* (i.e., messages provided by parents, peers, and so on) can be used to augment direct communication. *Enabling variables* include the availability, accessibility, and acceptability of resources required to perform the behavior. For many health-related behaviors, *community organization* is required to ensure such resources (e.g., ensuring that safety belts are installed in vehicles).

PRECEDE thus provides a generic framework within which more detailed theories might be integrated. The health belief model (e.g., Becker, 1974) might be used to delineate *predisposing* variables that account for the most variance in a given behavior such as use of seat belts (e.g., age, gender, socioeconomic status, and perceived susceptibility to and severity of a crash). *Reinforcing* variables might be delineated by theories posited by Fishbein and Ajzen (1975) (e.g., subjective norms, attitudes toward the behavior, behavioral intent), and by Bandura (1986) (e.g., self-efficacy, incentive motivators, vicarious motivators). Aday and Anderson's theories (1974) suggest that *enabling* variables include the availability, accessibility, and acceptability of resources required to perform the behavior (e.g., seat belts). Some combination of specific predisposing, reinforcing, and enabling variables that account for the most variance in the behavior might provide an eclectic, parsimonious model to guide the development of interventions.

Focusing on Priority Behaviors

Although a large number of behaviors influence the health of populations, a comparatively small number have a disproportionately great effect. The effectiveness and efficiency of health promotion programs might be increased by focusing on those priority health behaviors that most influence the health of target populations (Carter Center of Emory University, 1985).

A technique that generates important information for establishing health priorities is calculation of *population attributable risk* (PAR), i.e., the fraction of a disease in a population due to exposure to a given risk factor (Levin, 1953). If $P.$ represents the *proportion of the total population exposed to a risk factor,* and R the *relative risk* of developing the disease among those exposed in comparison to those not exposed, then:

$$\text{PAR} = P.(R - 1)/P.(R - 1) + 1$$

This technique can be used to estimate, and compare, the extent to which various behavioral risk factors contribute to mortality within populations. For example, as shown in Table 4, in 1983 32.4% of adults who lived in Michigan reported that they smoked cigarettes (i.e., the proportion of the population exposed to the risk factor). In comparison to nonsmokers, smokers are 1.7 times more likely to die from heart attacks, 10.8 times more likely to die from lung cancer, 6.1 times more likely to die from emphysema, etc. (i.e., the relative risk for death from each disease is 1.7, 10.8, 6.1, etc.). In 1983, 29,488 Michigan residents died from heart attacks, 4533 died from lung cancer, 2395 died from emphysema, etc. Thus, 18.5% (or 5451) of all heart attack deaths in Michigan in 1983 were attributable to smoking, as were 76.0% (or 3447) of all lung cancer deaths, 62.3% (or 1492)

TABLE 4. Deaths among Michigan Residents over 1 Year of Age in 1983 Attributable to Smoking

Risk factor/prevalence[a]	*R*	Deaths 1+ years	PAR	Attributable deaths	Lives saved[b]
Heart attack	1.7	29,488	18.5%	5,451	1,245
Lung cancer	10.8	4,533	76.0%	3,447	787
Emphysema	6.1	2,395	62.3%	1,492	341
Stroke	1.3	5,535	8.9%	490	112
Other cancer	1.3	11,679	8.9%	1,035	236
Flu and pneumonia	1.4	2,019	11.5%	232	53
Total		55,649	21.8%	12,147	2,774

[a] In 1983, 32.4% were current smokers.
[b] If the number of Michigan residents who smoked had been reduced by 25%.

of all emphysema deaths, etc. If the number of Michigan residents who smoke had been reduced by 25.0%, 1245 fewer people would have died from heart attacks that year, 787 fewer would have died from lung cancer, 341 fewer would have died from emphysema, etc. (Ad Hoc Medical and Health Provider Advisory Committee, 1984). More sophisticated techniques of population attributable risk analysis can be used to assess the effects of interaction, confounding, and observational error on attributable risk estimation (Walter, 1983).

Population attributable risk analyses, and other techniques increasingly are being used to help identify priority behaviors that most influence the health of a given population, and to focus health promotion interventions on those behaviors (Texas Department of Health, 1986). The Health Promotion and Disease Prevention Supplement to the National Health Interview Survey has been implemented to estimate the prevalence of important health behaviors among adults in the United States (National Center for Health Statistics, 1985). The Behavioral Risk Factor Surveillance System has been implemented to estimate the prevalence of important health behaviors among adults within individual States (Bradstock *et al.*, 1984).

Focusing on High-Risk Populations

Some populations are at higher risk for a given disease than are others. For example, it has been estimated that by 1991, 70% of all cases of AIDS in the United States will be diagnosed among homosexual or bisexual men, and 25% will be diagnosed among intravenous drug abusers (U.S. Public Health Service, 1986). In addition, minority populations are at higher risk for many diseases. For example, between 1979 and 1981, the relative risk of mortality from the following causes among black and white females aged 25–34 was: cardiovascular disease, 4.02; malignant neoplasms, 1.35; cerebrovascular disease, 3.50; accidents, 1.13; diabetes mellitus, 2.60; chronic liver diseases, 6.46; homicide, 6.00; suicide, 0.54 (U.S. Department of Health and Human Services, 1985a). Thus, research to improve the effectiveness of health education and health promotion programs increasingly is (1) targeting high-risk and minority populations, and (2) designing interventions specifically to address the needs and cultural characteristics of these populations (e.g., Galli *et al.*, 1987). Indeed, the first of eight recommendations made by the Secretary's Task Force on Black and Minority Health (US DHHS, 1985a,b) was that:

> The Department should launch an outreach campaign to disseminate health information

> and education materials and program strategies specifically designed for minority sectors of the population including Blacks, Hispanics, Asian/Pacific Islanders, and Native Americans . . . [and should focus on] those public health areas identified by the Task Force which have the greatest impact on death and disability among minority populations: cancer; cardiovascular disease; chemical dependency; diabetes; homicide, suicide, and unintentional injuries; and, infant mortality. (p. 9)

Basic research about cultural and ethnic determinants of health beliefs, attitudes, and behaviors will be valuable in increasing the effectiveness of these campaigns. A transcultural perspective, and the concept of "health culture" can help health professionals address the unique perceptions, beliefs, and perspectives of these target populations.

Policies

Policy might be defined as any plan or course of action adopted by an organization, designed to influence and determine decisions, actions, and other matters. By applying the third definition of health promotion, interventions might be defined as policies designed to influence and determine health-related behaviors of a population. Research increasingly is being conducted to assess the effects of various types of health promotion policies. These policies might be classified within three categories (Kolbe, Tolsma, & Katz, in press).

The first category includes *policies that either require or prohibit behaviors* that influence the health of populations. More specifically, this category might be dichotomized to include: (a) policies that require behaviors thought to maintain or improve the health of the individual required to perform the behavior, or of others; or (b) policies that prohibit behaviors thought to threaten the health of the individual prohibited from performing the behavior, or of others. Examples of the former include policies that require individuals to wear safety belts, owners to have pets vaccinated, and children to be immunized. Examples of the latter include policies that prohibit the use of illegal drugs, drinking and driving, and smoking in certain places. Others have written eloquently about establishing health promotion policies that expressly require or prohibit population behaviors (e.g., Davis & Ng, 1981; Faden & Faden, 1978; Green, 1981; Mico, 1978; Reizen, Ruff, & Danielson, 1978; Wikler, 1978).

A second category includes *policies that provide the mandate and resources for an organization to implement health promotion programs* specifically designed to enable populations to modify voluntarily behaviors that affect health. Examples include policies that established the Public Health Promotion Division at the Texas Department of Health, Center for Health Promotion and Education at the Centers for Disease Control, and Division of Information and Education for Health at the World Health Organization.

A third category includes *policies that directly or indirectly facilitate population behaviors* that affect health. Examples include policies that require automobile manufacturers to install safety belts in vehicles, that reduce insurance premiums to increase safety belt use, and that enforce safety belt use laws. Indeed, it is likely that health promotion programs to influence many health behaviors (such as use of seat belts) might be most effective if they combined policies that might require (category one) and/or facilitate (category three) a given health behavior; with health education interventions to encourage adoption of the behavior, and to engender public support for the establishment, continuation, and enforcement of relevant policies.

Knowledge generated from basic health behavior research could be useful in developing policies that will be most acceptable to, and thus least resisted by, target populations. Such knowledge would include information about how beliefs, social norms, social networks, and family practices, for example, support or discourage the policies being advocated. Research data on personal health-related values would be useful in providing an appropriate focus for such policies.

Combining Interventions

Complementary or synergistic effects might be achieved by simultaneously implementing diverse interventions to influence a given behavior within a target population. Illustratively, the impact of a school health promotion program might be increased by simultaneously implementing interventions to address a given health behavior through more than one of the eight components of the total school health promotion program depicted in Figure 2. For example, a *school health education* program to reduce tobacco use among students might be considerably more effective if it were accompanied by school policies that prohibit smoking by faculty as well as students in the *school environment* (e.g., Rashak, Olsen, Spears, & Haggerty, 1986). As a second example, a recent study suggested that elementary school students are provided roughly 50% more total fat, 250% more saturated fat, and 20% more sodium by the *school food service program* than they should receive; and that the *school physical education program* enables students to engage in aerobic fitness activities for only about 6% of the physical education class time provided (Parcel *et al.*, 1987). Schools thus might substantially reduce behavioral risks for cardiovascular disease and cancer by simultaneously educating students to avoid these risks, and modifying the school food service and school physical education program so that students actually can avoid the risks.

Again, increased basic knowledge about the determinants of a wide range of health behaviors, particularly the values and motives of the target population, could lead to increasing the effectiveness of these complementary programs.

HEALTH BEHAVIOR INDICATOR SYSTEMS

It is essential to have some means to monitor the prevalence of important health behaviors among populations over time in order to plan and assess the effectiveness of health promotion programs (e.g., Andrews, 1981; Murhaghan, 1981; WHO, 1981a,b). Indicators of population behaviors are especially important given the relatively long interim between the implementation of a given health promotion program and the modification of the specific population behaviors it was designed to influence; and the additional long interim between the modification of specific population behaviors and consequent reduction of disease in that population.

Since 1980, four comprehensive indicator systems for planning, monitoring, and managing national, state, and local health promotion programs have been implemented in the United States. Each system increasingly will drive the development of means and methodologies to measure the prevalence of important health behaviors over time, consequences of those behaviors, determinants of those behaviors, and the effectiveness of interventions implemented to influence those behaviors. Each of these systems is briefly described below.

The Objectives for the Nation

In 1979, the U.S. Public Health Service convened experts in 15 health priority areas to develop specific, measurable health objectives to be attained by 1990. It was reasoned that health promotion and disease prevention programs could achieve their greatest impact if: *preventive health services* primarily focused on objectives in (1) high blood pressure control, (2) family planning, (3) pregnancy and infant health, (4) immunization, and (5) sexually transmitted diseases; if *health protection* primarily focused on objectives in (6) toxic agent control, (7) occupational safety and health, (8) accident prevention and injury control, (9) fluoridation and dental health, and (10) surveillance and control of infectious diseases; and if *health promotion* programs primarily focused on objectives in (11) smoking and health, (12) misuse of alcohol and drugs, (13) nutrition, (14) physical fitness and exercise, and (15) control of stress and violent behavior.

Each of these 15 health priority areas includes health behavior objectives to be monitored over time. An example of a surveillance and evaluation objective from the Misuse of Alcohol and Drugs priority area (US DHHS, 1979) is:

> By 1990, a comprehensive data capability should be established to monitor and evaluate the status and impact of misuse of alcohol and drugs on: health status; motor vehicle accidents; accidental injuries in addition to those from motor vehicles; interpersonal aggression and violence; sexual assault; vandalism and property damage; pregnancy outcomes; and emotional and physical development of infants and children.

In addition, to monitor important behavioral Objectives for the Nation that are not being monitored by other data systems, the National Center for Health Statistics developed a Health Promotion and Disease Prevention Supplement to become part of the National Health Interview Survey. The 1985 Health Promotion and Disease Prevention Supplement was designed to provide national baseline data about: general health (including nutrition), injury control and child health, high blood pressure, stress, exercise, smoking, alcohol use, dental care, and occupational safety and health. Two types of data were generated from the supplement: data about the prevalence of certain health behaviors, and data about population knowledge related to certain health behaviors. The 1985 Supplement will be implemented again in 1990 to assess the nation's progress in improving knowledge about critical health behaviors, and to gauge the prevalence of those behaviors (National Center for Health Statistics, 1985).

The Cancer Control Objectives

In 1985 a second indicator system with important health behavior objectives was developed by the National Cancer Institute (1986). To achieve the goal of reducing age-adjusted cancer deaths fully by 25–50% before the year 2000, specific measurable Cancer Control Objectives for the Nation, to be attained by the years 1990 and 2000 respectively, were written in three areas: (1) *prevention* (principally by influencing tobacco use, consumption of dietary fat and fiber, and occupational exposures to carcinogens); (2) *screening* (primarily by influencing screening for breast cancer and cervical cancer); and (3) *treatment* (by accelerating dissemination of state-of-the-art cancer therapy to increase survival rates).

A *surveillance system* for monitoring progress toward achieving these objectives was framed to assess consequent and related changes in: the prevalence of various risk factors; medical practices affecting cancer outcomes; participation in cancer screening; access to medical care for cancer; behavior related to seeking medical care for cancer; knowledge, attitudes, and beliefs of the public and of professions related to cancer; as well as in mortality from specific cancers; incidence of specific cancers; cancer patient survival; facilities for the treatment of cancer; and financing and associated medical care for cancer.

The Behavioral Risk Factor Surveillance System

Between 1981 and 1983, the U.S. Centers for Disease Control (CDC) helped 28 interested states and the District of Columbia to survey the prevalence of several important health behaviors among their respective populations. In 1983, a supplemental survey of the same health behaviors in all remaining states except Hawaii was conducted by the University of North Carolina. Using a standardized core questionnaire, random digit dialing technique, and interviewing protocol, trained staff and interviewers in participating states collected information by telephone about health behaviors such as: cigarette smoking, hypertension treatment compliance, weight, seat belt usage, physical activity, acute and chronic alcohol use, and drinking and driving, in addition to collecting standard demographic information about age, race, sex, and education. The behaviors surveyed were selected because of their association with the 10 leading causes of premature death among adults in the United States (e.g., Bradstock *et al.,* 1984).

Because numerous states were interested in such data and used it for planning disease prevention programs, an ongoing Behavioral Risk Factor Surveillance System (BRFSS) was implemented in 1984 to regularly interview adults in 23 participating states. The BRFSS thus provides data about important health behaviors of 55% of the total adult population in the United States (U.S. Center for Health Promotion and Education, 1985).

This third health behavior indicator system is unlike the two described above in two important ways. First, the system provides state-level, in contrast to national-level, estimates; thus, it can be used for state disease prevention program planning, monitoring, and management. Second, the BRFSS is not designed to establish levels of the behavior to be attained within a given period of time (i.e., it is not designed to establish goals or objectives).

The Model Standards for Community Preventive Health Services

A fourth set of indicators for planning, monitoring, and managing health promotion and disease prevention programs is contained in *Model Standards: A Guide for Community Preventive Health Services* (e.g., American Public Health Association, 1985; Schaefer, 1985). Recognizing that each community has its own unique aggregation of health problems and resources, representatives of national, state, and local health officials collaborated to design a common set of model standards that could enable state and local health agencies (e.g., state health departments, local health departments, Health System Agencies, State Health Planning & Development Agencies) to work within and among their agencies to design disease prevention programs that would efficiently address the specific needs of their respective communities.

Among the 33 disease prevention program areas (e.g., abusive and violent behavior, air quality, health education, mental health, nutritional services, problems of aging and dependent populations, public health laboratory) are a number of objectives related to health behavior, e.g., elective abortions, unwanted pregnancies.

RESEARCH SYNTHESIS

As more research about health behaviors is conducted and accumulates, it will become increasingly important to aggregate and understand the combined results systematically. Findings from health behavior research often vary in confusing irregularity across behaviors, populations, types of interventions, and countless other factors. Sixty studies on the effects of smoking cessation interventions, for example, may defy simple summary. The ultimate meaning of these studies could no more be ascertained by a traditional narrative discursive review than one could ascertain the meaning of 60 test scores without the aid of specific techniques that have been developed to organize, depict, and interrelate the data (e.g., through statistical measures of central tendency and variance).

To comprehend the considerable accumulation of data generated by increasingly numerous health behavior research studies, more sophisticated forms of research synthesis are being developed and used. Mullen and Ramirez (1987), in a useful overview of research synthesis issues and methods, suggested that approaches to research synthesis can be characterized according to the type of analysis conducted (ranging from the purely quantitative to the purely qualitative), and according to the type of studies reviewed (including evaluation, correlational, epidemiologic, and descriptive studies). These authors suggested how a variety of approaches can be included under each category.

CONCLUSION

In the continuing evolution of disease and society, basic research about how behaviors affect the health of populations, and about factors that influence the occurrence of those behaviors, could markedly improve the well-being of existing and future populations. The achievement of such improvements, however, will depend on applied research: to design, evaluate, and disseminate interventions that can influence critical health behaviors; and to monitor those behaviors, and the health outcomes they affect. Accordingly, those trained and committed to conducting health behavior research together bear a considerable, though largely unacknowledged, responsibility.

REFERENCES

Aday, L., & Anderson, R. (1974). A framework for the study of access to medical care. *Health Services Research, 9*(4), 208–220.

Ad Hoc Medical and Health Provider Advisory Committee. (1984). *Health care cost containment: A preventive approach* (Final report to the Senate Committee to study health care cost containment). Lansing: Michigan Department of Health.

American Public Health Association. (1985). *Model standards for community preventive health services* (2nd ed.). Washington, DC: Author.

Andrews, F. M. (1981). Social indicators and health-for-all. *Social Science and Medicine, 15*(3), 219–223.

Bandura, A. (1986). *Social foundations of thought and action: A social cognitive theory*. Englewood Cliffs, NJ: Prentice–Hall.

Baric, L. (1969). Recognition of the "at-risk" role: A means to influence health behavior. *International Journal of Health Education, 18*(1), 2–12.

Bass, F. (1982). Invalidating tobacco. In R. Taylor, J. Ureda, & J. Denham (Eds.), *Health promotion: Principles and clinical application*. New York: Appleton–Century–Crofts.

Becker, M. (Ed.). (1974). *The health belief model and personal health behavior. Health Education Monographs, 2*(4).

Blair, S., Smith, M., Collingwood, T., Reynolds, R., Prentice, M., & Sterling, C. (1986). Health promotion for educators: Impact on absenteeism. *Preventive Medicine, 15,* 166–175.

Bradstock, M., Marks, J., Forman, M., Gentry, E., Hogelin, G., & Trowbridge, F. (1984). Behavioral risk factor surveillance, 1981–1983. *Morbidity and Mortality Weekly Reports Surveillance Summaries, 33,* 1–4.

Carter Center of Emory University. (1985). *Closing the gap health policy project: Interim summary*. Atlanta: Author.

Davis, D., & Ng, L. (1981). National policy issues for health promotion and disease prevention. In L. Ng & D. Davis (Eds.), *Strategies for public health: Promoting health and preventing disease* (pp. 1–31). Princeton, NJ: Van Nostrand–Reinhold.

Epp, L. (1986). *Achieving health for all: A framework for health promotion in Canada*. Toronto: Health and Welfare, Canada.

European Working Group on Concepts and Principles of Health Promotion. (1985). *Concepts and principles of health promotion.* Copenhagen: World Health Organization Regional Office for Europe.

Faden, R., & Faden, A. (1978). The ethics of health education as public health policy. *Health Education Monographs, 6*(2), 180–197.

Fishbein, M., & Ajzen, I. (1975). *Belief, attitude, intention and behavior: An introduction to theory and research.* Reading, MA: Addison–Wesley.

Galli, N., Greenberg, J., & Tobin, F. (1987). Health education and sensitivity to cultural, religious, and ethnic beliefs. *Journal of School Health, 57*(5), 177–180.

Gordon, N. (1986). Never smokers, triers, and current smokers: Three distinct target groups for school-based anti-smoking programs. *Health Education Quarterly, 13*(2), 163–180.

Green, L. (1979a). Health promotion policy and the placement of responsibility for personal health care. *Family and Community Health, 2,* 51–64.

Green, L. (1979b). National policy in the promotion of health. *International Journal of Health Education, 22*(3), 161–168.

Green, L. (1981). National policy in the promotion of health. In M. Hiller (Ed.), *Medical ethics and the law: Implications for public policy* (pp. 135–148). Cambridge, MA: Ballinger.

Green, L., Kreuter, M., Deeds, S., & Partridge, K. (1980). *Health education planning: A diagnostic approach.* Palo Alto, CA: Mayfield.

Kar, S. (1984). Psychosocial environment: A health promotion model. *International Quarterly of Community Health Education, 4*(4), 311–341.

Kasl, S., & Cobb, S. (1966a). Health behavior, illness behavior, and sick-role behavior: I. Health and illness behavior. *Archives of Environmental Health, 12*(2), 246–264.

Kasl, S., & Cobb, S. (1966b). Health behavior, illness behavior, and sick-role behavior: II. Sick-role behavior. *Archives of Environmental Health, 12*(4), 531–543.

Kolbe, L. (1984a). Improving the health status of children: Frameworks for behavioral research and development. In G. Campbell (Ed.), *Health education and youth: A review of research and developments.* Philadelphia: Falmer Press.

Kolbe, L. (1984b). Improving the health status of children: An epidemiological approach to establishing priorities for behavioral research. In G. Campbell (Ed.), *Health education and youth: A review of research and developments.* Philadelphia: Falmer Press.

Kolbe, L. (1985). Why school health education? An empirical point of view. *Health Education, 16*(2), 116–120.

Kolbe, L. (1986). Indicators for planning and monitoring school health programs. In S. Kar, E. Berkanovic, & S. Churgin (Eds.), *Proceedings of the Symposium on Indicators of Health Promotive Behaviors.* Los Angeles: University of California Press.

Kolbe, L., Green, L., Foreyt, J., Darnell, L., Goodrick, K., Williams, H., Ward, D., Korton, A. S., Karacan, I., Widmeyer, R., & Stainbrook, G. (1986). Appropriate functions of health education in schools: Improving health and cognitive performance. In N. Krasnegor, J. Arasteh, & M. Cataldo (Eds.), *Child health behavior: A behavioral pediatrics perspective.* New York: Wiley.

Kolbe, L., Tolsma, D., & Katz, M. (in press). International, national, state, and local health promotion policies. In *Advances in Health Education and Health Promotion, IV.* New York: Human Sciences Press.

Leventhal, H., & Cleary, P. (1980). The smoking problem: A review of the research and theory in behavioral risk modification. *Psychological Bulletin, 88*(2), 370–405.

Levin, M. (1953). The occurrence of lung cancer in man. *Acta Union Internationalis contra Cancrum, 9,* 531–541.

Mason, J., & Powell, K. (1985). Physical activity, behavioral epidemiology, and public health. *Public Health Reports, 100*(2), 113–115.

Mausner, J., & Kramer, S. (1985). *Epidemiology: An introductory text.* Philadelphia: Saunders.

Mico, P. (1978). An introduction to policy for health educators. *Health Education Monographs, 6*(Suppl. 2), 7–17.

Mullen, P., & Ramirez, G. (1987). Information synthesis and meta-analysis. In W. Ward, M. Becker, P. Mullen, & S. Simonds (Eds.), *Advances in health education and promotion.* Greenwich, CT: JAI Press.

Murhaghan, J. (1981). Health indicators information systems for the year 2000. *Annual Review of Public Health, 2,* 299–361.

National Cancer Institute. (1986). *Cancer control objectives for the nation, 1985–2000.* Washington, DC: National Institutes of Health.

National Center for Health Statistics. (1981). Prevention profile. In *Health United States, 1980.* Washington, DC: U.S. Department of Health and Human Services.

National Center for Health Statistics. (1985). *Provisional data from the health promotion and disease prevention supplement to the National Health Interview Survey: United States, January–March, 1985.* Washington, DC: U.S. Department of Health and Human Services.

Parcel, G., Simons-Morton, B., O'Hara, N., Baranowski, T., Kolbe, L., & Bee, (1987). School promotion of healthful diet and exercise behavior: An integration of organizational change and social learning theory interventions. *Journal of School Health, 57*(4), 150–156.

Rashak, N., Olsen, L., Spears, A., & Haggerty, J. (1986). Smoking policies of secondary schools in Arizona. *Journal of School Health, 56,* 180–183.

Reizen, M., Ruff, J., & Danielson, R. (1978). Policy development and implementation issues for health education. *Health Education Monographs, 6*(Suppl. 1), 74–90.

Rosen, T., & Shipley, R. 1983. The stage analysis of self-initiated smoking reductions. *Addictive Behaviors, 8,* 263–272.

Schaefer, M. (1985). Moving the standards movement. *American Journal of Public Health, 75*(6), 645–647.

Texas Department of Health. (1986). *Action plans for determining and attaining priority health objectives for Texas.* Austin: The John E. Fogarty International Center for Advanced Study in the Health Sciences & The American College of Preventive Medicine. (1976). *Health promotion and consumer health education.* New York: Prodist.

U.S. Center for Health Promotion and Education. (1985). *Behavioral risk factor surveillance system.* Atlanta: Centers for Disease Control.

U.S. Department of Health, Education and Welfare. (1978, September). *Disease prevention and health promotion: Federal programs and prospects* (Report of the Departmental Task Force on Prevention). Washington, DC: U.S. Government Printing Office.

U.S. Department of Health, Education and Welfare. (1979). *Healthy people: The surgeon general's report on health promotion and disease prevention.* Washington, DC: U.S. Department of Health and Human Services.

U.S. Department of Health and Human Services. (1985a). *Report of the secretary's task force on black and minority health: Executive summary, I.* Washington, DC: U.S. Government Printing Office.

U.S. Department of Health and Human Services. (1985b). *Report of the secretary's task force on black and minority health: Crosscutting issues in minority health, II.* Washington, DC: U.S. Government Printing Office.

U.S. Public Health Service. (1986). Coolfont Report: A PHS plan for prevention and control of AIDS and the AIDS virus. *Public Health Reports, 101*(4), 341.

Walter, S. (1983). Effects of interaction, confounding and observational error on attributable risk estimation. *American Journal of Epidemiology, 117,* 598–604.

Wikler, D. (1978). Persuasion and coercion for health: Ethical issues in government efforts to change lifestyles. *Milbank Memorial Fund Quarterly, 56*(3), 303–338.

World Health Organization. (1981a). Global strategy of health for all by the year 2000. *Health for all series* (No. 3). Geneva: Author.

World Health Organization. (1981b). Global strategy of health for all by the year 2000. *Health for all series* (No. 4). Geneva: Author.

CHAPTER 22

Chronic Illness Management

A Focus for Future Research Applications

Eugene B. Gallagher

This chapter aims to develop directions for health behavior research on the management of chronic illness. As the preceding chapters in this volume richly demonstrate, there has been an impressive structure of investigation within the field of health behavior research, which has elucidated how people feel, believe, and act in regard to their health. Particularly well known are the studies inspired by the health belief model.

Research generated by the health belief model has established health behavior as a topic for investigation in contemporary society which is of equal importance with other basic categories such as family relationships, religious belief, public opinion, and social class. Health behavior research has also demonstrated its relevance for public policy in various directions, for example by discerning the impact of attitudinal barriers to the achievement of community health goals (Koos, 1954).

Despite these singular accomplishments of the health behavior research tradition, it has been reluctant to examine behavior in the context of the management of *illness*—the attitudes, values, interactions, and behavioral stances which arise in the care and treatment of persons professionally designated as ill. This is not a trivial reluctance. This reluctance curtails an important contribution as our society continues to increase its desire and need for sophisticated medical care. Further, it amounts to a failure to test within the hospital, nursing home, and clinic those same concepts and methods of investigation which have proved applicable in the study of well persons as they face health risks in everyday life.

It would be erroneous to maintain that there has been no health behavior research whatsoever which has studied ill persons or those who, while not diagnosed as ill, have symptoms, i.e., are not well. A number of studies have examined how symptomatic individuals enter the health care system (timing of entry in relation to symptom severity, anticipated costs and benefits, type of resource utilized, and so forth), several studies have looked at patients with various diagnoses—arthritis (Oakes, Ward, Gray, Klauber, & Moody 1970), heart attack (Croog & Levine, 1982), rheumatic fever (Heinzelmann, 1962), chronic renal failure (Hartman & Becker, 1978)—focusing especially upon the patient's degree of compliance with medical regimens. These studies have employed concepts basic within the health behavior research tradition, such as the patient's sense of vulnerability, and weighing the advantages and disadvantages of various paths of action.

EUGENE B. GALLAGHER • Departments of Behavioral Science and Sociology, University of Kentucky, Lexington, Kentucky 40536.

In addition to these empirical thrusts into the domain of the unwell, health behavior research has at the semantic and conceptual level explicitly incorporated the unwell by expanding its purview from the "health behavior" (of well persons) to a more inclusive conception of "health-related behavior." This latter category presents a threefold categorization which commences (1) with concern for prevention or detection of illness among well persons, and then embraces (2) the behavior and attitudes of persons who have symptoms, and (3) the behavior and attitudes of persons who are defined as ill, i.e., professionally diagnosed as having a disease or other medical condition (Kasl & Cobb, 1966a,b; Becker & Maiman, 1983).

Though this categorization actually came as an early construction in the health behavior research tradition, it remains a largely unfulfilled attempt to embrace the illness domain. The great bulk of research and conceptualization has emphasized the situation and prospects of well persons.

The institutional and disciplinary matrix from which health behavior research developed provided a strong basis for its initial focus upon well individuals and for its continuation along this path. Schools of public health and departments of epidemiology or preventive medicine in medical schools constituted the base in which the leading health behavior researchers developed their ideas. Many of these researchers had received their own training in psychology, particularly social psychology. In academic health institutions, they turned their conceptual fecundity and rigor to the elaboration of psychological constructs derived from the relationships between behavior and attitudes, from Lewinian field theory, and from the effects of group norms and mass communications upon individual behavior. Such constructs were novel in schools of public health, the intellectual atmosphere of which was dedicated to concern for infectious disease, and they provided new vigor to public health theory and programs. They were the stimulus to fresh thinking about the individual's role in health and disease, in contrast with the earlier focus upon epidemics and contagion. The health belief model furnished paradigmatic energy to much of this conceptual development. However, other paradigms, drawn from cultural anthropology, behavioral medicine, ethnomedicine, and medical sociology, also figured in the broad reach of health behavior research.

THE ILLNESS MANAGEMENT SITUATION

This chapter will trace an analytic framework—*the illness management situation*—within which health behavior research can fashion questions and concepts which branch logically from its earlier roots. This framework will indicate points of continuity and contrast with the main lines of its previous development.

The illness management situation refers to persons who have been professionally diagnosed as ill or having a medical condition. This paradigm is further restricted here to persons having *chronic,* as opposed to acute, illness. The acute/chronic distinction is of course part of medical logic and terminology. A current medical dictionary defines "chronic" as "lingering, lasting, opposed to acute . . ." (Roper, 1978, p. 65) and "acute" as "short and severe; not long drawn out or chronic" (p. 5). Although the acute/chronic dichotomy is too sharp and not always satisfying even for medical purposes, it points to a distinction of general importance to health behavior research.

Health behavior research has been slow to turn its attention to chronic illness. Becker (1974) suggested that dependence upon conceptual categories and variables rising from the medical model (i.e., using biomedically derived and physician-imposed diagnostic labels) has not been productive in the study of health behavior. His reservations fall with particular weight upon patient characteristics which are "relatively enduring and unalterable" such as are found in chronic illness and where "little could be done to improve the situation" (p. 409). Not unlike the medical care system itself, which has tended to ignore the increasing burden of chronic illness in society, health behavior research has in its own way focused upon medical problems which, yielding to a behavioral or attitudinal change, hold the promise of a short-run positive outcome—a disease prevented or treated early to good effect. Further, it may well be that social scientists studying health behavior, like other scientists and intellectuals, avoid paradigms and cognitive structures which lie outside their own field, preferring to increase the power and reach of their own concepts.

Kasl (1974) examined gaps in the logical structure of health behavior research and remedies for these gaps. In establishing a conceptual structure suitable for health behavior research on chronic illness, he pointed out that new concepts may be necessary when behavior involves "longer contact with a health professional or with a treatment setting, and a partial or total withdrawal from one's usual social roles and obligations. Because of this, new determinants may become relevant: the nature of the treatment setting and of the interaction between the patient and health professionals, the relative attractiveness of the social roles which 'compete' with the sick role, and so on" (p. 435).

The sphere of chronic illness offers important problems for study to the field of health behavior research. For example, medical status as the possessor of a chronic or acute disease has implications for the kinds of professional services the patient receives and for the kinds of professional expectations and attitudes the patient encounters. Taken as an objective, externally based state, the patient's position on the chronic/acute dichotomy also has important implications for the self-concept and motivational state relative to illness. These two foci—the patient as the target of health professional expectations and the patient's self-concept as the bearer of illness—designate conceptual areas of potential interest to health behavior research and they are amenable to constructive dissection for the purpose of measurement.

In acute illness, the patient either dies or gets better within a short period of time. Sometimes the outcome is beyond medical help; everything depends upon the patient's constitution and powers of resistance. Even when medical intervention can make a difference, the acute ambience gives little room for fluctuations in the intensity and scope of treatment, or for differences in self-concept to affect the patient's dealings with the illness. In contrast, chronic, enduring illness requires ongoing adjustment and management which will be marked by phases when the patient controls the situation and other phases when medical help becomes desirable and the patient's reliance upon professionals increases. These fluctuations thus form an important feature of illness management.

The health behavior researcher can establish a continuum with one pole at the extreme of patient self-management and the other at the extreme of professional management. These questions then become important:

1. At a given time, what is the patient's position on the continuum?
2. What factors affect the patient's position at a given time?

We cannot assume a strict correlation between the patient's need for professional help and an exacerbation of the illness as objectively measured. Instead, health behavior research must allow for, and investigate, the interplay of psychological, situational, and medical factors in determining the patient's position on the continuum.

AUTHORITY AND COMMUNICATION WITHIN THE ILLNESS MANAGEMENT SITUATION

Fluctuations in the chronically ill patient's need for medical attention are related to two other ranges of variation which are of considerable interest to health behavior research.

These variations occur (1) in the exercise of the medical authority and (2) in the dynamics of communication.

The major basis for medical authority is the physician's expert knowledge and skill. His authority is expressed in the form of medical advice, decision-making, and action. In conveying knowledge, assessing the patient's condition and prospects, and providing counsel, the physician communicates with the patient from a position of authoritative expertise. However, medical authority is not self-validating—it lies in the respect and deference of the patient, who lacks expertise, toward the physician to deal with the affliction.

The chronic patient, unlike the acute one, often has a personal experiential understanding of the disease and its impact on the self. Medical advice may be questioned or ignored if it contradicts the patient's own experience; and medical expertise frequently fails to provide the patient with practical information on how to live with illness. In *Chronic Illness and the Quality of Life,* Strauss (1975) pointed out the adaptations which chronic patients must make in their daily life; emphysema sufferers and others with diminished breathing capacity, for example, detour around hills when walking. The knowledge of tolerable walking routes for the individual patient is clearly not medical knowledge, and the physician is in no better position than many others in contact with such a patient to provide that information. The physician might well not be able to formulate for the individual patient what the limits of exertion tolerance are. In contrast, pharmacology is an area of profound medical expertise. Even in that area a "senior" chronic patient might have strong opinions and preferences concerning particular drugs, though of course the patient relies upon the physician's prerogative to prescribe.

Just as medical authority is exercised putatively for the benefit of the patient, so also are physician–patient communications carried out for the benefit of the patient. This point requires emphasis because it provides an ultimate standard by which health behavior research can judge the effectiveness or appropriateness of communications.

There have been relatively few studies of physician–patient communication, owing to the difficulty of such research. One common approach has been to measure the amount of information which the patient has retained from the total conveyed by the physician (Ley, Bradshaw, Eaves, & Walker, 1973). One may question the value of retention of sheer information, emptied of its significance as the patient copes with the medical problem. Such research is open to the criticism that, in measuring what is easily available (medical facts, words appearing on transcripts of encounters between physician and patient, diagnostic or prognostic statements by the physician, and so forth), it conveniently avoids the search to understand how the patient influences the production of such information within the interview context, assimilates it once the physician enunciates it, and then integrates it into characteristic illness behavior. Whatever its limitations, such research does have potential value for uncovering standard trends in physician–patient communication, e.g., the balance of utterances between the physician and the patient, and the ratio of affectively toned statements to purely cognitive, informational statements. Even if the basic underlying forces which produce communication patterns are not known, such parameters can serve as reference values for identifying aberrant extremes when they occur, and for directing attention to communication episodes which invite special scrutiny and explanation.

The transmission of information is a vital part of illness management, and an important area for future health behavior research. Much research conducted under the health belief model analyzed the effects of messages dealing with preventive health practices and the value of diagnostic screening procedures, asking, for example, whether negative threat messages were more effective than positively toned messages in inducing desired health behavior. Such messages were analyzed as decontextualized psychological stimuli, abstracted from live settings and from the cumulative resonance which any single new or first-time message arouses in the life-experienced adult recipient.

None of the principles which govern health behavior, such as the actor's weighing of the relative benefits of various courses of action, are invalid within the management situation of the chronic patient. However, in order to specify their effect, it will be necessary to devise tools which explicitly recognize that the patient is neither an outsider nor a newcomer to the system of health care, and that many of the messages received in regard to the illness may have been heard many times before. Assessing the impact of a given message requires not only analyzing its literal stimulus value but also looking at contextual factors such as the patient's level of knowledge about the disease; the comparison and crediting of alternative sources of information; and the patient's self-concept and sense of well-being as these are affected by the medical condition.

CHRONIC ILLNESS AND ADULT MODES OF LEARNING

Beyond these established principles, an additional range of principles holds promise for increasing our understanding of the patient with chronic illness. Communications to the patient are embedded within an ongoing medical biography. The patient's illness behavior does not reflect a series of disjunctive impacts under discrete stimuli but rather a learning process with some cumulative features and other features which are transitory and extinguishable. Seligman's concept of learned helplessness (1975) catches the way in which a perception of threat beyond a person's control can gradually anchor and spread within the self-concept, leading to a sense of helplessness and depression. From the standpoint of clinical understanding and benefit, the question becomes that of the patient's adjustment to the irreducible exactions of the illness and adaptation to it in ways which maintain life quality, as opportunity and circumstance permit.

Concepts from the field of adult socialization and social learning may also be of great value. Though a chronic patient career can commence at a young age, most chronic patients enter their illness as adults. A chronic illness may entail, and the patient role impose, varying qualities of dependency that mimic childhood dependency. Nevertheless, more is involved than simple regression to a dependent status. The change of status which occurs is a complex process involving both a relinquishing of adult competencies and prerogatives, as well as the learning of the adaptations and compensations required by illness, disability, and treatment.

As an adult, the patient builds upon a repertoire of skills, needs, and expectations in the ongoing learning of the chronic illness situation. Is there a similarity between this kind of learning and the adult learning of a second language? It is known that second-language learning proceeds on the basis of the learner's having already mastered the first language in childhood. The adult has—although generally unaware of it—basic knowledge of grammatical categories which was absent in the child and which play an important part in learning a new language. Adults are not susceptible to the same rewards and fears that shaped a their learning as children. Indeed, a powerful driving force in all adult learning is precisely the desire to be treated with dignity, i.e., not like a child. Does this impair learning, which conventionally implies a superordinate, mature teacher and a childlike pupil of lesser status? Or does it imply, instead, a different, more complex form of learning? The phases of acquisition of the chronic patient role may be better comprehended if this process is analyzed with concepts applicable to other adult roles (Thornton & Nardi, 1974; Turner, 1978).

MEDICAL AUTHORITY AS A NEGOTIATED PROCESS

This discussion of medical authority has conveyed the idea that expert knowledge gives the physician authority. Medical authority, unlike the authority of the law or the authority of a military officer over subordinates, has no coercive power at its disposal and must base its claim upon the social prestige of the profession and its imputed desire to help the sick patient—upon rational appeal, influence, and persuasion with the individual patient. It quickly becomes artificial and abstract, to detach medical authority from the scenes and processes of its application. Thus, medical authority must be examined within the context of communications between physician and patient. What does the patient need that the doctor can provide? How does the physician convey to the patient a view of the situation and what is to be done about it? What is the patient's understanding of this and response to it?

Finding answers to these questions would reveal that medical authority is a negotiated property of the physician–patient relationship instead of an inherent attribute of the physician's role or an external constraint automatically imposed upon the situation. Such a conception might have implications for the study of patient compliance, which is of special importance in chronic illness. Many investigations of compliance have drawn uncritically upon popular and traditional images of medical authority which depict it as an absolute ("doctor's orders") that the patient is obliged to obey without hesitation or reflection.

In understanding how the patient is guided in the management of illness, it is necessary also to think of authority as having a flexible locus within the field of medical resources and personnel. In an earlier era when medical care was more limited and less effective, what physicians did constituted the whole of the medical care. The physician's activity and influence encompassed virtually the entire sphere of medical authority. In contemporary medical care, there are many categories of medical specialties and health workers, each category of which possesses some unique competencies and responsibilities and some which overlap with those of other categories. The conventional view is that nonphysician workers function on the delegated authority of the physician, but this view seems increasingly inadequate. It fails to capture the significance of vital interactions of patients with nurses and other health professionals, and the exposure of patients to advice from diverse physicians. It is especially inadequate for understanding chronic illness, where the balances between the patient's self-management, medical intervention, and services provided by nonmedical personnel shift from time to time.

Medical authority has been greatly affected by the expansion of channels for information about disease and treatment. What the physician recommends is evaluated by patients in the light of medical news in the mass media and of lay networks composed of patients' relatives and friends. Labeling this general phenomenon as "health consumerism," medical sociologists have come to believe that the questioning of medical expertise has become widespread in American society, especially among middle-class persons, and that many patients want to have information resources in order to make decisions, rather than to follow doctor's orders (Pratt, 1978; Reeder, 1972; Haug & Lavin, 1983) in simple compliance. Although much of the quest for medical information occurs among healthy persons in regard to preventing illness, much also occurs among chronic patients who want to formulate their own strategies for managing illness.

Health consumerism is a topic ripe for broader empirical study than it has received. Is it primarily healthy persons who can muster the emotional energy required to compare and question medical opinions? In the foxhole of *serious* illness, most patients may want an authority that they can confidently trust; but *chronic* illness, with its long plateaus, may engender greater self-reliance.

PSYCHOLOGY AND SOCIOLOGY IN THE STUDY OF ILLNESS MANAGEMENT

The ability of health behavior research to study chronic illness effectively depends in part upon whether it can disentangle and render researchable the complex of communication and authority factors which lie within the illness management paradigm. While other disciplines have contributed importantly to health behavior research, this task is primarily a challenge for both psychology and sociology.

While I do not wish to draw speciously precise lines between these two disciplines, psychologists are perhaps less inclined than sociologists to investigate medical phenomena that are shaped by professional roles in institutional settings, or phenomena such as chronic illness which have slow outcomes occurring over a long period of time. Psychology's intellectual drive to formulate precise manipulable or measurable mechanisms of human behavior is frustrated by having to take into account too many sources of variation. Sociologists generally seek an interpretive description of behavior occurring in social context, though at the price of less powerful explanation. Thus, the most comprehensive analyses of medical authority (Freidson, 1970; Field, 1972) have come from sociology, as has the analysis of health consumerism.

Whatever the factors which make chronic illness a difficult topic of study, both psychological and sociological formulations are needed. Consider, for example, the complementary enrichment which both disciplines can offer in studying the following two areas: the patient's self-concept, and the communications and authority complex.

Patient Self-Concept

The first area is the patient's self-concept. Do patients see themselves primarily as persons who have an illness, or primarily as patients? To what extent are their self-concepts dominated by their illness? I wish to pose these questions for serious inquiry and to avoid the glib supposition that all it takes is "right attitude" to cope with a chronic illness. Although it is acceptable at a semantic and heuristic level to ask, "Do they see themselves as persons with a chronic illness or as chronically ill patients?", realistic investigation must allow for patient responses which simultaneously stand on both sides of this dichotomy, i.e., which express a mix of the sense of positive, normal ability and the resigned sense of lasting damage or impairment. Similarly, practical efforts for the counseling or rehabilitation of patients, which may be guided by the results of such research, must allow psychological scope for the ambivalent feelings which patients may have toward incapacity. To take a simple example, the self-concept of a chronic renal patient receiving regular hemodialysis is bound to be influenced by the considerable constraints of the treatment. Two such patients may of course differ markedly in the impact which this life-maintaining treatment has upon their self-concept and activity levels, but it is a constraint which cannot be disregarded or wished away.

Psychological formulations about the setting of goals and level of aspiration seem relevant to conceptualizing these questions. For example, the mildly diabetic patient who establishes the goal of managing the illness through diet without resort to insulin may need to maintain a patient self-concept in order to mobilize the requisite degrees of self-discipline or vigilance. By contrast, the chronic renal failure patient who undergoes dialysis is already in an objective sense "yoked" to the dialysis machine. *That* patient might achieve a higher degree of autonomous existence by being rid of the patient self-concept.

Sociological formulations may be equally important, such as the symbolic interactionist perspective which allows for the incorporation into one's self-concept of the expectations and images projected from significant others. Thus, a family, from misguided support or protectiveness, may convey to the patient the sense of being less capable of self-management than is in fact the case.

The Communications–Authority Complex

The second area concerns the communications–authority complex within the illness management situation. Health behavior research in this area might productively draw from cognitive psychology and from sociology.

Earlier health behavior studies demonstrated the impact of various kinds of messages upon the preventive behavior of individuals. Such messages were characterized in terms of the nature of the appeal they conveyed and the affective valences which they aroused in recipients. The study of the patient's situation in chronic illness requires a similar effort, which is, however, affected by the fact that any particular message the patient receives is something that, considered as a decontextualized stimulus, has probably also been received earlier. Its potential for effect in illness management should be regarded as incremental rather than immediate. However, the ups and downs of chronic illness may also mean that the patient undergoes moments and phases of particular susceptibility (and resistance) to messages. There is increasing attention to this principle in public health and clinical medicine. For example, the approach of the 1960s and 1970s, aiming for broadside screening and health education of the public, has been refined by the realistic awareness that limited resources can be directed with greater effect to selected target groups, and to individuals at critical moments of illness, than to anybody at any time. Adult female smokers may, for example, be more motivated, and able, to stop smoking during pregnancy than at other times.

Further, messages which the patient receives must be characterized according to their authoritativeness. Heuristically, more credible or authoritative messages will have greater effect than those with less authoritativeness. But what actually gives messages their authoritative quality? One might assume that, in terms of their source, what the physician conveys is more credible than what nonphysicians convey. But other factors come into play. Advice concerning diet for a diabetic patient emanating from a healthy physician might be less convincing than advice from a friend who is also diabetic. Further, if messages are subject to informal empirical testing over time by the chronic patient, their confirmation or disconfirmation may affect their authoritativeness, for that patient, of future messages from the same source or with similar content.

The foregoing suggestions are perhaps too specific in their conceptualization. It seems likely, however, that the mixture of information and credibility which inheres continuously in communications concerning the management of chronic illness can be reduced to analyzable components by the application of sociological and psychological concepts to the patient's situation.

THE CHRONIC RENAL PATIENT

The foregoing formulation of the illness management situation can be illustrated by reference to chronic renal failure (also commonly designated as "end-stage renal disease"—ESRD). This illustration is selected in order to demonstrate those features of the formulation which have clearest applicability and also to point out areas where further conceptualization and research are needed.

Some 85,000 renal patients in the United States receive medical care which is substantially paid for by the federal ESRD program. The incidence and prevalence of ESRD can be expected to increase gradually as the population ages. This increase will be due both to primary renal failure and to secondary renal failure arising from other diseases such as hypertension and diabetes.

At present, there are two basic treatment modalities for ESRD: dialysis of the patient's blood, and renal transplantation. A successful renal transplant goes far to remove the patient from the chronic patient category. The transplant patient nevertheless must take immunosuppressive medications on a lifelong basis and is never completely free of the possibility of transplant failure, in which event there must be a resort to dialysis. Because the transplant patient is less of a full-fledged patient, the renal dialysis patient is of greater concern here.

The renal dialysis patient has been aptly described as "intermittently dying" (Beavert, 1974). This description refers to the physiological fact that, in between dialysis sessions, metabolic substances accumulate in the blood which would eventually—that is, without the periodic "rescue" by the dialysis process—lead to death from toxic uremia. Dialysis can be carried out in two modes: hemodialysis and peritoneal dialysis. The hemodialysis patient is connected with a dialysis apparatus three times a week for 4 to 5 hours; the connection occurs through the insertion of needles into a specially prepared site for access to the blood supply. The peritoneal patient is dialyzed steadily during most waking hours daily through a surgically created aperture leading through the peritoneum into the cavity.

In either mode, dialysis is a demanding treatment. In hemodialysis the patient receives treatment at a dialysis center, where professional personnel will probably conduct most of the treatment procedures, but the patient has the task of getting to the center on schedule three times a week. Peritoneal dialysis can be done at home or at work, according to the patient's own schedule. Although there is greater freedom in scheduling, the peritoneal patient has the burden of self-treatment; in particular, following exacting sterile procedures. Some hemodialysis patients also carry out this treatment at home, with similar advantages and hazards.

In addition to treatment demands, the dialysis patient is subject to continuous dietary restrictions set by the physician and nutritionist on the basis of periodic blood analyses. Various complications of treatment pose a further set of important contingencies on dialysis. Long-term dialysis leads, in many patients, to degenerative changes in bone composition which can be minimized by additional dietary precautions. The site of blood access, for both hemo- and peritoneal dialysis patients, is an inherent weak point in the treatment process, subjecting the skin surface to abrasion and infection. Many patients require a second surgery to redo the access site after 10 or more years on dialysis.

Many aspects of the chronic illness management situation can be seen in this sketch of the dialysis patient. An important variable is the extent to which the patient is subject to active physician intervention (as when the access site develops a persistent infection) because of a medical crisis, as compared with the more usual stable routine of treatment, which places the physician in a background role. Although renal failure is a chronic illness and dialysis is a chronic treatment, the situation of the patient fluctuates significantly in its medical acuteness from time to time. (It is for this reason that it was stated earlier that the acute/chronic dichotomy fails to capture the management situation for various kinds of chronic illness.) For temporary periods, the dialysis patient becomes an acute patient, losing customary autonomy for management. Individual patients vary in their transitions from autonomy to dependence upon medical intervention and in their subsequent return to autonomy.

Compliance with treatment impositions and restrictions can be examined in relation to the way the patient understands and attributes authority to professional communications. Certainly almost all dialysis patients realize that they have a potentially lethal condition. Nevertheless, many are lax about dietary compliance, particularly by exceeding their prescribed liquid intake. Although many patients violate, or experiment with their diet, they are more compliant with sterile procedures. Systematic analysis might reveal that the patient has more confidence in self-management of risks connected with food intake than those connected with the more arcane, invisible process of infection.

The foregoing discussion of the routines of dialysis conveys the picture of an ongoing illness management situation, in which the dialysis patient makes a continuing series of decisions concerning treatment with cumulatively consequential effects upon medical status and general well-being. The patient's attitude toward and understanding of treatment contingencies, and the patient's self-concept as a relatively sick or well person are issues which can be probed and empirically clarified through concepts and techniques of health behavior research.

CONCLUSION

This chapter has shown that the concepts of health behavior research can be applied to the management of patients with chronic illness. The example chosen—chronic renal failure—is of particular interest because it is a serious disease which, with careful management, can be stabilized over indefinitely long periods of time. Considerable study of patient adaptation to this disease and its treatment has already been carried out by psychologists, sociologists, and other social scientists, moving toward a critical formulation of basic issues which confront the dialysis patient (Evans *et al.,* 1985; Fox & Swazey, 1978; Holcomb & Macdonald, 1973). In general terms, it can be posited that the patient's response to these issues depends upon the personal mode of dealing with the constraints and dependencies of illness and treatment.

A widely accepted notion concerning the health status of the public is that many of the most serious diseases have behavioral origins and can be prevented by judicious behavior in regard to diet, exercise, and other components of life-style. Although mortal humans cannot prevent everything forever, there is nevertheless obvious value in postponing what cannot be ultimately prevented, and in pursuing the important contribution which health behavior research can play in formulating knowledge leading toward such postponement. The picture presented here of illness management deals with what happens when the patient is already afflicted with a chronic disease. Here too, health behavior research can contribute much of value, particularly in relation to modes of adult learning, patient self-concept, and communications with medical authority. Research application could begin by examining the most widespread chronic degenerative conditions—chronic heart disease, cancer, essential hypertension, and stroke (as well as chronic renal failure)—from the standpoint developed above, subjecting them to a systematic comparative analysis of illness management in each. What is presented here is a prolegomenon to establish a common ground between health behavior research and a useful social science perspective on illness management.

REFERENCES

Beavert, C. S. (1974). *Caretakers of the intermittent dying: Role strain of a hemodialysis team.* Master's thesis. Department of Sociology, University of Missouri, Columbia.

Becker, M. H. (1974). The health belief model and sick role behavior. In M. H. Becker (Ed.), *The health belief model and personal health behavior. Health Education Monographs, 2*(4), 409–420.

Becker, M. H., & Maiman, L. A. (1983). Models of health-related behavior. In D. Mechanic (Ed.),

Handbook of health, health care, and the health professions (pp. 539–568). New York: Free Press.

Croog, S. H., & Levine, S. (1982). *Life after a heart attack.* New York: Human Sciences Press.

Evans, R. W., Manninen, D. L., Garrison, L. P., Hart, L. G., Blagg, C. R., Gutman, R. A., Hull, A. R., & Lowrie, E. G. (1985). The quality of life in patients with end-stage renal disease. *New England Journal of Medicine, 312*(9), 553–559.

Field, M. G. (1972). The doctor–patient relationship in the perspective of "fee-for-service" and "third-party" medicine. In E. G. Jaco (Ed.), *Patients, physicians, and illness—A sourcebook in behavioral science and health* (2nd ed., pp. 222–232). New York: Free Press.

Fox, R. C., & Swazey, J. P. (1978). *The courage to fail.* Chicago: University of Chicago Press.

Freidson, E. (1970). *Professional dominance: The social structure of medical care.* New York: Atherton Press.

Hartman, P. E., & Becker, M. H. (1978). Non-compliance with prescribed regimen among chronic hemodialysis patients. *Dialysis and Transplantation, 7,* 978–989.

Haug, M., & Lavin, B. (1983). *Consumerism in medicine: Challenging physician authority.* Beverly Hills: Sage.

Heinzelmann, F. (1962). Factors in prophylaxis behavior in treating rheumatic fever: An exploratory study. *Journal of Health and Human Behavior, 3,* 73–81.

Holcomb, J., & Macdonald, R. W. (1973). Social functioning of artificial kidney patients. *Social Science and Medicine, 7,* 109–119.

Kasl, S. V. (1974). The health belief model and behavior related to chronic illness. In M. H. Becker (Ed.), *The health belief model and personal health behavior. Health Education Monographs, 2*(4), 433–454.

Kasl, S. V., & Cobb, S. (1966a). Health behavior, illness behavior, and sick role behavior. I. Health and illness behavior. *Archives of Environmental Health, 12,* 246–266.

Kasl, S. V., & Cobb, S. (1966b). Health behavior, illness behavior, and sick role behavior. II. Sick role behavior. *Archives of Environmental Health, 12,* 531–541.

Koos, E. (1954). *The health of Regionville.* New York: Columbia University Press.

Ley, P., Bradshaw, P. W., Eaves, D., & Walker, C. M. (1973). A method for increasing patients' recall of information presented by doctors. *Psychological Medicine, 3,* 217–220.

Oakes, T. W., Ward, J. R., Gray, R. M., Klauber, M. R., & Moody, P. M. (1970). Family expectations and arthritis patient compliance to a hand resting splint regimen. *Journal of Chronic Diseases, 22,* 757–764.

Pratt, L. V. (1978). Reshaping the consumer's posture in health care. In E. B. Gallagher (Ed.), *The doctor–patient relationship in the changing health scene* (U.S. Department of Health, Education and Welfare (NIH) Publication No. 78–183, pp. 197–214). Washington, DC: U.S. Government Printing Office.

Reeder, L. G. (1972). The patient-client as consumer: Some observations on the changing professional–client relationship. *Journal of Health and Social Behavior, 13,* 402–416.

Roper, N. (1978). *New American pocket dictionary.* Edinburgh: Churchill Livingstone.

Seligman, M. E. P. (1975). *Helplessness: On depression, development, and death.* San Francisco: Freeman.

Strauss, A. L. (1975). *Chronic illness and the quality of life.* St. Louis: Mosby.

Thornton, R., & Nardi, P. M. (1974). The dynamics of role acquisition. *American Journal of Sociology, 80,* 870–885.

Turner, R. H. (1978). The role and the person. *American Journal of Sociology, 84,* 1–23.

CHAPTER 23

Health Behavior Research

Present and Future

David S. Gochman

This chapter begins with an overview of some conceptual advances that characterize the emergence of contemporary, late 1980s–early 1990s, health behavior research. It continues with a discussion of issues related to health behavior's identity, and describes an agenda for future research, including meta issues, substantive areas for research, and searching for meaning. A summary concludes the chapter.

THE PRESENT: LATE 1980s–EARLY 1990s

Together, the preceding chapters document the history of health behavior research during the three-decade period from the late 1950s to the late 1980s. From varied perspectives, the contributors attest to a period and process of continuous conceptual advancement involving refinement and refocusing. In numerous contexts, health behavior research has moved away from simplistic paradigms, to more complex, more thoughtful ones; from sketchily differentiated variables to more articulated conceptions providing greater precision and specificity; from predictions based on single variables, or one level of variable, to predictions based on pluralistic conceptions and multivariate designs; from naive measures to instrumentation that reflects advanced statistical techniques and factor analyses. Space does not permit systematic treatment of all of these, but a discussion of some of these conceptual advances provides a way of summarizing an appreciable portion of the preceding material.

CONCEPTUAL ADVANCES

The process of continuous conceptual advancement, involving refinement and refocusing, can be readily seen in the models (or paradigms, or "theories") used to predict health behaviors, as well as in the behaviors themselves.

DAVID S. GOCHMAN • Raymond A. Kent School of Social Work, University of Louisville, Louisville, Kentucky 40292.

Models

Examples of conceptual refinement are most obvious in the health belief and locus of controls models; in the models of social organization; in role models; and in the models of client–professional interaction.

The Health Belief Model. The health belief model has been transformed from a simple paradigm, in which a single, medically or professionally sanctioned "preventive behavior" was predicted from three relatively simply construed and simply measured perceptions, to a model, which as Kirscht's chapter demonstrates, takes into account a range of social and environmental factors and makes predictions about a wider range of health behaviors. In early health belief model research, for example, perceived susceptibility was generally considered solely in terms of a single health concern (e.g., cancer or tuberculosis). Later research expanded the concept to embrace a variety of health problems and demonstrated that it was a consistent individual attribute: respondents who had high (low) levels of expecting to encounter one health problem had similarly high (low) levels of expecting others (e.g., Gochman, 1970, 1971). This consistent personal characteristic was termed "perceived vulnerability" to distinguish it from the single-problem expectation. Research further established that the perceptual variables were empirically independent of the motivational components that were initially presumed to inhere within them (e.g., Gochman, 1977).

Additional studies (e.g., Eisen, Zellman, & McAlister, 1985) enriched the conceptualization of perceived benefits and developed ways of measuring this variable with greater precision, and in the decade between the mid-1970s and the mid-1980s perceived benefits replaced perceived susceptibility as the most heuristic of the model's dimensions (Janz & Becker, 1984).

Locus of Control. Similarly, research based on locus of control has moved away from using a general model toward using one that is specific to health. Moreover, as Lau's chapter reveals, the conceptualization now takes account of the distinction between one's desire for control and the belief that one has it, the multidimensionality of beliefs about control, and the "value" component of the initial "value-expectancy" theory that had been missing from earlier research.

Social Organization. Research dealing with social organization variables has moved away from the simple parochial–cosmopolitan dichotomy proposed by Suchman, through refinements that separated socioeconomic status from social integration (e.g., Moody & Gray, 1972), toward conceptions that embrace cultural norms, as Geertsen's chapter shows, as well as more precise understandings of social linkages and their role in the influence process, as the chapters by both Geertsen and Ritter reveal. Moreover, Weidman's chapter on the transcultural perspective especially sensitizes researchers to the importance of understanding the "health culture" of diverse social groupings and social organization variables within a cultural context.

Roles. Increasing conceptual complexity can be seen in changes in gender-role and sick-role formulations.

The general questions that Nathanson raised (1975) in her seminal work about gender-role issues and health behavior have become transformed into specific, testable hypotheses about fixed roles (e.g., Marcus, Seeman, & Telesky, 1983); multiple roles (e.g., Verbrugge, 1983); and nurturant roles (e.g., Gove, 1984). Moreover, Waldron's chapter reveals that gender roles have important culture-specific components and that these are reflected in cultural differences in gender-related health behaviors.

Increased complexity can also be seen in the development of concepts related to the sick role. Parsons' initial sick-role formulation (1951), which related the behaviors involved in "being sick" to the needs, values, and expectations of the larger social unit, has been reconceptualized, as the chapters by Arluke, Segall, and Wolinsky as an aggregate note, to embrace the behavior of persons with chronic conditions, to explain personal failure, and to include societal and professional responsiveness to changing economic and employment indicators, demographic differences in beliefs about the sick role, individual variability in enacting appropriate sick-role behaviors, the need to understand the differential impact of sick role on individuals, and the distinction between sick role and patient role.

Client–Professional Interaction. Closely related to reconceptualization of sick role, particularly in relation to the patient–physician relationship, is the reconceptualization of client–professional interaction. Conceptions of this interaction have begun to move away from the traditional (but nonetheless still typical) hierarchical model, in which a patient with a specifically defined medical problem seeks consultation, diagnosis, and treatment from a traditional, orthodox physician, and toward considering models such as those proposed by Szasz and Hollender (1956/1975) in which there is greater egalitarianism, greater sharing of information, and greater negotiation of reality.

Conceptions of the patient role have developed away from passivity to greater assertiveness; away from the seeking solely of medical technology, toward the seeking of caring and relief from the anxiety generated both by the illness and by the uncertainty about the effectiveness of the treatment and about the recovery. Moreover, as Herzlich and Pierret (1985) noted, there has been a change in the status of the patient: the patient's view is increasingly commanding respect and is no longer thought to be only a distortion and simplification, but as having a logic of its own and as worthy of being understood on its own terms. The chapters by Roter and Ben-Sira deal with different but complementary ways in which the complexity of this interaction has been studied, and Haug's chapter identifies ways in which the underlying power dynamics of this interaction have changed.

Behaviors

Three examples of behaviors that demonstrate the ongoing and continuous striving for increased conceptual refinement are preventive behavior, utilization behaviors, and compliance.

Preventive Behavior. Refinement of the concept of preventive behavior is observed in the chapters by Kirscht, Ritter, and Kolbe, in which behavior is dimensionalized in terms of its repetitiveness, of whether it is to be acquired or eliminated, or of its phases. Additional reconceptualization is provided in Langlie's (1977) observations of empirically distinct direct-risk preventive behaviors, behaviors which have direct or immediate potential for inducing injury or disease, e.g., reckless driving, jaywalking, exposing oneself to germs or smoke; and indirect risk behaviors, the enactment (or nonenactment) of which does not present an immediate potential hazard, e.g., having routine medical or dental checkups, using seat belts, getting routine immunizations.

Michela and Brady's (1984) use of multidimensional scaling procedures identified important ways in which persons differentiate health actions. Among these are whether the action has long-term or short-term, or beneficial or harmful effects; whether the actions are influenced by who the respondent is with; whether they are engaged in by the respondent's friends; and whether the enactments depend on "ability." All of these dimensions are considered to have implications for the performance or nonperformance of the preventive behaviors.

Utilization. The conception of utilization of services has moved beyond use of a single preventive service (e.g., early health belief model research), or of an enumeration of visits to physicians during some specified period (Suchman, 1965/1972), to include consideration of whether the use (or nonuse) of service was appropriate, and to acknowledge that nonuse might actually be desirable (e.g., Ross & Duff, 1982); the rationale for choosing a physician (e.g., Kasteler, Kane, Olsen, & Thetford, 1976); and whether services were sought as a way of dealing with stress and/or disequilibrium (Zola, 1973). Furthermore, nonuse of services can now be seen to reflect system barriers resulting from organizational policies and practices, as Greenley and Davidson's chapter suggests. Levin (1976) even argued that self-care—laypersons serving as their own primary care providers—be considered as an integral component of the health care system, and that the legitimacy of "ownership" of all functions of professional health care workers be considered as open to challenge.

Compliance. The concept of compliance was initially narrowly considered in terms of how closely a patient followed a medically prescribed regimen, e.g., taking medication for hypertension, with no allowance either for the patient's participation in the process or for questioning of the suitability of, or rationale for, the regimen. Early research, as Stimson (1974) and Hulka, Cassel, Kupper, and Burdette (1976), among others, have carefully noted, primarily represented notably unsuccessful attempts to identify personal and/or demographic characteristics of "noncompliers," with little or no consideration given to the dynamics of the interaction between the professional and the patient. The conceptualization of compliance now embraces the awareness that nonacceptance of a regimen may be beneficial, if the diagnostic and prescription processes are flawed (e.g., Lipton & Hershaft, 1985); the legitimacy of the rationale underlying the patient's decision not to accept the regimen (e.g., Stimson & Webb, 1975); the dynamics of the interaction and communication process; the role of negotiation processes in relation to diagnosis, treatment, and adherence (Anderson & Helm, 1979; Sorenson, 1974); and, as the chapter by Cole, Berger, and Garrity clearly specifies, adherence to programs designed to improve occupational safety, that are far removed from medical regimens.

PRESENT INTO FUTURE: ISSUES OF IDENTITY

Because health behavior has not yet solidly achieved its own identity, there are few institutional arrangements, i.e., departments or programs, that serve to attract numbers of "health behaviorists." Accordingly, most health behaviorists work in relative isolation from one another and do not have the opportunity for the face-to-face interaction that generates conceptual breadth and enhances methodological strengths. Health behavior often "falls between the cracks," institutionally and organizationally. Issues related to health behavior's identity must thus be satisfactorily resolved for it to move productively into the future. Among these issues are its relationship with behavioral medicine and medical schools, its interdisciplinary nature, its ideological neutrality, and its independence of political cooptation.

Health Behavior and Medicine

Behavioral Medicine. Health behavior research and behavioral medicine differ not only in their "substantive" definitions, as discussed in Chapter 1, but in their "directional" definitions as well. Directional definitions have labeling qualities, which guide or impel movement along selected paths (e.g., Gochman, 1982). Behavioral medicine is an attractive and potent "label" with the capacity to "direct" research activities selectively. Researchers identifying with behavioral medicine are thus increasingly likely to accept and build upon the medical model, to conduct research addressing medical problems, and to subordinate *basic* research interests to those with immediately discernible *medical applications*.

Unquestionably, the practical and human value of such activities is worthwhile. But they do not routinely advance *basic* health behavior research—knowledge about the behavior itself. Basic research in health behavior will be productively developed and conducted to the degree that it can resist being labeled as "behavioral medicine."

Medical School Settings. Programs generating health behavior research, regardless of how they are labeled, are often located within medical schools, usually in departments of community or behavioral medicine, or behavioral science. Often, such programs have produced research of high quality and great practical value. Research of similar quality and value is often conducted in professional schools of dentistry, nursing, and public health. Understandably, the primary objectives—the clinical instruction and research needs—of schools of medicine (and dentistry, nursing, and public health) are often incongruent, or in conflict with the objectives and needs of nonclinical, academic departments and programs. To the degree that such incongruence, or institutionally generated conflict, exists, the objectives and needs of nonclinical academic departments, especially those perceived as "soft science," are likely to be subordinated to those of the clinical departments, particularly those involved in high-technology medicine. This will be true regardless of the ultimate practical value for training and practice of the knowledge generated by such basic research. Instances of some of the effects of this subordinate status can be found in the chapter by Baumgart and Costello.

Questions thus arise about the sustained effects of locating health behavior research within medical (and other professional) schools. For example, what are the effects of health behavior research's subordinate status in relation to clinical programs on allocation of funds, personnel, and space? What are the effects of subordinate status on the vitality of basic health behavior research? Despite some impressive research track records, What might the productivity of such programs have been if they were located elsewhere? Such questions are more salient for health behavior than for programs such as biochemistry and microbiology because these have no similar need to establish their identities. Yet even in medical sociology, a field with an established identity, serious questions have been raised about the negative impact of sustained involvement in medically defined interests on the essential scientific activities of developing theory and generating knowledge (Wolinsky, 1988, Chapter 2).

Although it may be argued that locating health behavior research in medical school settings fosters the integration of health behavior knowledge into medical curricula, the continued low priority of such content and its lack of meaningful incorporation in the training of physicians, as the chapter by Baumgart and Costello relates, makes this argument unconvincing.

Although there sometimes are expedient reasons (e.g., political, economic, funding) for some health behavior research activities to be embraced by a "behavioral medicine" label and to be conducted in medical school settings, their continuation in these settings provides an arena for institutionally generated conflict between the legitimate requirements of behavioral medicine and the needs of health behavior research to establish basic knowledge and understanding for its own sake.

Health Behavior Research Is Interdisciplinary

Health behavior research is not the exclusive "turf" or domain of any one discipline or profession. Health behavior research has already been distinguished from behavioral medicine and, in Chapter 1, from behavioral health. Health behavior research is, furthermore, distinct from health psychology, medical sociology, ethnomedicine, medical anthropology, and any other similarly discrete discipline. Health behavior research is and must be interdisciplinary. It must be conducted collaboratively by scientists in (in alphabetical order) anthropology, dentistry, health and physical education, medicine, nursing, nutrition, psychiatry, psychology, public health, social work, and sociology. Each of these fields offers unique perspectives, skills, and interests. Productive, rigorous, basic health behavior research requires borrowing among, and sharing the broad spectrum of theories, concepts, and methods. Such interdisciplinary collaboration enhances the likelihood of increasing basic health behavior knowledge.

Academic Programs in Health Behavior. Basic health behavior research thus requires organizational and institutional structures that encourage interdisciplinary efforts, facilitate the interaction of researchers representing relevant disciplines and professions, and establish and reinforce health behavior's identity. *Ideally,* such institutional structures would be departments or programs of "health behavior" made up of persons from several of these disciplines and professions who are engaged in and committed to basic health behavior research. *Ideally,* their interdisciplinary research activities would be recognized as essentially scholarly in nature rather than as adjuncts to community service or to solving personal or community health and medical problems. *Ideally,* such structures would be located within the basic arts and sciences units of universities, with strong linkages to scholarly, substantive doctoral programs in relevant areas, as well as to professional training programs in dentistry, medicine, nursing, and social work.

In settings such as these, basic research would go hand in hand with graduate level instruction both in doctoral programs in health behavior and in the disciplines that participate in it. Establishment of such programs would reduce the isolation that health behaviorists experience. Relatively few such programs exist. Many more are needed.

Being located elsewhere than in medical schools, especially if linked to rigorous doctoral programs, could very possibly increase the status accorded to health behavior research, and could thus increase the likelihood of health behavior knowledge being integrated into the training programs of medical and other health professionals.

Furthermore, the "administrative identity" that would result from acknowledging such a department or program would foster its recognition and increase its visibility as a basic interdisciplinary activity. Moreover, its intellectual respectability would increase to the degree that it is seen as overlapping with and representing basic, traditional academic disciplines rather than as an adjunct of medicine, or as an essentially applied science. Such recognition, visibility, and academic respectability would appreciably strengthen its identity.

Interdisciplinary Publication. Health behavior as an interdisciplinary research activity needs its own scholarly journal. Several journals of superb quality publish reports of health behavior investigations, but these journals—*Social Science and Medicine, Journal of Health and Social Behavior, American Journal of Public Health,* and *Health Psychology*—do not have domains that are coterminous with that of health behavior as a basic interdisciplinary research discipline. They each contain much that is not relevant to health behavior, and each has a special focus that precludes publishing much basic interdisciplinary research. A scholarly journal dedicated to basic, interdisciplinary health behavior research would not only provide a suitable vehicle for publishing, but would further solidify health behavior's identity.

Health Behavior and "Ideology"

Although partisans of one model or another (e.g., health belief model, locus of control, cosmopolitanism–parochialism) have emerged from time to time in the history of health behavior research, such partisanship has never assumed the "Holy War" proportions of the dogmatic debates in related disciplines (i.e., behaviorism versus psychoanalysis versus gestalt theory within psychology; Marxism versus structural–functionalism within sociology). Basic research is rarely served by such polemics. The viability and productivity of health behavior research will be enhanced to the degree that such ideological overkill can continue to be avoided in the future.

Moreover, the ideological neutrality mentioned in Chapter 1 in relation to individual responsibility for health, must similarly be demonstrated in relation to social, societal, and cultural factors, and to policy factors that determine health behaviors. The research process must not be prevented from developing new knowledge about the personal factors that determine health actions, on the political grounds that such knowledge might be used to excuse the failure of governmental structures or private agencies to adopt or change social policies related to health care and health services.

However, much health behavior research, even those studies conducted with a large system focus, *has* focused on inducing changes in individuals, or on generating knowledge that ultimately increases the likelihood of such individual change. Borrowing and generalizing from Bynder and New's analysis (1976) of the imbalance between micro- and macrosociological concepts in disability research, one can argue that health behavior research must not accept the "therapeutic" role of improving technology simply to change the individual, rather than of developing knowledge to change the professions and policies *themselves* that have traditionally sought to change the individual.

Nor must research be prevented from developing new knowledge of the role of social, policy, and structural variables, on the moral or religious grounds that such knowledge might be used to excuse the reluctance or failure of individuals to assume responsibility for their own actions.

On the other hand, the knowledge of individual determinants of health actions—particularly in relation to behavioral consistency and stability—can be taken into account in the formulation of policy in order to improve estimates of the eventual impact of policy changes, and thus improve the effectiveness of the policies themselves. Similarly, knowledge about the social and institutional context of individual behavior can improve the effectiveness of programs designed to increase the likelihood that individuals *can* assume responsibility for their behavior, and thus increase the effectiveness of programs designed to generate behavioral changes.

Political Cooptation

Kinston's analysis (1983) of health services research in Great Britain described how ideology and political interests have had a chilling and nullifying effect on basic research processes. Health behavior researchers should be increasingly sensitized to such pressures, and not be coopted by the political process to advance any single presumed correct perspective or approach. To the degree that such political cooptation occurs, it will place scientific research values in a subordinate position, and will ultimately devalue and destroy the credibility of the research process.

Political cooptation can take another, less insidious form: subordination to funding sources. Much funding of health behavior research comes from federal and state governments which are continually reassessing (a polite way of saying "changing") their own priorities in the light of changing political climates, regardless of whether these are in the public interest or not.

Such linkage of health behavior investigations with fluctuating governmental priorities raises questions about the degree to which the scientific process is subordinated to political interests. Questions must also be raised about the impact of continually changing governmental policies and priorities on basic *longitudinal* research. Moreover, hurrying research proposals toward premature completion to meet new and trendy priorities raises additional questions about their thoroughness, thoughtfulness, and clarity of concepts, for example, all of which relate to their essence as *basic* investigations.

THE FUTURE: A RESEARCH AGENDA

The future agenda for health behavior research can be discussed under three headings: meta issues, substantive areas, and searches for meaning.

Meta Issues

The need for more and better research exists in any area at any time, reflecting the tentativeness of all scientific "knowledge." It is thus redundant to say that more and better research is needed in health behavior. Yet failure to acknowledge this could be construed as oversight, negligence, or gross lack of understanding. There is a standard litany that appears in critical evaluative reviews, that declares the need for: larger, more representative samples; greater precision in measurement; more controlled research designs; increasingly complex multivariate design; and more frequent replications. Having dutifully stated this, the chapter can go on to consider four issues more specific to health behavior research: clarity and precision of conceptual formulations; theoretical linkages; greater integration of approaches; and increased logical positivism.

Conceptual Clarity. Against the background of increasing conceptual complexity and refinement is the thorny issue of lack of conceptual precision and clarity. Seldom in health behavior research are variables derived systematically from carefully constructed theoretical concepts. As Bruhn and Parcel (1982) noted, particularly in the area of cognitive systems, "concepts need to be sharper and clearer and they need to be integrated with theory" (p. 151). For example, "perceived susceptibility" or "perceived vulnerability" is sometimes defined as the expectancy that health problems will be encountered (e.g., Gochman, 1977), and sometimes as the amount of worrying done about such problems (e.g., Lewis & Lewis, 1982). It is quite possible that one can have a high expectancy that a problem will occur, but not worry unduly about it; and conversely, worry a great deal about a problem, but not expect it to happen.

The family is another area where increased conceptual clarity is greatly needed. Researchers rarely define what model or concept of the family they are using, Pratt's work (1976) being a notable exception. More detailed discussion on the need for increased conceptual clarity in health behavior research is provided in Gochman's (1985) assessment of the state of research on family and children's health-related concepts. Increased conceptual clarity in the future is necessary to improve health behavior research.

Linkage with Theory. Several of the chapters identify the need for increased linkage with theory. The lack of conceptual clarity is itself related to the often-absent linkage of health behavior research with broader theoretical frameworks in psychology, sociology, and anthropology. Although the health-belief and locus of control models, and research on the development of health beliefs, for example, can be broadly related to psychological theories (e.g., Gochman, 1985), seldom are the specific relationships delineated, and rarely is health behavior research used to demonstrate systematically the validity of these theories. The same is true of the relationship between health behavior research and sociological and anthropological theories. The development and strengthening of explicit theoretical linkages in the future is necessary to improve health behavior research.

Integration of Approaches. Collaborative efforts, and the sharing of concepts and methods inhere in health behavior's interdisciplinary character and thus in its identity. Yet few studies to date have reflected such collaboration. Mechanic's (1979) discussion of the failure of much research on illness behavior to yield appreciable findings attests to the lack of such collaborative efforts. Mechanic identified two rather distinct "literatures": theoretical studies of sociocultural, organizational, and psychosocial factors which use small, intensively interviewed samples, and which pay attention to subjective experiences; and multivariate, cross-sectional studies, which use less detailed measures, but more powerful statistical techniques and large samples. Mechanic urged future research that combines these two broad approaches to maximize the likelihood of nontrivial findings.

Similarly, Eckert and Goldstein (1983) urged an integration that would combine the broad concepts derived from anthropology, for example, with the methodological precision of the techniques of psychology. Increased conceptual and methodological integration in the future, and the synergism that is likely to result when researchers from several disciplines bring their varied perspectives together are necessary to improve health behavior research.

Logical Positivism. Amid the increasing empiricism of the last three decades, and the availability of a larger number of measures and techniques of data analysis, there remain vestiges of armchair theorizing that has not been linked to empirical observations. This is the analytic or "logical" component of logical positivism, which has been accepted as a basic paradigm of science. Through the various chapters in this book, there are hints of not-yet-tested models, concepts, and frames of reference. However intriguing these may be, however they capture the imagination, they remain only half useful if they are not coordinated with empiricism, the "positivism" component, and thus translated into empirically testable and tested hypotheses. Although this is perhaps more widespread in analyses of larger social systems, it remains a problem for health behavior as a basic research enterprise. Increased empiricism in the future, appropriately coupled with conceptually derived hypotheses, is necessary for health behavior to achieve and retain its identity as a basic scientific enterprise.

Research Areas

Four substantive areas are particularly relevant and critical for future health behavior research: the origins and development of health behavior; the role of the family in health behavior; health-relevant motivation; and coping.

Origins and Development of Health Behavior. Lau's chapter calls attention to the general lack of knowledge about the origins of beliefs about health locus of control. Such a lack is representative of a much broader gap in health behavior knowledge. Little is known about the roots of health beliefs and health actions in general. Much research has been undertaken to shape and modify them, but few investigations have attempted systematically to explore their origins.

Coupled with the need for greater knowledge and understanding about the origins of health beliefs and behaviors, is the need for greater knowledge and understanding about how such beliefs and actions develop, as Bruhn's chapter suggests. Although some attempts have been made to explore the development of health-related concepts in young populations, for example, Gellert's analyses of the development of beliefs about body parts (1962, 1978); Nagy's studies of beliefs about causes of illness (1951, 1953); Natapoff's Piagetian examination of beliefs about being healthy (1982); and Gochman's examination of perceived vulnerability, perceived benefits, health motivation, and preventive attitudes (1986); a consensus exists that there is a dearth of well-conducted, rigorous research in this area (e.g., Bruhn & Parcel, 1982; Gochman, 1985; Kalnins & Love, 1982). Bush and Holmbeck's Children's Health Care Attitudes Questionnaire (1987), which uses verbal as well as nonverbal responses, promises to be an important assessment tool in future developmental studies.

Questions arise about the importance of a range of factors in the origins and development of such beliefs and behaviors: the family, friends, peer groups, social relationships, and societal and cultural values and institutions. The path-analysis methodology discussed in the chapter by Bush and Iannotti offers a useful technique for analyzing the multifaceted data that such future research will generate, and for comparing the predictive value of different models that account for them.

Basic research into the origins of health beliefs and actions, and how they develop is thus a major challenge for future health behavior research.

The Family and Health Behavior. Although the family is presumed to be a major determinant, and although Campbell (1978), for example, identified some maternal value determinants of youngsters' conceptions of the sick role, reviews of the literature (e.g., Baranowski & Nader, 1985; Gochman, 1985) indicate a virtual absence of knowledge about relationships between family characteristics and children's health beliefs and behaviors. Baranowski and Nader described this relationship as "almost ignored" (p. 53), and the chapter by Sallis and Nader notes the paucity of documentation of mechanisms of family influence on health behavior. Moreover, Dielman, Leech, Becker, Rosenstock, and Horvath (1982), noting that studies relating parental and youngsters' health beliefs have been "relatively rare," were unable in their own investigation to demonstrate any relationships: "Child health beliefs are scarcely influenced by parental characteristics" (p. 63).

Possibly, the failure to discover the roots of childrens' health behavior in family characteristics reflects a combination of inadequate conceptualization of "the family" together with a very small number of studies conducted in this area. Research has seldom looked at the family as family. More often than not, research has considered "family" in terms of some personal or demographic characteristic of one or both parents, or in terms of its size.

Future health behavior research could productively examine the family in terms of its characteristics as an integral social unit, i.e., its roles, its norms, its values, and its patterns of communication, for example. Pratt (1976) developed one of the few conceptual models available that considers the family in this way, and studies based on her model are sorely needed. Furthermore, in addition to building upon the important work described by Sallis and Nader in their chapter analyzing the family as a determinant of risk behaviors, such as smoking and improper diet, future research could productively analyze family characteristics as determinants of a broad spectrum of health behaviors.

Health-Relevant Motivation. A third area for future research is health-relevant motivation. Few studies have been conducted on "health" or the "desire for health" or "the wish to possess good health" as motives, or on their relationship to overt health behaviors.

Possibly, health in itself may not be a potent motive for eliciting health behaviors. It has not been observed to be a potent motive in young populations (Gochman, 1975, 1986) and little research has been done to demonstrate its potency in adults, although Lau, Hartman, and Ware (1986) began important research in this area.

Moreover, it may be increasingly important to differentiate between health as a motive and other motives which can effectively be drawn upon to generate health behavior, what might be termed health-relevant, or health-germane, motivation. Thus, a more basic question for future health behavior research might be: What are the motives that can be used to generate health behavior? The desires to be physically or socially active, occupationally and professionally useful or successful, or responsible to family and friends may turn out to be more relevant to health behavior than "health" itself.

Moreover, health behavior research must address issues such as those raised by Burt (1984), of whether health is perceived as juxtaposed with pleasure, indicating that actions considered to be healthy are often thought to be unappealing, distasteful, and otherwise noxious; and those raised in the chapter by Bruhn about the conflict between personal risk and other motives and values, and about the "trade-offs" involved in changing behavior.

Few instruments exist to measure health as a motive. Future research will require methodological advancement in this area.

Coping. Nearly all of the specific behaviors that have been the focus of health behavior research have been considered in relation to specific conditions, specific risk factors, and specific acts of utilization, for example. In contrast, a literature is emerging that focuses upon general coping mechanisms, i.e., ways in which people deal with problems, stresses, and disequilibria, that suggests that patterns of coping are relevant to health status (e.g., Ben-Sira & Padeh, 1978; Pearlin & Schooler, 1978). Such mechanisms would include how people respond to the demands and challenges posed by their desires for remaining healthy and safe, or their desires for any of the other goals or values that require good health. Among these coping mechanisms are cognitive responses that control or modify the meaning of stress-inducing situations.

In a related analysis, Antonovsky's conception of the "sense of coherence" as a factor in salutogenesis (1984) includes as an important component an individual's ability to set boundaries selectively around some events that are stress producing by declaring that these problems do not have much priority, do not matter sufficiently, and thus need not be made manageable. Such skills in establishing priorities and boundaries appear to be similar to what Pearlin and Schooler identified as responses that control the meaning of stressful experiences.

To the degree that such patterns of coping behavior are related to health status, they are health behaviors. If so, their origins and determinants, the ways in which they relate to other health and safety actions and risk behaviors, use of services, and acceptance of regimens, for example, are areas for health behavior research and expand the conception of health behavior.

The Search for Meaning

Health as a motive, motives relevant to health, and cognitive responses that have the capacity to change the meaning of situations, lead to questions about the salience or meaning of health and of terms related to it: the meaning of illness, the meaning of treatment, and the meaning of the health care environment. Although these could be discussed as areas for future research, they represent a distinctly different way of looking at research areas, and thus warrant consideration under a separate heading.

Meaning of Illness. The profession of social work has a tradition of borrowing from a variety of disciplines (e.g., Bartlett, 1961). Yet, in one very critical area, it can claim proper "ownership." In health settings, particularly hospitals and clinics, it is the particular responsibility of the professional social worker on the interdisciplinary care team to explore, understand, and work with the "meaning" of an illness or a condition for the patient and the patient's family (Bartlett, 1961, pp. 134–135). In such a context, "meaning" differs from what illness means in general, and as it is treated in Chapter 1. In such a context, the "meaning" of illness represents its salience and implications for the patient and/or the patient's family and significant others. What the illness experience means in these terms has important implications for a range of health behavior—including preventive activities, acceptance of a regimen, giving up the sick role, and acceptance of rehabilitation.

Ben-Sira (1977) addressed the meaning of illness in his study of the person's "image" of an illness, or "involvement" with a disease, and devised a way of incorporating elements of the health belief model into a single measure of the "salience" of an illness to the patient. He further related such meaning, or salience, to preventive behavior. Moreover, the chapter by Ben-Sira further amplifies the role of the meaning of illness through discussion of "lay-intelligible explanations," and of the importance of relief from the illness-generated anxiety as an objective in the patient's interactions with a health care practitioner. Stimson and Webb (1975, p. 2) also pointed out how patients attempt to make sense out of what has happened to them.

Meaning of Treatment. In the context of their analysis of how pressures for reputation in persons and institutions lead to increased technological interventions, Fox and Swazey (1978) raised critical questions about the meaning of treatment and about whether treatment must be employed simply because it is available. They ask, for example, "Is it medically and morally proper to dialyze or transplant *all* these patients because monies are available, whether or not they will benefit from treatment?" (p. 379). The meaning of treatment is juxtaposed with the question of the quality of life.

Similarly, Elinson (1985) raised the question of the meaning of treatment by pointing to the potential conflict between therapeutic goals aimed at increasing the quality of life and those aimed at increasing its quantity. Such conflicts are likely to increase in older populations, whose values may not always be deferent to medical technology, and whose concern for quality of life may transcend acceptance of "good" medical care, particularly when evidence is accumulating that an acceptable quality of life can be maintained even during the terminal stages of illness (Morris, Suissa, Sherwood, Wright, & Greer, 1986).

Furthermore, as the chapters by Ben-Sira and Roter make clear, the affective components of treatment—what the treatment means in terms of the feelings and emotional needs of the patient—in contrast to the instrumental or technical components, are increasingly important areas for systematic future research.

Moreover, compliance studies are increasingly identifying what the medication means to the patient. Conrad (1985), for example, showed that compliance can be a reminder that the patient has a stigmatized condition (e.g., epilepsy).

Thus, the meaning of treatment in relation to personal needs, to personal values, and to personal conceptions of what constitutes quality of life appears to be an important factor in reconsidering definitions of "compliance," "adherence," or "acceptance" of treatment, and is thus a promising area for future health behavior research.

Meaning of Environment. The chapter by Whitehead, Fusillo, and Kaplan urges that the way in which laypersons—patients, clients, consumers—attempt to make sense out of their physical environments be investigated systematically. Specifically, the chapter notes the importance of movement, contours, bulk, and simplicity as determinants of ability to remember a location; the role of graphic displays in making settings comprehensible and thus maximally useful; and some hypothesized relationships between these physical dimensions of the environment and the degree to which clients feel that the environment is manageable and predictable, and that they are being treated as responsible persons.

The manner in which more general aspects of space and time generate meanings also has subtle implications for health behavior. In the context of analyzing social constructions of space and time, Armstrong systematically examined (1985) changes in the spatial and temporal arrangements of British medical practice, and how these changes have modified conceptions about the meaning of the treatment process and about how professionals and patients relate to one another. According to Armstrong, the traditional British "surgery" was part of the physician's "smoke room" and not partitioned or separated from it in any way. Thus, medical space was not divorced from domestic space. The traditional British surgery did not have distinct areas for specialized medical functions, i.e., for testing, diagnosis, and treatment. Medical space, however, eventually became differentiated from domestic space; at first, through the establishment of a separate surgery, possibly with its own entrance; and later, through the establishment of clinics and health centers as sites for primary care practice. As a consequence of such physical separation, it became less likely for physicians to visit patients at home, solidifying the separation of medical and domestic spaces. Such changes are interpreted as having powerful implications for divorcing medical problems, issues, and practices from the total life of the patient and the community. Further spatial separation of functions within modern clinics and practice settings is seen to be related to the fragmentation of the treatment process.

Parallel with, and related to spatial changes were changes in the social construction of the temporal aspects of practice. Armstrong noted that the separation of the medical from the domestic established and strengthened the boundaries between the physician's own personal life and the physician's professional activities. Physicians could now have "off-duty time" that they previously lacked. It also led to setting of appointments, and to other forms of "time management" that are related to fragmentation of the interactions between physicians and patients.

So far, such social constructions of the meanings of space and time have received little attention, yet they present an important area for future health behavior research.

SUMMARY

Health behavior research has made appreciable strides in developing increased conceptual complexity in its models and in the behaviors it observes. If it is to develop and mature as a basic area of interdisciplinary study, it must resolve some issues related to its identity, particularly in relation to behavioral medicine and to being located within medical schools. Ideally, distinct health behavior research programs should be located within arts and sciences units of universities, and should be linked with basic scientific disciplines as well as with the helping professions. Such distinct programs, together with an interdisciplinary journal that would publish basic health behavior research findings, would strengthen the identity of health behavior.

Such interdisciplinary programs have important future research tasks, particularly in relation to the origins and development of health behavior, the family as a determinant of health behavior, health-relevant motivation, coping mechanisms, and searches for the meaning of illness, treatment, and the health care environment.

REFERENCES

Anderson, W. T., & Helm, D. T. (1979). The physician–patient encounter: A process of reality negotiation. In E. G. Jaco (Ed.), *Patients, physicians and illness* (3rd ed.). New York: Free Press.
Antonovsky, A. (1984). The sense of coherence as a determinant of health. In J. D. Matarazzo, S. M. Weiss, J. A. Herd, N. E. Miller, & S. M. Weiss (Eds.), *Behavioral health: A handbook of health enhancement and disease prevention.* New York: Wiley.
Armstrong, D. (1985). Space and time in British general practice. *Social Science and Medicine, 20,* 659–666.
Baranowski, T., & Nader, P. R. (1985). Family health behavior. In D. C. Turk & R. D. Kerns (Eds.), *Health, illness, and families: A life-span perspective.* New York: Wiley.
Bartlett, H. M. (1961). *Social work practice in the health field.* New York: National Association of Social Workers.
Ben-Sira, Z. (1977). Involvement with a disease and health-promoting behavior. *Social Science and Medicine, 11,* 165–173.
Ben-Sira, Z., & Padeh, B. (1978). "Instrumental coping" and "affective defense": An additional perspective in health promoting behavior. *Social Science and Medicine, 12,* 163–168.
Bruhn, J. G., & Parcel, G. S. (1982). Current knowledge about the health behavior of young children: A conference summary. In D. S. Gochman & G. S. Parcel (Eds.), Children's health beliefs and health behaviors [Special issue]. *Health Education Quarterly, 9,* 142–166.
Burt, J. J. (1984). Metahealth: A challenge for the future. In J. D. Matarazzo, S. M. Weiss, J. A. Herd, N. E. Miller, & S. M. Weiss (Eds.), *Behavioral health: A handbook of health enhancement and disease prevention.* New York: Wiley.
Bush, J. P., & Holmbeck, G. N. (1987). Children's attitudes about health care: Initial development of a questionnaire. *Journal of Pediatric Psychology, 12,* 429–443.
Bynder, H., & New, P. K.-M. (1976). Time for a change: From micro-to macro-sociological concepts in disability research. *Journal of Health and Social Behavior, 17,* 45–52.
Campbell, J. D. (1978). The child in the sick-role: Contributions of age, sex, parental status, and parental values. *Journal of Health and Social Behavior, 19,* 35–51.
Conrad, P. (1985). The meaning of medications: Another look at compliance. *Social Science and Medicine, 20,* 29–37.
Dielman, T. E., Leech, S. L., Becker, M. H., Rosenstock, I. M., & Horvath, W. J. (1982). Parental and child health beliefs and behavior. In D. S. Gochman & G. S. Parcel (Eds.), Children's health beliefs and health behaviors [Special issue]. *Health Education Quarterly, 9,* 60–77.
Eckert, J. K., & Goldstein, M. C. (1983). An anthropological approach to the study of illness behavior in an urban community. *Urban Anthropology, 12,* 125–139.
Eisen, M., Zellman, G. L., & McAlister, A. L. (1985). A health belief model approach to adolescents' fertility control: Some pilot program findings. *Health Education Quarterly, 12,* 185–210.
Elinson, J. (1985). The end of medicine and the end of medical sociology. *Journal of Health and Social Behavior, 26,* 268–275.
Fox, R. C., & Swazey, J. P. (1978). *The courage to fail: A social view of organ transplants and dialysis* (2nd ed., rev.). Chicago: University of Chicago Press.
Gellert, E. (1962). Children's conceptions of the content and functions of the human body. *Genetic Psychology Monographs, 61,* 293–405.
Gellert, E. (1978). What do I have inside me? How children view their bodies. In E. Gellert (Ed.), *Psychosocial aspects of pediatric care.* New York: Grune & Stratton.
Gochman, D. S. (1970). Children's perceptions of vulnerability to illness and accidents. *Public Health Reports, 85,* 69–73.
Gochman, D. S. (1971). Children's perceptions of vulnerability to illness and accidents: A replication, extension and refinement. *HSMHA Health Reports, 86,* 247–252.
Gochman, D. S. (1975). The measurement and development of dentally relevant motives. *Journal of Public Health Dentistry, 35,* 160–164.
Gochman, D. S. (1977). Perceived vulnerability and its psychosocial context. *Social Science and Medicine, 11,* 115–120.
Gochman, D. S. (1982). Labels, systems and motives: Some perspectives for future research. In D.

S. Gochman & G. S. Parcel (Eds.), Children's health beliefs and health behaviors [Special issue]. *Health Education Quarterly, 9,* 167–174.

Gochman, D. S. (1985). Family determinants of children's concepts of health and illness. In D. C. Turk & R. D. Kerns (Eds.), *Health, illness, and families: A life-span perspective.* New York: Wiley.

Gochman, D. S. (1986). *Youngsters' health cognitions: Cross-sectional and longitudinal analyses.* Louisville, KY: Health Behavior Systems.

Gove, W. R. (1984). Gender differences in mental and physical illness: The effects of fixed roles and nurturant roles. *Social Science and Medicine, 19,* 77–84.

Herzlich, C., & Pierret, J. (1985). The social construction of the patient: Patients and illnesses in other ages. *Social Science and Medicine, 20,* 145–151.

Hulka, B. S., Cassel, J. C., Kupper, L. L., & Burdette, J. A. (1976). Communication, compliance, and concordance between physicians and patients with prescribed medications. *American Journal of Public Health, 66,* 847–853.

Janz, N. K., & Becker, M. H. (1984). The health belief model: A decade later. *Health Education Quarterly, 11,* 1–47.

Kalnins, I., & Love, R. (1982). Children's concepts of health and illness—and implications for health education: An overview. In D. S. Gochman & G. S. Parcel (Eds.), Children's health beliefs and health behaviors [Special issue]. *Health Education Quarterly, 9,* 8–19.

Kasteler, J., Kane, R. L., Olsen, D. M., & Thetford, C. (1976). Issues underlying prevalence of "doctor-shopping" behavior. *Journal of Health and Social Behavior, 17,* 328–339.

Kinston, W. (1983). Pluralism in the organisation of health services research. *Social Science and Medicine, 17,* 299–313.

Langlie, J. K. (1977). Social networks, health beliefs, and preventive health behavior. *Journal of Health and Social Behavior, 18,* 244–260.

Lau, R. R., Hartman, K. A., & Ware, J. E., Jr. (1986). Health as a value: Methodological and theoretical considerations. *Health Psychology, 5,* 25–43.

Levin, L. S. (1976). The layperson as the primary health care practitioner. *Public Health Reports, 91,* 204–210.

Lewis, C. E., & Lewis, M. A. (1982). Children's health-related decision-making. In D. S. Gochman & G. S. Parcel (Eds.), Children's health beliefs and health behaviors [Special issue]. *Health Education Quarterly, 9,* 129–141.

Lipton, J. P., & Hershaft, A. M. (1985). On the widespread acceptance of dubious medical findings. *Journal of Health and Social Behavior, 26,* 336–351.

Marcus, A. C., Seeman, T. E., & Telesky, C. W. (1983). Sex differences in reports of illness and disability: A further test of the fixed role hypothesis. *Social Science and Medicine, 17,* 993–1002.

Mechanic, D. (1979). Correlates of physician utilization: Why do major multivariate studies of physician utilization find trivial psychosocial and organizational effects? *Journal of Health and Social Behavior, 20,* 387–396.

Michela, J. L., & Brady, P. (1984, August). *Perceived distinctions among behaviors that promote health and safety.* Paper presented at the meeting of the American Psychological Association, Toronto.

Moody, P. M., & Gray, R. M. (1972). Social class, social integration, and the use of preventive health services. In E. G. Jaco (Ed.), *Patients, physicians and illness: A sourcebook in behavioral science and health* (2nd ed.). New York: Free Press.

Morris, J. N., Suissa, S., Sherwood, S., Wright, S. M., & Greer, D. (1986). Last days: A study of the quality of life of terminally ill cancer patients. *Journal of Chronic Diseases, 39,* 47–62.

Nagy, M. H. (1951). Children's ideas on the origin of illness. *Health Education Journal, 9,* 6–12.

Nagy, M. H. (1953). The representation of "germs" by children. *Journal of Genetic Psychology, 83,* 227–240.

Natapoff, J. N. (1982). A developmental analysis of children's ideas of health. In D. S. Gochman & G. S. Parcel (Eds.), Children's health beliefs and health behaviors [Special issue]. *Health Education Quarterly, 9,* 34–45.

Nathanson, C. A. (1975). Illness and the feminine role: A theoretical review. *Social Science and Medicine, 9,* 57–62.

Parsons, T. (1951). *The social system.* Glencoe: Free Press.

Pearlin, L. I., & Schooler, C. (1978). The structure of coping. *Journal of Health and Social Behavior, 19,* 2–21.

Pratt, L. (1976). *Family structure and effective health behavior: The energized family*. Boston: Houghton Mifflin.

Ross, C. E., & Duff, R. S. (1982). Returning to the doctor: The effect of client characteristics, type of practice, and experience with care. *Journal of Health and Social Behavior, 23,* 119–131.

Sorenson, J. R. (1974). Biomedical innovation, uncertainty, and doctor–patient interaction. *Journal of Health and Social Behavior, 15,* 366–374.

Stimson, G. V. (1974). Obeying doctor's orders: A view from the other side. *Social Science and Medicine, 8,* 97–104.

Stimson, G., & Webb, B. (1975). *Going to see the doctor: The consultation process in general practice*. London: Routledge & Kegan Paul.

Suchman, E. A. (1972). Social patterns of illness and medical care. In E. G. Jaco (Ed.), *Patients, physicians and illness: A sourcebook in behavioral science and health* (2nd ed.). New York: Free Press. (Reprinted from *Journal of Health and Human Behavior,* 1965, *6,* 2–16)

Szasz, T. S., & Hollender, M. H. (1975). A contribution to the philosophy of medicine: The basic models of the doctor–patient relationship. In T. Millon (Ed.), *Medical behavioral science*. Philadelphia: Saunders. (Reprinted from *Archives of Internal Medicine,* 1956, *97,* 585–592)

Verbrugge, L. M. (1983). Multiple roles and physical health of women and men. *Journal of Health and Social Behavior, 24,* 16–30.

Wolinsky, F. D. (1988). *The sociology of health: Principles, practitioners, and issues* (2nd ed.). Belmont, CA: Wadsworth.

Zola, I. K. (1973). Pathways to the doctor—from person to patient. *Social Science and Medicine, 7,* 677–689.

Index

The reader should also consult the Contents, which identifies all major chapter headings.